Exam Prep Manual

Pharmacology

First South Asian Edition

As per NMC's Revised Competency-Based Medical Education Curriculum 2024

Based on Board Review Series (BRS)

Exam Prep Manual
Pharmacology

First South Asian Edition

As per NMC's Revised Competency-Based Medical Education Curriculum 2024

SAE Editors

Ashok K. Shenoy MBBS, MD
Professor and Former HOD
Department of Pharmacology
Kasturba Medical College
Mangalore (A constituent unit of Manipal Academy of Higher Education, Manipal)

Ashwin Kamath MBBS, MD
Associate Professor
Department of Pharmacology
Kasturba Medical College
Mangalore (A constituent unit of Manipal Academy of Higher Education, Manipal)

Preethi J. Shenoy MBBS, MD
Additional Professor
Department of Pharmacology
Kasturba Medical College
Mangalore (A constituent unit of Manipal Academy of Higher Education, Manipal)

Sheetal D. Ullal MBBS, MD
Professor and HOD
Department of Pharmacology
Kasturba Medical College
Mangalore (A constituent unit of Manipal Academy of Higher Education, Manipal)

International Author

Sarah Lerchenfeldt PharmD
Assistant Professor
Department of Foundational Medical Studies
Oakland University William Beaumont School of Medicine
Rochester, Michigan

This work is an adaptation of *BRS Pharmacology, Seventh Edition*. Authorized for sale only in South Asia.

Wolters Kluwer

Publishing Manager: Ruchi Chawla
Development Editor: Megha Saini
Asstt Manager, Manufacturing: Sumit Johry

3rd Floor, Tower B, Building No. 10, Phase – II, DLF Cyber City, Gurgaon, Haryana – 122002

Print ISBN: 9788197099588
E-ISBN: 9788196949174

Published by Wolters Kluwer (India) Pvt. Ltd., New Delhi
Compositor: Design Modus, New Delhi (www.designmodus.in)
Printed and bound at SDR Printers, Trans Delhi Signature City Ghaziabad (U.P.)

To download our latest price list or contact us, please visit https://www.wolterskluwer.com/en-in/solutions/lwwindia. For any other queries, email us at ggm-india.support@wolterskluwer.com.

Preface to the South Asian Edition

Exam Prep Manual Pharmacology, Ist South Asian Edition of the popular International Board Review Series in Pharmacology has been written for undergraduate medical students and other health profession students, specifically designed to support students and educators in the context of new and previous Competency-Based Medical Education (CBME) of National Medical Commission of India. This book is primarily designed as a book for quick reading, be it for familiarizing oneself with a chapter before in-depth reading of the classical textbooks or preparing for competitive examinations. The book presents the subject matter in a concise and lucid form, focusing on drug information that is expected to be known and understood by an Indian Medical Graduate. Most of the competencies in Pharmacology, as per the Competency-Based Medical Education (CBME) curriculum 2019, have been covered; however, in keeping with the character of the original series, the emphasis has been on presenting the information succinctly rather than a detailed coverage of all the competencies. In addition to preparing for the year-end, NEET, and NExT examinations in India, the book is also helpful in preparing for the international licensing examinations. Also, although the book is primarily written keeping in mind the requirements of the medical undergraduates, the concise format of the book is also likely to be helpful for dental, nursing, and physiotherapy students in preparing for their pharmacology examination.

Organization

The South Asian edition begins with a chapter devoted to the general principles of drug kinetics and dynamics, followed by chapters concerned with drugs acting on the major body systems. Each chapter includes a presentation of specific drugs with a discussion of their general properties, mechanism of action, pharmacologic effects, therapeutic uses, and adverse effects. A drug list, tables, and figures summarize essential drug information included in all chapters. Drugs relevant to the Indian context have been presented. In addition, some important newer drugs acting via novel mechanisms/targets and those mentioned in international treatment guidelines/recommendations have also been mentioned although they may not be currently available locally.

Clinically oriented, examination-style review questions and answers with explanations follow each chapter to help students assess their understanding of the information. Similarly, a comprehensive examination question list with answers is included at the end of the book. These questions serve as a self-assessment tool to help students determine their knowledge and understanding of the subject as well as comprehend a given clinical case scenario from a pharmacological perspective and arrive at the right answers.

Acknowledgments

We sincerely thank Dr. *Sarah Lerchenfeldt, the author of the seventh edition of BRS Pharmacology, and* Dr. Gary C. Rosenfeld and Dr. David S. Loose, who authored the first six editions of *this book*. The content and format in this book are largely due to their thinking and efforts.

We would also like to thank Ms. Sheenam Aggarwal, Associate Director, Content Management & Publishing at Wolters Kluwer India, and her team for their meticulous attention to detail, tireless work ethic, and dedication to excellence. We extend our thanks to Ms Ruchi Chawla, Content and Publishing Consultant, for her incredible support and understanding. Similarly, we deeply value the dedication, passion, hard work of Ms Megha Saini, Content Management Analyst.

Ashok K. Shenoy
Ashwin Kamath
Preethi J. Shenoy
Sheetal D. Ullal

Preface to the International Edition

This concise review of medical pharmacology is designed for health professions students, including medical students, dental students, and those enrolled in physician assistant or nurse practitioner programs. It is intended primarily to help students prepare for course examinations and licensing examinations, including the United States Medical Licensing Examination (USMLE) Step 1. This book presents condensed and succinct descriptions of relevant and current board-driven information pertaining to pharmacology without the usual associated details. It is not meant to be a substitute for the comprehensive presentation of information and difficult concepts found in standard pharmacology texts.

ORGANIZATION

The seventh edition begins with a chapter devoted to the general principles of drug action, followed by chapters concerned with drugs acting on the major body systems. Other chapters discuss anti-inflammatory and immunosuppressive agents, drugs used to treat anemia and disorders of hemostasis, infectious diseases, cancer, and toxicology.

Each chapter includes a presentation of specific drugs with a discussion of their general properties, mechanism of action, pharmacologic effects, therapeutic uses, and adverse effects. A drug list, tables, and figures summarize essential drug information included in all chapters.

Clinically oriented, USMLE-style review questions and answers with explanations follow each chapter to help students assess their understanding of the information. Similarly, a comprehensive examination consisting of USMLE-style questions is included at the end of the book. This examination serves as a self-assessment tool to help students determine their fund of knowledge and diagnose any weaknesses in pharmacology.

KEY FEATURES

- Updated with current drug information
- End-of-chapter review tests feature updated USMLE-style questions
- Several tables and figures summarize essential information for quick recall
- Updated drug lists for each chapter
- Additional USMLE-style comprehensive examination questions and explanations

Sarah Lerchenfeldt, PharmD

Contents

Competency Mapping*

Competency-Based Undergraduate Curriculum 2019 Topics: Chapter-Wise Coverage

Competency Number	Topic	Chapter Number	Page Number
PH1.1	Define and describe the principles of pharmacology and pharmacotherapeutics	1	1
PH1.2	Describe the basis of evidence based medicine and therapeutic drug monitoring evidence based medicine	1	21, 22–23
PH1.4	Describe absorption, distribution, metabolism and excretion of drugs pharmacokinetics (PK)	1	9–10, 11, 12–14
PH1.5	Describe general principles of mechanism of drug action pharmacodynamics	1	1–8
PH1.6	Describe principles of pharmacovigilance and ADR reporting systems	1	22
PH1.7	Define, identify and describe the management of adverse drug reactions (ADR)	1	21
PH1.9	Describe nomenclature of drugs i.e. generic, branded drugs	1	8
PH1.11	Describe various routes of drug administration, e.g., oral, SC, IV, IM, SL	1	10–11
PH1.13	Describe mechanism of action, types, doses, side effects, indications and contraindications of adrenergic and anti-adrenergic drugs	2	30–35, 43–50
PH1.14	Describe mechanism of action, types, doses, side effects, indications and contraindications of cholinergic and anticholinergic drugs	2	30–35, 36–43
PH1.15	Describe mechanism/s of action, types, doses, side effects, indications and contraindications of skeletal muscle relaxants	2	50–53
PH1.16	Describe mechanism/s of action, types, doses, side effects, indications and contraindications of the drugs which act by modulating autacoids, including: anti-histaminics, 5-HT modulating drugs, NSAIDs, drugs for gout, anti-rheumatic drugs, drugs for migraine	3	64–79
PH1.17	Describe the mechanism/s of action, types, side effects, indications and contraindications of local anesthetics	2	53–55
PH1.18	Describe the mechanism/s of action, types, side effects, indications and contraindications of general anesthetics, and preanesthetic medications	4	108–111
PH1.19	Describe the mechanism/s of action, types, side effects, indications and contraindications of the drugs which act on CNS	4	85–108, 112–117
PH1.20	Describe the effects of acute and chronic ethanol intake	4	118–120
PH1.21	Describe the symptoms and management of methanol and ethanol poisonings	4	120
PH1.22	Describe drugs of abuse (dependence, addiction, stimulants, depressants, psychedelics, drugs used for criminal offences)	4	117–126
PH1.24	Describe the mechanism/s of action, types, doses, side effects, indications and contraindications of the drugs affecting renal systems including diuretics, antidiuretics – vasopressin and analogues	5, 10	132–139, 228–229
PH1.25	Describe the mechanism/s of action, types, doses, side effects, indications and contraindications of the drugs acting on blood, like anticoagulants, antiplatelets, fibrinolytics, plasma expanders	7	177–186
PH1.26	Describe mechanism of action, types, doses, side effects, indications and contraindications of the drugs modulating the renin-angiotensin and aldosterone system	6	145–147, 152
PH1.27	Describe the mechanism s of action, types, doses, side effects, indications and contraindications of antihypertensive drugs and drugs used in shock	6	144–151
PH1.28	Describe the mechanism s of action, types, doses, side effects, indications and contraindications of the drugs used in is chemic heart disease (stable, unstable angina and myocardial infarction), peripheral vascular disease	6	154–157
PH1.29	Describe the mechanisms of action, types, doses, side effects, indications and contraindications of the drugs used in congestive heart failure	6	151–154

*Reference: National Medical Commission. Competency Based Undergraduate Curriculum for the Indian Medical Graduate, Vol. 1 (2019).

Competency Number	Topic	Chapter Number	Page Number
PH1.30	Describe the mechanisms of action, types, doses, side effects, indications and contraindications of the antiarrhythmics	6	157–162
PH1.31	Describe the mechanisms of action, types, doses, side effects, indications and contraindications of the drugs used in the management of dyslipidemias	6	162–165
PH1.32	Describe the mechanism/s of action, types, doses, side effects, indications and contraindications of drugs used in bronchial asthma and COPD	8	192–198
PH1.33	Describe the mechanism of action, types, doses, side effects, indications and contraindications of the drugs used in cough (antitussives, expectorants/mucolytics)	8	199–200
PH1.34	Describe the mechanism/s of action, types, doses, side effects, indications and contraindications of the drugs used as below: 1. Acid-peptic disease and GERD 2. Antiemetics and prokinetics 3. Antidiarrhoeals 4. Laxatives 5. Inflammatory bowel disease 6. Irritable bowel disorders, biliary and pancreatic disorders	9	204–216
PH1.35	Describe the mechanism/s of action, types, doses, side effects, indications and contraindications of drugs used in hematological disorders like: 1. Drugs used in anemias 2. Colony Stimulating factors	7	172–177
PH1.36	Describe the mechanism of action, types, doses, side effects, indications and contraindications of drugs used in endocrine disorders (diabetes mellitus, thyroid disorders and osteoporosis)	10	241–254
PH1.37	Describe the mechanisms of action, types, doses, side effects, indications and contraindications of the drugs used as sex hormones, their analogues and anterior pituitary hormones	10	225–237
PH1.38	Describe the mechanism of action, types, doses, side effects, indications and contraindications of corticosteroids	10	237–241
PH1.39	Describe mechanism of action, types, doses, side effects, indications and contraindications the drugs used for contraception	10	233–235
PH1.40	Describe mechanism of action, types, doses, side effects, indications and contraindications of: 1. Drugs used in the treatment of infertility, and 2. Drugs used in erectile dysfunction	10	231, 236–237
PH1.41	Describe the mechanisms of action, types, doses, side effects, indications and contraindications of uterine relaxants and stimulants	10	229, 67
PH1.42	Describe general principles of chemotherapy	11	261–262
PH1.43	Describe and discuss the rational use of antimicrobials including antibiotic stewardship program	11	262
PH1.44	Describe the first line antitubercular dugs, their mechanisms of action, side effects and doses	11	275–276
PH1.45	Describe the drugs used in MDR and XDR tuberculosis	11	276–277
PH1.46	Describe the mechanisms of action, types, doses, side effects, indications and contraindications of antileprotic drugs	11	277–278
PH1.47	Describe the mechanisms of action, types, doses, side effects, indications and contraindications of the drugs used in malaria, KALA-AZAR, amebiasis and intestinal helminthiasis	11	280–284
PH1.48	Describe the mechanisms of action, types, doses, side effects, indications and contraindications of the drugs used in UTI/STD and viral diseases including HIV	11	284–289
PH1.49	Describe mechanism of action, classes, side effects, indications and contraindications of anticancer drugs	12	296–312
PH1.51	Describe occupational and environmental pesticides, food adulterants, pollutants and insect repellants	13	318–324
PH1.52	Describe management of common poisoning, insecticides, common sting and bites	13	327–329
PH1.53	Describe heavy metal poisoning and chelating agents	13	324–327
PH1.58	Describe drugs used in ocular disorders	13	329–330

Competency Mapping*

Competency-Based Undergraduate Curriculum 2024
Topics: Chapter-Wise Coverage

Competency Number	Topic	Chapter Number
PH1.1	Describe the principles of pharmacology, pharmacotherapeutics and define various terms in pharmacology.	1
PH1.2	Describe evidence-based medicine and rational use of drugs and discuss why these are relevant to therapeutics.	1
PH1.3	Describe nomenclature of drugs i.e., generic, branded drugs and scheduled drugs, explaining the utility of the nomenclature, cost effectiveness and use.	1
PH1.6	Describe salient features of absorption, distribution, metabolism and excretion of drugs with emphasis on various routes of drug administration.	1
PH1.7	Describe various principles of mechanism of action of drugs.	1
PH1.10	Describe changes in pharmacology of drugs in geriatric, pediatric and special situations such as Pregnancy, lactation, hepatic and renal disorders and adjust the drug treatment accordingly.	1
PH1.11	Define Adverse Drug Reactions (ADRs) and their types. Identify the ADRs in the given case scenario and assess causality.	1
PH1.12	Define Pharmacovigilance its principles and demonstrate ADR reporting.	1
PH2.1	Describe types, salient pharmacokinetics, pharmacodynamics, therapeutic uses, adverse drug reactions of adrenergic and antiadrenergic drugs	2
PH2.2	Describe types, salient pharmacokinetics, pharmacodynamics, therapeutic uses, adverse drug reactions of cholinergic and anticholinergic drugs and demonstrate OPC poisoning management	2
PH2.3	Explain the rationale and demonstrate the emergency use of various sympathetic and parasympathetic drug agonists/antagonists (like Noradrenaline/ Adrenaline/Dopamine/ Dobutamine, Atropine) in case-based scenarios	2
PH2.4	Explain salient pharmacokinetics, pharmacodynamics, therapeutic uses, adverse drug reactions of skeletal muscle relaxants	2
PH2.5	Explain types, salient pharmacokinetics, pharmacodynamics, therapeutic uses, adverse drug reactions of local anaesthetics (LA) and demonstrate various methods of administration of LA	2
PH2.6	Explain types, salient pharmacokinetics, pharmacodynamics, therapeutic uses, adverse drug reactions of anti-histaminics and explain management of common cold and allergic rhinitis.	3
PH2.7	Define pain and enumerate drugs used for pain. Explain salient pharmacokinetics, pharmacodynamics, therapeutic uses, adverse drug reactions of analgesics including NSAIDs (except opioids)	3
PH2.8	Devise management plan for a case of gout, arthritis and migraine using appropriate drugs	3
PH3.1	Describe types, salient pharmacokinetics, pharmacodynamics, therapeutic uses, adverse drug reactions of General anaesthetics, and pre-anaesthetic medications.	4
PH3.2	Describe types, salient pharmacokinetics, pharmacodynamics, therapeutic uses, adverse drug reactions of different sedative and hypnotic agents and explain pharmacological basis of selection and use of different sedative and hypnotic agents.	4
PH3.3	Describe types, salient pharmacokinetics, pharmacodynamics, therapeutic uses, adverse drug reactions of drugs used in epilepsy and devise management plan for a case of uncontrolled seizure.	4
PH3.4	Describe types, salient pharmacokinetics, pharmacodynamics, therapeutic uses, adverse drug reactions of drugs of opioid analgesics and explain the special instructions for use of opioids.	4
PH3.5	Describe types, salient pharmacokinetics, pharmacodynamics, therapeutic uses, adverse drug reactions of drugs used for depression and psychosis, devise management plan for depressive and psychotic disorders.	4
PH3.6	Describe types, salient pharmacokinetics, pharmacodynamics, therapeutic uses, adverse drug reactions of drugs used in anxiety disorders. Discuss about general goals of Pharmacotherapy for the management of above disorders.	4

*As per the 2024 Revised Guidelines for Competency Based Medical Education (CBME) Curriculum by the Under Graduate Medical Education Board (UGMEB), National Medical Commission (NMC). Competency Based Undergraduate Curriculum for the Indian Medical Graduate, Vol. 1 (2024).

Competency Number	Topic	Chapter Number
PH3.7	Explain types, salient pharmacokinetics, pharmacodynamics, therapeutic uses, adverse drug reactions of drugs used for Parkinsonism and other neurodegenerative disorders. Write a prescription to manage a case of drug induced parkinsonism.	4
PH3.8	Identify and manage methanol poisoning and chronic ethanol Intoxication	4
PH3.9	Describe the drugs that are abused and cause addiction (dependence, addiction, stimulants, depressants, psychedelics, drugs used for criminal offences). Explain the process and steps for management of drug de addiction	4
PH4.1	Explain types, salient pharmacokinetics, pharmacodynamics, therapeutic uses, adverse drug reactions of drugs used for different anaemias and thrombocytopenia.	6
PH4.2	Explain types, salient pharmacokinetics, pharmacodynamics, therapeutic uses, adverse drug reactions of drugs acting on coagulation system (Coagulants/anticoagulants) and devise a plan to monitor therapy and management of adverse effects.	6
PH4.3	Describe types, salient pharmacokinetics, pharmacodynamics, therapeutic uses, adverse drug reactions of Fibrinolytics and Antifibrinolytic agents.	6
PH4.4	Explain types, salient pharmacokinetics, pharmacodynamics, therapeutic uses, adverse drug reactions of Antiplatelets agents.	6
PH4.5	Explain types, salient pharmacokinetics, pharmacodynamics, therapeutic uses, adverse drug reactions of Diuretics, antidiuretics- vasopressin and analogues	7
PH4.6	Explain salient pharmacokinetics, pharmacodynamics, therapeutic uses, adverse drug reactions of drugs modulating renin angiotensin aldosterone system.	5
PH4.7	Explain types, salient pharmacokinetics, pharmacodynamics, therapeutic uses, adverse drug reactions of drugs used for the management of hypertension Devise plan for pharmacologic management of hypertension with Diabetes, Pregnancy induced hypertension and hypertensive emergency and urgency	5
PH4.8	Describe types, salient pharmacokinetics, pharmacodynamics, therapeutic uses, adverse drug reactions of drugs used for the management of ischemic heart disease (stable, unstable angina and myocardial infarction), peripheral vascular disease and devise management plan for a patient of acute myocardial Infarction	5
PH4.9	Explain salient pharmacokinetics, pharmacodynamics, therapeutic uses, adverse drug reactions of drugs used for the management of heart failure. Devise management plan for heart failure patients and describe the strategies to prevent long term complications of heart failure.	5
PH4.10	Explain salient pharmacokinetics, pharmacodynamics, therapeutic uses, adverse drug reactions of drugs used for cardiac arrhythmias. Devise a plan to manage a patient with supraventricular, ventricular arrhythmias, cardiac arrest and fibrillations	5
PH4.11	Explain salient pharmacokinetics, pharmacodynamics, therapeutic uses, adverse drug reactions of drugs used for the management of dyslipidaemias and enumerate drugs leading to dyslipidaemias	5
PH5.1	Devise management of various stages of Bronchial asthma, COPD. Explain salient pharmacokinetics, pharmacodynamics, therapeutic uses, adverse drug reactions of drugs used for the management of Bronchial asthma, COPD and Rhinitis.	8
PH5.2	Explain types, salient pharmacokinetics, pharmacodynamics, therapeutic uses, adverse drug reactions of drugs used for cough management. Describe management of dry and productive cough	8
PH6.1	Explain types, salient pharmacokinetics, pharmacodynamics, therapeutic uses, adverse drug reactions of drugs used in Acid peptic diseases including Peptic Ulcers, GERD and devise a management plan for a case of peptic ulcer.	9
PH6.2	Describe types, salient pharmacokinetics, pharmacodynamics, therapeutic uses, adverse drug reactions of prokinetics and drugs used for emesis and antiemetics.	9
PH6.3	Describe salient pharmacokinetics, pharmacodynamics, therapeutic uses, adverse drug reactions of drugs used for the management of diarrhoea and devise pharmacotherapeutic plan to manage acute and chronic diarrhoea in adults and children.	9
PH6.4	Describe salient pharmacokinetics, pharmacodynamics, adverse drug reactions of drugs used for the management of constipation and devise management plan for a case of constipation	9
PH6.5	Describe salient pharmacokinetics, pharmacodynamics, adverse drug reactions of drugs used for the management of Inflammatory Bowel Disease and Irritable Bowel Disorders	9
PH7.1	Describe the types, kinetics, dynamics, adverse drug reactions of drugs used in diabetes mellitus and devise management for an obese and non-obese diabetic patient and also comment on prevention of complications of the diabetes.	10

Competency Number	Topic	Chapter Number
PH7.2	Describe the types, kinetics, dynamics, therapeutic uses, adverse drug reactions of drugs used in osteoporosis and devise management plan for a female and male patient with osteoporosis.	10
PH7.3	Describe the types, kinetics, dynamics, adverse drug reactions of drugs used in thyroid Disorders and devise a management plan for a case with thyroid Disorder.	10
PH7.4	Describe the types, mechanisms of action, adverse effects, indications and contraindications of the drugs which modify the release of Anterior Pituitary Hormones	10
PH7.5	Explain the types, kinetics, dynamics, adverse effects, indications and contraindications of corticosteroids and communicate to patient the appropriate use of corticosteroids	10
PH7.6	Describe the types, kinetics, dynamics, adverse effects, indications and contraindications of Androgens and drugs used of Erectile Dysfunction	10
PH7.7	Explain the types, kinetics, dynamics, adverse effects, indications and contraindications of drugs which modify Female Reproductive Functions including contraceptives. Explain the important instruction for use of female and male contraceptives	10
PH7.8	Explain the types, kinetics, dynamics, adverse effects, indications and contraindications of uterine relaxants and stimulants.	10
PH7.9	Describe drugs used for treatment of Infertility	7
PH8.1	Discuss general principles of chemotherapy with emphasis on antimicrobial resistance.	11
PH8.2	Discuss rational use of antimicrobials and describe antibiotic stewardship program of your institute.	11
PH8.3	Explain the kinetics, dynamics, adverse effects, indications of the following antibacterial drugs: Sulphonamides Quinolones, Betalactams, Macrolides, Tetracyclines, Aminoglycosides, and newer antibacterial drugs.	11
PH8.5	Explain the types, kinetics, dynamics, therapeutic uses and adverse effects of drugs used in tuberculosis. Devise management plan for tuberculosis treatment in various categories.	11
PH8.6	Discuss the types, Kinetics, dynamics, adverse effects for drugs used for Leprosy and outline management of Lepra reactions.	11
PH8.7	Discuss the types, Kinetics, dynamics, adverse effects of drugs used for following Protozoal / Vector borne diseases: 1. Amoebiasis 2. Kala-azar 3. Malaria 4. Filariasis	11
PH8.8	Explain the types, kinetics, dynamics, adverse effects of drugs used for fungal infections.	11
PH8.9	Discuss the types, kinetics, dynamics, adverse effects of drugs used for Intestinal Helminthiasis.	11
PH8.10	Discuss the types, kinetics, dynamics, adverse effects, indications and contraindications of drugs used for viral diseases including HIV.	11
PH8.11	Describe the types, kinetics, dynamics, adverse effects, indications and contraindications of anti-cancer drugs. Devise plan for amelioration of anticancer drug induced toxicity.	12
PH9.1	Describe the types, kinetics, dynamics, therapeutic uses, adverse drug reactions of immunomodulators	3
PH9.2	Describe management of common drug poisonings, insecticides, common stings and bites	13
PH9.3	Describe chelating agents and make a plan for management of heavy metal poisoning	13
PH9.7	Describe drugs used in glaucoma and other ocular disorders including topical (ocular) drug delivery systems	13

Chapter 1

Fundamental Principles of Pharmacology

Competencies Addressed: PH1.1, PH1.2, PH1.4–PH1.7, PH1.9, PH1.11

I. DEFINITIONS

A. Pharmacology: It is a branch of science that deals with actions and mechanisms of action of drugs and other chemical substances on living organisms.

B. Drug: According to the World Health Organization (WHO), a drug is any substance or product that is used or intended to be used to modify or explore physiologic systems or pathologic states for the benefit of the recipient.

C. Pharmacotherapeutics: It refers to the practice of monitoring and optimizing pharmacotherapy to ensure the overall treatment plan for patients.

D. Pharmacokinetics: Pharmacokinetics is concerned with the way the body handles drugs, that is, the movement of drugs throughout the body, including absorption, distribution, metabolism, and elimination.

E. Pharmacodynamics: Pharmacodynamics is concerned with the **effect of drugs on the body**, including the biochemical, cellular, and physiologic effects of drugs with their mechanisms of action.

F. Clinical pharmacology: It is a multidisciplinary field that encompasses various aspects of the relationship between drugs and humans, aiming to optimize pharmacotherapy at both individual and population levels.

II. SOURCES OF DRUGS

A. Natural: Plants, animals, minerals, microorganisms

B. Synthetic: Produced in the laboratory

C. Semisynthetic: Combination of natural and synthetic elements

III. DOSE–RESPONSE RELATIONSHIPS

A. Drug effects. Drug effects are produced by altering the normal functions of cells and tissues in the body via one of the four general mechanisms:

1. ***Interaction with receptors***
   - **a.** Receptors are naturally occurring target macromolecules that mediate the effects of endogenous physiologic substances such as neurotransmitters or hormones.

b. Figure 1.1 illustrates the four major classes of drug–receptor interactions, using specific examples of endogenous ligands.

(1) Ligand-activated ion channels. Figure 1.1A illustrates acetylcholine interacting with a nicotinic receptor that is a nonspecific Na^+/K^+ transmembrane ion channel. Interaction of a molecule of acetylcholine with each subunit of the channel produces a conformational change that permits the passage of sodium (Na^+) and potassium (K^+). Other channels that are targets for various drugs include specific calcium (Ca^{2+}) and K^+ channels.

(2) G-protein-coupled receptors (Fig. 1.1B–D). G-protein–coupled receptors compose the largest class of receptors. All the receptors have seven transmembrane segments, three intracellular loops, and an intracellular carboxy-terminal tail. The biologic activity of the receptors is mediated via interaction with a number of G (guanosine triphosphate [GTP] binding) proteins.

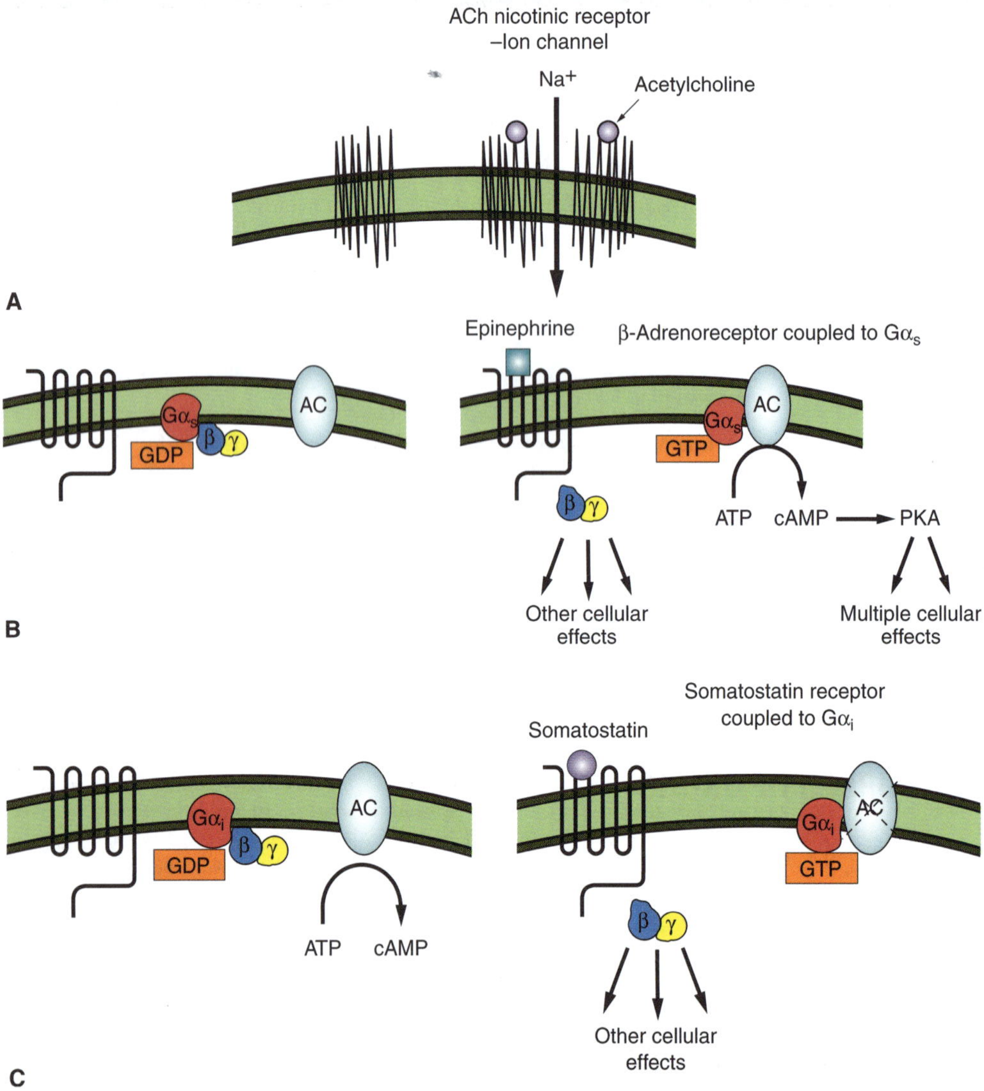

FIGURE 1.1. Four major classes of drug–receptor interactions, with specific examples of endogenous ligands. **A.** Acetylcholine interaction with a nicotinic receptor, a ligand-activated ion channel. **B–D.** G-protein-coupled receptors. **B.** Epinephrine interaction with a $G\alpha_s$-coupled β-adrenoceptor. **C.** Somatostatin interaction with a $G\alpha_i$ ($G\alpha_{inhibitory}$)-coupled receptor. **D.** Serotonin interaction with a G_q (and G_{11})-coupled receptor. **E.** Insulin interaction with a receptor-activated tyrosine kinase. **F.** Cortisol interaction with an intracellular nuclear receptor. ATP, adenosine triphosphate; cAMP, cyclic AMP; DAG, diacylglycerol; GDP, guanosine diphosphate; GTP, guanosine triphosphate; IP3, inositol 1,4,5-triphosphate; PIP2, phosphatidylinositol 4,5-bisphosphate; PLC, phospholipase C.

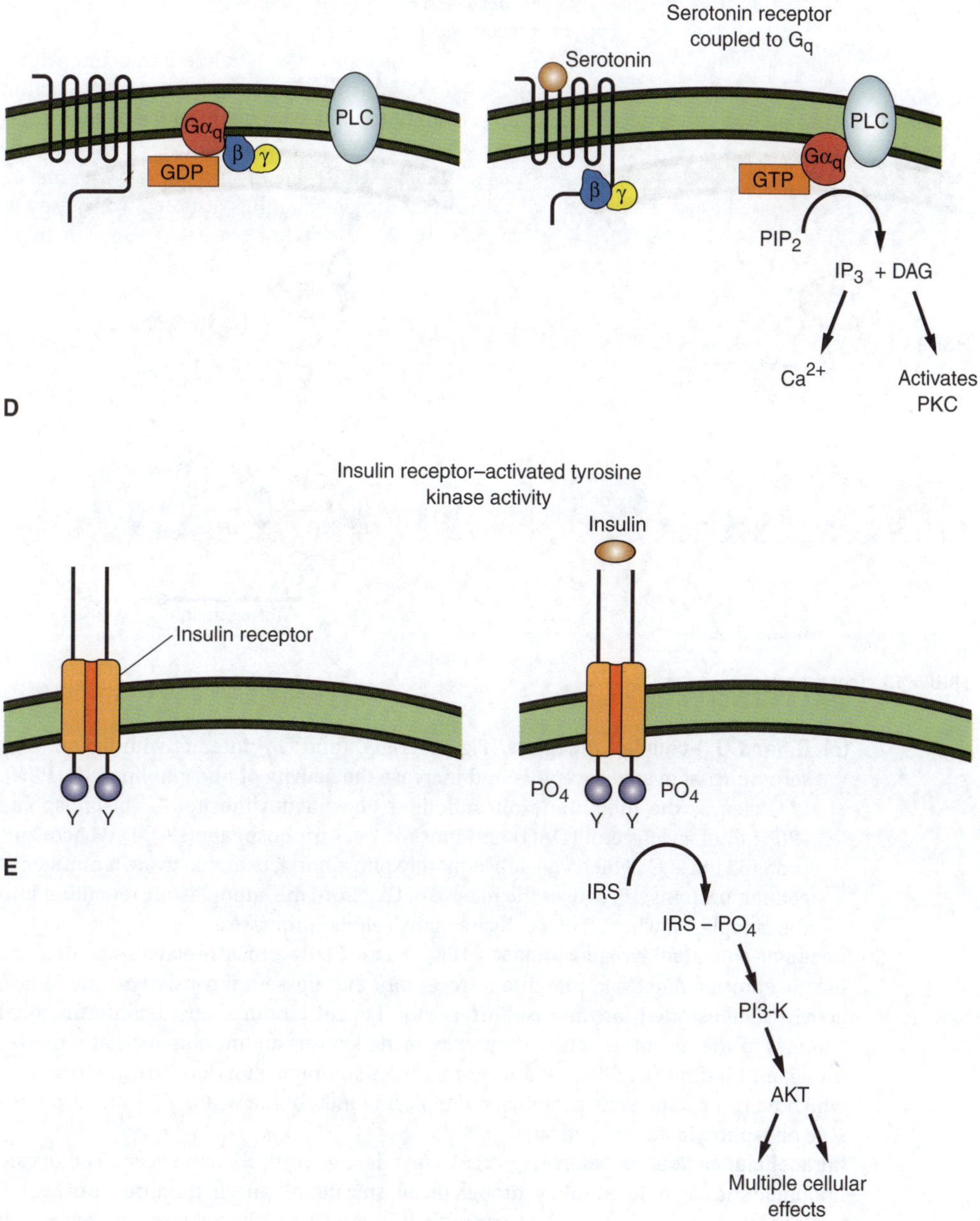

FIGURE 1.1. *(continued)*

(a) $G\alpha_s$-coupled receptors. Figure 1.1B illustrates that a β-adrenoceptor, which when activated by ligand binding (e.g., epinephrine), exchanges GDP for GTP. This facilitates the migration of $G\alpha_s$ ($G\alpha_{stimulatory}$) and its interaction with adenylyl cyclase (AC). $G\alpha_s$-bound AC catalyzes the production of cyclic AMP (cAMP) from adenosine triphosphate (ATP); cAMP activates protein kinase A, which subsequently acts to phosphorylate and activate a number of effector proteins. The βγ dimer may also activate some effectors. Hydrolysis of the GTP bound to the Gα to guanosine diphosphate (GDP) terminates the signal.

(b) $G\alpha_i$ ($G\alpha_{inhibitory}$)-coupled receptors (Fig. 1.1C). Ligand binding (e.g., somatostatin) to $G\alpha_i$-coupled receptors similarly exchanges GTP for GDP, but $G\alpha_i$ inhibits AC, leading to reduced cAMP production.

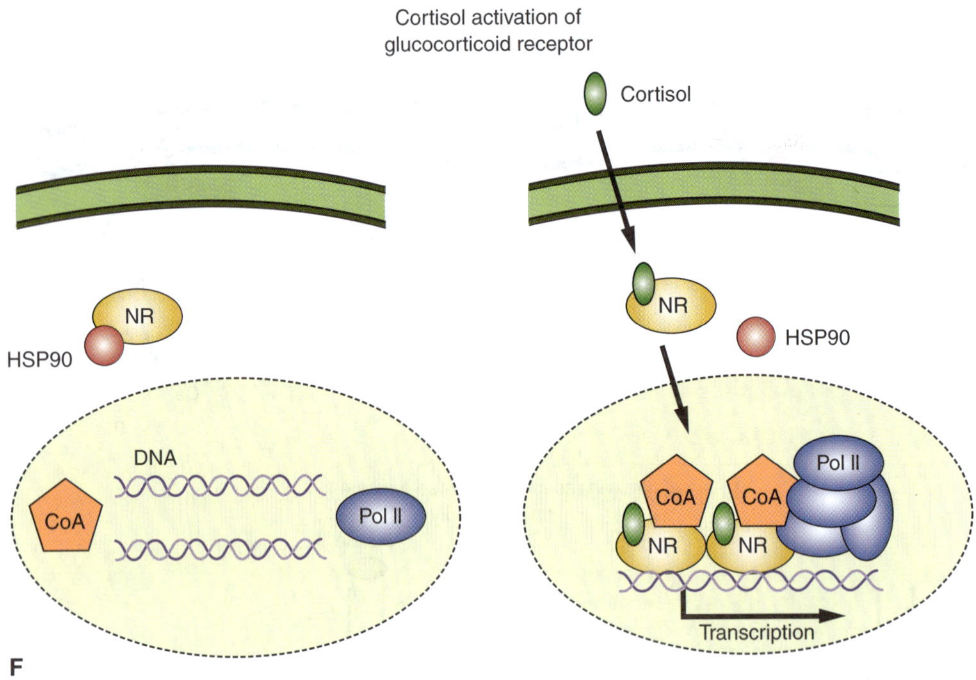

FIGURE 1.1. *(continued)*

(c) G_q (and G_{11})-coupled receptors (Fig. 1.1D). G_q (and G_{11}) interact with ligand (e.g., serotonin)-activated receptors and increase the activity of phospholipase C (PLC). PLC cleaves the membrane phospholipid phosphatidylinositol 4,5-bisphosphate (PIP_2) to diacylglycerol (DAG) and inositol 1,4,5-triphosphate (IP_3). DAG activates protein kinase C, which can subsequently phosphorylate and activate a number of cellular proteins; IP_3 causes the release of Ca^{2+} from the endoplasmic reticulum into the cytoplasm, where it can activate many cellular processes.

(3) Receptor-activated tyrosine kinases (Fig. 1.1E). Many growth-related signals (e.g., insulin) are mediated via membrane receptors that possess intrinsic tyrosine kinase activity as illustrated for the insulin receptor. Ligand binding causes conformational changes in the receptor; some receptor tyrosine kinases are monomers that dimerize on ligand binding. The liganded receptors then autophosphorylate tyrosine residues, which recruit cytoplasmic proteins to the plasma membrane where they are also tyrosine phosphorylated and activated.

(4) Intracellular nuclear receptors (Fig. 1.1F). Ligands (e.g., cortisol) for nuclear receptors are lipophilic and can diffuse rapidly through the plasma membrane. In the absence of ligand, nuclear receptors are inactive because of their interaction with chaperone proteins such as heat-shock proteins like HSP-90. Binding of ligand promotes structural changes in the receptor that facilitate dissociation of chaperones, entry of receptors into the nucleus, hetero- or homodimerization of receptors, and high-affinity interaction with the DNA of target genes. DNA-bound nuclear receptors are able to recruit a diverse number of proteins called coactivators, which subsequently act to increase transcription of the target gene.

2. ***Alteration of the activity of enzymes*** by activation or inhibition of the enzyme's catalytic activity
3. ***Antimetabolite action***, in which the drug, acting as a nonfunctional analogue of a naturally occurring metabolite, interferes with normal metabolism
4. ***Nonspecific chemical or physical interactions***, such as those caused by antacids, osmotic agents, or chelators

B. The graded dose–response curve. The graded dose–response curve expresses an individual's response to increasing doses of a given drug. The magnitude of a pharmacologic response is

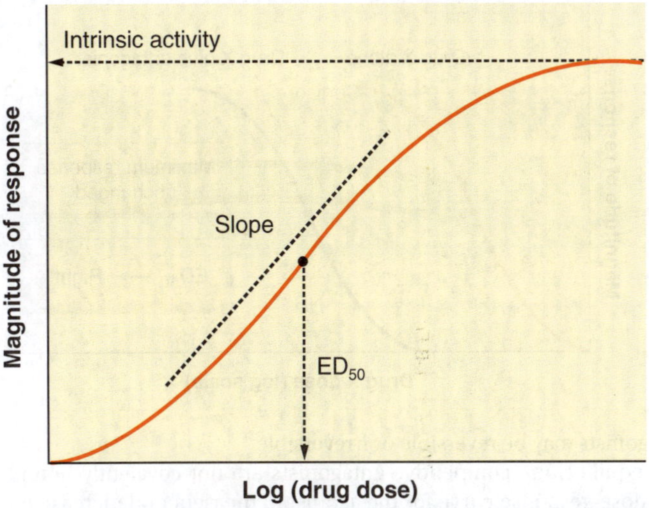

FIGURE 1.2. Graded dose–response curve. ED_{50}, median effective dose.

proportional to the number of receptors with which a drug effectively interacts (Fig. 1.2). The graded dose–response curve includes the following parameters:

1. ***Magnitude of response*** is graded; it continuously increases with the dose up to the maximal capacity of the system and is often depicted as a function of the logarithm of the dose administered (to see the relationship over a wide range of doses).
2. ***Median effective dose (ED_{50})*** is the dose that produces the half-maximal response; the threshold dose is that which produces the first noticeable effect.
3. ***Intrinsic activity*** is the ability of a drug, once bound, to activate the receptor.
   a. **Agonists** are drugs capable of binding to, and activating, a receptor.
      (1) **Full agonists** occupy receptors to cause maximal activation.
         (a) Intrinsic activity = 1
      (2) **Partial agonists** can occupy receptors but cannot elicit a maximal response.
         (a) Intrinsic activity <1 (Fig. 1.3; drug C)
   b. **Antagonists** bind to the receptor but do not initiate a response; they block the action of an agonist or endogenous substance that works through the receptor.
      (1) **Competitive antagonists** combine with the same site on the receptor but their binding does not activate the receptor.
         (a) Intrinsic activity = 0.
         (b) They may inhibit the actions of endogenous substances or other drugs.

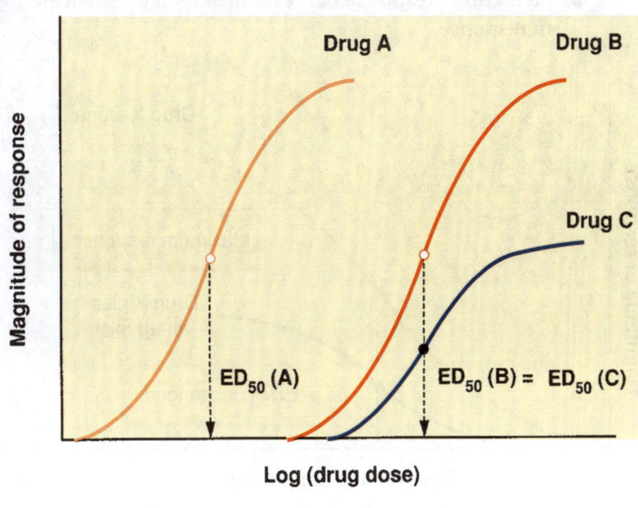

FIGURE 1.3. Graded dose–response curves for two agonists (**A** and **B**) and a partial agonist (**C**). ED_{50}, median effective dose.

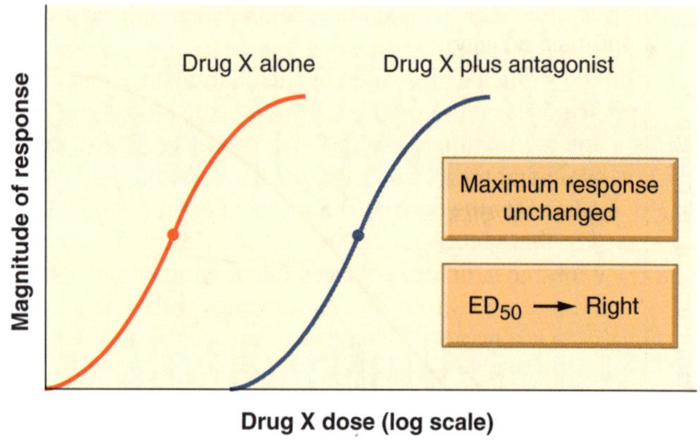

FIGURE 1.4. Graded dose–response curves illustrating the effects of competitive antagonists. ED_{50}, median effective dose.

(c) Competitive antagonists may be reversible or irreversible.

i. Reversible, or equilibrium, competitive antagonists are not covalently bound. They shift the dose–response curve for the agonist to the right and increase the ED_{50}, in which more agonist is required to elicit a response in the presence of the antagonist (Fig. 1.4). Because higher doses of agonist can overcome the inhibition, the maximal response can still be obtained.

(2) Noncompetitive antagonists bind to the receptor at a site other than the agonist-binding site (Fig. 1.5) and either prevent the agonist from binding correctly or prevent it from activating the receptor. Consequently, the effective amount of receptor is reduced. Receptors unoccupied by antagonist retain the same affinity for agonist, and the ED_{50} is unchanged.

4. ***Potency of a drug*** is the relative measure of the amount of a drug required to produce a specified level of response (e.g., 50%) compared with other drugs that produce the same effect via the same receptor mechanism.
   - **a.** The potency of a drug is determined by the **affinity** of a drug for its receptor and the amount of administered drug that reaches the receptor site.
   - **b.** The relative potency of a drug can be demonstrated by comparing the ED_{50} values of two full agonists; the drug with the lower ED_{50} is more potent (e.g., in Fig. 1.3, drug A is more potent than drug B).
5. ***The efficacy of a drug*** is the ability of a drug to elicit the pharmacologic response.
   - **a.** Efficacy may be affected by such factors as the number of drug–receptor complexes formed, the ability of the drug to activate the receptor once it is bound (i.e., the drug's intrinsic activity), and the status of the target organ or cell.
6. ***Slope*** is measured at the midportion of the dose–response curve.
   - **a.** The slope varies for different drugs and different responses.
   - **b.** Steep dose–response curves indicate that a small change in dose produces a large change in response.

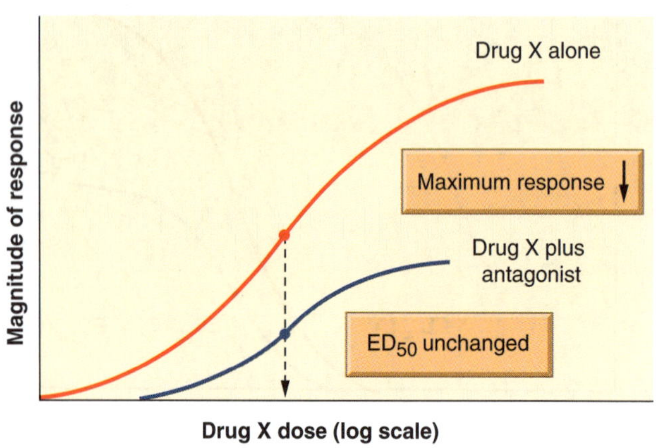

FIGURE 1.5. Graded dose–response curves illustrating the effects of noncompetitive antagonists. ED_{50}, median effective dose.

7. ***Variability*** reflects the differences between individuals in response to a given drug.

8. ***Therapeutic index (TI)*** relates the desired therapeutic effect to undesired toxicity; it is determined using data provided by the quantal dose–response curve.

   a. The TI is defined as TD_{50}/ED_{50} (i.e., the ratio of the dose that produces a toxic effect in half of the population to the dose that produces the desired effect in half of the population).

   b. Note that the TI should be used with caution in instances when the quantal dose–response curves for the desired and toxic effects are not parallel.

   c. The **therapeutic range** (therapeutic window) is the range of serum concentration of the drug required to **achieve desired therapeutic effects without toxicity.**

      (1) Serum concentrations for drugs with a **narrow therapeutic range** must be monitored closely; **small changes** in dose or organ dysfunction may lead to either **therapeutic failure or toxicity.**

C. The quantal dose–response curve

1. The quantal dose–response curve (Fig. 1.6A and B) relates the dosage of a drug to the frequency with which a designated response will occur within a population.

   a. The response may be an "all-or-none" phenomenon (e.g., individuals either do or do not fall asleep after receiving a sedative) or a predetermined intensity of effect.

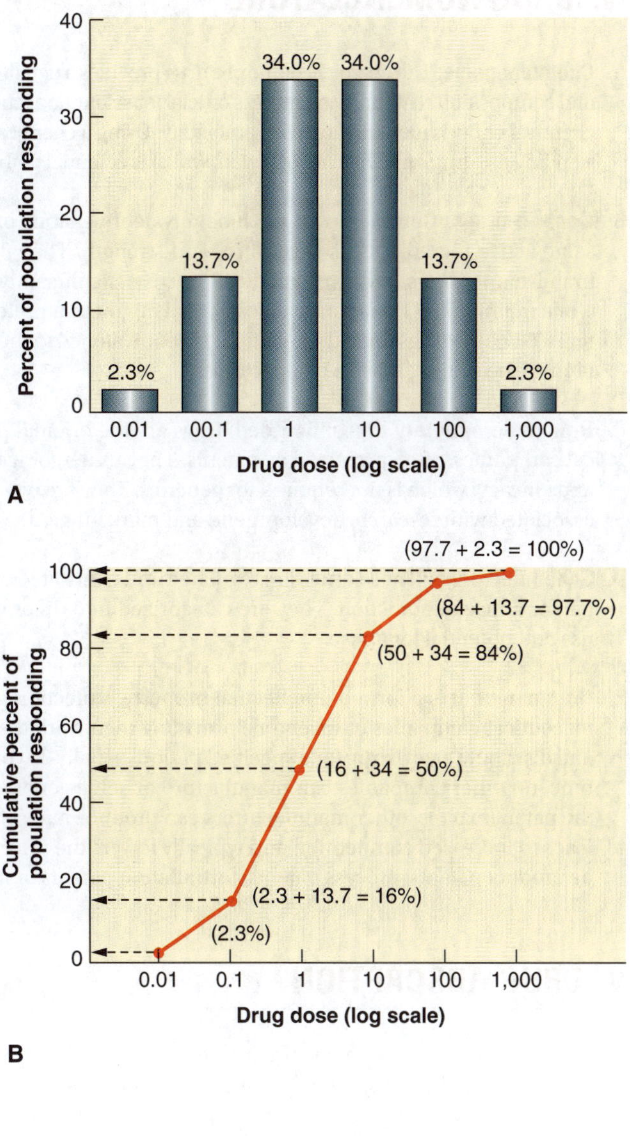

FIGURE 1.6. A. Frequency distribution plot. Number of individuals (as percentage of the population) who require the indicated drug dose to exhibit an identical response. As illustrated, 2.3% of the population requires 0.01 unit to exhibit the response, 13.7% requires 0.1 unit, and so on. **B.** Quantal dose–response curve. The cumulative number of individuals (as a percentage of the population) who will respond if the indicated dose of drug is administered to the entire population.

2. It is obtained via transformation of the data used for a frequency distribution plot to reflect the cumulative frequency of a response.
3. In the context of the quantal dose–response curve, ED_{50} indicates the dose of a drug that produces the response in half of the population. (Note that this differs from the meaning of ED_{50} in a graded dose–response curve.)
   a. For example, in Figure 1.6B, the ED_{50} would be 1. The TD_{50} for a drug would be determined from the midpoint of a similar curve indicating the cumulative percent of the population showing a toxic response to a drug.
4. Receptor upregulation refers to an increase in the number of receptors for a specific ligand in response to various stimuli.
   a. Chronic administration of β-blocker can upregulate β-receptor density, leading to severe hypertension and tachycardia on abrupt withdrawal.
5. Receptor downregulation involves a decrease in in the number of receptors on the cell surface in response to repeated stimulation.
   a. Clonidine causes downregulation of α-receptors, which can result in a hypertensive crisis if the drug is rapidly withdrawn.

IV. DRUG NOMENCLATURE

A. Chemical name: The chemical name of a drug provides a detailed description of its molecular structure and composition. This nomenclature is crucial for scientific accuracy and clarity, ensuring that the exact chemical entity is identified without ambiguity. Using a chemical-based nomenclature helps in understanding the drug's mechanism of action, which is essential for both clinical and research purposes.

B. Generic drugs: Generic drugs are bioequivalent versions of brand-name drugs, containing the same active ingredients, dosage form, and strength. They provide a cost-effective alternative to brand-name drugs, reducing medication costs significantly. They offer significant cost savings while maintaining therapeutic efficacy, making them a preferred choice in many healthcare systems. Generic drugs must demonstrate bioequivalence to the brand-name counterpart but do not require the same extensive clinical trials.

C. Branded/proprietary drugs: Branded drugs are the original products developed by pharmaceutical companies, often protected by patents. They undergo rigorous clinical trials to establish safety and efficacy, which is not required for generics. They are typically more expensive due to the costs associated with research, development, and marketing.

D. Scheduled drugs: These drugs are regulated and controlled by the government due to their potential for abuse or addiction. They are categorized into different schedules based on their medical use and potential for abuse.

E. Drug patent: It is a form of intellectual property protection granted by the governments to pharmaceutical companies or inventors, providing them with the exclusive right to manufacture, sell, and distribute a new drug for a specified period, usually 20 years from the date of filing. During this time, no other companies can manufacture or sell a generic version of the patented drug. Once the patent expires, other manufacturers can produce and sell generic versions of the drug, which leads to increased competition and typically lowers the price of the medication. Drug patents can be product patents, process patents, formulation patents or method of use patents.

V. DRUG ABSORPTION

Drug absorption is the movement of a drug from its site of administration into the bloodstream. In many cases, a drug must be transported across one or more biologic membranes to reach the bloodstream.

A. Drug transport across membranes

1. ***Diffusion of unionized drugs*** is the most common and most important mode of traversing biologic membranes.
   a. Drugs diffuse passively down their concentration gradient.
   b. Diffusion can be influenced significantly by the **lipid–water partition coefficient** of the drug, which is the ratio of solubility in an organic solvent to solubility in an aqueous solution.
      (1) In general, **absorption increases as lipid solubility (partition coefficient) increases.**
   c. Other factors that can also influence diffusion include the concentration gradient of the drug across the cell membrane and the surface area of the cell membrane.
2. ***Diffusion of drugs that are weak electrolytes***
   a. Only the **unionized** form of a drug **can diffuse** to any significant degree across biologic membranes.
   b. The degree of ionization of a weak acid or base is determined by the **p*K* of the drug and pH of its environment** according to the **Henderson-Hasselbalch equation.**
      (1) For a weak acid (A):

$$HA \rightleftarrows H^+ + A^-,$$
$$pH = pK + \log[A^-]/[HA], \text{ and}$$
$$\log[A^-]/[HA] = pH - pK$$

where HA is the concentration of the protonated, or unionized, form of the acid and A^- is the concentration of the ionized, or unprotonated, form.

      (2) For a weak base (B):

$$BH^+ \rightleftarrows H^+ + B,$$
$$pH = pK + \log[B]/[BH^+], \text{ and}$$
$$\log[B]/[BH^+] = pH - pK$$

where BH^+ is the concentration of the protonated form of the base and B is the concentration of the unprotonated form.

   c. When the p*K* of a drug equals the pH of the surroundings, 50% ionization occurs, in which equal numbers of ionized and unionized species are present.
      (1) A lower p*K* reflects a stronger acid.
      (2) A higher p*K* corresponds to a stronger base.
   d. Drugs with different p*K* values will diffuse across membranes at different rates.
   e. The pH of the biologic fluid in which the drug is dissolved affects the degree of ionization and, therefore, the rate of drug transport.
   f. **Ion trapping** occurs when a drug that is a weak acid or weak base **moves between fluid compartments with different pHs,** for example, when an oral drug is absorbed from the stomach (pH of 1–2) to the plasma (pH of 7.4).
      (1) The drug will tend to **accumulate** in the fluid compartment in which it is most **highly ionized.**
         (a) Weak acids tend to accumulate in the fluid with the higher pH.
         (b) Weak bases tend to accumulate in the fluid with the lower pH.
3. ***Active transport*** is an energy-dependent process that can move drugs against a concentration gradient through **protein-mediated transport systems.**
   a. Active transport occurs in only one direction and is saturable.
   b. It is usually the mode of transport for drugs that resemble actively transported endogenous substances such as sugars, amino acids, and nucleosides.
   c. Some transport systems increase drug transport and entry into cells to increase drug effects. Others cause active efflux of drugs from target cells and decrease their activity.
4. ***Filtration*** is the bulk flow of solvent and solute through channels in the membrane.
   a. It is seen with small molecules (usually with a molecular weight <100 Da) that can pass through the channels (pores).
   b. Some substances with a greater molecular weight, like certain proteins, can be filtered through intercellular channels.
   c. Concentration gradients affect the rate of filtration.
5. ***Facilitated diffusion*** is movement of a substance down a concentration gradient.
   a. It is carrier mediated, specific, and saturable; it does not require energy.

B. Routes of administration

1. *Oral administration*

a. **Sites of absorption**

(1) **Stomach**

(a) **Lipid-soluble drugs** and **weak acids**, which are normally unionized at the low pH of gastric contents, may be absorbed directly from the stomach.

(b) **Weak bases** and **strong acids** (pK = 2–3) are not normally absorbed from this site since they tend to exist as ions that carry either a positive or a negative charge, respectively.

(2) **Small intestine**

(a) The small intestine is the **primary site of absorption** of most drugs because of the very large surface area across which drugs, including partially ionized weak acids and bases, may diffuse.

(b) Acids are normally absorbed more extensively from the small intestine than from the stomach, even though the intestine has a higher pH of 5–7.

b. The **bioavailability of a drug** is the fraction of drug (administered by any route) that reaches the systemic bloodstream unaltered (bioavailability = 1 or 100% for intravenous [IV] administration). Bioequivalence refers to the condition in which the plasma concentrations versus time profiles of two drug formulations are identical.

(1) The **first-pass effect** influences drug absorption by metabolism in the liver or by biliary secretion. After absorption from the stomach or small intestine, a drug must pass through the liver before reaching the general circulation and its target site.

(a) If the capacity of liver metabolic enzymes to inactivate the drug is great, only limited amounts of active drug will escape the process.

i. During the first pass, the liver metabolizes some drugs so extensively that it precludes their use.

(2) Other factors that may alter absorption from the stomach or small intestine include the following:

(a) Gastric emptying time and passage of drug to the intestine may be influenced by **gastric contents** and **intestinal motility**.

i. A **decreased emptying time** generally **decreases the rate of absorption** because the intestine is the major absorptive site for most orally administered drugs.

(b) **Gastrointestinal (GI) blood flow** plays an important role in drug absorption by continuously maintaining the concentration gradient across epithelial membranes.

i. The absorption of small, very lipid-soluble molecules is "blood flow limited," whereas highly polar molecules are "blood flow independent."

(c) **Stomach acid** and enzyme inactivation may destroy certain drugs. Enteric coating prevents breakdown of tablets by the acidic pH of the stomach.

(d) **Interactions** with food, drugs, and other constituents of the gastric milieu may influence absorption.

(e) **Inert ingredients** in oral preparations may alter absorption.

2. *Parenteral administration*

Parenteral administration includes three major routes: **IV, intramuscular (IM)**, and **subcutaneous (SC)**. Parenteral administration generally results in more predictable bioavailability than oral administration.

a. With **IV** administration, the drug is injected directly into the bloodstream (100% bioavailable). It represents the most rapid means of introducing drugs into the body and is particularly useful in the treatment of emergencies.

b. After **IM** and **SC** administration, many drugs can enter the capillaries directly through pores between endothelial cells.

3. *Other routes of administration*

a. **Inhalation** results in **rapid absorption** because of the large surface area and rich blood supply of the alveoli.

(1) It is frequently used for gaseous anesthetics and for other drugs that act on the airways, such as the glucocorticoids used to treat bronchial asthma.

b. **Sublingual administration** is useful for drugs with **high first-pass metabolism**, since hepatic metabolism is bypassed.

c. **Intrathecal administration** is useful for drugs that do not readily cross the blood–brain barrier.
d. **Rectal administration** minimizes first-pass metabolism. It may be useful when oral drugs cannot be taken due to nausea and vomiting,
e. **Topical administration** is used widely when a local effect is desired or to **minimize systemic effects**, especially in dermatology and ophthalmology.

VI. DRUG DISTRIBUTION

Drug distribution is the movement of a drug from the bloodstream to the various tissues of the body.

A. **Distribution of drugs.** Distribution of drugs is the process by which a drug leaves the bloodstream and enters the extracellular fluids and tissues. A drug must diffuse across cellular membranes if its site of action is intracellular. In this case, lipid solubility is important for effective distribution.

1. ***Importance of blood flow***
   a. In most tissues, drugs can leave the circulation readily by diffusion across or between capillary endothelial cells. Thus, the **initial rate of distribution** of a drug **depends heavily on blood flow** to various organs (brain, liver, kidney > muscle, skin > fat, bone).
   b. At **equilibrium**, or **steady state**, the amount of drug in an organ is related to the mass of the organ and its properties, as well as the properties of the specific drug.
2. ***Volume of distribution (V_d)*** is the **volume of total body fluid** into which a drug appears to distribute after it reaches equilibrium in the body. It is determined by administering a known dose of drug (expressed in units of mass) intravenously and measuring the initial plasma concentration (expressed in units of mass/volume):

$$V_d = \frac{\text{Amount of drug administered (mg)}}{\text{Initial plasma concentration (mg/L)}}$$

   Volume of distribution is expressed in units of volume. In most cases, the initial plasma concentration, C_0, is determined by extrapolation from the elimination phase.
   a. **Standard values** of volumes of fluid compartments in an average 70-kg adult are as follows: plasma, 3 L; extracellular fluid, 12 L; and total body water 41 L.
   b. **Features** of volume of distribution
      (1) The use of V_d values is primarily conceptual, in which **drugs that distribute extensively have relatively large V_d values** and vice versa.
         (a) A low V_d value may indicate extensive plasma protein binding of the drug.
         (b) A high V_d may indicate that the drug is extensively bound to tissue sites.
      (2) Among other variables, V_d may be influenced by age, sex, weight, and disease processes (e.g., edema, ascites).
3. ***Drug redistribution*** describes when the relative distribution of a drug in different tissues or fluid compartments of the body changes with time. This is usually seen with highly lipophilic drugs, such as thiopental, that initially enter tissues with high blood flow (e.g., the brain) and then quickly redistribute to tissues with lower blood flow (e.g., skeletal muscle and adipose tissue).
4. ***Barriers to drug distribution***
   a. Blood–brain barrier
      (1) **Ionized** or **polar drugs distribute poorly to the CNS**, because they must pass through, rather than between, endothelial cells.
      (2) **Inflammation**, such as that resulting from meningitis, may increase the ability of ionized, poorly soluble drugs to cross the blood-brain barrier.
      (3) The blood–brain barrier may not be fully developed at the time of birth.
   b. Placental barrier
      (1) **Lipid-soluble drugs** cross the placental barrier more easily than polar drugs.
      (2) Drugs with a molecular weight of <600 Da pass the placental barrier more readily than larger molecules.
      (3) The possibility that drugs administered to the mother may cross the placenta and reach the fetus is always an important consideration in therapy.

B. Binding of drugs by plasma proteins

1. Drugs in the plasma may exist in the free form or may be bound to plasma proteins or other blood components, such as red blood cells.
2. ***General features of plasma protein binding***
   a. The extent of plasma protein binding is **highly variable**; depending on the drug, it may range from 0% to more than 99% bound. Binding is generally reversible.
   b. Only free drug is small enough to pass through the spaces between the endothelial cells that form the capillaries; extensive binding slows the rate at which the drug reaches its site of action and may prolong duration of action.
   c. Some plasma proteins bind many different drugs, whereas other proteins bind only one or a limited number. For example, **serum albumin tends to bind many acidic and neutral drugs**, whereas α_1-acid glycoprotein tends to bind many basic drugs.
   d. Highly bound drugs are restricted to plasma and tend to have lower volumes of distribution and longer duration of action.
   e. Binding is selective and not exclusive, for example, albumin has got multiple binding sites for different drugs. Drugs can compete for the same binding sites, which can lead to displacement reactions and drug–drug interactions.

VII. METABOLISM (BIOTRANSFORMATION) OF DRUGS

A. General properties

1. Most drugs undergo biotransformation, or metabolism, after they enter the body.
   a. It almost always produces metabolites that are more polar than the parent drug, often terminating the pharmacologic action and increasing removal of the drug from the body (via excretion).
   b. **Metabolites carry ionizable groups** and are often **more charged and more polar** than the parent compounds.
      (1) This increased charge may lead to a more rapid rate of clearance because of possible secretion by acid or base carriers in the kidney; it may also lead to decreased tubular reabsorption.
   c. Possible consequences of biotransformation include the production of the following:
      (1) **Inactive metabolites** (most common)
      (2) Metabolites with increased or decreased potencies
         (a) The active parent drugs may be metabolized to active metabolites.
         (b) **Prodrugs** are inactive compounds that are metabolized to active drugs.
      (3) Metabolites with qualitatively different pharmacologic actions
      (4) Toxic metabolites
2. Many drugs undergo several sequential biotransformation reactions, which are catalyzed by specific enzyme systems.
3. The **liver is the major site of metabolism**, although specific drugs may undergo biotransformation in other tissues.
4. Drug metabolism can be affected by many parameters, including the following:
   a. **Drugs** (drug–drug interactions) and **diet** (food–drug interactions)
   b. Organ function and various disease states
      (1) **Decreased liver function** may lead to decreased metabolism of certain drugs.
      (2) Drug metabolism may decrease in cardiac and pulmonary disease.
   c. **Age** and **developmental status**
      (1) Very young children and elderly individuals may be more sensitive to drugs due to undeveloped or decreased levels of drug-metabolizing enzymes.
      (2) Hormonal status and genetics may also affect drug metabolism.

B. Classification of biotransformation reactions

1. ***Phase I (nonsynthetic) reactions*** involve enzyme-catalyzed biotransformation of the drug without any conjugations.
   a. They often convert the parent drug to a more polar (water-soluble) compound.
      (1) They frequently introduce a **polar functional group, such as –OH, –SH, or –NH_2**, which serves as the active center for sequential conjugation in phase II reactions.

(2) These include **oxidations, reductions**, and **hydrolysis reactions.**

b. Although phase I products may be excreted, in many cases, they undergo phase II reactions.

c. Enzymes catalyzing phase I include **cytochrome P450 (CYP)**, aldehyde and alcohol dehydrogenase, deaminases, esterases, amidases, and epoxide hydratases.

2. ***Phase II (synthetic) reactions*** include **conjugation reactions**, which involve the enzyme-catalyzed combination of a drug with an endogenous substance.

a. The polar functional group of phase I products is often combined with glucuronic acid (**glucuronidation**), acetic acid (**acetylation**), or sulfuric acid (sulfation).

b. The final product is a highly polar conjugate that can be readily eliminated.

c. Enzymes catalyzing phase II biotransformation reactions include glucuronyl transferase (glucuronide conjugation), sulfotransferase (sulfate conjugation), transacylases (amino acid conjugation), acetylases, ethylases, methylases, and glutathione transferase.

C. Cytochrome P450 monooxygenase (mixed function oxidase)

1. **General features**

a. CYP monooxygenase plays a central role in drug biotransformation.

(1) This enzyme system is the one most frequently involved in **phase I reactions.**

(2) It catalyzes numerous reactions, including aromatic and aliphatic hydroxylations; dealkylation at nitrogen, sulfur, and oxygen atoms; heteroatom oxidations at nitrogen and sulfur atoms; reductions at nitrogen atoms; and ester and amide hydrolysis.

b. There are many types of CYP enzymes.

c. Each type catalyzes the biotransformation of a unique spectrum of drugs, although there is some overlap with substrate specificities. The CYP families are referred to using Arabic numerals (e.g., CYP1, CYP2).

(1) Each family has a number of subfamilies denoted by an uppercase letter (e.g., CYP2A, CYP2B).

(2) The individual enzymes within each subfamily are denoted by another Arabic numeral (e.g., CYP3A1, CYP3A2).

d. The **CYP2C, CYP2D, and CYP3A** enzymes are responsible for the metabolism of most drugs.

(1) **CYP3A4 is the most abundant hepatic enzyme** and is involved in the metabolism of more than half of clinically important drugs.

2. The **primary location** of CYP is the **liver**, although significant levels are also found in the small and large intestines.

a. CYP450 activity is also found in many other tissues, including the adrenals, ovaries, and testis, and tissues involved in steroidogenesis and steroid metabolism.

b. The enzyme's subcellular location is the **endoplasmic reticulum.**

c. Lipid membrane location facilitates the metabolism of lipid-soluble drugs.

3. **Mechanism of reaction**

a. In the overall reaction, the drug is oxidized and oxygen is reduced to water.

b. Reducing equivalents are provided by **nicotinamide adenine dinucleotide phosphate (NADPH)**, and generation of this cofactor is coupled to **CYP reductase.**

c. The overall reaction for aromatic hydroxylation can be described as follows:

$$\text{Drug} + O_2 + \text{NADPH} + H^+ \rightarrow \text{Drug} - \text{OH} + \text{NADP}^+ + H_2O$$

4. **Genetic polymorphism** of several clinically important CYPs, particularly **CYP2C** and **CYP2D**, is a source of variable metabolism in humans, including differences among racial and ethnic groups. These enzymes have substantially different properties (V_{max} or K_m).

5. **Induction**

a. Enzyme induction may occur due to **drugs** and **endogenous substances**, such as hormones; they can preferentially induce one or more forms of CYP450.

b. When caused by drugs, induction is pharmacologically important as a major source of **drug interactions.** A drug may induce its own metabolism (metabolic tolerance) or that of other drugs.

(1) Induction can be caused by a wide variety of drugs, such as quinidine, phenytoin, **phenobarbital, rifampin**, and **carbamazepine.**

(2) Environmental agents, such as **tobacco smoke**, may also induce CYP450 enzymes.

c. Some of the same drugs that induce CYP3A4 can induce the drug efflux transporter P-glycoprotein, such as rifampin and St. John's wort.

6. **Inhibition**
   a. Competitive or noncompetitive (clinically more likely) inhibition of CYP450 enzyme activity can result in the **reduced metabolism of other drugs** or endogenous substrates, such as **testosterone**.
   b. Enzyme inhibition is a **major source of drug–drug interactions**. It is caused by a number of commonly used drugs, including **cimetidine, fluconazole, fluoxetine**, and **erythromycin**. **Environmental or dietary agents (e.g., grapefruit juice)** can also cause enzyme inhibition.
   c. Some of the same drugs that inhibit CYP3A4 can inhibit the drug efflux transporter P-glycoprotein, including amiodarone, clarithromycin, erythromycin, and ketoconazole.

D. Glucuronyl transferase

1. General features
   a. Glucuronyl transferase is a set of enzymes with unique, but overlapping, specificities that are involved in **phase II reactions**.
   b. It catalyzes the conjugation of glucuronic acid to a variety of active centers, including –OH, –COOH, –SH, and $–NH_2$.
2. Location and induction
   a. Glucuronyl transferase is located in the **endoplasmic reticulum**.
   b. It is the only phase II reaction that is **inducible by drugs** and is a possible site of drug interactions.

E. Hepatic extraction of drugs

1. General extraction by the liver occurs because of the liver's large size (1,500 g) and high blood flow (1 mL/g/min).
2. The **extraction ratio** is the amount of drug removed in the liver divided by the amount of drug entering the organ; a drug completely extracted by the liver would have an extraction ratio of 1. Highly extracted drugs can have a hepatic clearance approaching 1,500 mL/min.
3. **First-pass effect.** Drugs taken orally pass across membranes of the GI tract into the portal vein and through the liver before entering the general circulation.
   a. **Bioavailability** of orally administered drugs is **decreased** by the fraction of drug removed by the first pass through the liver. For example, a drug with a hepatic extraction ratio of 1 would have 0% bioavailability; a drug such as lidocaine, with an extraction ratio of 0.7, would have 30% bioavailability.
   b. In the presence of hepatic disease, drugs with a high first-pass extraction may reach the systemic circulation in higher than normal amounts, and dose adjustment may be required.

VIII. DRUG ELIMINATION AND TERMINATION OF ACTION

A. Mechanisms of drug elimination and termination of action

1. In most cases, the action of a drug is terminated by **enzyme-catalyzed conversion** to an inactive (or less active) compound and/or **elimination from the body** via the kidney or other routes.
2. Redistribution of drugs from the site of action may terminate the action of a drug, although this occurs infrequently. For example, the action of the anesthetic **thiopental** is terminated largely by its redistribution from the brain (where it initially accumulates as a result of its high lipid solubility and the high blood flow to that organ) to the more poorly perfused adipose tissue.

B. Routes of excretion

1. Routes of excretion may include urine, feces (e.g., unabsorbed drugs and drugs secreted in bile), saliva, sweat, tears, milk (with possible transfer to neonates), and lungs (e.g., alcohols and anesthetics).
2. Any route may be important for a given drug, but the **kidney is the major site of excretion** for most drugs.
3. Some drugs are secreted by liver cells into the bile, pass into the intestine, and are eliminated in the feces (e.g., rifampin, indomethacin, estradiol).
4. Some drugs undergo **enterohepatic circulation** (reabsorbed from the intestine); in this case, the drug effect may be prolonged.

C. General principles for drug clearance (CL)

1. Conceptually, clearance is a measure of the capacity of the body to remove a drug.
2. Mathematically, clearance is the proportionality constant that relates the rate of drug elimination to the plasma concentration of the drug.
   - **a.** The units of clearance are volume/time.
   - **b.** Drugs with high clearance are rapidly removed from the body.
   - **c.** Drugs with low clearance are removed slowly from the body.
3. ***Specific organ clearance*** is the capacity of an individual organ to eliminate a drug. It may be due to metabolism (e.g., hepatic clearance by the liver) or excretion (e.g., renal clearance by elimination in the urine).

$$\text{Rate of elimination by organ} = CL_{\text{organ}} \times [\text{Drug}]_{\text{plasma perfusing organ}}$$

or

$$CL_{\text{organ}} = \frac{\text{Rate of elimination by organ}}{[\text{Drug}]_{\text{plasma perfusing organ}}}$$

4. ***Whole body clearance*** is the capacity of the body to eliminate the drug by all mechanisms. Therefore, whole body clearance is equal to the sum of all of the specific organ clearance mechanisms by which the active drug is eliminated from the body:

$$CL_{\text{whole body}} = CL_{\text{organ 1}} + CL_{\text{organ 2}} + CL_{\text{organ } N}$$

The term "clearance" generally refers to whole body clearance unless otherwise specified. In this case,

$$\text{Rate of elimination from body} = CL_{\text{whole body}} \times [\text{Drug}]_{\text{plasma}}$$

and

$$CL = \frac{\text{Rate of elimination by body}}{[\text{Drug}]_{\text{plasma}}}$$

5. ***Plasma clearance*** is numerically the same as whole body clearance, but this terminology is sometimes used because clearance may be viewed as the volume of plasma that contains the amount of drug removed per unit time (recall that the units of clearance are volume/time).
   - **a.** If not specified, this term refers to the volume of plasma "cleared" of drug by all bodily mechanisms (i.e., whole body clearance).
   - **b.** The term may also be applied to clearance by specific organs; for example, renal plasma clearance is the volume of plasma containing the amount of drug eliminated in the urine per unit time.

D. Net renal excretion of drugs

1. ***Net renal excretion*** of drugs is the result of **three separate processes:** (1) the amount of drug filtered at the glomerulus, (2) plus the amount of drug secreted by active transport mechanisms in the kidney (3) minus the amount of drug passively reabsorbed throughout the tubule.
   - **a. Filtration**
     - **(1)** Most drugs have low molecular weights and are freely filtered from the plasma at the glomerulus.
     - **(2)** Serum protein binding reduces filtration since plasma proteins are too large to be filtered.
     - **(3)** Compared with adults, the glomerular filtration rate (GFR) is 30%–40% lower during a child's first year of life.
   - **b. Secretion**
     - **(1)** The kidney proximal tubule contains **two transport systems** that may secrete drugs into the ultrafiltrate, one for **organic acids** (organic acid transporters [OATs]) and a second for **organic bases** (organic base transporters [OBTs]).
       - **(a)** There are multiple OATs and OBTs with specificities for different organic molecules in the tubule.

(b) They **require energy for active transport** against a concentration gradient.

(c) They are also a site for potential **drug–drug interactions**; drugs may compete with each other for binding to the transporters.

(2) Plasma protein binding does not normally have a large effect on secretion because the affinity of the transport systems for most drugs is greater than the affinity of plasma-binding proteins.

c. **Reabsorption**

(1) Reabsorption may occur throughout the tubule; some compounds, including endogenous compounds such as glucose, are actively reabsorbed.

(2) Reabsorption of the **unionized form** of drugs that are weak acids and bases can occur by simple **passive diffusion**, the rate of which depends on the lipid solubility and pK of the drug, as well as the concentration gradient of the drug between the urine and the plasma.

(3) Reabsorption may be affected by **alterations of urinary pH**, which affects elimination of weak acids or bases by altering their ionization (i.e., **ion trapping**).

(a) For example, alkalinization of the urine will result in a higher proportion of the ionized form of an acidic drug that will decrease its reabsorption and hence increase its elimination.

2. ***Renal clearance of drugs***

a. Renal clearance measures the volume of plasma that is cleared of drug per unit time:

$$\mathrm{CL}\,(\mathrm{mL/min}) = U \times \frac{V}{P}$$

where ***U*** is the concentration of drug per milliliter of **urine,** ***V*** **the volume** of the urine excreted per minute, and ***P*** the concentration of drug per milliliter of **plasma**.

(1) A drug excreted by **filtration alone** will have a clearance equal to the GFR (125–130 mL/min).

(2) A drug excreted by **filtration and complete secretion** will have a clearance equal to renal plasma clearance (650 mL/min).

(3) Clearance values between 130 and 650 mL/min suggest that a drug is **filtered, secreted, and partially reabsorbed**.

b. A variety of factors influence renal clearance, including age, other drugs, and disease.

c. In the presence of **renal failure**, the clearance of a drug may be reduced significantly, resulting in higher plasma levels (dose reductions may be required).

IX. CHANGES IN PHARMACOLOGY OF DRUGS IN SPECIAL POPULATION

A. **Geriatric considerations:** The pharmacokinetic parameters such as absorption, distribution, metabolism, and excretion can be altered due to physiological changes associated with aging. Slower gastric emptying and reduced blood flow can delay drug absorption. Increased body fat leads to a longer half-life for lipophilic (fat-soluble) drugs. Decreased water content results in higher concentrations of polar (water-soluble) drugs. Reduced plasma proteins (like albumin) can increase the free fraction of drugs that bind to protein, leading to potential toxicity. Decreased renal function can lead to prolonged drug half-lives, necessitating dose adjustments. Existence of multiple comorbidities often leads to polypharmacy, increasing the risk of drug–drug interactions and adverse reactions. It is prudent to start with a low dose and titrate up slowly to avoid adverse effects, monitor renal/hepatic function and attempt to avoid polypharmacy. Regular medication reviews using criteria like Beers can help identify potentially inappropriate medications (PIMs) and reduce adverse effects.

B. **Pediatric considerations:** Children are not just small adults. Neonates have high gastrointestinal pH and immature liver and kidney function, affecting drug absorption and clearance. Infants have higher water content and lower fat content affecting distribution of drugs. Renal function is immature in neonates and infants. Pediatric dosing often requires calculations based on weight or body surface area. The long-term impact of medications on growth and development must be considered, particularly for chronic conditions.

C. **Pregnancy and lactation:** Physiological changes during pregnancy and lactation may affect drug absorption, distribution, metabolism, and excretion, requiring adjustments in dose, duration, or frequency of medication administration. Increased blood volume and changes in body fat can alter drug distribution, while increased renal blood flow and glomerular filtration rate enhance the clearance may necessitate higher doses of certain medications. Changes in serum protein levels can affect drug binding, potentially increasing free drug concentrations. Some drugs are contraindicated in pregnancy and lactation due to teratogenic effects, and caution is advised for using others as drugs may pass through the placenta to the fetus and cause teratogenic effects. Drugs can transfer into breast milk, with varying degrees of concentration. For example, lamotrigine shows significant transfer, while others like quetiapine have lower milk/serum ratios. Understanding these changes is essential for optimizing maternal and fetal health and guiding drug therapy in pregnant and lactating women.

D. **Hepatic and renal disorders:** Liver function significantly affects drug metabolism. Drugs that undergo extensive first-pass metabolism may require dosage adjustments in patients with hepatic impairment to prevent toxicity. Liver diseases like cirrhosis reduce the liver's ability to clear drugs, leading to higher drug concentrations and potential toxicity. Decreased activity of enzymes such as CYP2E1 and CYP3A4 is common, affecting drug metabolism and increasing the risk of drug interactions. Both phase I (oxidation) and phase II (conjugation) metabolic pathways are impaired, altering drug metabolism. Impaired production of drug-binding proteins alters drug distribution and increases free drug concentrations. Lower doses and extended dosing intervals are often necessary to prevent drug accumulation and toxicity.

Kidney disorders significantly impact the pharmacology of drugs, necessitating careful consideration in drug dosing and selection to avoid adverse effects and ensure therapeutic efficacy. Impaired kidney function can reduce drug absorption due to delayed gastric emptying and gut edema, alteration of drug distribution due to changes in extracellular fluid volume, plasma protein binding, and tissue binding, reduced glomerular filtration, tubular secretion, and reabsorption, necessitating dosage adjustments based on creatinine clearance. Reducing the dose or increasing the dosing interval, or both, to maintain therapeutic drug levels may be necessary (e.g., digoxin, aminoglycosides) along with regular monitoring of serum creatinine and GFR to guide dose adjustments.

X. PHARMACOKINETIC PRINCIPLES

A. General pharmacokinetic principles

1. Pharmacokinetics describes changes in plasma drug concentration over time.
2. Although it is ideal to determine the amount of drug that reaches its site of action as a function of time after administration, it is usually impractical or not feasible.
   a. The plasma drug concentration is measured since the amount of drug in the tissues is generally related to plasma concentration.

B. Distribution and elimination

1. ***One-compartment model*** (Fig. 1.7)
   a. The drug appears to distribute instantaneously after IV administration of a single dose. If the mechanisms for drug elimination, such as biotransformation by hepatic enzymes and renal secretion, are not saturated following the therapeutic dose, a semi-log plot of plasma concentration versus time will be **linear**.
   b. Drug elimination is **first order**, in which a **constant fraction** of drug is eliminated per unit time.
      (1) For example, one-half (50%) of the drug is eliminated every 8 hours.
      (2) Elimination of most drugs is a first-order process.

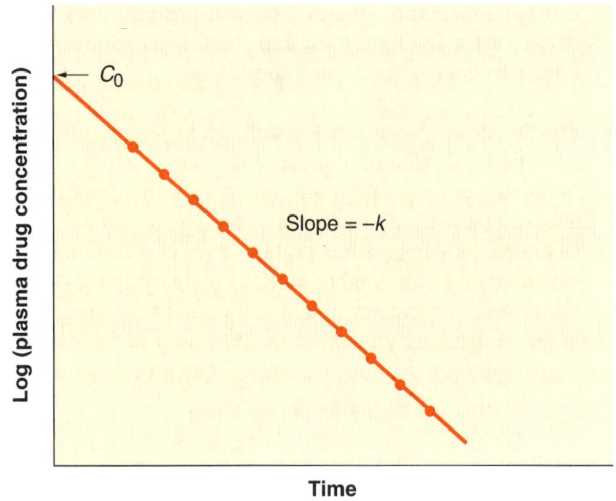

FIGURE 1.7. One-compartment model of drug distribution.

c. The slope of the semi-log plot is **−*k*,** where ***k* is the rate constant of elimination** and has units of time, and the intercept on the *y* axis is C_0. (*Note:* C_0 is used to calculate V_d for drugs that obey a one-compartment model.)

d. The **plasma drug concentration (C_t) relative to the initial concentration (C_0)** at any time (t) after administration is given by

$$\ln C_t = \ln C_0 - kt$$

and the **relationship of the plasma concentrations** at any two points in time is given by

$$\ln C_2 = \ln C_1 - k(t_2 - t_1)$$

2. *Two-compartment model* (Fig. 1.8)

a. The two-compartment model is a **more common model for distribution and elimination** of drugs.

b. Initial rapid decreases in the plasma concentration of a drug are observed because of a **distribution phase,** which is the time required for the drug to reach an **equilibrium** distribution between a central compartment, such as the plasma space, and a second compartment, such as the aggregate tissues and fluids to which the drug distributes.

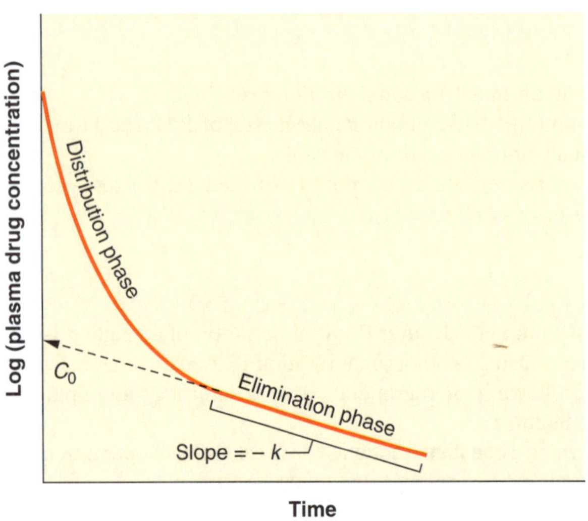

FIGURE 1.8. Two-compartment model of drug distribution.

(1) During this phase, plasma drug concentrations decrease very rapidly because the drug is being eliminated from the body (e.g., by metabolism and renal elimination), as well as exiting the plasma space as it distributes to other tissues and fluid compartments.

c. After distribution, a linear decrease in the log drug concentration is observed if the **elimination phase** is first order. The curve is less steep in this phase because there is no longer a net decrease in plasma levels of drug due to distribution to the tissues (which has been completed).

d. For drugs that obey a two-compartment model, the value of C_0 obtained by extrapolation of the elimination phase is used to calculate V_d, and the elimination rate constant, k, is obtained from the slope of the elimination phase.

e. The expressions for ln C_t and clearance (CL) shown above for a one-compartment model also apply during the elimination phase for drugs that obey a two-compartment model.

3. ***First-order elimination***

a. The elimination of **most drugs** at therapeutic doses is **first order**, where a **constant fraction of drug is eliminated per unit time.**

(1) It occurs when the drug does not saturate elimination systems.

(2) The rate of elimination is a **linear function** of the plasma drug concentration.

b. The rate of elimination depends on the concentration of drug in the plasma and is equal to the plasma concentration of the drug multiplied by a **proportionality constant:**

$$\text{Rate of elimination from body (mass/time)} = \text{Constant} \times [\text{Drug}]_{\text{plasma}} \text{ (mass/vol)}$$

Because the rate of elimination is given in units of mass/time and concentration is in units of mass/volume, the units of the constant are volume/time. This constant is referred to as the clearance of the drug.

c. As the constant percentage of the drug is eliminated in unit time, the predictability is better in terms of dose adjustments.

d. The drug's half-life remains constant and is independent of drug concentration.

e. The decline in the concentration of drug on a semi-log paper appears as a straight line.

4. ***Zero-order elimination***

a. **Zero-order** elimination occurs when a **constant amount of the drug is eliminated per unit time**; it does **not depend on plasma concentration.**

(1) It may occur when **therapeutic doses of drugs exceed the capacity of elimination mechanisms** (the mechanism by which the body eliminates the drug, such as hepatic metabolism or kidney secretion, is saturated), leading to saturation kinetics or capacity-limited elimination, also known as Michaelis–Menten elimination.

b. In this model, the plot of the log of the plasma concentration versus time will decrease in a concave upward manner (e.g., 10 mg of drug will be eliminated every 8 hours). (Note that after an interval of time sufficient to reduce the drug level below the saturation point, first-order elimination occurs.)

c. Examples of drugs removed by zero-order kinetics include phenytoin and ethanol.

d. The drug's half-life is not constant and varies with the drug concentration.

e. Drugs obeying zero-order kinetics pose a risk of accumulation and toxicity. A small hike in the dosage can result in disproportionate elevation of plasma concentration. This warrants monitoring and proper dose adjustments especially when saturation occurs.

C. Half-life ($t_{1/2}$)

1. Half-life is the time it takes for the **plasma drug concentration to be reduced by 50%.** This concept applies only to drugs eliminated by **first-order kinetics.**

2. Half-life is determined by the following:

a. Log plasma drug concentration versus time profile for drugs fitting a one-compartment model.

b. Elimination phase for drugs fitting the two-compartment model.

c. If the dose administered does not exceed the capacity of the elimination systems (i.e., the dose does not saturate those systems), the half-life will remain constant.

3. The half-life is related to the **elimination rate constant (*k*)** by the equation $t_{1/2} = 0.693/k$ (i.e., for a steep decrease in concentration, k is high; therefore, $t_{1/2}$ is short).

4. It is related to the **volume of distribution (V_d)** and **clearance (CL)** by the equation $t_{1/2} = 0.693\ V_d/CL$.

a. This relationship emphasizes that drugs that are widely distributed in the body (i.e., a high V_d) will take longer to be eliminated and drugs for which the body has a high capacity to remove (i.e., a high CL) will take a short time to be eliminated.

5. In most cases, more than 95% of the drug will be **eliminated in a time interval equal to five half-lives**; this applies for therapeutic doses of most drugs.

6. Half-life generally determines dosing frequency. Drugs with shorter half-lives need to be administered more frequently and vice versa, this impacting dosing regimens. The duration of action of a drug, time to reach steady-state plasma concentration, and time to washout are determined by the drug's half-life.

D. Multidose kinetics

1. ***Infusion and multidose repeat administration***
   a. If a drug is given by continuous IV infusion at a constant dose rate and elimination is first order, it will eventually reach a constant steady-state plasma concentration.
      (1) The **steady-state concentration** occurs when the **rate of elimination is equal to the rate of administration.**
   b. If a drug that is eliminated by first-order kinetics is administered repeatedly (e.g., one tablet or injection every 8 hours), the *average* plasma concentration of the drug will increase until a *mean* steady-state level is reached.
      (1) This will not occur for drugs that exhibit zero-order elimination.
   c. The **time required to reach steady state is equal to five half-lives** regardless of whether administration is via continuous infusion or repeated administration.
      (1) Whenever a dose rate is changed, it will take five half-lives for a new steady-state level to be reached for any route of administration.

2. ***Steady state after repeat administration***
   a. Some fluctuation in plasma concentration will occur even at steady state.
   b. Levels will be at the high point of the steady-state range shortly after a dose is administered; levels will be at the low point immediately before administration of the next dose. Hence, **steady state designates an average plasma concentration** and the range of fluctuations above and below that level.
   c. The magnitude of fluctuations can be controlled by the **dosing interval**.
      (1) A shorter dosing interval decreases fluctuations, and a longer dosing interval increases them.
   d. On cessation of multidose administration, more than 95% of the drug will be eliminated in a time interval equal to five half-lives if first-order kinetics applies.

3. ***Maintenance dose rate***
   a. The **maintenance dose rate** is the dose of a drug required per unit time to **maintain a desired steady-state level** in the plasma to sustain a specific therapeutic effect.
   b. To determine the dose rate required to maintain an average steady-state plasma concentration of drug, multiply the desired plasma concentration by the CL:

$$\text{Maintenance dose rate} = \text{Desired}\left[\text{drug}\right]_{\text{plasma}} \times \text{Clearance (CL)}$$
$$(\text{amount/time}) = (\text{amount/volume}) \times (\text{volume/time})$$

   This yields dose rate in units of amount per time (e.g., mg/h).
      (1) To remain at steady state, the **dose rate must equal the elimination rate.**
         (a) The rate at which the drug is added to the body must equal the rate at which it is eliminated.
      (2) The elimination rate = CL × $[\text{Drug}]_{\text{plasma}}$; therefore, because the dose rate must equal the elimination rate to be at steady state, the dose rate also equals CL × Desired $[\text{drug}]_{\text{plasma}}$.
   c. If the drug is administered at the maintenance dose rate, a steady-state plasma concentration will be reached in four to five half-lives. (*Note:* This is four to five half-lives, not four to five doses!)

4. ***Loading dose***
   a. For certain drugs, an initial loading dose may be given to achieve rapid levels and earlier therapeutic effects; this may be useful in potentially life-threatening situations, such as a severe infection (e.g., aminoglycosides, vancomycin) or pulmonary embolism (e.g., heparin).

b. To calculate the loading dose, the desired plasma concentration of drug can be multiplied by the V_d:

$$\text{Loading dose} = \text{Desired}\,[\text{drug}]_{\text{plasma}} \times V_d$$
$$(\text{amount or mass}) = (\text{mass/volume}) \times (\text{volume})$$

c. After administration of the loading dose (which rapidly achieves the desired plasma concentration of drug), the drug is administered at the maintenance dose rate to maintain the drug concentration at the desired steady-state level.

E. Therapeutic drug monitoring (TDM)

1. Involves measuring drug concentrations in serum or plasma and interpreting these levels to optimize drug therapy for individual patients.
2. Plays a crucial role in personalized medicine by optimizing drug dosing, monitoring patient compliance, and evaluating drug interactions.
3. Indicated for drugs with narrow margin of safety (low TI), drugs exhibiting high interindividual pharmacokinetic variability, and drugs that have the potential for severe adverse effects if not monitored properly. Drugs must demonstrate a definite relationship between plasma concentration and clinical response.
4. Drugs commonly monitored include antiepileptics (phenytoin, carbamazepine, valproate), antimanic drugs (lithium), immunosuppressants (cyclosporine, tacrolimus), digoxin, theophylline, aminoglycoside antibiotics, etc.
5. Few drugs do not require TDM: Drugs with high TI (amoxicillin, ibuprofen, ciprofloxacin), over-the-counter medications, drugs with predictable pharmacokinetics (penicillin, statins), drugs with minimal risk of toxicity and used for short term, and when clinical/other laboratory parameters are easily monitored than plasma concentrations (blood pressure with antihypertensives, blood glucose with antidiabetics).
6. Requires specialized laboratory equipment such as high performance liquid chromatography (HPLC), thereby increasing healthcare costs. Timings of sample collections have to be precise for an effective and accurate interpretation.

F. Methods to prolong the duration of drug action

1. Long-acting formulations (sustained-release systems, controlled-released systems, extended-release systems), for example, nifedipine, metformin, and contraceptives.
2. Prodrugs (e.g., enalapril which gets converted to enalaprilat) provide prolonged antihypertensive effects.
3. Esterification (e.g., testosterone esters like testosterone enanthate) provides long-lasting replacement therapy.
4. Implants (e.g., levonorgestrel) provide long-term contraception through slow release of drugs.
5. Transdermal patches (e.g., nicotine patch) provide steady release over a long time.
6. Depot injections (e.g., medroxyprogesterone acetate) provide long-lasting effects for months together.
7. PEGylation (e.g., peginterferon alpha-2a) extends the half-life and reduces dosing frequency.
8. Use of drug carriers such as hydrogels, microspheres, and nanotubes prolongs the drug action.

G. Adverse drug reaction

It refers to response to a medicinal product which is noxious and unintended, and which occurs at doses normally used in humans for prophylaxis, diagnosis, therapy of disease, or for the modification of physiologic function. It can be:

1. Type A (augmented reactions): Predictable, dose dependent, and extensions of the known pharmacologic actions of drugs, for example, hypoglycemia from insulin and hemorrhage from heparin
2. Type B (bizarre) reactions: Unpredictable, dose independent, idiosyncratic, and unrelated to the drug's known pharmacologic actions, for example, anaphylaxis from penicillin G, agranulocytosis from clozapine, and Stevens-Johnson syndrome from sulfonamides
3. Type C (continuing or chronic) reactions: Associated with long-term drug therapy which might be due to cumulative effects, for example, osteoporosis from glucocorticoids and renal toxicity from nonsteroidal anti-inflammatory drugs

4. Type D (delayed) reactions: Occur after some time including after the discontinuation of drug at times, e.g., pulmonary fibrosis from amiodarone and carcinogenicity
5. Type E (end of use) reactions: Due to drug withdrawal, e.g., rebound hypertension from clonidine and acute adrenal insufficiency from corticosteroid withdrawal

XI. PHARMACOVIGILANCE

1. It refers to science and activities related to the detection, assessment, understanding, and prevention of adverse effects or any other drug-related problems. It is required to improve patient care and safety in the use of all drugs and medical interventions, contributing to the scientific understanding of the benefits, harms, and risks of medicines, thus contributing to the safe and rational use of medicines.
2. Methods of pharmacovigilance include spontaneous reporting of adverse drug events, active surveillance, case-control studies, cohort studies, randomized controlled clinical trials, meta-analyses and systematic reviews, database and registry studies, various scientific literature, postmarketing surveillance, and pharmacoepidemiologic studies.
3. Pharmacovigilance Programme of India (PvPI): It is an initiative to ensure drug safety and monitor adverse drug effects launched by the Ministry of Health and Family Welfare, Government of India, in 2010 and supervised by the Central Drugs Standard Control Organization (CDSCO) in collaboration with the Indian Pharmacopoeia Commission (IPC), Ghaziabad (National Coordination Center). All the medical colleges in the country serve as ADR monitoring centers apart from other healthcare facilities which collect the adverse drug reactions and report to the IPC through VigiFlow, the pharmacovigilance software.
4. A signal refers to a potential association between drugs and adverse effects that is unknown or incompletely understood. Signal detection involves data mining of various pharmacovigilance methods. After detection, the signal is validated, assessed, and prioritized, and regulatory action is recommended (updating product labels, issuing safety warnings, withdrawing the drug from the market). The new safety information is communicated to the healthcare professionals and consumers.

XII. ORPHAN DRUG

It refers to a drug intended to treat a condition affecting no more than 5 lakh persons in India or 2 lakh persons in the United States.

Pharmaceutical companies are often hesitant to invest in development of orphan drugs because the return on development is uncertain. Governments often provide incentives such as tax breaks, research grants and extended market exclusivity to encourage orphan drug development. Repurposing existing drugs for common conditions has emerged as a potential solution which can be more cost-effective and quicker to implement. Examples for orphan drugs include Ivacaftor in cystic fibrosis, alglucosidase alfa in Pompe disease, miglustat in Niemann-Pick disease type C, Idursulfase in Hunter syndrome (Mucopolysaccharidosis II), ruxolitinib in myelofibrosis, eculizumab in paroxysmal nocturnal hemoglobinuria etc.

XIII. EVIDENCE-BASED MEDICINE

Conscientious, explicit, and judicious use of current best evidence in making decisions about the care of individual patients. The typical processes are structured as follows: formulating a research question, searching for evidence, appraising the evidence (quality and applicability), applying the evidence, and assessing the outcomes. Various types of clinical studies are the following:

A. Experimental studies

1. Randomized controlled trials (RCTs): Participants are randomly assigned to the test or control group. It can involve placebo too. It minimizes bias and confounding variables and identifies potential causation between an intervention and an outcome.
2. Crossover trials: Participants receive both the intervention and the control in a sequential manner, thereby serving as their own control reducing variability in outcomes.
3. Adaptive trials: These allow modifications to the study procedures (e.g., sample size, allocation of treatment) based on interim results.

B. Observational studies

1. Case-control studies: They compare participants with a defined outcome (case) with those without (control) looking back to determine exposure levels. They are useful in studying rare diseases with long latent periods and outbreak investigations.
2. Cohort studies: They involve following up a group of individuals over time to measure outcomes based on an exposure to a potential cause. They can measure incidence and disease progression but require substantial time and funding. They can be prospective or retrospective too.
3. Cross-sectional studies: They assess a population at a single point in time measuring both exposure and outcome simultaneously providing a snapshot of the population. They can assist in hypothesis generation and establishment of association and prevalence but not of causation. These are faster and less expensive.
4. Descriptive studies: They include case reports and case series.
5. Ecological studies: They analyze data at the population level rather than at the individual level.

C. Others

1. Quasiexperimental studies: They are nonrandomized experiments used to evaluate the association between an intervention and an outcome. They establish causal relationships when RCTs are not feasible due to ethical or practical reasons.
2. Systematic reviews and meta-analyses: They are not primary studies but rather synthesize findings from multiple studies to provide a comprehensive overview of a particular research question. They are powerful tools for summarizing existing literature and offer the highest levels of evidence—crucial for informing clinical practice, developing guidelines, and making health policy decisions.

Review Test

Directions: Select the best answer for each question.

1. Somatostatin interacts with which of the following receptors?

(A) G_i-protein-coupled receptor
(B) G_q-protein-coupled receptor
(C) Intracellular nuclear receptor
(D) Ligand-activated ion channel
(E) Receptor-activated tyrosine kinase

2. What characteristic gives cortisol the ability to target intranuclear receptors?

(A) Diffuses through lipid membranes
(B) Interacts with adenylyl cyclase
(C) Interacts with G-protein-coupled receptors
(D) Recruits intracellular kinases
(E) Undergoes autophosphorylation

3. A 66-year-old man is admitted to the hospital with confusion, nausea, and blurred vision. He is currently on digoxin for the treatment of heart failure. On physical exam ination, his heart rate is 120 bpm. Further evaluation reveals a digoxin level of 5.3 ng/mL (normal range: 0.5–2 ng/mL). The doctor believes that his symptoms are due to digoxin toxicity. Which parameter is used to indicate the ability of digoxin to produce the desired effect relative to a toxic effect?

(A) Bioavailability
(B) Efficacy
(C) Intrinsic activity
(D) Potency
(E) Therapeutic index

4. A 64-year-old woman presents to the emergency room with severe abdominal pain and feculent emesis. She has a history of multiple abdominal surgeries due to Crohn disease. Further evaluation reveals a small bowel obstruction. A few hours later, she undergoes surgery for lysis of adhesions and resection of the small bowel. Why should the use of oral medications be avoided in this patient?

(A) Decreased passage of drug through the intestine
(B) Decreased gastrointestinal blood flow
(C) Destruction of drug by stomach acid
(D) Increased first-pass effect
(E) Increased protein binding of the drug

5. An 82-year-old woman is admitted to the hospital for management of a heart failure exacerbation. She has peripheral edema and ascites due to the exacerbation. Further evaluation also reveals a urinary tract infection requiring antibiotic treatment. Due to her history of heart failure, changes in what pharmacodynamic parameter should be considered prior to choosing the most appropriate antibiotic dose?

(A) Impaired blood flow to the intestine
(B) Increased protein binding of various drugs
(C) Increased volume of distribution
(D) Increased drug elimination

6. Which of the following terms is used to describe the elimination rate via metabolism catalyzed by alcohol dehydrogenase when the enzyme is saturated?

(A) Biotransformation
(B) Clearance
(C) First-order elimination
(D) Redistribution
(E) Zero-order kinetics

7. Which of the following statements is true in regard to glucuronidation reactions?

(A) Considered phase I reactions
(B) Include the enzymatic activity of alcohol dehydrogenase
(C) Require an active center as the site of conjugation
(D) Require nicotinamide adenine dinucleotide phosphate

8. A 38-year-old woman presents to her psychiatrist for the management of depression. She feels that her current treatment is ineffective and would like to switch medications. The patient reveals that she drinks alcohol every night to relieve her feelings of sadness and guilt. Blood work is positive for elevated liver enzymes. The doctor starts imipramine, which has an extensive first-pass metabolism. How would this drug be affected?

(A) Decreased half-life
(B) Decreased absorption
(C) Decreased solubility
(D) Increased concentration
(E) Increased pH

9. A 24-year-old female is prescribed erythromycin for gastroparesis. It is prescribed four times daily due to its short half-life. What is the rationale for such a frequent dosing?

(A) Achieve the steady-state plasma concentration of the drug
(B) Aid more complete distribution of the drug
(C) Avoid the toxicity of the drug because of its low therapeutic index
(D) Ensure that the drug concentration remains constant over time
(E) Inhibit the first-pass metabolism of the drug

10. A 78-year-old woman is started on digoxin for the management of congestive heart failure. Her initial dose is 0.25 mg. The C_0, obtained by extrapolation of the elimination phase, is determined to be 0.05 mg/L. What is the patient's estimated volume of distribution?

(A) 0.0125 L
(B) 0.2 L
(C) 0.5 L
(D) 1 L
(E) 5 L

11. A drug has a volume of distribution of 50 L. At plasma concentrations greater than 2 mg/L, it undergoes zero-order elimination at a rate of 2 mg/h. If a patient is brought to the emergency room with a plasma concentration of 4 mg/L of the drug, how long will it take (in hours) for the plasma concentration to decrease by 50%?

(A) 1
(B) 2
(C) 10
(D) 25
(E) 50

12. A 100-mg tablet of drug X is given to a patient every 24 hours to achieve an average steady-state plasma concentration of 10 mg/L. If the dosing regimen is changed to one 50-mg tablet every 12 hours, what will be the resulting average plasma concentration (in mg/L) of the drug after five half-lives?

(A) 2.5
(B) 5
(C) 10
(D) 20
(E) 40

13. A 35-year-old woman is started on ceftriaxone as empiric therapy for meningitis. Following intravenous administration, the initial rates of drug distribution to different tissues depend primarily on which of the following parameters?

(A) Active transport of the drug out of different cell types
(B) Blood flow to the tissues
(C) Degree of ionization of the drug in the tissues
(D) Fat content of the tissues
(E) Specific organ clearances

14. A drug is administered in the form of an inactive prodrug. The prodrug increases the expression of a cytochrome P450, which converts it to its active form. With chronic, long-term administration of the prodrug, which of the following will be observed?

(A) Efficacy will decrease.
(B) Efficacy will increase.
(C) Potency will decrease.
(D) Potency will increase.

15. Which subfamily of cytochrome P450s is responsible for the highest fraction of clinically important drug interactions resulting from metabolism?

(A) CYP1A
(B) CYP2A
(C) CYP3A
(D) CYP4A
(E) CYP5A

16. If the oral dosing rate of a drug is held constant, what will occur if the bioavailability is increased?

(A) Decreased first-order elimination rate constant
(B) Decreased total body clearance
(C) Increased half-life for first-order elimination
(D) Increased steady-state plasma concentration
(E) Increased volume of distribution

17. A 45-year-old man is given an oral maintenance dose of drug calculated to achieve a steady-state plasma concentration of 5 μg/L.

After dosing the patient for a sufficient amount of time to reach steady state, the average plasma concentration of drug is 10 μg/L. A decrease in which of the following parameters may explain the higher-than-anticipated plasma drug concentration?

(A) Bioavailability
(B) Clearance
(C) Half-life
(D) Volume of distribution

18. Administration of an intravenous loading dose of drug X yields an initial plasma concentration of 100 μg/L. The following table illustrates the plasma concentration of drug X as a function of time after the initial loading dose:

Time (h)	Plasma Concentration (μg/L)
0	100
1	50
5	25
9	12.5

What is the half-life (in hours) of drug X?

(A) 1
(B) 2
(C) 4
(D) 5
(E) 9

19. Which of the following factors will determine the number of drug–receptor complexes formed?

(A) Half-life of the drug
(B) Rate of renal secretion
(C) Receptor affinity for the drug
(D) Therapeutic index of the drug

20. Which of the following is an action of a noncompetitive antagonist?

(A) Alters the mechanism of action of an agonist
(B) Alters the potency of an agonist
(C) Binds to the same site on the receptor as the agonist
(D) Decreases the maximum response to an agonist
(E) Shifts the dose–response curve of an agonist to the right

21. The renal clearance of a drug is 10 mL/min. The drug has a low molecular weight and is 20% bound to plasma proteins. It is most likely that renal excretion of this drug involves which of the following mechanisms?

(A) Active tubular secretion only
(B) Glomerular filtration only
(C) Glomerular filtration and active tubular secretion
(D) Glomerular filtration and passive tubular reabsorption
(E) Passive tubular reabsorption only

22. Which of the following is the primary goal of therapeutic drug monitoring?

(A) To assess the possible adverse effects of drugs
(B) To evaluate the cost-effectiveness of drugs
(C) To ensure that the plasma levels are within the therapeutic range
(D) To determine which patient responds better
(E) To understand genetic variations in drug response

23. Which of the following activity is NOT performed under pharmacovigilance?

(A) Detection of adverse drug reactions
(B) Understanding the causality of adverse reactions
(C) Prevention of the adverse drug reactions
(D) Evaluating the efficacy of the drug
(E) Detecting the signal

Answers and Explanations

1. **The answer is A.** Somatostatin binds to a G_i-coupled protein receptor, initiating exchange of GTP for GDP, which inhibits AC and leads to reduced cAMP production. The G_q-protein-coupled receptor is an example of the PLC pathway, in which interaction with the ligand leads to increased PLC activity and eventual activation of protein kinase C via the PIP_2 and IP_3 pathway. This is exemplified by interaction of epinephrine with its receptor. The ligand-activated ion channel is an example of interaction of specific ligand with an ion channel, which permits passage of ions through the channel. Acetylcholine is an example of such an interaction. Receptor-activated tyrosine kinase is exemplified by insulin, where binding of ligand activates specific tyrosine kinase, leading to a cascade of reactions within the cell. Finally, an intracellular nuclear receptor is exemplified by cortisol, which binds to it and exerts its effects on DNA replication.
2. **The answer is A.** The ability to target intracellular receptors depends on the ligand's ability to cross lipid barriers, such as the nuclear envelope. Recruitment of intracellular kinases is characterized by some receptor-activated tyrosine kinases. Autophosphorylation is a feature of many different kinases. Interactions with G-protein and AC are characteristics of membrane receptors.
3. **The answer is E.** Digoxin is an example of a drug with a very low therapeutic index (TI), which requires frequent monitoring of the plasma level to achieve the balance between the desired effect and untoward toxicity. Potency of the drug is the amount of drug needed to produce a given response. Intrinsic activity of the drug is the ability to elicit a response. Efficacy of the drug is the maximal drug effect that can be achieved in a patient under a given set of conditions. Bioavailability of the drug is the fraction of the drug that reaches the bloodstream unaltered.
4. **The answer is A.** Adequate passage of drug through the small intestine is required to observe the effects of the drug, because most of the absorption takes place in the small intestine. After extensive abdominal surgery, especially that involving a resection of a portion of the small bowel, the passage may be slowed, or even stopped, for a period of time. Abdominal surgery rarely results in reduced blood flow to the intestine, nor does such an operation influence protein binding, or the first-pass effect. Destruction of drug by stomach acid does not depend on intra-abdominal surgery.
5. **The answer is C.** Because of the patient's edema and ascites from heart failure, the apparent volume of distribution will be increased, which may require small adjustments in the usual medication doses. Edematous states do not influence gastrointestinal (GI) blood flow, nor do they affect drug–protein interactions. Drug elimination may be slowed with a congestive heart failure (CHF) exacerbation, not increased. Drug kinetics are generally not changed by edematous states.
6. **The answer is E.** Alcohol (ethanol) is one of the few drugs that follow zero-order kinetics (i.e., higher drug concentrations are not metabolized because the enzyme that is involved in the process is saturable). In first-order elimination, the rate of elimination actually depends on the concentration of the drug, multiplied by the proportionality constant. Clearance is a measure of the capacity of the body to remove the drug. Biotransformation refers to the general mechanism of a particular drug's elimination. Redistribution is one of the possible fates of a drug, which usually terminates drug action.
7. **The answer is C.** Glucuronidation reactions, which are considered phase II reactions, require an active center (a functional group) as the site of conjugation. Phase I reactions are biotransformation reactions, not conjugation reactions. Alcohol dehydrogenase is an example of a phase I reaction. Nicotinamide adenine dinucleotide phosphate (NADPH) is required for aromatic hydroxylation, an example of a phase I reaction.
8. **The answer is D.** First-pass metabolism simply means passage through the portal circulation before reaching the systemic circulation. In the face of liver dysfunction, drug levels may reach higher concentrations. Bioavailability of drugs is decreased, not increased, by the fraction removed after the first pass through the liver. Drugs are usually less rapidly metabolized when hepatic enzymes are elevated (which indicates hepatic dysfunction). Solubility of drugs is not associated with hepatic damage.

9. **The answer is A.** Dosing schedules of drugs are adjusted according to their half-lives to achieve steady-state plasma concentration. Attempting to avoid the toxicity of the drug because of its low therapeutic index (TI) represents an unlikely scenario, since to reduce toxicity of a drug with a low TI, one would reduce the dosing schedule, not increase it. Distribution of the drug is generally not affected by dosing schedule, nor is dose scheduling affected by first-pass metabolism. Some fluctuation in plasma concentration occurs even at steady state; it is the average concentration over time that is the goal of steady state.

10. **The answer is E.** To calculate the volume of distribution, use the formula in which the dose of the drug is divided by the plasma concentration. In this case, 0.25 mg is divided by 0.05 mg/L, giving the result of 5 L for volume of distribution.

11. **The answer is E.** For the plasma concentration of drug to decrease by 50%, half the drug present in the body initially must be eliminated. The amount of drug in the body initially is the volume of distribution × the plasma concentration (50 L × 4 mg/L = 200 mg). When the plasma concentration falls to 2 mg/L, the body will contain 100 mg of drug (50 L × 2 mg/L = 100 mg). Since the body eliminates the drug at a rate of 2 mg/h, it will require 50 hours for 100 mg of the drug to be eliminated.

12. **The answer is C.** A 100-mg tablet every 24 hours is a dose rate of 4.17 mg/h (100/24 = 4.17), which is the same dose rate as one 50-mg tablet every 12 hours (50/12 = 4.17). Thus, the average plasma concentration will remain the same, but *decreasing both* the dose and the dose interval will decrease the peak to trough variation of plasma concentration.

13. **The answer is B.** The *initial rate* of distribution of a drug to a tissue depends primarily on the rate of blood flow to that tissue. At longer times, however, a drug may undergo redistribution among various tissues, for example, a very lipophilic drug may become concentrated in adipose tissue with time.

14. **The answer is D.** The induction of the cytochrome P450 following chronic administration will increase the conversion of the inactive prodrug to its active form. This will shift the dose–response curve of the prodrug to the left (i.e., increase its potency) without changing its efficacy.

15. **The answer is C.** The CYP3A subfamily is responsible for roughly 50% of the total cytochrome P450 activity present in the liver and is estimated to be responsible for approximately half of all clinically important untoward drug interactions resulting from metabolism.

16. **The answer is D.** If the oral dosing rate is constant but the bioavailability increases, the fraction of the administered dose that reaches the general circulation unaltered increases. This, in turn, will increase the steady-state plasma concentration.

17. **The answer is B.** Steady-state plasma concentration of drug = (dose rate)/(clearance). Thus, a decrease in clearance will increase the plasma drug concentration, whereas an increase in any of the other three parameters will *decrease* the steady-state plasma concentration.

18. **The answer is C.** Inspection of the plasma concentration values indicates that the half-life of drug does not become constant until 1–9 hours after administration. The drug concentration decreases by half (from 50 to 25 μg/L) between 1 and 5 hours (a 4-hour interval) and again decreases by half (from 25 to 12.5 μg/L) between 5 and 9 hours (again, a 4-hour interval). This indicates that the half-life of the drug is 4 hours. The rapid decrease in plasma concentration between 0 and 1 hour, followed by a slower decrease thereafter (and the constant half-life thereafter), indicates that this drug obeys a two-compartment model with an initial distribution phase followed by an elimination phase. The half-life is always determined from the elimination phase data.

19. **The answer is C.** Receptor affinity for the drug will determine the number of drug–receptor complexes formed. Efficacy is the ability of the drug to activate the receptor after binding has occurred. Therapeutic index (TI) is related to safety of the drug. Half-life and secretion are properties of elimination and do not influence the formation of drug–receptor complexes.

20. **The answer is D.** A noncompetitive antagonist decreases the magnitude of the response to an agonist but does not alter the agonist's potency (i.e., the ED_{50} remains unchanged). A competitive antagonist interacts at the agonist-binding site.

21. **The answer is D.** This drug will undergo filtration and passive reabsorption. Since the molecular weight of the drug is small, free drug will be filtered. Because 20% of the drug is bound to plasma

proteins, 80% of it is free and available for filtration, which would be at a rate of 100 mL/min (i.e., 0.8 × 125 mL/min; 125 mL/min is the normal glomerular filtration rate [GFR]). A clearance of 10 mL/min must indicate that most of the filtered drug is reabsorbed.

22. **The answer is C.** Therapeutic drug monitoring does not evaluate the adverse effects of drugs. Instead, it is performed for drugs that have the potential for severe adverse effects. It involves neither pharmacoeconomics nor pharmacogenetics. It assesses whether the plasma concentrations of drug are within the particular range or not. It does not compare who responds better.

23. **The answer is D.** Pharmacovigilance is the science and activities related to the detection, assessment, understanding, and prevention of adverse effects or any other drug-related problems. Signal detection is the objective of such activities. Pharmacovigilance does not aim to evaluate the efficacy of the drug.Rate of elimination by organ

Chapter 2

Drugs Acting on the Autonomic Nervous System, Peripheral Nervous System, and Local Anesthetics

Competencies Addressed: PH1.13–PH1.15, PH1.17

I. THE NERVOUS SYSTEM

A. General overview of the nervous system

1. The nervous system is divided into the:
   a. Central nervous system (CNS)
      (1) Brain
      (2) Spinal cord
   b. Peripheral nervous system
      (1) Neuronal tissues outside the CNS
2. The motor (efferent) portion of the nervous system can be divided into two major subdivisions.
   a. Autonomic (unconscious control): Controls visceral functions (such as cardiac output or digestion).
      (1) Sympathetic division: Fight or flight response
      (2) Parasympathetic division: Rest or digest response
      (3) Enteric nervous system
   b. Somatic (conscious control): Controls voluntary movements.
   c. Both systems have important afferent (sensory) inputs that provide information regarding the internal and external environments. They also modify motor output.

II. THE PERIPHERAL EFFERENT NERVOUS SYSTEM

A. The autonomic nervous system (ANS) controls involuntary activity

(Fig. 2.1; Table 2.1)

1. **Parasympathetic nervous system (PNS)**
   a. Long preganglionic axons originate from neurons in the cranial and sacral areas of the spinal cord and, with few exceptions, synapse on neurons in ganglia located close to or within the innervated organ.
   b. Short postganglionic axons innervate cardiac muscle, bronchial smooth muscle, and exocrine glands.
   c. Parasympathetic innervation predominates over sympathetic innervation of salivary glands, lacrimal glands, and erectile tissue.
2. **Sympathetic nervous system (SNS)**
   a. Short preganglionic axons originate from neurons in the thoracic and lumbar areas of the spinal cord and synapse on neurons in ganglia located outside of, but close to, the spinal cord. The adrenal medulla, anatomically considered a modified ganglion, is innervated by sympathetic preganglionic axons.
   b. Long postganglionic axons innervate many of the same tissues and organs as the PNS.

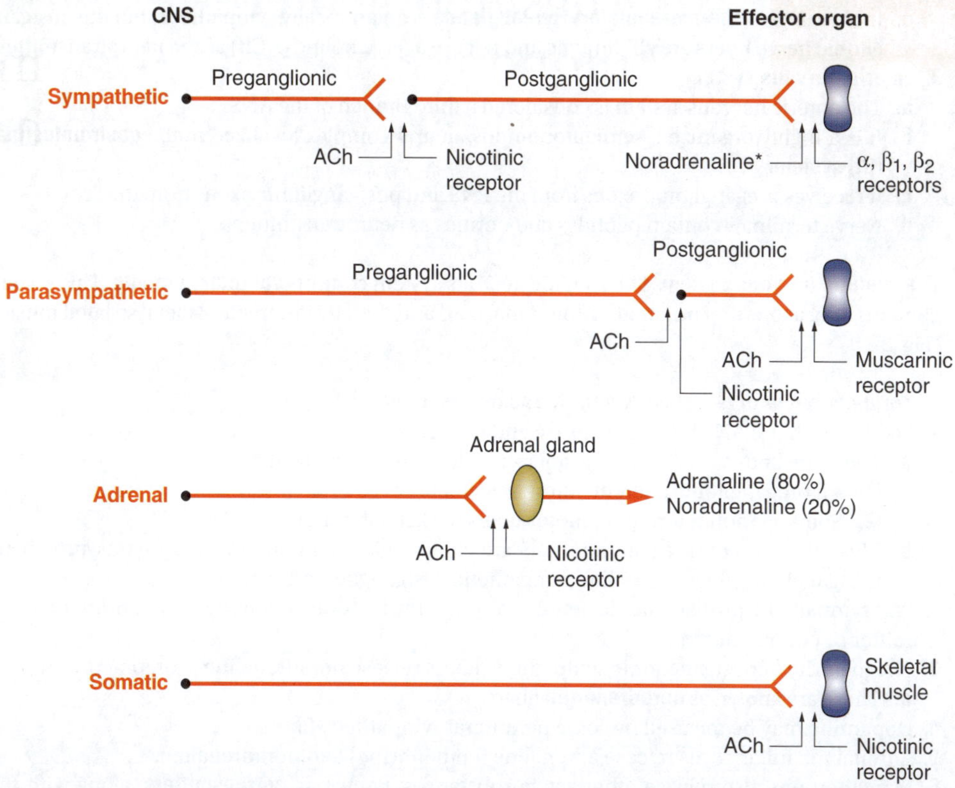

FIGURE 2.1. Organization of the autonomic nervous system. (*) Except sweat glands, which use ACh. ACh, acetylcholine.

TABLE 2.1 Actions of the Autonomic Nervous System on Selected Effector Organs

Effector	Action of Sympathetic (Thoracolumbar) Division	Action of Parasympathetic (Craniosacral) Division
Eye (pupil)	Dilation (ex)	Constriction (ex)
Heart		
Rate	Acceleration (ex)	Slowing (in)
Contractility	Increased (ex)	Decreased (in)
Arterioles		
Skin and most others	Constriction (ex)	—
Skeletal muscle	Dilation (ex)	—
Glands		
Salivary	Viscid secretion (ex)	Watery secretion (ex)
Lacrimal	—	Secretion (ex)
Sweat	Secretion (ex)	—
Bronchial muscle	Relaxation (in)	Contraction (ex)
GI tract		
Muscle wall	Relaxation (in)	Contraction (ex)
Sphincters	Contraction (ex)	Relaxation (in)
Urinary bladder		
Fundus	Relaxation (in)	Contraction (ex)
Trigone; sphincter	Contraction (ex)	Relaxation (in)
Penis	Ejaculation (ex)	Erection (in)
Uterus	Relaxation (in)	—
Metabolism		
Liver	Gluconeogenesis (ex)	—
	Glycogenolysis (ex)	—
Kidney	Renin secretion(ex)	—
Fat cells	Lipolysis (ex)	

ex, excitatory; GI, gastrointestinal; in, inhibitory; —, no functionally important innervation.

c. Innervation of **thermoregulatory sweat glands** is anatomically sympathetic, but the postganglionic nerve fibers are cholinergic and release acetylcholine (ACh) as the neurotransmitter.

3. **Enteric nervous system**
   a. The enteric nervous system is considered a third branch of the ANS.
   b. It is a highly organized, semiautonomous, neural complex localized in the **gastrointestinal (GI) system.**
   c. It receives preganglionic axons from the PNS and postganglionic axons from the SNS.
   d. Nerve terminals contain peptides and purines as neurotransmitters.

B. The somatic nervous system. The somatic nervous system controls **voluntary activity**. This system contains long axons that originate in the spinal cord and directly innervate skeletal striated muscle (Fig. 2.1).

C. General overview of the primary neurotransmitters of the ANS

1. Many peripheral ANS fibers synthesize and release ACh.
   a. These are known as cholinergic fibers, and include the following:
      (1) All preganglionic efferent autonomic fibers
      (2) Somatic (nonautonomic) motor fibers to skeletal muscle
   b. Most efferent fibers leaving the CNS are cholinergic, in addition to most parasympathetic postganglionic fibers and some sympathetic postganglionic fibers.
2. Parasympathetic postganglionic neurons also use nitric oxide or peptides as the primary transmitter or cotransmitters.
3. The majority of postganglionic sympathetic fibers release noradrenaline (norepinephrine).
   a. These are known as **noradrenergic** fibers.
4. Dopamine may be released by some peripheral sympathetic fibers.
5. Adrenal medullary cells release adrenaline (epinephrine) and noradrenaline.
6. Many neurons also release other active substances, known as **cotransmitters**, along with the primary neurotransmitter.
   a. May be stored in the same vesicle along with the primary neurotransmitter or in a separate vesicle.
   b. May modulate the effects of the primary neurotransmitter or have independent effects.
   c. Example: Cholinergic nerves contain vasoactive intestinal polypeptide and adrenergic nerves contain ATP as the cotransmitter.

D. Neurotransmitters of the autonomic and somatic nervous systems (Fig. 2.1)

1. **Acetylcholine**
   a. Biosynthesis
      (1) ACh is synthesized in nerve terminals by the cytoplasmic enzyme choline acetyltransferase, which catalyzes the transfer of an acetate group from acetyl coenzyme A to choline.
      (2) Synthesized ACh is transported from cytoplasm to vesicle-associated transporters.
   b. Storage, release, and termination
      (1) It is stored in nerve terminal vesicles and released by nerve action potentials through calcium-dependent exocytosis.
      (2) On release (a step blocked by **botulinum toxin**), **ACh is rapidly hydrolyzed and inactivated by tissue acetylcholinesterase (AChE)** and by **nonspecific butyrylcholinesterase** (pseudocholinesterase) to choline and acetate.
   c. ACh is the neurotransmitter across synapses:
      (1) At the ganglia of the SNS and PNS
      (2) In tissues innervated by the PNS and the somatic nervous system
   d. It is not administered parenterally for therapeutic purposes because it is hydrolyzed nearly instantly by butyrylcholinesterase.
2. **Noradrenaline and adrenaline**
   a. Noradrenaline and adrenaline are **catecholamines**; they possess a catechol nucleus and an ethylamine side chain.
   b. Biosynthesis (Fig. 2.2)
      (1) In prejunctional nerve endings, tyrosine is hydroxylated by tyrosine hydroxylase, the rate-limiting enzyme in the synthesis of catecholamines, to form dihydroxyphenylalanine (dopa).
      (2) Dopa is decarboxylated by dopa decarboxylase to form dopamine.

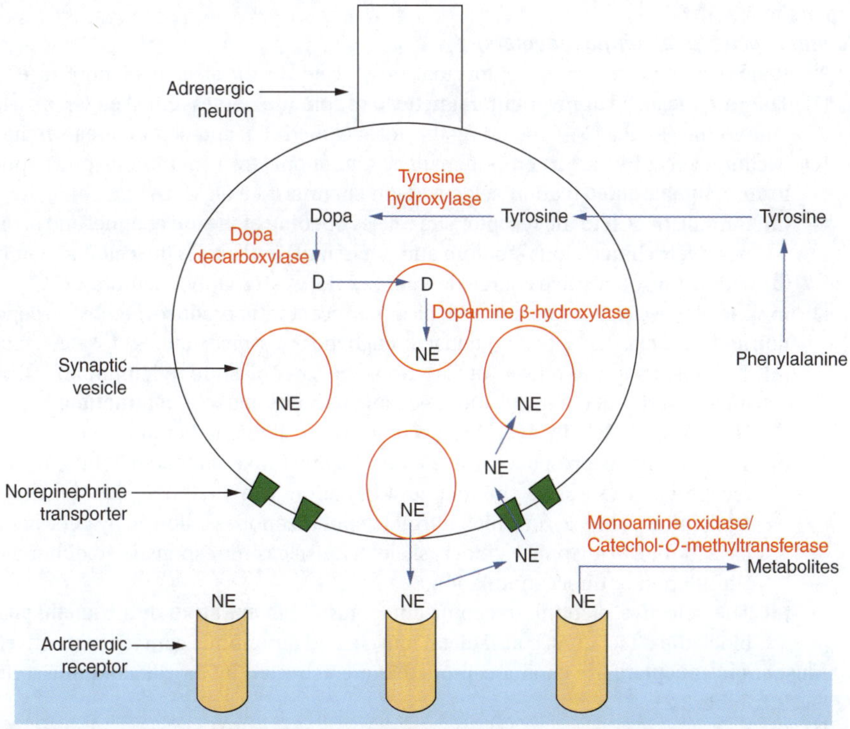

FIGURE 2.2. Biosynthesis of noradrenaline. D, dopamine; dopa, dihydroxyphenylalanine; NE, norepinephrine.

- **(3)** Dopamine is transported into vesicles (a step blocked by **reserpine**), where it is hydroxylated on the side chain by dopamine β-hydroxylase to form noradrenaline.
- **(4)** In certain areas of the brain and in the adrenal medulla, noradrenaline is methylated on the amine group of the side chain by phenylethanolamine-*N*-methyltransferase (PNMT) to form adrenaline.

c. Storage and release

- **(1)** Noradrenaline is stored in vesicles that, through a calcium-dependent process, release their contents by exocytosis from nerve terminals at postganglionic nerve endings of the SNS (except at thermoregulatory sweat glands, where ACh is the neurotransmitter).
- **(2)** Noradrenaline also exists in a nonvesicular cytoplasmic pool that is released by indirectly acting sympathomimetic amines (e.g., **tyramine, amphetamine, ephedrine**) by a process that is not calcium dependent.
- **(3)** Noradrenaline and some adrenaline are released from adrenergic nerve endings in the brain.
- **(4)** In the periphery, adrenaline is the major catecholamine released from adrenal medullary chromaffin cells into the general circulation, where it functions as a hormone. Some noradrenaline is also released.

d. Termination

- **(1)** The action of **noradrenaline** is primarily terminated by **active transport** from the cytoplasm into the nerve terminal by a noradrenaline transporter (**uptake 1**).
  - **(a)** This process is inhibited by **cocaine** and **tricyclic antidepressants**.
  - **(b)** **Noradrenaline** is then transported by a second carrier system into storage vesicles, as are **dopamine** and **serotonin** (a process also blocked by **reserpine**).
- **(2)** Another active transport system (**uptake 2**) is located on glia and smooth muscle cells.
- **(3)** There is also some simple **diffusion** away from the synapse.
- **(4)** Noradrenaline and adrenaline are also oxidatively **deaminated by mitochondrial monoamine oxidase (MAO)** in nerve terminals and effector cells, notably in the liver and intestine.
- **(5)** Nerve cells and effector cells contain **catechol-*O*-methyltransferase (COMT),** which metabolizes catecholamines.

E. Receptors of the ANS

1. *Cholinoceptors (cholinergic receptors)*

a. **Nicotinic receptors** are cholinoceptors that are activated by the alkaloid nicotine (see Fig. 2.1).

(1) They are localized at myoneural junctions of somatic nerves and skeletal muscle (N_M); autonomic ganglia (N_G), including the adrenal medulla; and certain areas in the brain.

(2) Nicotinic receptors are a component of postjunctional transmembrane polypeptide that forms a **ligand-gated** (cation-selective) ion channel (see Fig. 1.1A).

(a) Binding of ACh to the receptor site causes opening of the ion channel and an influx of positively charged ions (sodium and potassium) and across the cellular membrane.

(b) This influx of positive charge depolarizes the postsynaptic membrane.

(3) In skeletal muscle, ACh interacts with nicotinic receptors to produce membrane depolarization and a propagated action potential through the transverse tubules of skeletal muscle.

(a) This results in the release of Ca^{2+} from the sarcoplasmic reticulum and, through a further series of chemical and mechanical events, **muscle contraction.**

(b) Hydrolysis of ACh by AChE results in muscle cell repolarization.

(c) The continued presence of a nicotine agonist, like **succinylcholine,** at nicotinic receptors, or excessive cholinergic stimulation, can lead to a **"depolarizing blockade"** (phase I block), in which normal depolarization is followed by persistent depolarization. During phase I block, skeletal muscle is unresponsive to either neuronal stimulation or direct stimulation.

(d) The selective nicotinic receptor antagonists, **tubocurarine** and **trimethaphan,** can block the effect of ACh at skeletal muscle and autonomic ganglia, respectively.

b. **Muscarinic receptors** are cholinoceptors that are activated by the alkaloid muscarine (see Fig. 2.1; Table 2.2).

(1) Muscarinic receptors are localized on numerous autonomic effector cells, including cardiac atrial muscle and cells of the sinoatrial (SA) and atrioventricular (AV) nodes, smooth muscle, exocrine glands, and vascular endothelium (mostly arterioles), although the latter does not receive parasympathetic innervation, as well as certain areas in the brain.

(2) They consist of at least five **receptor subtypes (M_1–M_5).**

(a) M_1 receptors are found in sympathetic postganglionic neurons.

(b) M_2 receptors are found in cardiac and smooth muscles.

(c) M_3 receptors are found in glandular cells (e.g., gastric parietal cells), and the vascular endothelium and vascular smooth muscle.

(d) M_5 receptors are found in the vascular endothelium.

(e) All receptor subtypes are found in CNS neurons.

(3) ACh interacts with **M_1, M_3, and M_5** muscarinic cholinoceptors to increase **phosphatidylinositol (PI) turnover** and **Ca^{2+} mobilization** (see Fig. 1.1D; Table 2.2).

(a) By activation of the **G protein (G_q)**, the interaction of ACh with M_1 and M_3 muscarinic cholinoceptors stimulates **polyphosphatidylinositol phosphodiesterase (phospholipase C),** which hydrolyzes PI to **inositol trisphosphate (IP_3)** and **diacylglycerol (DAG).**

(b) **IP_3 mobilizes intracellular Ca^{2+}** from the endoplasmic and sarcoplasmic reticula, and activates Ca^{2+}-regulated enzymes and cell processes.

TABLE 2.2 Effects of Cholinergic and Adrenergic G-Protein-Coupled Receptors

Receptor Type	G-Protein-Coupled Receptor	Effect
α_1	G_q coupled	Increase phospholipase C → increase IP_3, DAG, Ca^{2+}
α_2	G_i coupled	Decrease adenylyl cyclase → decrease cAMP
β_1, β_2	G_s coupled	Increase adenylyl cyclase → increase cAMP
Muscarinic-1, muscarinic-3, and muscarinic-5	G_q coupled	Increase phospholipase C → increase IP_3, DAG, Ca^{2+}
Muscarinic-2 and muscarinic-4	G_i coupled	Decrease adenylyl cyclase → decrease cAMP

cAMP, cyclic AMP; DAG, diacylglycerol; IP3, inositol trisphosphate.

(c) **DAG activates protein kinase C,** which results in phosphorylation of cellular enzymes and other protein substrates and the **influx of extracellular calcium** that results in activation of contractile elements in smooth muscle.

(4) ACh also interacts with **M_2 and M_4** muscarinic cholinoceptors to **activate G proteins (G_i),** which leads to **inhibition of adenylyl cyclase** activity with decreased levels of cyclic AMP (cAMP) and to **increased potassium (K^+) conductance** with effector cell hyperpolarization (Table 2.2).

(5) Cholinergic agonists act on **M_3** muscarinic receptors of **endothelial cells** to promote the release of **nitric oxide (NO),** which diffuses to the **vascular smooth muscle** to activate guanylyl cyclase and **increase cyclic GMP** (cGMP), and to produce **relaxation.**

2. ***Adrenoceptors***

a. **α-Adrenoceptors** (see Fig. 2.1)

(1) α-Adrenoceptors are classified into two major receptor subgroups (there are subtypes of each group).

(a) **α_1-Receptors** are located in **postjunctional** effector cells, notably vascular smooth muscle, where responses are mainly excitatory.

(b) **α_2-Receptors** are located primarily in **prejunctional** adrenergic nerve terminals, and also in fat cells and in the β cells of the pancreas.

(2) They mediate many functions, including the following:

(a) Vasoconstriction (α_1)

(b) GI relaxation (α_1)

(c) Mydriasis (α_1)

(d) Prejunctional inhibition of release of noradrenaline and other neurotransmitters (α_2)

(e) Inhibition of insulin release (α_2)

(f) Inhibition of lipolysis (α_2)

(3) α-Adrenoceptors are distinguished from β-adrenoceptors by their interaction (in descending order of potency), with the adrenergic agonists **adrenaline = noradrenaline >> isoprenaline,** and by their interaction with relatively selective antagonists such as **phentolamine.**

(4) **α_1-Adrenoceptors,** like muscarinic M_1 cholinoceptors, **activate guanine nucleotide-binding proteins (Gq)** in many cells, which results in activation of **phospholipase C** and stimulation of phosphoinositide hydrolysis that leads to increased formation of **IP_3**, mobilization of intracellular stores of Ca^{2+}, increased **DAG**, and activation of protein kinase C.

(5) **α_2-Adrenoceptors,** like muscarinic M_2-cholinoceptors, **activate inhibitory guanine nucleotide-binding proteins (G_i), inhibit adenylyl cyclase** activity, and decrease intracellular cAMP levels and the activity of cAMP-dependent protein kinases (see Fig. 1.1C).

b. **β-Adrenoceptors** (see Fig. 2.1)

(1) β-Adrenoceptors, located mostly in postjunctional effector cells, are classified into two major receptor subtypes, β_1-receptors (primarily excitatory) and β_2-receptors (primarily inhibitory).

(a) **β_1-Receptor subtype**

i. β_1-Receptors mediate increased contractility and conduction velocity, and renin secretion in the kidney.

ii. The β_1-receptor subtype is defined by its interaction (in descending order of potency) with the adrenergic agonists **isoprenaline > adrenaline = noradrenaline** and by its interaction with relatively selective antagonists such as **atenolol.**

(b) **β_2-Receptor subtype**

i. β_2-Receptors mediate vasodilation and intestinal, bronchial, and uterine smooth muscle relaxation.

ii. The β_2-receptor subtype is defined by its interaction (in descending order of potency) with the adrenergic agonists **isoprenaline = adrenaline >> noradrenaline.**

(2) **β-Receptor activation**

(a) β-Receptors activate **guanine nucleotide-binding proteins** (G_s) (see Fig. 1.1B; Table 2.2).

(b) Activation **stimulates adenylate cyclase** activity and increases intracellular cAMP levels and the activity of cAMP-dependent protein kinases.

(c) Adrenoceptor-mediated changes in the activity of protein kinases (and also levels of intracellular Ca^{2+}) bring about changes in the activity of specific enzymes and structural and regulatory proteins, resulting in modification of cell and organ activity.

III. PARASYMPATHOMIMETIC DRUGS

A. Direct-acting muscarinic cholinoceptor agonists

1. *Mechanism of action and chemical structure*

a. Direct-acting parasympathomimetic drugs act at muscarinic cholinoceptors to mimic many of the physiologic effects that result from stimulation of the parasympathetic division of the ANS (see Fig. 2.1).

b. Bethanechol and methacholine are choline esters with a quaternary ammonium group that are structurally similar to ACh.

c. They have substantially reduced activity at nicotinic receptors and are more resistant to hydrolysis by AChE.

2. *Pharmacologic effects* (Tables 2.3 and 2.4)

a. **Eye**

(1) Direct-acting muscarinic cholinoceptor agonists **contract the circular smooth muscle fibers of the ciliary muscle and iris to produce** a spasm of accommodation and an increased outflow of aqueous humor into the canal of Schlemm, respectively. This results in a **reduction in intraocular pressure (IOP).**

(2) These drugs contract the sphincter pupillae to cause **miosis.**

b. **Cardiovascular system**

(1) Direct-acting muscarinic cholinoceptor agonists produce a **negative chronotropic effect** (reduced SA node activity).

(2) These drugs **decrease conduction velocity** through the AV node.

TABLE 2.3 Actions of Muscarinic Agonists

Effector	Effects of Muscarinic Agonists
Heart (rate, conduction velocity)[a]	Decrease
Arterioles (tone)	Decrease
Blood pressure	Decrease
Pupil size	Decrease
Salivation	Increase
Lacrimation	Increase
Bronchial tone	Increase
Intestine (motility)	Increase
GI secretions	Increase
Urinary bladder	
Body (tone)	Increase
Sphincter	Decrease

GI, gastrointestinal.

[a]Responses (e.g., heart rate) may be affected by reflexes.

TABLE 2.4 Effects of Muscarinic Cholinoceptor Agonists and Antagonists and Adrenoceptor Agonists on Smooth Muscles of the Eye

Type of Drug	Muscle	Effect	Result
Muscarinic agonist	Iris circular (constrictor)	Contraction	Miosis
	Ciliary circular	Contraction	Accommodation
Muscarinic antagonist	Iris circular (constrictor)	Relaxation	Mydriasis
	Ciliary circular	Relaxation	Cycloplegia
α-Adrenergic agonist	Iris radial (dilator)	Contraction	Mydriasis
	Ciliary circular	None	None

(a) They have no effect on force of contraction because there are no muscarinic receptors on (or parasympathetic innervation of) ventricles.

(3) Direct-acting muscarinic cholinoceptor agonists produce **vasodilation** that results primarily from their action on endothelial cells to promote the release of **NO,** which diffuses to the vascular smooth muscle and produces relaxation.

(a) Vascular smooth muscle has muscarinic receptors but no parasympathetic innervation.

(b) The decrease in blood pressure can result in a reflex increase in heart rate.

c. GI tract

(1) Direct-acting muscarinic cholinoceptor agonists increase smooth muscle contractions and tone, with increased **peristaltic activity and motility**.

(2) These drugs **increase salivation and acid secretion.**

d. Urinary tract

(1) Direct-acting muscarinic cholinoceptor agonists **increase contraction of the ureter and bladder smooth muscle.**

(2) These drugs increase **sphincter relaxation**.

e. Respiratory system

(1) These drugs can cause **bronchoconstriction** with increased resistance and increased bronchial secretions.

f. Other effects

(1) They can increase the secretion of tears from lacrimal glands and increase sweat gland secretion.

(2) These drugs produce tremor and ataxia.

3. ***Specific drugs and their indications***

a. These drugs are used primarily for diseases of the eye, GI tract, urinary tract, the neuromuscular junction, and the heart (Table 2.5).

b. Bethanechol

(1) This agent increases bladder muscle tone and causes contractions to initiate urination. It also stimulates GI motility and can help restore peristalsis. It has limited distribution to the CNS.

(2) It is approved for the management of postoperative and postpartum urinary retention and neurogenic bladder.

(3) It has the potential to cause a reflux infection if the patient has bacteriuria (when the sphincter fails to relax as bethanechol contracts the bladder).

c. Methacholine

(1) This agent is only used to **diagnose bronchial airway hyperreactivity** in patients with no clinically apparent asthma.

(2) Since severe bronchoconstriction and reduced respiratory function may occur, it should not be used in patients with clinically apparent asthma, wheezing, or a low baseline pulmonary function test.

d. Pilocarpine

(1) Pilocarpine is a tertiary amine that is well absorbed from the GI tract and enters the CNS.

(2) It is occasionally used topically for **open-angle glaucoma,** either as eye drops or as a sustained-release ocular insert.

(a) When used before surgery to treat **acute narrow-angle glaucoma** (a medical emergency), pilocarpine is often given in a synergistic combination with an indirectly acting muscarinic agonist, such as **physostigmine.**

(3) Orally, pilocarpine is used to increase salivary secretion (sialogogue); it used to treat xerostomia associated with **Sjögren syndrome**.

TABLE 2.5 Selected Indications of Selected Direct-Acting Cholinoceptor Agonists

Agent	Conditions/Disorders
Bethanechol	Prevents urine retention; postoperative abdominal distension; gastric atony
Methacholine	Diagnostic for bronchial hypersensitivity
Pilocarpine	Open-angle glaucoma; acute narrow-angle glaucoma; Sjögren syndrome

e. **Cevimeline** is used for the treatment of xerostomia associated with Sjögren syndrome.
f. **Carbachol** is used rarely as a treatment for open-angle glaucoma. It is also approved to cause miosis during ophthalmic surgery.

4. ***Adverse effects***
   a. The **adverse effects** associated with direct-acting muscarinic cholinoceptor agonists are extensions of their pharmacologic activity.
   b. Adverse effects may include nausea, vomiting, diarrhea, sweating, and salivation. More serious effects include **bronchoconstriction** and **decreased blood pressure.** These effects can be reversed by atropine.
   c. Systemic effects are minimal for drugs applied topically.
5. ***Precautions***
   a. Caution must be used in patients with **asthma** and **cardiac disease**.
      (1) They are not recommended in hyperthyroidism since they predispose patients to arrhythmias.
   b. They are also not recommended when there is mechanical obstruction of the GI or urinary tract.

B. Acetylcholinesterase inhibitors (indirect-acting parasympathomimetic agents)

1. ACh interacts with AChE at two sites (Fig. 2.3).
   a. The N⁺ of choline (ionic bond) binds to the anionic site, and the acetyl ester binds to the esteratic site (serine residue).
   b. As ACh is hydrolyzed, the serine-OH side chain is acetylated and free choline is released.
   c. Acetylserine is hydrolyzed to serine and acetate.
   d. The half-life ($t_{1/2}$) of acetylserine hydrolysis is 100–150 microseconds.
2. Phosphoric acid esters (**organophosphates**)
   a. ***Specific agents***
      (1) Insecticides: Parathion and malathion
      (2) Nerve gases: Sarin and tabun
   b. ***Mechanism of action.*** These drugs **bind to AChE** and **render the enzyme nonfunctional**; this leads to **increased ACh at the neuronal synapses** at the neuromuscular junction.
      (1) They bind to AChE and undergo prompt hydrolysis.
      (2) The phosphate ion is released slowly from the enzyme active site, preventing the binding and hydrolysis of endogenous ACh.
      (3) Compared with the carbamates, the organophosphates are long-acting drugs that form a very stable phosphate complex with AChE.

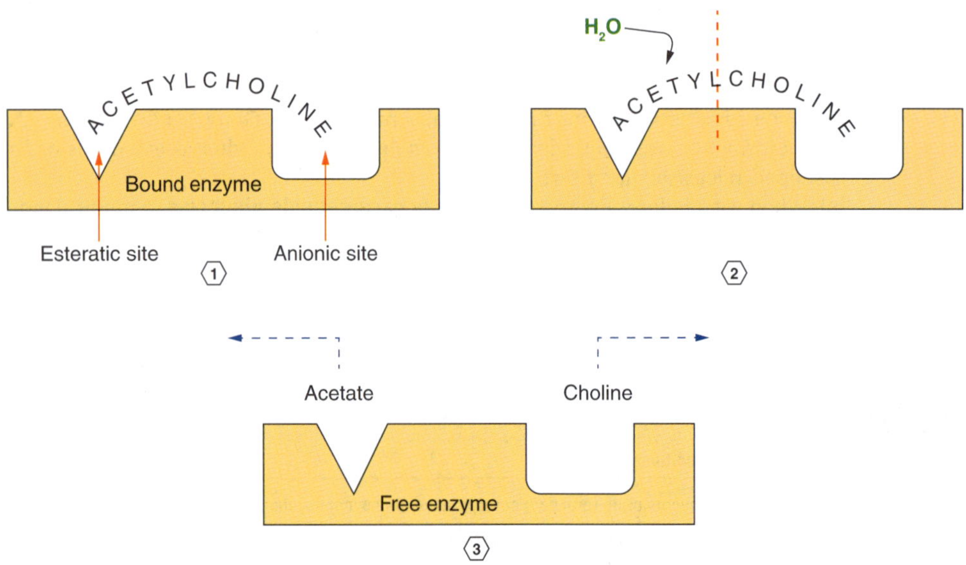

FIGURE 2.3 Interaction of acetylcholine with cholinesterase enzyme.

(a) They undergo **a conformational change known as "aging,"** causing AChE to become **irreversibly resistant to reactivation by the antidote (pralidoxime).**

(4) They prolong the peripheral and central effects of ACh.

c. ***Indications.*** These agents are not used in a clinical setting. They are pesticides that are used in agriculture and nerve agents that may be used in terrorism or chemical warfare.

(1) **Echothiophate** is an irreversible and toxic organophosphate cholinesterase inhibitor; it results in **phosphorylation of AChE** rather than in acetylation. It is an ophthalmic agent approved for the treatment of elevated IOP.

d. ***Adverse effects***

(1) Parathion is a very dangerous insecticide, which can cause all parasympathetic effects, including muscle paralysis and coma (malathion is much safer).

(2) Toxicity occurs due to cholinergic excess.

(3) *DUMBBELLS* is a commonly used medical mnemonic used to identity adverse effects from an overdose or poisoning due to a cholinergic agent:

Diarrhea
Urination
Miosis (pupil constriction)
Bradycardia
Bronchospasm/bronchorrhea
Emesis
Lacrimation
Lethargy
Salivation

(4) ACh stimulation of nicotinic receptors at the neuromuscular junction may cause fasciculations, muscle weakness, and paralysis, similar to the depolarizing effect of succinylcholine in producing neuromuscular blockade.

(5) Since sweat glands are regulated through sympathetic activation of postganglionic muscarinic receptors, patients may experience diaphoresis.

e. Management of organophosphate poisoning (see Chapter 13, Toxicology).

(1) Patients will most likely require 100% oxygen and endotracheal intubation.

(2) Succinylcholine should not be used since it is metabolized by AChE, leading to prolonged neuromuscular blockade.

(3) **Atropine** is an anticholinergic agent that competes with ACh at muscarinic receptors. It is used to **reverse symptoms of cholinergic poisoning**, including bronchorrhea and bronchoconstriction.

(a) **It does not have an effect on the nicotinic receptors responsible for muscle weakness and paralysis.**

(4) **Pralidoxime (2-PAM)** is helpful in the management of symptoms due to muscarinic and nicotinic receptor activation.

(a) It **reactivates cholinesterase** that had been inactivated by phosphorylation due to exposure to organophosphates by displacing the enzyme from its receptor sites.

i. It binds the anionic site and reacts with the P=O group of alkylphosphorylated serine to cause hydrolysis of the phosphoserine bond.

(b) It **must be administered soon after exposure** (within minutes); if "aging" has occurred, this agent will not work.

i. This drug is most effective at the neuromuscular junction.

ii. It is ineffective in the CNS and against carbamylated AChE.

(c) Pralidoxime produces few adverse effects in normal doses.

3. Carbamic acid esters (carbamates)

a. ***Specific agents*** include neostigmine, physostigmine, and pyridostigmine.

b. ***Mechanism of action***

(1) These agents **inhibit AChE**; they inhibit the destruction of ACh, causing an **increase** in **ACh levels** at both muscarinic and nicotinic cholinoceptors.

(a) Similar to the organophosphates, they bind to cholinesterase and undergo prompt hydrolysis.

(b) The carbamate ion is slowly released from the enzyme active site, preventing the binding and hydrolysis of endogenous ACh.

(c) They mimic many of the physiologic effects that result from increased ACh in the synaptic junction and stimulation of cholinoceptors of the parasympathetic division of the ANS.

(d) They prolong the peripheral and central effects of ACh.

(e) Unlike organophosphates, these agents are **transient** cholinesterase inhibitors; they usually hydrolyze from the enzymatic site within 48 hours.

c. ***Pharmacologic properties***

(1) **Neostigmine** and **pyridostigmine** are **quaternary ammonium** cations (positively charged); therefore, they are **poorly absorbed** from the GI tract and have negligible distribution into the CNS.

(2) **Physostigmine** is a tertiary amine; it is not charged and is **well absorbed** and **enters the CNS**.

d. ***Indications***

(1) Myasthenia gravis is an **autoimmune disease** in which antibodies complex with nicotinic receptors at the neuromuscular junction to cause skeletal muscle weakness and fatigue.

(a) AChE inhibitors are used to increase ACh levels at the neuromuscular junction to fully activate the remaining receptors.

(b) Neostigmine and pyridostigmine are used for the symptomatic control of myasthenia gravis.

(2) Neostigmine and pyridostigmine are also used to reverse effects due to nondepolarizing neuromuscular blocking agents.

(3) Physostigmine is used to reverse toxic, life-threatening delirium caused by anticholinergic toxicity.

e. ***Adverse effects*** may include nausea, vomiting, diarrhea, and urinary urgency, due to an increase in parasympathetic effects.

(1) Compared with organophosphates, carbamate toxicity tends to be of a shorter duration.

4. Central AChE inhibitors (agents for Alzheimer disease) (see Chapter 5)

a. ***Specific agents*** include rivastigmine, galantamine, and donepezil.

b. ***Mechanism of action.*** They reversibly **inhibit** centrally active **AChE** and **increase concentrations of ACh** available for synaptic transmission in the CNS.

c. ***Adverse effects*** may include nausea, diarrhea, weight loss, and **sleep disturbances**, including insomnia and vivid dreams. Bradycardia and hypotension may occur due to enhanced vagal tone.

IV. ANTICHOLINERGIC DRUGS

A. Muscarinic-receptor antagonists (antimuscarinic agents)

1. ***Mechanism of action*** (Table 2.6)

a. Muscarinic-receptor antagonists are competitive antagonists of ACh at all muscarinic cholinoceptors.

2. ***Pharmacologic effects***

a. **Eye** (see Table 2.4)

(1) Muscarinic-receptor antagonists produce **cycloplegia** by blocking parasympathetic tone, leading to paralysis of the ciliary muscle and loss of accommodation.

(2) They produce **mydriasis** by blocking parasympathetic tone to the iris circular (constrictor) muscle. Unopposed sympathetic stimulation of the radial muscle results in dilation of the pupil (passive mydriasis).

b. **Cardiovascular system**

(1) These agents **increase heart rate** due to cholinergic blockade at the SA node.

c. **Gastrointestinal tract**

(1) Muscarinic-receptor antagonists **decrease salivation.**

TABLE 2.6 Properties of Selected Cholinoceptor-Blocking Agents

Agent	Action	Receptors: Muscarinic	Receptors: Nicotinic	Comments
Atropine	Competitive antagonist	+		Prototype muscarinic cholinoceptor-blocking agent
Scopolamine	Competitive antagonist	+		Actions similar to those of atropine
Propantheline	Competitive antagonist	+		Peripheral-acting cholinoceptor blocking agent
Trimethaphan	Competitive, nondepolarizing antagonist		+	Peripheral-acting ganglionic blocking agent
Cisatracurium	Competitive, nondepolarizing antagonist at motor end plate		+	Neuromuscular junction blocking agent
Succinylcholine	Depolarizing agonist at motor end plate		+	Neuromuscular junction blocking agent

(2) They **reduce peristalsis,** resulting in prolonged gastric emptying and intestinal transit.
(3) In addition, these agents reduce gastric acid secretion.

d. **Respiratory system**
(1) They can cause **bronchodilation** and decrease mucus secretion.

e. **Urinary tract**
(1) These agents relax the ureters and bladder and constrict the urinary sphincter.

f. **Other effects**
(1) Tertiary amines can produce restlessness, headache, excitement, hallucinations, and delirium.
(2) **Anhidrosis** and dry skin may occur due to the inhibition of sympathetic cholinergic innervation of the sweat glands.

3. ***Pharmacologic properties***
a. Most tertiary muscarinic-receptor antagonists are well absorbed across the GI tract or mucosal surfaces; they distribute well throughout the body, including the brain.

4. ***Specific agents and their indications*** (Table 2.7)
a. ***Eye***
(1) Homatropine, cyclopentolate, **tropicamide**
(a) These agents prevent cholinergic stimulation at the sphincter muscle of the iris and the muscle of the ciliary body.
(b) They produce dilation and prevent accommodation.
(c) They are administered topically as eye drops or ointments for **refractive measurements** and for **ophthalmoscopic examination** of the retina and other structures of the eye.
(d) α-Adrenoceptor agonists, such as **phenylephrine,** are used for simple funduscopic examination without cycloplegia.

TABLE 2.7 Selected Indications of Muscarinic Cholinoceptor Antagonists

Organ/System	Therapeutic Use
Eye	Refractive measurement; ophthalmologic examination, uveitis and iritis
Heart	Heart block
Bladder	Urinary urgency
Lung	Surgical anesthesia to suppress secretions; COPD; asthma
CNS	Motion sickness (scopolamine); Parkinson disease
Multiple organs/systems	Cholinergic poisoning

CNS, central nervous system; COPD, chronic obstructive pulmonary disease.

(2) Longer-acting muscarinic-receptor antagonists, such as homatropine, are generally preferred as adjuncts to phenylephrine to prevent synechia formation in anterior uveitis and iritis.

b. ***Cardiovascular system***

(1) Atropine is used for symptomatic sinus bradycardia and AV nodal block (see Chapter 4).

c. ***Urinary tract***

(1) Anticholinergic agents can be used for the management of overactive bladder.

(a) Nonselective agents: Oxybutynin, tolterodine, trospium, fesoterodine

(b) M_3-selective: Solifenacin, darifenacin

(2) These agents antagonize parasympathetic control of the bladder; they act on muscarinic receptors of the detrusor muscle to increase capacity of the bladder and decrease intravesicular pressure and frequency of contractions.

(3) Fewer CNS effects occur with the M_3-selective agents and trospium (quaternary amine).

d. ***Central nervous system***

(1) **Parkinson disease**

(a) **Benztropine,** orphenadrine, and trihexyphenidyl.

(b) These drugs **block muscarinic receptors** and **suppress overactivity of cholinergic interneurons** in the striatum (see Chapter 5).

(2) Motion sickness

(a) **Scopolamine** prevents **motion sickness** by blocking muscarinic receptors in the vestibular system and in the CNS (see Chapter 8).

e. ***Respiratory system***

(1) **Atropine** and **scopolamine** can be used to suppress bronchiolar secretions during **surgical and spinal anesthesia** and to prevent the muscarinic effects of AChE inhibitors used to reverse muscle paralysis at the end of surgery.

(2) **Ipratropium** and **tiotropium** are used to treat reactive airway disease such as asthma and chronic obstructive pulmonary disease (COPD) (see Chapter 9).

f. **Gastrointestinal system** (see Chapter 8)

g. **Uterus**

(1) **Valethamate** is an anticholinergic with smooth muscle relaxant properties. It is used for dilation of the cervix during labor. It is also used as an antispasmodic in intestinal and urinary/biliary tract disorders.

5. ***Adverse effects***

a. The adverse effects of muscarinic-receptor antagonists are extensions of their pharmacologic activity.

b. Effects may include the following:

(1) Mydriasis, cycloplegia (blind as a bat)

(2) Dry eyes and mouth (dry as a bone)

(3) Elevated temperature (hot as a hare)

(4) Flushing (red as a beet)

(5) Urinary retention (full as a flask)

(6) Agitation, hallucinations, delirium (mad as a hatter)

(7) Tachycardia

The classic description of anticholinergic toxicity is: "Red as a beet, dry as a bone, hot as a hare, blind as a bat, mad as a hatter, full as a flask."

c. Symptomatic treatment is recommended.

d. **Neostigmine** may be used to treat poisoning with quaternary muscarinic-receptor antagonists.

6. ***Precaution*** must be used in narrow-angle glaucoma and prostatic hypertrophy.

7. ***Drug interactions.*** Additive effects may occur when administered with other drugs that have antimuscarinic activity, including certain antidepressants, antipsychotics, and antihistamines.

B. Antinicotinic agents

1. Ganglion-blocking drugs

a. ***Specific agent.*** **Mecamylamine.**

b. ***Mechanism of action.*** Ganglionic-blocking drugs **inhibit the effect of ACh at nicotinic receptors** by acting competitively (**nondepolarizing blockade**) at both sympathetic and parasympathetic autonomic ganglia (N_n receptors). In particular, mecamylamine inhibits ACh at the autonomic ganglia, which causes a decrease in blood pressure.

c. ***Indications.*** They are used for the treatment of severe hypertension and in uncomplicated malignant hypertension. Due to the lack of selectivity and numerous adverse effects, they are used rarely in the clinical setting.

d. ***Adverse effects*** can be severe since both sympathetic and parasympathetic systems are blocked. Orthostatic hypotension and CNS effects, including dizziness and tremor, may occur. Patients are often unable to tolerate ganglionic-blocking agents for long-term use.

V. SYMPATHOMIMETIC DRUGS

A. Mechanism of action

1. These drugs are **direct, indirect, or mixed-acting; they activate** postjunctional and prejunctional **adrenoceptors** and **mimic** the effects of **endogenous catecholamines**, such as noradrenaline and adrenaline.
   a. Their actions can generally be predicted from the type and location of the receptors with which they interact and whether or not they cross the blood–brain barrier to enter the CNS (Table 2.8).
2. Indirectly acting agents can have several different actions, for example, amphetamine.
   a. They can act within nerve endings to **increase the release of stored catecholamines.**
   b. Some agents act at the prejunctional membrane to **block the reuptake of catecholamines** that have been released from nerve endings.
   c. They may act **enzymatically to prevent catecholamine biotransformation.**
3. Mixed-acting drugs act both directly and indirectly, for example, mephentermine.

B. Pharmacologic effects (Table 2.8)

1. ***Cardiovascular system***
   a. **β_1-Receptor agonists**, through an increased calcium influx in cardiac cells, increase the rate (chronotropic effect) and force (inotropic effect) of myocardial contraction and increase the conduction velocity (dromotropic effect) through the AV node, with a decrease in the refractory period.

TABLE 2.8 Direct Effects of Adrenoceptor Agonists

Effector	α_1	α_2	β_1	β_2
Heart				
Rate			Increase	
Force			Increase	
Arterioles (most)	Constrict			Dilate
Blood pressure	Increase			Decrease
Intestine				
Wall	Relax	Relax		Relax
Sphincters	Contract			
Salivation				
Volume	Increase			
Amylase			Increase	
Pupil	Dilate			
Bronchial smooth muscle				Relax
Urinary bladder				
Body	Constrict			Relax
Sphincter	Constrict			
Release of NE from nerves		Decrease		

NE, noradrenaline.

b. **β_2-Receptor agonists** cause relaxation of vascular smooth muscle that may invoke a reflex increase in heart rate.

c. **α_1-Receptor agonists** constrict smooth muscle of resistance blood vessels (e.g., in the skin and splanchnic beds), causing increased peripheral resistance usually with an increase in blood pressure.

(1) In normotensive patients (less effect in those with hypotension), the increased blood pressure may invoke a reflex baroreceptor vagal discharge and a slowing of the heart, with or without an accompanying change in cardiac output.

d. **α_2-Receptor agonists** reduce blood pressure by a prejunctional action on neurons in the CNS to inhibit sympathetic outflow.

2. ***Eye*** (see Table 2.4)

a. **α-Receptor agonists** contract the radial muscle of the iris and dilate the pupil (mydriasis). These drugs also increase the outflow of aqueous humor from the eye.

b. **β-Receptor antagonists** decrease the production of aqueous humor.

3. ***Respiratory system***

a. Effects include **β_2-receptor agonist**–induced relaxation of bronchial smooth muscle and decreased airway resistance.

4. ***Metabolic and endocrine effects***

a. **β-Receptor agonists** increase liver and skeletal muscle glycogenolysis and increase lipolysis in fat cells. **α_2-Receptor agonists** inhibit lipolysis.

b. **β-Receptor agonists** increase, and **α_2-receptor agonists** decrease, insulin secretion.

5. ***Genitourinary tract effects*** include **α-receptor agonist** contraction of the bladder wall, urethral sphincter, prostate, seminal vesicles, and ductus deferens.

C. Specific sympathomimetic agents and their indications (Table 2.9)

1. ***Adrenaline and noradrenaline***

a. Adrenaline and noradrenaline are poorly absorbed from the GI tract and do not enter the CNS to any appreciable extent.

(1) Absorption of adrenaline from subcutaneous sites is slow because of local vasoconstriction.

b. Enzymes in the liver, such as COMT and MAO, metabolize adrenaline and noradrenaline.

c. Adrenaline and noradrenaline actions at neuroeffector junctions are terminated primarily by **simple diffusion** away from the receptor site and by **active uptake** into sympathetic nerve terminals and subsequent active transport into storage vesicles. Actions are also partially terminated at neuroeffector junctions by metabolism by extraneuronal COMT and intraneuronal MAO.

(1) **Adrenaline**

(a) Adrenaline can activate **β_1-, β_2-, α_1-, and α_2-receptors.**

i. Adrenaline administration in humans **increases systolic pressure** as a result of positive inotropic and chronotropic effects on the heart (β_1-receptor activation).

ii. It generally results in **decreased total peripheral resistance** and **decreased diastolic pressure due to vasodilation** in the vascular bed of skeletal muscle (β_2-receptor activation) that overcomes the vasoconstriction produced in most other vascular beds, including the kidney (α-receptor activation).

iii. The mean arterial pressure may increase slightly, decrease, or remain unchanged, depending on the balance of effects on systolic and diastolic pressure.

(b) Dose-dependent effects

i. At low doses, adrenaline activates **β_1**- and **β_2**- receptors (similar to isoprenaline).

(i) **β_1** activation causes an increase in heart rate, stroke volume, cardiac output, and pulse pressure.

(ii) **β_2** activation causes decreased total peripheral resistance and blood pressure.

ii. At medium doses, it can activate **β_1-, β_2-, and α_1-receptors** (similar to dobutamine).

(i) **β_1** activation causes an increase in heart rate, stroke volume, cardiac output, and pulse pressure.

(ii) **β_2** activation causes decreased total peripheral resistance and blood pressure, whereas **α_1** activation has the exact opposite effect.

TABLE 2.9 Selected Therapeutic Uses of Adrenoceptor Agonists

Clinical Condition/Application	Agonist	Receptor
Hypotensive emergency	Phenylephrine; methoxamine; noradrenaline	α_1
Chronic, orthostatic hypotension	Ephedrine; midodrine, phenylephrine	α_1
Anaphylactic shock	Adrenaline	α and β
Heart block, cardiac arrest	Isoprenaline; adrenaline	β_1
Congestive heart failure	Dobutamine	β_1
Infiltration nerve block	Adrenaline	α_1
Hay fever and rhinitis	Phenylephrine; OTC[a]	α_1
Asthma	Orciprenaline; terbutaline; salbutamol	β_2

[a]Over-the-counter preparations.

1. Due to the physiologic antagonism with β_2 and α_1, they can cancel each other's effects; for example, blood pressure will not change.
2. Only β_1 activity remains, leading to increased contractility and tachycardia.

iii. At high doses, adrenaline activates **β_1-, β_2-, and α_1-receptors, but the effect on the α_1-receptor predominates (similar to noradrenaline).**

(c) Blood pressure will increase due to increased vasoconstriction; there is also the potential for reflex tachycardia. Adrenaline **increases coronary blood flow** as a result of increased cardiac workload; it may precipitate **angina** in patients with coronary insufficiency.

(d) Adrenaline **increases the drainage of aqueous humor** (α-receptor activation) and reduces pressure in **open-angle glaucoma.** It **dilates the pupil** (mydriasis) by contraction of the radial muscle of the eye (α-receptor activation).

(e) Adrenaline **relaxes bronchial smooth muscle** (β_2-receptor activation).

(2) Adrenaline is used for the **management of type I allergic reactions**, including **anaphylactic reactions**. It is also used for the management of cardiogenic or septic shock. It may be used for mydriasis during intraocular surgery.

(3) **Noradrenaline** is used as a pressor agent in shock. It **activates β_1-receptors** and **α-receptors**. It has little activity at β_2-receptors.

2. *Dopamine*

a. Dopamine activates peripheral **β_1-adrenoceptors** to increase heart rate and contractility.

b. It also **activates** prejunctional and postjunctional dopamine **D_1 receptors** in the renal, coronary, and splanchnic vessels to reduce arterial resistance and increase blood flow. Prejunctionally, dopamine inhibits noradrenaline release.

c. At **low doses,** it stimulates **dopamine receptors** to **produce renal and mesenteric vasodilation.**

d. At **medium doses,** it activates dopamine and β_1-receptors, which leads to renal vasodilation and cardiac stimulation.

e. At **very high doses**, it stimulates **α_1-receptors** to cause **vasoconstriction**, with a reflex decrease in heart rate.

f. It is used for **hemodynamic support** as an adjunct in the treatment of shock.

3. *β-Adrenoceptor agonists*

a. Dobutamine

(1) Dobutamine activates **α-receptors** and **β-receptors.** It does not affect dopamine receptors.

(a) It is an agonist at **β_1-receptors**, which results in increased cardiac contractility and heart rate.

(b) It also acts on **β_2- and α_1-receptors** in the vasculature; oftentimes, the β_2 effects are more predominant, leading to vasodilation.

(2) Overall, dobutamine increases cardiac output, with limited vasodilating effects and reflex tachycardia.

(3) It is used for the management of patients with **cardiac decompensation**, including cardiogenic shock, and for inotropic support in heart failure.

b. **Isoprenaline**
   (1) This agent stimulates β_1- and β_2-receptors resulting in relaxation of bronchial, GI, and uterine smooth muscle.
   (2) It also causes increased heart rate and contractility and vasodilation of peripheral vasculature.
   (3) It is used for the management of bradyarrhythmias, including AV nodal block.

c. **β_2-Receptor agonists,** such as salbutamol, **relax bronchial smooth muscle**. They are used for the treatment of asthma; because of their selectivity for the β_2-receptor, they have fewer cardiac effects (see Chapter 9).

4. ***α-Adrenoceptor agonists***
   a. **Phenylephrine**
      (1) This drug causes **direct α_1-receptor stimulation** that results in vasoconstriction, increased total peripheral resistance, and increased systolic and diastolic pressure.
      (2) It can be used for the management of cardiogenic shock and hypotension during anesthesia. It is also used as a nasal decongestant.
      (3) It facilitates **examination of the retina** because of its mydriatic effect. It is also used for minor allergic hyperemia of the conjunctiva.
   b. **Oxymetazoline** is a selective α_{1A}-receptor agonist that produces vasoconstriction. Topically, it is used for the treatment of persistent facial erythema associated with rosacea. The intranasal form is used for nasal congestion.
   c. Methyldopa, guanfacine, and clonidine are **α_2-adrenergic agonists.** They are **centrally acting vasodilators** used for the management of hypertension (see Chapter 4).

5. ***Other sympathomimetic agents***
   a. **Ephedrine**
      (1) This agent releases tissue stores of noradrenaline leading to α- and β-receptor stimulation.
      (2) It has a longer duration of action and similar effects to those of **adrenaline,** but is less potent.
         (a) It has a longer duration of action because it is resistant to metabolism by COMT and MAO.
      (3) Unlike catecholamines, it penetrates the brain and can produce CNS stimulation.
      (4) **Ephedrine** is found in the herbal medication **ma huang.**
      (5) After continued use, **tachyphylaxis** may develop due to ephedrine's peripheral effects.
      (6) It is approved for anesthesia-induced hypotension.
   b. **Pseudoephedrine** is an isomer of ephedrine used as a decongestant (see Chapter 9).
   c. **Modafinil** is a CNS stimulant. The mechanism is unclear. It may increase dopamine in the brain by blocking dopamine transporters, in addition to other effects. It is used for the treatment of **narcolepsy**, shift work sleep disorder, and obstructive sleep apnea.
   d. **Dextroamphetamine** promotes the release of dopamine and noradrenaline from their storage sites in the presynaptic nerve terminals. It is a CNS stimulant used for the management of narcolepsy.
   e. **Methamphetamine** is a CNS stimulant used for obesity.
   f. **Methylphenidate** is used for **attention-deficit/hyperactivity disorder** (ADHD) (see Chapter 5).
      (1) It is well absorbed, enters the CNS readily, and has marked stimulant activity.
   g. **Fenoldopam** is a selective dopamine **D_1-receptor agonist** used to treat severe hypertension.

D. Adverse effects and toxicity

1. The adverse effects of sympathomimetic drugs are generally extensions of their pharmacologic activity.
2. Overdose with **adrenaline** or other pressor agents may result in **severe hypertension,** with possible **cerebral hemorrhage, pulmonary edema,** and **cardiac arrhythmia.** Milder effects include headache, dizziness, and tremor. Increased cardiac workload may result in angina or myocardial infarction in patients with coronary insufficiency.
3. Phenylephrine should not be used to treat closed-angle glaucoma before iridectomy as it may cause **increased IOP.**
4. Sudden discontinuation of a centrally acting **α_2-adrenoceptor agonist** may cause **withdrawal symptoms** that include headache, tachycardia, and a rebound rise in blood pressure.
5. Drug abuse may occur with amphetamine and amphetamine-like drugs.

E. Drug interactions

1. **Tricyclic antidepressants** block catecholamine reuptake and may potentiate the effects of noradrenaline and adrenaline.
2. Some **halogenated anesthetic agents** and **digitalis** may sensitize the heart to β-receptor stimulants, resulting in ventricular arrhythmias.

VI. ADRENERGIC RECEPTOR ANTAGONISTS

These drugs interact with either α- or β-adrenoceptors to prevent or reverse the actions of endogenously released noradrenaline or adrenaline or exogenously administered sympathomimetic agents.

A. α-Adrenoceptor antagonists

1. ***Pharmacologic effects***
   a. The pharmacologic effects of α-adrenoceptor antagonists are predominantly cardiovascular and include **lowered peripheral vascular resistance and blood pressure.** These agents prevent pressor effects of α-receptor agonists.
   b. α_1-Adrenoceptor antagonists can also antagonize sympathetic control of the bladder; they relax smooth muscle in the bladder neck, prostate capsule, and prostatic urethra and decrease resistance to outflow of urine.
2. ***Specific agents and their indications*** (Table 2.10)
   a. **Phentolamine** is a short-acting competitive antagonist at both α_1- and α_2-receptors. It reduces peripheral resistance and decreases blood pressure.
      (1) It is approved for the diagnosis of **pheochromocytoma** and for the prevention and management of hypertensive episodes associated with pheochromocytoma.
         (a) Pheochromocytoma is a **tumor of the adrenal medulla that secretes excessive amounts of catecholamines**. Symptoms include hypertension, tachycardia, and arrhythmias.
         (b) β-Receptor antagonists are often used to prevent the cardiac effects of excessive catecholamines after an α-receptor blockade is established.
      (2) It can be infiltrated locally to prevent dermal necrosis by reversing the vasoconstrictor effects of extravasated noradrenaline and dopamine.
      (3) To treat hypertensive emergency due to clonidine withdrawal, amphetamine overdosage, cocaine toxicity, etc.
   b. **Phenoxybenzamine**
      (1) Phenoxybenzamine is a noncompetitive, irreversible antagonist with some selectivity for α_1-receptors.
      (2) Phenoxybenzamine binds covalently, resulting in a long-lasting blockade.
      (3) It is used to treat sweating and hypertension associated with pheochromocytoma.
   c. Prazosin, terazosin, doxazosin, tamsulosin, silodosin, and alfuzosin are selective α_1-antagonists.
      (1) Prazosin, **terazosin,** and **doxazosin** are used for the management of hypertension.
      (2) **Terazosin, doxazosin, alfuzosin, tamsulosin,** and **silodosin** are used for the management of **benign prostatic hyperplasia (BPH).**
         (a) **Tamsulosin** and **silodosin** are **α_{1A}-selective agents**, which have **less effect on blood pressure.**
      (3) Prazosin can also be used to reduce symptoms associated with post-traumatic stress disorder (PTSD)–related nightmares by blocking excessive responsiveness to noradrenaline stimulation at postsynaptic α_1-adrenergic receptors.
      (4) Prazosin is also used for the management of Raynaud phenomenon.
   d. **Labetalol** and **carvedilol** (see Chapter 4)
      (1) These agents are **competitive antagonists** (partial agonist) at the α_1-receptors. In addition, they block β-receptors.
      (2) They reduce heart rate and myocardial contractility, decrease total peripheral resistance, and lower blood pressure.
      (3) These agents are used for hypertension and heart failure.

TABLE 2.10 Therapeutic Uses of Selected Adrenoceptor Antagonists

Drug	Receptor	Features	Major Uses
Phentolamine[a]	α_1 and α_2	Short duration of action (1–2 hours)	Hypertension of pheochromocytoma
Phenoxybenzamine[a]		Long duration of action (15–50 hours)	Hypertension of pheochromocytoma
Prazosin[a]	α_1	Minimal reflex tachycardia	Mild-to-moderate hypertension (often with a diuretic or a β-adrenoceptor antagonist)
Terazosin			Mild-to-moderate hypertension
Doxazosin			Mild-to-moderate hypertension
Propranolol[a]	β_1 and β_2	Local anesthetic activity	Hypertension; angina; pheochromocytoma, cardiac arrhythmias; migraine headache; hypertrophic subaortic stenosis
Timolol			Hypertension; glaucoma
Metipranolol			Glaucoma
Levobunolol			Glaucoma
Nadolol		Long duration of action (15–25 hours)	Hypertension; angina
Pindolol		Partial β_2-receptor agonist activity[b]	Hypertension; angina
Penbutolol		Partial β_2-receptor agonist activity[b]; mild-to-moderate hypertension	Hypertension; angina
Carteolol		Partial β_2-receptor agonist activity[b]; excreted unchanged	Hypertension; angina; glaucoma
Metoprolol[a]	$\beta_1 > \beta_2$	Patient bioavailability is variable; extended-release form available	Hypertension; angina
Atenolol		Eliminated by the kidney	Hypertension; angina
Esmolol		Ultrashort acting (10 minutes)	Supraventricular tachycardia
Betaxolol		Long duration of action (15–25 hours)	Glaucoma; hypertension
Acebutolol		Partial agonist[b]	Hypertension; ventricular arrhythmias
Labetalol[a]	β_1, β_2, and α_1	Partial agonist[b]; rapid blood pressure reduction; local anesthetic activity	Mild-to-severe hypertension; hypertensive emergencies

[a]Drugs listed in **boldface type** are considered prototype drugs.
[b]Lower blood pressure without significant reduction in cardiac output or resting heart rate; also do not elevate triglyceride levels or decrease high-density lipoprotein cholesterol.

3. ***Adverse effects***
   a. α_1-Antagonists such as **prazosin, terazosin,** and **doxazosin** produce postural hypotension and bradycardia on initial administration; these drugs produce no significant tachycardia. The α_{1A}-selective agents have less effect on blood pressure.
   b. **Phentolamine** and **phenoxybenzamine** can cause postural hypotension as well as tachycardia.

B. β-Adrenoreceptor antagonists

1. ***Pharmacologic effects***
   a. **Cardiovascular system** (see Chapter 4)
      (1) β-Adrenoreceptor antagonists **lower blood pressure;** this is most likely due to their combined effects on the heart, the renin–angiotensin system, and the CNS.
      (2) These drugs **reduce** sympathetic-stimulated increases in **heart rate, contractility**, and **cardiac output.**
      (3) They **lengthen AV conduction time and refractoriness**. They also **suppress automaticity.**
      (4) Initially, these drugs may increase peripheral resistance. However, long-term administration results in decreased peripheral resistance in patients with hypertension.
      (5) β-Adrenoreceptor antagonists reduce renin release.
   b. **Respiratory system**
      (1) β-Adrenoreceptor antagonists **increase airway resistance** as a result of β_2-receptor blockade.

(2) Nonselective β-antagonists prevent bronchodilation due to their effects on bronchial β_2 receptors; this may lead to increased airway resistance.

c. **Eye**

(1) β-Adrenoreceptor antagonists decrease the production of aqueous humor (β_2), resulting in **reduced IOP**.

d. **Other pharmacologic effects**

(1) β-Adrenoreceptor antagonists **inhibit lipolysis** (β_3).

(2) These drugs **inhibit glycogenolysis** (β_2) in the liver (they may impede recovery from the hypoglycemic effect of insulin).

(3) These decrease high-density lipoprotein levels.

2. ***Specific drugs*** (see Chapter 4) (Table 2.10)

a. Propranolol

(1) This agent is a competitive antagonist at β_1- and β_2-receptors.

(2) It is used in **long-term treatment of hypertension.**

(3) This drug is used to treat **supraventricular and ventricular arrhythmias.** It can also be used in the prevention of migraine headaches.

b. **Metoprolol, atenolol, acebutolol,** and **esmolol**

(1) These drugs are selective **β_1-receptor antagonists** (cardioselective β-blockers).

(2) They may offer some advantage over nonselective β-adrenoceptor antagonists to treat cardiovascular disease in asthmatic patients, although cautious use is still warranted.

(3) **Esmolol** is **ultrashort acting** ($t_{1/2}$ = 10 minutes) because of extensive hydrolysis by plasma esterases; it is administered by **intravenous infusion.**

c. **Labetalol** and **carvedilol**

(1) Labetalol is a partial agonist that blocks β-receptors and α_1-receptors (3:1 to 7:1 ratio).

(2) Carvedilol also has mixed activity but is equiactive at β-receptors and α_1-receptors.

(3) They reduce heart rate and myocardial contractility, decrease total peripheral resistance, and lower blood pressure.

d. **Pindolol, carteolol,** and **penbutolol** are nonselective antagonists with partial β_2-receptor agonist activity.

e. **Acebutolol** and **pindolol** have **intrinsic sympathomimetic activity (ISA).** They are partial agonists and provide low-level β-stimulation at rest, but full β-receptor blockade at times of high sympathetic activity.

(1) They **cause less bradycardia** and may be useful in patients with diminished cardiac reserve or a tendency for bradycardia.

3. ***Indications*** (see Table 2.10)

a. **Cardiovascular system** (see also Chapter 4)

(1) β-Blockers have many indications. They are used in the management of hypertension, **angina** and **myocardial infarction, arrhythmias,** and **heart failure.**

b. **Eye**

(1) Topical application of **timolol, betaxolol,** and **carteolol** reduces IOP in **glaucoma.**

(2) In some cases, these agents can be systemically absorbed, and may lead to increased airway resistance and decreased heart rate and contractility.

c. **Other uses**

(1) β-Blockers can be used to decrease symptoms of hyperthyroidism that are due to increased β-adrenergic tone, such as tachycardia, tremor, and anxiety.

(a) In high doses, propranolol can inhibit 5′-monodeiodinase and prevent the conversion of thyroxine (T_4) to triiodothyronine (T_3).

(2) Other indications for propranolol include essential tremor, anxiety disorder, and migraine headache prophylaxis.

4. ***Adverse effects and contraindications***

a. General side effects may include dizziness and drowsiness.

b. They may cause **decreased heart rate, blood pressure, contractility,** and **AV node conduction.**

c. Acute withdrawal can be dangerous and lead to exacerbation of ischemic symptoms, including angina or myocardial infarction. **Tapered withdrawal** is recommended.

d. Nonselective agents may increase airway resistance and exacerbate peripheral artery disease (due to β_2 blockade).
e. β_2-Adrenoceptor blockade also decreases catecholamine-induced glycogenolysis. They may also mask tachycardia associated with hypoglycemia.

VII. SKELETAL MUSCLE RELAXANTS

Skeletal muscle relaxants are broadly classified into the peripherally (neuromuscular blockers) and centrally acting (spasmolytics) drugs. Some other drugs, such as dantrolene and quinine, act directly on the skeletal muscles but their use is similar to those of centrally acting muscle relaxants.

1. Nondepolarizing neuromuscular blockers (skeletal muscle relaxants)
a. ***Mechanism of action***
(1) Nondepolarizing agents **competitively inhibit the effect of ACh** at the postjunctional membrane **nicotinic receptor** of the neuromuscular junction (N_m receptors). There is some prejunctional inhibition of ACh release.
(2) These agents **prevent depolarization of the muscle** and propagation of the action potential.
b. ***Pharmacologic properties***
(1) Nondepolarizing agents are administered parenterally and are generally used for **long-term motor paralysis.** Paralysis and muscle relaxation usually occur within 1–5 minutes.
(2) The duration of action for these agents generally ranges from 20 to 90 minutes.
(a) Intermediate-acting agents, such as **rocuronium** or **vecuronium**, are more commonly used than long-acting agents like D-tubocurarine.
(3) Most nondepolarizing agents are metabolized by the liver or are excreted unchanged. The duration of action may be prolonged by hepatic or renal disease.
c. ***Specific drugs*** (Table 2.11)
(1) **Tubocurarine** (prototype) is seldom used clinically at this time.
(2) **Metocurine** is a derivative of tubocurarine.
(a) It has the same properties, but less histamine release; therefore, it causes less hypotension and bronchoconstriction.
(b) It has a long duration of action (>40 minutes).
(3) **Atracurium**
(a) Atracurium causes some histamine release.

TABLE 2.11 Properties of Selected Skeletal Muscle Relaxants

	Duration of Action	Ganglion Blockade	Histamine Release	Cardiac Muscarinic Receptors	Comments
Nondepolarizing agent					
Tubocurarine[a]	Long	+	++	—	Prototype
Atracurium[a]	Intermediate	—	+	—	Inactivated spontaneously in plasma; laudanosine, a breakdown product, may cause seizures
Cisatracurium[a]	Intermediate	—	—	—	Less laudanosine formed than atracurium
Mivacurium[a]	Short	—	++	—	Hydrolyzed by plasma cholinesterase
Pancuronium[b]	Long	—	—	++	Increased heart rate
Vecuronium[b]	Intermediate	—	—	—	Metabolized by liver
Depolarizing agent					
Succinylcholine	Very short	++	+	++	Hydrolyzed by cholinesterase; malignant hyperthermia is a rare, potentially fatal complication

[a]Isoquinoline derivative.
[b]Steroid derivative.

(b) It is **inactivated spontaneously in plasma** by nonenzymatic hydrolysis (Hoffmann elimination) that is delayed by acidosis.
(c) Its duration of action is reduced by hyperventilation-induced respiratory alkalosis.
(d) **Laudanosine,** a breakdown product of atracurium, may accumulate to cause **seizures**.

(4) **Cisatracurium**
(a) This agent is a stereoisomer of atracurium with less histamine release and less laudanosine formation.
(b) It has **replaced atracurium** use in clinical practice.

(5) **Mivacurium**
(a) This is a short-acting (10–20 minutes) agent that is rapidly hydrolyzed by plasma cholinesterase.
(b) It has a slow onset of action relative to succinylcholine.
(c) This agent produces moderate histamine release at high doses.

(6) **Vecuronium**, **rocuronium**, and **pancuronium**
(a) These are steroid derivatives with **minimal histaminic or ganglion-blocking activity.**
(b) Vecuronium and rocuronium have intermediate durations of action (20–40 minutes).
(c) Pancuronium has a longer duration of action (120–180 minutes) and is used less frequently than the others.

d. ***Indications***
(1) Nondepolarizing agents are used during surgery as adjuncts to general anesthetics to **induce muscle paralysis and muscle relaxation**.
(a) The order of muscle paralysis is small, rapidly contracting muscles (e.g., extrinsic muscles of the eye) before slower contracting muscle groups (e.g., face and extremities), followed by intercostal muscles, and then the diaphragm.
(b) Recovery of muscle function is in reverse order, and respiration often must be assisted.
(2) These agents are also used for muscle paralysis in patients when it is **critical to control ventilation**, such as ventilatory failure from pneumonia, for **endotracheal intubation**, and to control muscle contractions during electroconvulsive therapy.

e. ***Reversal of nondepolarizing drug blockade***
(1) AChE inhibitors, such as **neostigmine,** are administered for pharmacologic antagonism to reverse residual postsurgical nicotinic receptor blockade and avoid inadvertent hypoxia or apnea.
(2) Sugammadex is an agent that forms a complex with rocuronium and vecuronium, which helps in reversal of their action.

f. ***Adverse effects and contraindications***
(1) Cardiovascular system
(a) Tubocurarine, atracurium, mivacurium, pancuronium, and metocurine may cause **hypotension** or **increased heart rate** due to histamine release, ganglionic-blocking activity, or vagolytic activity.
(2) Respiratory system
(a) Some nondepolarizing agents can produce **bronchospasm** due to histamine release.
(b) Agents that release histamine are contraindicated for asthmatic patients and patients with a history of anaphylactic reactions.

g. ***Drug interactions***
(1) **General inhalation anesthetics,** particularly **isoflurane**, increase the neuromuscular blocking action of nondepolarizing agents. Dose reduction of the neuromuscular junction–blocking drug may be necessary.
(2) **Aminoglycoside antibiotics** inhibit prejunctional ACh release and potentiate the effect of nondepolarizing and depolarizing neuromuscular junction–blocking drugs.

2. Depolarizing neuromuscular blockers (skeletal muscle relaxants)
a. ***Specific agent.*** Succinylcholine (Table 2.8).
b. ***Mechanism of action***
(1) Succinylcholine is a **nicotinic (N_m) receptor agonist** that acts at the motor end plate of the neuromuscular junction to produce **persistent stimulation and depolarization of the muscle**, thus preventing stimulation of contraction by ACh.

(2) Initial muscle contractions or **fasciculations** occur quickly (in the first 30–60 seconds); they may be masked by general anesthetics.

(3) Since succinylcholine is metabolized more slowly than ACh at the neuromuscular junction, the muscle cells remain depolarized (**depolarizing or phase I block**) and unresponsive to further stimulation, resulting in a **flaccid paralysis** (5–10 minutes).

(4) The muscle cells repolarize with continuous long-term exposure (45–60 minutes). However, they cannot depolarize again while succinylcholine is present; therefore, they remain unresponsive to ACh (**desensitizing or phase II block**).

(5) AChE inhibition will enhance the initial phase I block by succinylcholine, but can reverse phase II block.

c. ***Pharmacologic properties***

(1) Succinylcholine has a rapid onset and short duration of action, due to rapid **hydrolysis by plasma and liver cholinesterase.**

(2) Reduced plasma cholinesterase synthesis in end-stage hepatic disease or reduced activity following the use of irreversible AChE inhibitors may increase the duration of action.

d. ***Indications.*** It is used as an **adjunct in surgical anesthesia** to obtain muscle relaxation while using lower levels of general anesthetic, to induce **brief paralysis in short surgical procedures,** and to **facilitate intubation.**

e. ***Adverse effects***

(1) **Postoperative muscle pain** at higher doses

(2) **Hyperkalemia**

(a) Hyperkalemia results from loss of tissue potassium during depolarization.

(b) Risk of hyperkalemia is enhanced in patients with burns, muscle trauma, or spinal cord transections.

(c) It can be life threatening, leading to **cardiac arrest** and circulatory collapse.

(3) **Malignant hyperthermia**

(a) Malignant hyperthermia is a rare but potentially fatal complication in susceptible patients that results from a **rapid increase in muscle metabolism.**

i. Patients who experience this condition are genetically predisposed, with mutations in the **skeletal muscle Ca^{2+}-release channel of the sarcoplasmic reticulum (ryanodine receptor, RYR1).**

(b) Malignant hyperthermia is most likely to occur when succinylcholine is used with the general anesthetic **halothane.**

(c) Early signs include hypercarbia, **sinus tachycardia**, and **muscle rigidity**. Later signs include **hyperthermia**, ventricular tachycardia or fibrillation, and **myoglobinuria**.

(d) It can be treated with **dantrolene**, a skeletal muscle relaxant that binds to the RYR1 receptor to inhibit the release of calcium from the sarcoplasmic reticulum.

(4) **Prolonged paralysis** may result in apnea (succinylcholine apnea) in a small percentage of patients with genetically atypical or low levels of plasma cholinesterase. Mechanical ventilation is necessary.

(5) **Bradycardia** from direct muscarinic cholinoceptor stimulation is prevented by atropine.

(6) **Increased IOP** may result from extraocular muscle contractions; use of succinylcholine may be contraindicated for penetrating eye injuries.

(7) Succinylcholine produces increased intragastric pressure, which may result in fasciculations of abdominal muscles and a danger of aspiration.

3. **Spasmolytic agents for acute use**

a. ***Specific agents*** include **cyclobenzaprine, metaxalone, methocarbamol,** orphenadrine, and chlorzoxazone.

b. ***Mechanism of action***

(1) These agents are sedatives or act in the brainstem.

(a) They are centrally active drugs; in many cases, the mechanisms are not well understood.

(b) Metaxalone, methocarbamol, carisoprodol, chlorzoxazone, and thiocolchicoside cause depression of the nervous system.

(c) Cyclobenzaprine works in the brainstem to reduce tonic somatic motor activity influencing both α and γ motor neurons.

c. ***Indications***

(1) These agents are used for short-term use of muscle spasms due to acute, painful musculoskeletal conditions, including muscle injury or strains.

d. ***Adverse effects*** may include CNS depression. Cyclobenzaprine can cause anticholinergic effects and may cause confusion or hallucinations.

4. **Spasmolytic agents for chronic use**

a. ***Specific agents*** include **baclofen, diazepam, tizanidine, dantrolene, and quinine.**

b. ***Mechanism of action***

(1) These agents act to reduce abnormal muscle tone without paralysis.

(2) Baclofen ($GABA_B$), benzodiazepines ($GABA_A$), and tizanidine (α_2) act in the spinal cord and **reduce tonic output of the spinal motor neurons.**

(a) **Baclofen** is a **$GABA_B$ agonist** that leads to membrane hyperpolarization.

i. Presynaptic receptors: They reduce calcium influx and decrease the release of glutamic acid (excitatory transmitter).

ii. Postsynaptic receptors: They facilitate the inhibitory action of GABA.

(b) **Tizanidine** is an **α_2 agonist** that reinforces presynaptic inhibition in the spinal cord. It reduces muscle spasm with less muscle weakness than do other agents.

(c) **Diazepam** acts on the spinal cord and CNS to facilitate GABA activity at **$GABA_A$** receptors (see Chapter 5).

(3) **Dantrolene** acts directly on skeletal muscle to reduce contractions. It **interferes with Ca^{2+} release from the sarcoplasmic reticulum**; benefit may not be apparent for a week or more. Quinine also acts directly on the skeletal muscles and can be used for nocturnal leg cramps.

c. ***Indications***

(1) **They reduce increased muscle tone** associated with a variety of nervous system disorders, including **cerebral palsy, multiple sclerosis, spinal cord injury, and stroke.**

(a) These conditions result in loss of supraspinal control and hyperexcitability of α- and γ-motoneurons in the spinal cord, causing abnormal skeletal muscle, bowel, and bladder function.

(b) They are often associated with a high reflex activity that may result in painful muscle spasms.

d. ***Adverse effects include*** sedation. Dantrolene causes significant muscle weakness, although it has fewer effects on sedation. Tizanidine can cause xerostomia and hypotension.

e. **Botulinum toxin**

(1) Botulinum toxin acts by **inhibiting the release of ACh from motor nerve terminals.**

(2) It is used to treat local muscle spasms, spastic disorders like **cerebral palsy**, and blepharospasm- and strabismus-associated dystonia.

(3) It is also used for **chronic migraines** and cosmetic reduction of **facial wrinkles.**

VIII. LOCAL ANESTHETICS

A. Overview of local anesthetics

1. Local anesthetics produce a transient and **reversible loss of sensation** in a **circumscribed region** of the body **without loss of consciousness.**

a. Local anesthesia occurs when sensory transmission from a local area of the body to the CNS is blocked.

b. As a general rule, smaller nonmyelinated dorsal root type C nerve fibers that carry pain and temperature sensations are blocked before larger, myelinated type A fibers transmit sensory proprioception and motor functions.

B. Classification and chemistry of local anesthetics

1. Most available local anesthetics are classified as either **esters** or **amides.**

a. They generally consist of a lipophilic aromatic group connected to a hydrophilic, ionizable tertiary amine.

2. Most are **weak bases** with pK_a values between 7 and 9, and at physiologic pH, they are primarily in the charged, cationic form.
3. The **potency** of local anesthetics is **positively correlated** with their **lipid solubility** and **negatively correlated** with their **molecular size**.
4. They are selected for use on the basis of the duration of drug action (short, 20 minutes; intermediate, 1–1.5 hours; long, 2–4 hours), effectiveness at the administration site, and potential for toxicity.

C. Mechanism of action

1. Local anesthetics act by **blocking sodium channels** and the conduction of action potentials along sensory nerves.
2. The **nonionized** form of the drug is important for **reaching the receptor** site, and the **ionized** form is important for causing the **effect**.
   a. The drug must cross the lipid membrane to reach the cytoplasm; therefore, the more lipid-soluble (*nonionized, uncharged*) form reaches effective intracellular concentrations more rapidly than the ionized form.
   b. Once inside, the *ionized (charged)* form of the drug is the *more effective* blocking entity. After penetration into the cytoplasm, equilibration leads to the formation and binding of the charged cation at the sodium channel, leading to the production of a clinical effect.
3. Blockade is voltage and time dependent.
   a. At rest, the voltage-dependent sodium (Na^+) channels of sensory nerves are in the resting (closed) state. Following the action potential, the Na^+ channel becomes active (open) and then converts to an inactive (closed) state that is insensitive to depolarization.
   b. During excitation, the **ionized (charged) form** preferentially interacts with the **inactivated state** of the Na^+ channels to **block sodium current** and **increase the threshold for excitation**.
      (1) This results in a dose-dependent decrease in impulse conduction and in the rate of rise and amplitude of the action potential.

D. Pharmacologic properties

1. **Administration**
   a. Local anesthetics are administered topically by subcutaneous infiltration into tissues to bathe local nerves or by injection directly around nerves or into epidural or subarachnoid spaces.
   b. In clinical practice, **coadministration of a vasoconstrictor**, such as **adrenaline**, with a local anesthetic **reduces local blood flow** and systemic absorption.
      (1) This can prolong the duration of action and reduce systemic absorption and potential toxicity.
      (2) Adrenaline should not be coadministered for nerve block in areas such as fingers and toes that are supplied with end arteries, as it may cause ischemia or necrosis.
      (3) This combination can also delay wound healing, tissue edema, and necrosis due to increased oxygen consumption.
2. **Absorption**
   a. Many factors influence the rate and extent of absorption, including vascularity of the delivery site and drug concentration.
   b. **Lipid-soluble anesthetics** are usually **more potent** and have a **longer duration** of action. They may take longer to achieve the desired effect.
   c. Local anesthetics are **less effective** when they are injected into **infected tissues** because the **low extracellular pH favors** the **charged form** (ionized), with less of the neutral base available for diffusion across the membrane.
      (1) The physiologic pH is 7.4, but often times with inflamed or infected tissue, the pH may be as low as 6.4.
      (2) Most local anesthetics are weak bases, in which the pK_a is between 8.0 and 9.0.
3. **Metabolism**
   a. **Ester-type** local anesthetics that enter the bloodstream are metabolized by **plasma butyrylcholinesterase** and thus have very short plasma half-lives.
      (1) The plasma level of these anesthetics may be higher than usual in patients with decreased or genetically atypical cholinesterase.
   b. **Amide-type** local anesthetics are metabolized at varying rates and extents by **hepatic microsomal enzymes**.

4. Excretion

a. Local anesthetics are converted to water-soluble metabolites and excreted in urine.

(1) **Acidification** of **urine** promotes the ionized form for more **rapid elimination**.

E. Specific local anesthetics and their indications

1. Amides include **lidocaine** (prototype), **mepivacaine**, **prilocaine**, **dibucaine, ropivacaine**, and **bupivacaine.**

a. Lidocaine and mepivacaine have a rapid onset and intermediate duration of action.

(1) Both are used for peripheral nerve block and spinal anesthesia. Lidocaine is also used for infiltration block and for epidural anesthesia.

b. Prilocaine has an intermediate onset and intermediate duration of action.

(1) It is used for spinal anesthesia and is widely used for obstetrical analgesia.

c. **Eutectic lignocaine/prilocaine (EMLA):** It is used to anesthetize intact skin after surface application; it is obtained by mixing in equal proportion at 25°C to lower the melting point of the two solids; it is applied as occlusive dressing before IV cannulation and split skin graft harvest.

d. Bupivacaine has a slow onset and long duration of action. It is used for infiltration, regional, epidural, and spinal anesthesia; it is preferred for obstetrical anesthesia as it produces minimal motor blockade and neonatal depression; cardiotoxicity is a major limitation.

e. Levobupivacaine has less cardiotoxicity and seizure-inducing propensity.

f. Ropivacaine is long acting with less cardiotoxicity; it is employed for epidural and nerve blocks.

g. Dibucaine is the longest acting but highly toxic; hence, it is preferred only for surface anesthesia.

2. Esters include **procaine**, **chloroprocaine**, **cocaine**, **benzocaine**, and **tetracaine.**

a. Chloroprocaine has a more rapid onset of action than procaine and a short duration of action. It is very rapidly metabolized by plasma cholinesterase.

(1) It is used for obstetrical anesthesia.

b. Procaine has a medium onset and short duration of action.

(1) Procaine is used with benzylpenicillin as it forms a poorly soluble salt and hence prolongs its duration.

c. Cocaine has a medium onset and medium duration of action.

(1) Clinical use is limited due to the potential for adverse effects including CNS stimulation, tachycardia, restlessness, tremors, seizures, and arrhythmias.

d. Tetracaine has very slow onset of action (>10 minutes) and is long acting.

(1) It is used primarily for spinal anesthesia and for ophthalmologic use.

e. Benzocaine can cause methemoglobinemia; it is used for surface anesthesia in stomatitis or superficial ulcers.

f. Oxethazine is a topical anesthetic used for anesthetizing gastric mucosa for symptomatic relief in gastritis.

F. Adverse effects and toxicity

1. Adverse effects of local anesthetics are generally the result of overdose or inadvertent injection into the vascular system.

2. Systemic effects are most likely to occur with administration of the amide class.

3. CNS effects

a. Adverse CNS effects include **light-headedness**, **dizziness**, restlessness, tinnitus, tremor, and visual disturbances.

(1) Lidocaine and procaine may cause sedation.

b. At high blood concentrations, they may produce nystagmus, shivering, tonic–clonic seizures, respiratory depression, coma, and death.

4. Cardiovascular effects

a. Adverse cardiovascular effects develop at relatively higher plasma levels than do adverse CNS effects.

b. **Bradycardia** develops as a result of the block of cardiac sodium channels and the depression of pacemaker activity.

c. Hypotension develops from arteriolar dilation and decreased cardiac contractility.

d. Cardiac arrhythmias and cardiovascular collapse can also occur.

5. Prilocaine and benzocaine can cause methemoglobinemia.

6. Ester-linked local anesthetics can also cause hypersensitivity reactions.

DRUG SUMMARY TABLE

Direct-Acting Cholinoceptor Agonists
Acetylcholine intraocular solution
Bethanechol
Carbachol
Cevimeline
Methacholine
Pilocarpine

Indirect-Acting Cholinoceptor Agonists
Donepezil
Echothiophate
Galantamine
Neostigmine
Physostigmine
Pyridostigmine
Rivastigmine
Nerve gases and insecticides
Malathion
Parathion
Sarin
Tabun

Cholinesterase Regenerator
Pralidoxime

Muscarinic Cholinoceptor Antagonists
Atropine
Clidinium with chlordiazepoxide
Cyclopentolate
Darifenacin
Dicyclomine
Fesoterodine
Flavoxate
Glycopyrrolate
Homatropine
Ipratropium
Mepenzolate
Oxybutynin
Propantheline
Scopolamine
Solifenacin
Tiotropium
Tolterodine
Tropicamide
Trospium

Ganglion-Blocking Drugs
Mecamylamine

Skeletal Muscle Relaxants
Neuromuscular Blocking Drugs
Atracurium
Cisatracurium
Mivacurium
Pancuronium
Rocuronium
Succinylcholine
Vecuronium

Spasmolytic Drugs
Baclofen
Botulinum toxin—type A (OnabotulinumtoxinA)
Botulinum toxin—type B (RimabotulinumtoxinB)
Cyclobenzaprine
Dantrolene
Diazepam
Metaxalone
Methocarbamol
Orphenadrine
Tizanidine

Sympathomimetic Drugs
Adrenaline
Albuterol
Apraclonidine
Brimonidine ophthalmic
Clonidine
Dexmedetomidine
Dextroamphetamine
Dobutamine
Dopamine
Ephedrine
Fenoldopam
Formoterol
Guanabenz
Guanfacine
Hydroxyamphetamine (with tropicamide)
Isoproterenol
Levalbuterol
Metaproterenol (orciprenaline)
Methamphetamine
Methyldopa
Methylphenidate
Midodrine
Modafinil
Norepinephrine (noradrenaline)
Oxymetazoline
Phenylephrine
Pseudoephedrine
Salmeterol
Terbutaline
Tetrahydrozoline

Adrenergic Receptor Antagonists
Alfuzosin
Doxazocin
Phenoxybenzamine
Phentolamine
Prazosin
Silodosin
Tamsulosin
Terazosin

β-Receptor Blockers
Acebutolol
Atenolol
Bisoprolol
Carvedilol
Esmolol
Labetalol
Metoprolol
Nadolol
Timolol
Penbutolol
Pindolol
Timolol

Local Anesthetics
Amides
Lidocaine
Mepivacaine
Prilocaine
Bupivacaine
Esters
Chloroprocaine
Cocaine
Procaine
Tetracaine

Review Test

Directions: Select the best answer for each question.

1. A 42-year-old woman presents to her neurologist for the management of chronic migraines. She complains of headaches that occur over 15 days per month. After trying many interventions for migraine treatment and prevention, the neurologist decides to administer botulinum toxin type A. What is the mechanism of action for this medication?

(A) Blocks release of acetylcholine from storage vesicles
(B) Blocks the synapse at ganglia
(C) Blocks transport of choline into neurons
(D) Inhibits acetylcholinesterase
(E) Inhibits choline acetyltransferase

2. A 21-year-old man presents to the emergency room with difficulty breathing. On physical examination, the physician notices that the patient is unable to speak in full sentences. In addition, he is tachypneic with a heart rate of 120 beats/min, and is using his accessory muscles on inspiration. The patient is diagnosed with a severe asthma attack and started on a β_2-receptor agonist. What is the intracellular effect for this medication?

(A) Activates G_i-protein, resulting in inhibition of adenylyl cyclase
(B) Activates G_q-protein, resulting in increase of phosphatidylinositol and calcium mobilization
(C) Activates G_s-protein, resulting in stimulation of adenylyl cyclase
(D) Allows passage of sodium through a ligand-gated ion channel
(E) Binds to μ-receptors in specific areas of the brain

3. A 50-year-old man is started on a new medication for the management of acute postoperative urinary retention. The medication also stimulates gastrointestinal motility. What is the mechanism of action for the new medication?

(A) α-Agonist
(B) β_1-Antagonist
(C) β_2-Agonist
(D) Muscarinic agonist
(E) Nicotinic antagonist

4. A 38-year-old man is brought to the emergency room by his wife with symptoms of sudden difficulty breathing, sweatiness, and anxiety. He is a farmer and was spraying insecticide when the symptoms started to occur. According to his wife, the symptoms started around 25 minutes prior to their arrival. Aside from atropine, what other medication should be administered?

(A) Pancuronium
(B) Phenylephrine
(C) Physostigmine
(D) Pralidoxime
(E) Propranolol

5. A 63-year-old woman is started on a new medication for the management of overactive bladder. Potential adverse effects include dry eyes and dry mouth. What is the mechanism of action for this medication?

(A) α_1-Antagonist
(B) β_2-Agonist
(C) Inhibits acetylcholinesterase
(D) Muscarinic antagonist
(E) Neuromuscular blocker

6. A 78-year-old man with Parkinson disease experiences worsening of his symptoms. He is already taking levodopa. The addition of which medication may help alleviate the patient's symptoms?

(A) Benztropine
(B) Doxazocin
(C) Reserpine
(D) Timolol
(E) Tubocurarine

7. A 66-year-old woman with a long history of heavy smoking presents to her doctor with complaints of shortness of breath and chronic coughing for about 2 years. She says that her symptoms have been worsening in frequency. The doctor prescribes a bronchodilator with minimal cardiac side effects. Which medication is most likely prescribed?

(A) Albuterol
(B) Atenolol
(C) Ipratropium
(D) Prazosin
(E) Pseudoephedrine

8. A 34-year-old man presents to the emergency room after an accident in which he inadvertently chopped off the tip of his index finger. He undergoes surgery for reattachment of the digit, and after sedation, a local anesthetic without adrenaline is administered around the site of the injury. Why cannot adrenaline be used?

(A) Causes hypotension when administered with sedative agents
(B) Causes vasoconstriction and vascular ischemia
(C) Is contraindicated in emergency surgery
(D) Increases risk of blood loss during surgery
(E) Increases swelling of the tissues

9. A 7-year-old boy is brought to the pediatrician by his parents for complaints of hyperactivity at school. He is also inattentive and impulsive at home. After a detailed interview, the physician prescribes an amphetamine-containing medication for presumed attention-deficit hyperactivity disorder. How does this medication work?

(A) Blocks effects of noradrenaline
(B) Directly acts on cholinoreceptors
(C) Indirectly acts on noradrenaline receptors
(D) Inhibits adrenaline reuptake
(E) Inhibits serotonin reuptake

10. A 69-year-old man is started on terazosin for the management of benign prostatic hyperplasia. Which of the following adverse effects should the patient be counseled about?

(A) Bronchospasm
(B) Drug abuse
(C) Heart failure
(D) Postural hypotension
(E) Sedation

11. A hospital nurse informs the cardiologist about a patient with chest pain. The patient describes the pain as tight pressure and is demonstrably sweating and gasping for air. The electrocardiogram shows acute ST-segment elevations in inferior leads and the patient is diagnosed with a myocardial infarction. The patient is given oxygen, sublingual nitroglycerin, and morphine. What additional class of medication should the doctor prescribe?

(A) α-Agonist
(B) β-Blocker
(C) Dopamine agonist
(D) Muscarinic agonist
(E) Neuromuscular blocker

12. A 35-year-old woman presents to her primary care practitioner for a regular checkup. Her only complaint is recurrent migraine headaches, which have increased in frequency over the past year. On examination, her blood pressure is elevated at 150/70 mm Hg. The doctor prescribes a medication that will help to prevent migraines and treat hypertension. Which medication did the doctor most likely prescribe?

(A) Clonidine
(B) Hydrochlorothiazide
(C) Prazosin
(D) Propranolol
(E) Amlodipine

13. Intravenous administration of adrenaline to a patient results in a severe decrease in diastolic pressure and an increase in cardiac output. Which of the following drugs might the patient have previously taken that could account for this unexpected effect?

(A) Atropine
(B) Phenylephrine
(C) Prazosin
(D) Propranolol
(E) Pyridostigmine

14. A 32-year-old woman presents to the emergency room with ptosis, diplopia, and limited facial expressions. Further examination leads to a diagnosis of myasthenia gravis. Which medication can help manage the patient's symptoms?

(A) Atropine
(B) Cyclopentolate
(C) Pralidoxime
(D) Pyridostigmine
(E) Tropicamide

15. A 42-year-old woman experiences prolonged apnea following the administration of succinylcholine. The anesthesiologist attributes the prolonged effects to a hereditary deficiency of which of the following enzymes?

(A) Acetylcholinesterase
(B) Cytochrome P4503A
(C) Glucose-6-phosphate dehydrogenase
(D) Monoamine oxidase
(E) Plasma cholinesterase

16. A 32-year-old woman is given succinylcholine with halothane during a procedure. Shortly after, she begins to experience hypercarbia, hyperthermia, sinus tachycardia, and muscle rigidity. Later, symptoms include hyperthermia. How would dantrolene help manage the patient's condition?

(A) Acts centrally to reduce fever
(B) Blocks Ca^{2+} release from sarcoplasmic reticulum
(C) Induces contraction of skeletal muscle
(D) Increases the rate of succinylcholine metabolism
(E) Inhibits succinylcholine binding to nicotinic receptors

17. A 62-year-old man is started on a new medication for the management of hypertension. The new drug acts at prejunctional α_2-adrenoceptors. Which of the following medications was prescribed?

(A) Clonidine
(B) Dobutamine
(C) Dopamine
(D) Orciprenaline
(E) Phenylephrine

18. Drug X causes an increase in blood pressure and a decrease in heart rate when administered to a patient intravenously. If an antagonist at ganglionic nicotinic receptors is administered first, drug X causes an increase in blood pressure and an increase in heart rate. Which of the following medications acts similarly to drug X?

(A) Curare
(B) Isoproterenol
(C) Noradrenaline
(D) Propranolol
(E) Terbutaline

19. A 26-year-old woman presents to the emergency room with poisoning from an insecticide containing an acetylcholinesterase inhibitor. Which of the following agents would help manage her symptoms?

(A) Atropine
(B) Bethanechol
(C) Physostigmine
(D) Pilocarpine
(E) Propranolol

20. A 75-year-old woman arrives at the emergency room with shortness of breath, fatigue, swollen legs, and a weight gain of 10 lb over a few days. After further examination, she is diagnosed with a heart failure exacerbation. Emergency treatment is best managed with which of the following drugs?

(A) Dobutamine
(B) Isoproterenol
(C) Metaproterenol
(D) Noradrenaline
(E) Phenylephrine

21. A 43-year-old man attends an appointment with his ophthalmologist. The doctor instills eye drops to produce mydriasis and cycloplegia. Which one of the following agents was most likely administered?

(A) Atropine
(B) Carbachol
(C) Phenylephrine
(D) Prazosin
(E) Physostigmine

22. A 71-year-old woman is started on dobutamine for the short-term management of cardiac decompensation. The direct cardiac effects of dobutamine would be blocked by which one of the following agents?

(A) Clonidine
(B) Isoprenaline
(C) Metoprolol
(D) Prazosin
(E) Salbutamol

23. A 23-year-old man presents to the pharmacy with complaints of a bad cold. He asks for a medication that will offer temporary relief of nasal congestion. The pharmacist recommends phenylephrine nasal spray. What is the mechanism of action for this medication?

(A) Blocks β-adrenoceptors for vasodilation
(B) Stimulates α-adrenoceptors for vasoconstriction
(C) Blocks nicotinic cholinoceptors for vasodilation
(D) Stimulates muscarinic cholinoceptors for vasoconstriction
(E) Decreases histamine release.

24. An 82-year-old male has been diagnosed with Alzheimer disease following a history of episodic memory loss for 6 months. A drug suitable for this patient is:

(A) Atropine
(B) Galantamine
(C) Pilocarpine
(D) Physostigmine
(E) Trihexyphenidyl

25. A 36-year-old female has an overactive bladder following an abdominal surgery. Which of the following drugs is likely to be prescribed by the physician?

(A) Benztropine
(B) Hyoscine
(C) Pilocarpine
(D) Terazosin
(E) Tolterodine

26. A 40-year-old patient with bronchial asthma is well controlled with intermittent salbutamol therapy. Which of the following medications is best avoided in this patient?

(A) Adrenaline
(B) Ephedrine
(C) Glycopyrrolate
(D) Prazosin
(E) Timolol

27. A 70-year-old man was prescribed a β-blocker for hypertension that also has action on the α-adrenergic receptors. The drug prescribed is:

(A) Atenolol
(B) Esmolol
(C) Labetalol
(D) Pindolol
(E) Propranolol

28. A 15-year-old boy presents with complaints of blocked nose following common cold. Which of the following drugs can be prescribed to relieve the nasal blockade?

(A) Formoterol
(B) Isoxsuprine
(C) Methamphetamine
(D) Noradrenaline
(E) Oxymetazoline

29. A 38-year-old man has an appointment with his otolaryngologist for the management of recurrent sinusitis. A week after his appointment, the patient undergoes surgical debridement of the scarred sinus tissue, in which a local anesthetic with vasoconstrictive properties was used. Which of the following agents was most likely administered?

(A) Cocaine
(B) Lidocaine
(C) Mepivacaine
(D) Procaine
(E) Tetracaine

Answers and Explanations

1. **The answer is A.** Botulinum toxin blocks calcium-dependent exocytosis of acetylcholine from storage vesicles, producing paralysis. It can be injected around pain fibers that are involved in headaches. Botox enters the nerve endings near the injection site and blocks the release of chemicals involved in pain transmission; this can prevent activation of pain networks in the brain. Common sources of botulinum toxin include canned home goods and, in cases of infant botulism, honey. The condition is life threatening, and urgent care is necessary. Choline acetyltransferase is an enzyme that catalyzes synthesis of acetylcholine from an acetate and choline. Sodium-dependent transport of choline can be blocked by hemicholinium. Enzyme acetylcholinesterase is responsible for catalyzing hydrolysis of acetylcholine. Acetylcholine synapses at the ganglia of many neurons and tissues, and this step is not blocked by botulinum toxin.

2. **The answer is C.** β_2-Agonists, like albuterol, activate the G_s-protein, which results in stimulation of adenylyl cyclase, with subsequent increase in intracellular cAMP. This allows for relaxation of bronchial smooth muscle and decreased airway resistance. Passage of sodium via ligand-gated ion channel is manifested by nicotinic acetylcholine receptors. Activation of G_q-protein resulting in increase in phosphatidylinositol and calcium mobilization refers to the mechanism of action of muscarinic receptor types M_1 and M_3, as well as α_1-adrenoceptors. Activation of G_q-protein resulting in increase in phosphatidylinositol and calcium mobilization refers to mechanism of action of M_2-cholinoceptors and α_2-adrenoceptors. Finally, binding to μ-receptors in the specific areas of the brain describes the action of opioid agents.

3. **The answer is D.** Bethanechol is a type of muscarinic receptor agonist that is used clinically to ameliorate urinary retention. Nicotinic blockers such as trimethaphan are rarely used in clinical practice because of the lack of selectivity. α-Agonists such as adrenaline can be used in the management of acute bronchospasm (anaphylaxis). β_1-Blockers do not have direct effects on bronchial smooth muscle. β_2-Agonists such as albuterol are used for the treatment of asthma.

4. **The answer is D.** An acetylcholinesterase reactivator, like pralidoxime, must be given within 30 minutes of exposure to the insecticide. Due to the effects of "aging" (i.e., strengthening of the alkylphosphoryl–serine bond formed between AChE and organophosphate), it must be administered immediately. Physostigmine is a cholinesterase inhibitor that is occasionally used in atropine or scopolamine poisoning. Propranolol is a β-blocker used for hypertension as well as other indications. Phenylephrine is an α-agonist used for hypotensive emergencies. Pancuronium is a nondepolarizing inhibitor of acetylcholine that is used for muscle paralysis.

5. **The answer is D.** Oxybutynin, tolterodine, trospium, and fesoterodine are indicated for overactive bladder. They work by binding to muscarinic receptors located on the detrusor muscle of the bladder, suppressing involuntary contraction of the muscle. Neuromuscular blockers such as succinylcholine are used for anesthesia. α_1-Antagonists such as terazosin are used for benign prostatic hypertrophy. β_2-Agonists such as terbutaline can be used to suppress premature labor.

6. **The answer is A.** Benztropine, an antimuscarinic agent, is used as an adjunct for the treatment of Parkinson disease. Reserpine is a noradrenaline uptake inhibitor occasionally used for the treatment of hypertension. Doxazocin, an α-blocker, is used for benign prostatic hyperplasia. Timolol is a β-blocker used for glaucoma. Tubocurarine is a neuromuscular blocker used in anesthesia.

7. **The answer is C.** Ipratropium bromide is used extensively for chronic obstructive pulmonary disease (COPD), which is the most likely diagnosis in this case. It acts by antagonizing muscarinic receptors in bronchial smooth muscle, thereby causing bronchodilation. Albuterol is also used for the treatment of COPD; however, it can cause adverse cardiac effects such as tachycardia. Prazosin is an α-blocker used for benign prostatic hypertrophy. Atenolol is a β-blocker used for hypertension. Pseudoephedrine is an α-agonist used for nasal congestion.

8. **The answer is B.** Adrenaline is contraindicated as an anesthetic adjuvant for surgeries involving most facial structures, digits, and the penis, because of the risk of vascular compromise. This agent causes decreased blood loss for most other surgeries because of vasoconstriction. Although local anesthetic agents such as Marcaine or Xylocaine can cause mild local tissue swelling, adrenaline does not; either way, it is not a contraindication for hand surgery. Adrenaline causes elevated blood pressure when administered systemically; however, it has no systemic side effects when administered locally.
9. **The answer is C.** Amphetamine and similar compounds are stimulants used for the treatment of attention-deficit/hyperactivity disorder (ADHD) in which they are thought to act centrally to increase attention span. Currently, there are no approved medications that inhibit reuptake of adrenaline. Blocking the effects of noradrenaline will not alleviate symptoms of ADHD. Direct-acting cholinoceptor agonists are not used in the treatment of ADHD. Serotonin reuptake inhibitors are used for depression and some other conditions.
10. **The answer is D.** α_1-Adrenoceptor agonists, such as terazosin, may cause significant postural hypotension and should be prescribed carefully in the elderly population. Bronchospasm is a possible side effect of β-blockers. β-Blockers can also produce heart failure in some patients. Sedation is common with the use of some agents such as propranolol. Drug abuse can be observed in patients using centrally acting adrenoreceptor agonists such as amphetamine.
11. **The answer is B.** β-Blockers such as atenolol are an important part of management of acute myocardial infarction, along with oxygen, nitroglycerin, and morphine. They reduce sympathetic activity and heart contractility, thereby reducing the oxygen demand. α-Agonists such as phenylephrine are used in the management of hypotension due to shock. Muscarinic agonists such as pilocarpine can be used in the management of glaucoma. Neuromuscular blockers such as atracurium are used in anesthesia. Dopamine agonists are used in the management of Parkinson disease.
12. **The answer is D.** The β-blocker propranolol is a good choice for an antihypertensive medication; however, it is also successfully used for other indications, such as prophylaxis of migraine headaches, situational anxiety, and hyperthyroidism-induced palpitations. The other choices are all acceptable antihypertensive medications, but from this list, only propranolol is used for migraine prophylaxis.
13. **The answer is C.** Prazosin is the only drug listed that blocks postjunctional α_1-adrenoceptors and inhibits adrenaline-mediated vasoconstriction.
14. **The answer is D.** Acetylcholinesterase inhibitors are often considered the first line of treatment of myasthenia gravis due to their safety and ease of use. Pyridostigmine is the usual drug of choice. Neostigmine is also available but not commonly used. Acetylcholinesterase inhibitors provide only symptomatic therapy and may not be sufficient in the management of generalized myasthenia gravis.
15. **The answer is E.** Plasma cholinesterase is responsible for the rapid inactivation of succinylcholine. Reduced plasma cholinesterase synthesis in end-stage hepatic disease or reduced activity following the use of irreversible AChE inhibitors may increase the duration of action.
16. **The answer is B.** The patient most likely has malignant hyperthermia, a rare but potentially fatal complication in susceptible patients that results from a rapid increase in muscle metabolism. Patients who experience this condition are genetically predisposed, with mutations in the skeletal muscle Ca^{2+}-release channel of the sarcoplasmic reticulum (ryanodine receptor, RYR1). Malignant hyperthermia is most likely to occur when succinylcholine is used with the general anesthetic halothane. It can be treated with dantrolene, a skeletal muscle relaxant that binds to the RYR1 receptor to inhibit the release of calcium from the sarcoplasmic reticulum.
17. **The answer is A.** Clonidine acts at prejunctional α_2-adrenoceptors and is used to treat hypertension. Orciprenaline is a selective β_2-adrenoceptor agonist. Dobutamine is a relatively selective β_1-adrenoceptor agonist. Dopamine activates both prejunctional and postjunctional dopamine receptors and also β_1-adrenoceptors. Phenylephrine is an alpha-1 adrenergic receptor agonist which increases blood pressure.

18. The answer is C. In the absence of a nicotinic receptor antagonist, noradrenaline may result in a reflex baroreceptor-mediated increase in vagal activity. The presence of such an agent unmasks the direct stimulant effect of noradrenaline on heart rate.

19. The answer is A. Atropine blocks the effects of increased acetylcholine resulting from cholinesterase inhibition. Physostigmine indirectly activates cholinoceptors; bethanechol and pilocarpine directly activate cholinoceptors. Propranolol is a β-adrenoceptor antagonist.

20. The answer is A. Dobutamine, a relatively selective β_1-adrenoceptor agonist, increases cardiac output and lowers peripheral resistance. Metaproterenol has a relatively more selective action on the respiratory system than on the cardiovascular system. Phenylephrine and noradrenaline increase peripheral resistance. Isoproterenol increases heart rate.

21. The answer is A. Atropine produces both mydriasis and cycloplegia (the inability to accommodate for near vision). Phenylephrine causes mydriasis without cycloplegia. Carbachol causes pupillary constriction. Prazosin is an α-adrenoceptor antagonist.

22. The answer is C. The β_1-adrenoceptor antagonist metoprolol blocks the β_1-adrenoceptor activity of dobutamine.

23. The answer is B. Phenylephrine activates α-adrenoceptors, producing vasoconstriction and resulting in nasal decongestion.

24. The answer is B. Galantamine is a cerebroselective anticholinesterase which increases acetylcholine levels in the brain. Pilocarpine and physostigmine are cholinergic drugs which can act in the brain but are not cerebroselective. Atropine and trihexyphenidyl are anticholinergic and not useful in this case.

25. The answer is E. Tolterodine is an anticholinergic with some selectivity to the urinary bladder. Benztropine and hyoscine are also anticholinergics but not suitable options in this case. Pilocarpine is a cholinergic drug. Terazosin is an α_1-selective adrenergic receptor antagonist useful in the treatment of benign hypertrophy of prostate.

26. The answer is E. All the other drugs listed, except homatropine, are used topically to decrease the intraocular pressure. However, in acute angle-closure glaucoma, which is an ophthalmic emergency, mannitol administered intravenously helps to significantly lower the intraocular pressure and preserve vision. The topical drugs can be used to supplement the action of mannitol and for long-term control of intraocular pressure.

27. The answer is C. Labetalol is a nonselective β-blocker that also blocks the α-adrenergic receptors; the latter contributes to its vasodilatory action. Atenolol and esmolol are β_1-selective blockers (cardioselective). Propranolol is a nonselective β-blocker. Pindolol is also nonselective but with intrinsic sympathomimetic activity.

28. The answer is E. All the listed drugs are sympathomimetics. Oxymetazoline is an α-agonist used as a nasal decongestant. Formoterol is a bronchodilator. Isoxsuprine is used as a uterine relaxant. Methamphetamine is used to treat attention-deficit/hyperactivity disorder. Noradrenaline is used to treat shock.

29. The answer is A. Cocaine is ideal for such surgery because of its topical activity; it does not require the addition of epinephrine, as it has intrinsic vasoconstrictive activity that aids in hemostasis. Similar to cocaine, both procaine and tetracaine are ester-type compounds; however, procaine is not topically active, and tetracaine is used primarily for spinal anesthesia and ophthalmologic procedures. Lidocaine is an amide anesthetic preferred for infiltrative blocks and epidural anesthesia. Mepivacaine is another amide local anesthetic, although not topically active, which, like all such agents, acts by blocking sodium channels.

Chapter 3 Autocoids, Ergots, Anti-inflammatory Agents, and Immunosuppressive Agents

Competencies Addressed: PH1.16

I. HISTAMINE AND ANTIHISTAMINES

A. Histamine

1. ***Biosynthesis and distribution***
   a. Histamine is produced by decarboxylation of the amino acid histidine.
      (1) It is **synthesized** in the **mast cells** and **basophils** of the immune system, in the **enterochromaffin-like cells** (ECL) of the gastric mucosa, and in different neurons of the central nervous system (CNS).
         (a) Mast cells and basophils store histamine in secretory granules. Its release is induced by immunoglobulin E (IgE) fixation to mast cells (sensitization) and subsequent exposure to a specific antigen.
            i. Allergic processes or anaphylaxis can trigger degranulation.
         (b) ECL cells and histaminergic CNS neurons continuously release histamine as required for gastric acid secretion and neurotransmission, respectively.
2. ***Physiologic actions of histamine***
   a. All four receptor subtypes (H_1, H_2, H_3, and H_4) are G protein-coupled receptors (GPRCs).
   b. **Histamine (H_1) receptors**
      (1) These receptors are located in the smooth muscle, vascular endothelium, and brain.
      (2) They are **G_q** coupled and activate the second messengers **inositol triphosphate** (IP_3) and **diacylglycerol** (DAG).
      (3) H_1 receptors commonly mediate inflammatory and allergic reactions. Activation in the:
         (a) **Lungs** can lead to **bronchoconstriction** and asthma-like symptoms
         (b) **Vascular smooth muscle** may cause vasodilation of the postcapillary venule bed, leading to **erythema**
         (c) **Vascular endothelium** can lead to **edema**
         (d) **Peripheral nerves** can lead to **itchiness** and **pain**
   c. **Histamine (H_2) receptors**
      (1) These receptors are commonly found in **parietal cells** and **cardiac muscle**.
      (2) They are **G_s** coupled and lead to the activation of **adenylyl cyclase** and **increased cyclic AMP** (cAMP) production.
      (3) Activation of H_2 receptors
         (a) Increases **gastric acid production**, potentially leading to increased risk of peptic ulcer disease or heartburn
         (b) May also cause minor increases in heart rate
   d. H_3 and H_4 receptors are located in the brain, hematopoietic cells, and thymus.
      (1) There are no approved drugs that act through these receptors.

B. Histamine (H_1)-receptor antagonists

1. **Mechanism of action.** These drugs are **competitive inhibitors** at the **H_1 receptor.**
   a. They **relax histamine-induced contraction of bronchial smooth muscle** and have some use in allergic bronchospasm.
   b. They block the vasodilator action of histamine and inhibit histamine-induced increases in capillary permeability.
   c. They do not affect the release of histamine from secretory granules and are more effective when given prior to histamine release.
2. **First-generation agents**
   a. As a class, these agents are **lipid soluble**, readily cross the **blood–brain barrier**, and have **significant CNS actions**, mediated in large part by their **anticholinergic** activity.
      (1) Their structures are similar to those of antimuscarinic agents.
   b. ***Specific agents*** include chlorpheniramine, dimenhydrinate, **diphenhydramine**, doxylamine, cinnarizine, **meclizine**, and promethazine.
   c. ***Indications.*** These agents are commonly used for management of **allergic symptoms**, **insomnia**, **motion sickness**, and **nausea and vomiting**.
   d. ***Adverse effects*** may include **sedation** (synergistic with alcohol and other depressants; patients should be cautioned not to drive or operate machinery), dizziness, and anticholinergic effects (**dry mouth**, **blurred vision**, and **urine retention**).
3. **Second-generation agents**
   a. These agents are **lipophobic** and were developed to **avoid the sedation** and anticholinergic activity of the first-generation drugs.
   b. ***Specific agents*** include **loratadine**, **cetirizine**, levocetirizine, olopatadine, rupatadine, and **clemastine**. Metabolites of second-generation drugs are sometimes referred to as third-generation agents. These include **fexofenadine** and **desloratadine**.
   c. ***Indications.*** These agents are preferred over first-generation agents for the treatment of **allergic rhinitis and chronic idiopathic urticaria**, as they have similar efficacy and less CNS effects. Topical formulations of olopatadine are used for allergic rhinitis and allergic conjunctivitis.
   d. ***Adverse effects*** are significantly reduced with second-generation agents.

C. Histamine (H_2)-receptor antagonists (see Chapter 8)

1. ***Mechanism of action.*** These agents are **competitive antagonists** at the **H_2 receptor** in the gastric parietal cell; they **inhibit gastric acid secretion.**
2. ***Specific agents*** include **cimetidine**, **ranitidine**, **famotidine**, and **nizatidine**.
3. ***Indications.*** They are used in the treatment of **heartburn** and acid-induced indigestion. They promote the healing of **gastric and duodenal ulcers** and are used in the management of gastroesophageal reflux disease (GERD).
4. ***Adverse effects.*** H_2 antagonists are very safe drugs, and adverse effects are rare.
   a. **Cimetidine** is an **androgen-receptor antagonist** and may cause gynecomastia and impotence.
5. ***Drug interactions.*** **Cimetidine** is also a **potent cytochrome P450 (CYP450) inhibitor** and has the potential for many drug interactions.

D. Mast cell stabilizers (see Chapter 9)

1. ***Mechanism of action.*** Mast cell stabilizers **inhibit the release of histamine** and other autocoids from mast cells.
2. ***Specific agents*** include **cromolyn** and **nedocromil**.
3. ***Indications***
   a. **Cromolyn** is available in several dosage forms:
      (1) Oral solution for systemic mastocytosis
      (2) Oral inhalation (nebulization) for asthma and prevention of bronchospasm
      (3) Nasal spray for **allergic rhinitis**
      (4) Ophthalmic solution for **conjunctivitis** and keratitis
   b. **Nedocromil** is available as an ophthalmic solution for **allergic conjunctivitis**.
4. ***Adverse effects*** include headache, dry mouth, and dry eyes.

II. SEROTONIN AGONISTS AND ANTAGONISTS

A. Serotonin (5-hydroxytryptamine [5-HT])

1. *Biosynthesis and distribution*

a. Serotonin is **synthesized from the amino acid tryptophan** by hydroxylation and decarboxylation, in a two-step pathway.

b. Most serotonin is synthesized in the **ECL cells** of the gastrointestinal (GI) tract. It is also found in platelets and neurons of the CNS and enteric nervous system.

(1) In the CNS, cells in the raphe nuclei of the brainstem predominantly synthesize serotonin.

c. Serotonin is also a precursor of melatonin.

2. *Physiologic actions of serotonin*

a. There are multiple 5-HT-receptor subtypes that mediate a wide variety of physiologic effects.

b. **5-HT$_1$** receptors are **G$_i$** coupled and inhibit adenylyl cyclase and **decrease cAMP**.

(1) These receptors are located in the brain and smooth muscle tissues.

c. **5-HT$_2$** receptors are **G$_q$** coupled and **increase phospholipase C activity**.

(1) These receptors are located in the CNS and mediate hallucinogenic effects.

(2) Stimulation can also cause contraction of vascular and intestinal smooth muscle, increase microcirculation and vascular permeability, and lead to platelet aggregation.

d. **5-HT$_3$** receptors are **ligand-gated sodium and potassium ion channels**.

(1) Stimulation in the area postrema causes **nausea and vomiting**.

(2) Stimulation of peripheral sensory neurons causes **pain**.

e. **5-HT$_4$** receptors are **G$_s$** coupled and stimulate adenylyl cyclase and **increase cAMP**.

(1) In the GI tract, they mediate an increase in **secretion** and **peristalsis**.

B. Serotonin agonists (Table 3.1)

1. **Buspirone** (see Chapter 5)

a. ***Mechanism of action.*** Buspirone is a **5-HT$_{1A}$-selective partial agonist**. It also has weak dopamine receptor antagonism.

b. ***Indication.*** It is used for the management of **generalized anxiety disorder**.

(1) It may take 2 weeks for beneficial effects to appear.

(2) It does not affect GABA receptors; therefore, it is **not addictive** and causes **less sedation** than other antianxiety medications like benzodiazepines.

c. ***Adverse effects*** may include **dizziness**, **drowsiness**, and **nausea**.

2. 5-HT$_{1B/1D}$-receptor agonists (triptans)

a. ***Mechanism of action.*** The triptans are **5-HT$_{1B/1D}$-receptor agonists**. They cause **vasoconstriction** and reduce inflammation in **intracranial blood vessels** and sensory nerves of the trigeminal system.

b. ***Specific agents*** include **sumatriptan**, rizatriptan, eletriptan, **zolmitriptan**, almotriptan, frovatriptan, and **naratriptan**.

(1) All are available as oral agents. Some are also available as nasal sprays and subcutaneous injection.

TABLE 3.1 Examples of Drugs that Interact with Serotonin Receptors

Drug	Receptor	Action
Buspirone	5-HT$_{1a}$ agonist	Anxiolytic
Sumatriptan	5-HT$_{10,1B,1F}$ agonist	Acute migraine
Almotriptan	5-HT$_{10,1B,1F}$ agonist	Acute migraine
Dolasetron	5-HT$_3$ antagonist	Antiemetic
Granisetron	5-HT$_3$ antagonist	Antiemetic
Ondansetron	5-HT$_3$ antagonist	Antiemetic
Alosetron	5-HT$_3$ antagonist	Severe irritable bowel syndrome

5-HT, 5-hydroxytryptamine.

c. ***Indications.*** They are commonly used for the treatment of **acute migraines** and **cluster headaches.**

(1) About 50%–80% of patients report relief from pain within 2 hours.

d. ***Adverse effects*** may include **dizziness, drowsiness,** flushing, and **chest pain.**

(1) They can **cause coronary vasospasm** and are **contraindicated** in patients with **coronary artery disease (CAD)** or **angina.**

3. Treatment of an episode of migraine involves the use of nonsteroidal anti-inflammatory drugs (NSAIDs), antiemetics, triptans, or ergot alkaloids. For prophylaxis in individuals with frequent episodes, the following drugs are used: β-blockers (propranolol), calcium channel blockers (CCBs) (verapamil, flunarizine), antidepressants (amitriptyline, venlafaxine), anticonvulsants (valproate, topiramate, gabapentin), and calcitonin gene–related peptide antagonists (monoclonal antibodies: erenumab, galcanezumab; small-molecule CGRP antagonists: rimegepant, atogepant).

C. Serotonin antagonists (Table 3.1) (see Chapter 8)

1. 5-HT$_3$-receptor antagonists

a. ***Mechanism of action.*** **5-HT$_3$-receptor antagonists** block serotonin centrally in the **chemoreceptor trigger zone** and peripherally on vagal nerve terminals.

b. ***Specific agents*** include **ondansetron, granisetron, dolasetron,** and **palonosetron.**

c. ***Indications.*** They are used for the **prevention of nausea and vomiting** due to **chemotherapy** and **radiation** therapy. They are also used to prevent **postoperative** nausea and vomiting.

d. ***Adverse effects*** include **headache** and **constipation.** They also have the potential to cause **QTc prolongation** and arrhythmias.

e. **Alosetron** is a 5-HT$_3$ antagonist approved for **diarrhea-predominant irritable bowel syndrome** in **women.** It may cause serious GI side effects, including **ischemic colitis** and severe constipation.

D. Other serotonergic agents. Certain antidepressants and second-generation antipsychotic drugs also act on serotonin receptors. More information about these drugs can be found in Chapter 5.

III. ERGOT ALKALOIDS

A. Physiologic effects

1. **Ergots alkaloids** are produced by *Claviceps purpurea,* a fungus that infects grasses and grains, such as rye. They are structurally similar to the neurotransmitters norepinephrine, dopamine, and serotonin.

a. Ergots display **varying degrees** of **agonist or antagonist activity** in three receptor types: **α-adrenoceptors, dopamine receptors,** and **serotonin receptors.**

(1) Many agents exhibit partial agonist activities and thus can cause either stimulatory or inhibitory effects.

(2) The pharmacologic use of ergots is determined by the relative affinity and efficacy of the individual agents for these receptor systems.

B. Indications

1. *Postpartum hemorrhage*

a. **Methylergometrine** is a uterine-selective agent. It produces **sustained contractions** of the **uterine smooth muscle,** which shortens the third stage of labor and decreases blood loss. It should *not* be used to induce labor as it causes contraction of both upper and lower segments of the uterus, potentially causing fetal distress and uterine rupture.

2. *Migraine*

a. **Ergotamine** and **dihydroergotamine** are **5-HT$_{1B/1D}$-receptor agonists,** which result in **vasoconstriction** of intracranial blood vessels.

b. They are most effective when administered in the early (prodromal) stages of migraine to reverse rebound vasodilation.

c. They are frequently combined with caffeine, which may increase absorption.

d. Adverse effects may include GI distress. A more serious side effect is **prolonged vasospasm**.
   (1) Similar to the triptans, they are **contraindicated** in patients with **CAD**.
e. Serious and life-threatening peripheral ischemia may occur when administered with potent cytochrome P450 3A4 (CYP3A4) inhibitors.

3. ***Hyperprolactinemia***
   a. **Bromocriptine** and **cabergoline** (ergot derivatives) are dopaminergic agonists that **inhibit prolactin secretion**.
      (1) **Elevated prolactin** secretion can induce **infertility** and **amenorrhea** in women, **galactorrhea** in men and women, and **gynecomastia** in men.
      (2) **Used to treat acromegaly due to small pituitary tumors.**
   b. **Adverse effects** may include headache, dizziness, and nausea.

IV. EICOSANOIDS

A. Biosynthesis (Fig. 3.1)

1. Eicosanoids are a large group of autocoids with potent effects on many tissues in the body. The eicosanoids include the prostaglandins, thromboxanes (TXA_2), leukotrienes, hydroperoxyeicosatetraenoic acids (HPETEs), and hydroxyeicosatetraenoic acids (HETEs).
2. **Arachidonic acid** is the most common precursor of the eicosanoids. It is formed by two pathways:
   a. **Phospholipase A_2**-mediated production from membrane phospholipids; this pathway is inhibited by glucocorticoids by the action of annexin A1.
   b. **Phospholipase C** in concert with diglyceride lipase can also produce free arachidonate.
3. **Eicosanoids** are synthesized by **two pathways**:
   a. **Cyclooxygenase (COX)** pathway (there are two forms of COX)
      (1) The **COX-1** enzyme is located in the kidney, GI tract, and platelets, as well as many other locations.
         (a) It is expressed at fairly **constant levels** and provides **protective actions** on gastric mucosa, the endothelium, and in the kidney.

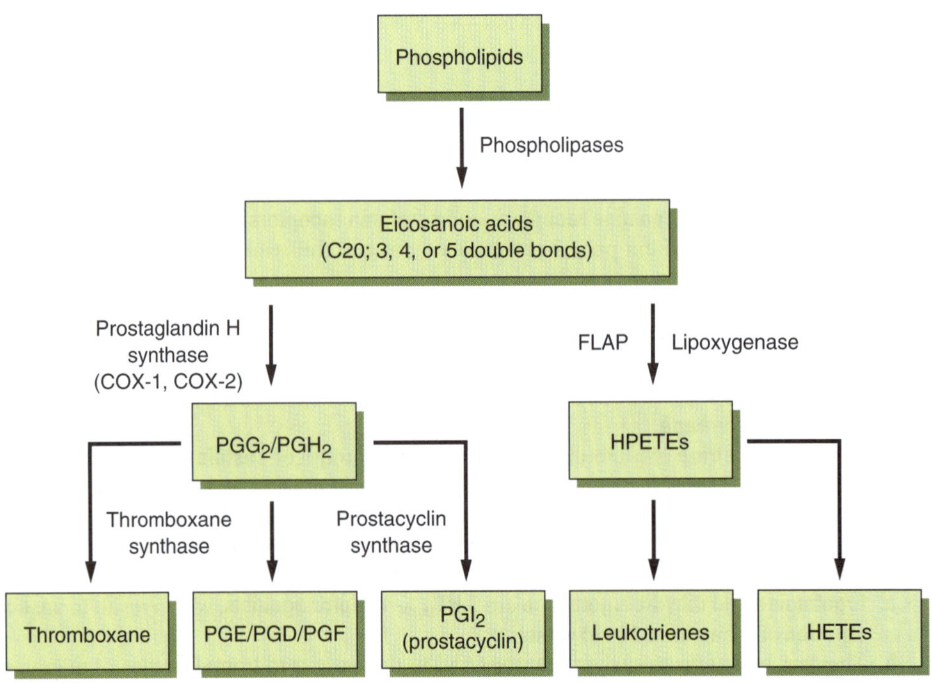

FIGURE 3.1. Biosynthesis of eicosanoids. COX, cyclooxygenase; HETEs, hydroxyeicosatetraenoic acids; HPETEs, hydroperoxyeicosatetraenoic acids; PGD, prostaglandin D; PGE, prostaglandin E; PGF, prostaglandin F.

TABLE 3.2 Location and Physiologic Actions of Eicosanoids

Vascular smooth muscle	TXA_2	Vasoconstriction
	PGI_2 and PGE_2	Vasodilation
Bronchial smooth muscle	PGF	Smooth muscle contraction
	PGE	Smooth muscle relaxation
	TXA_2 and leukotrienes	Potent bronchoconstriction
Uterine smooth muscle	PGE_2 and $PGF_{2\alpha}$	Contraction in pregnant women
Platelets	TXA_2	Enhance aggregation
	PGI_2	Decrease aggregation
Gastrointestinal tract	PGE_2	Increase the rate of longitudinal contraction, increase mucus production, and decrease acid secretion
Inflammation	PGI_2 and PGE_2	Increase blood flow and promote edema formation, enhance leukocyte infiltration
	HETEs and leukotrienes	Cause chemotaxis of neutrophils and eosinophils

HETEs, hydroxyeicosatetraenoic acids; PGE, prostaglandin E; PGF, prostaglandin F; PGI_2, prostacyclin; TXA_2, thromboxane

(2) The **COX-2** enzyme is found in great abundance in connective tissues, in the kidney, and in the endothelium. It is highly **inducible** by numerous factors associated with **inflammation**.

(3) The COX pathway produces **thromboxane** (TXA_2), **prostaglandin E** (PGE), **prostaglandin F** (PGF), **prostaglandin D** (PGD), and **prostacyclin** (PGI_2).

b. Lipoxygenase (LOX) pathway

(1) 5-LOX in association with 5-LOX–activating protein (FLAP) produces 5-HPETEs, which are subsequently converted to 5-HETEs and then to leukotrienes.

4. Eicosanoids are synthesized throughout the body (often tissue specific) and have various physiologic effects (Table 3.2).

a. $\mathbf{PGI_2}$ is synthesized in endothelial and vascular smooth muscle cells.

b. $\mathbf{TXA_2}$ synthesis occurs primarily in platelets.

c. HPETEs, **HETEs**, and the **leukotrienes** are synthesized predominantly in mast cells, white blood cells, airway epithelium, and platelets.

B. Indications

1. *Cervical ripening*

a. Dinoprostone (PGE_2) and gemeprost (PGE_1) reduce the collagen network within the cervix.

(1) They soften the cervix and relax the smooth muscle, allowing dilation and passage of the fetus through the birth canal.

2. *Termination of pregnancy*

a. Carboprost tromethamine ($PGF_{2\alpha}$) and **dinoprostone** stimulate uterine contractions similar to natural labor contractions.

b. Currently, these prostaglandins are combined with **mifepristone**, an antiprogestin, which blocks the effects of progesterone to cause contraction-inducing activity in the myometrium.

c. Dinoprost ($PGF_{2\alpha}$) and gemeprost are also used for abortion.

3. *Maintenance of ductus arteriosus*

a. Alprostadil (PGE_1) will maintain patency of the ductus arteriosus, which may be desirable before surgery.

4. *NSAID-induced ulcers*

a. Misoprostol (PGE_1 analogue) replaces the protective prostaglandins (gastromucosal defense mechanisms) consumed with prostaglandin-inhibiting therapies, such as NSAIDs.

5. *Erectile dysfunction*

a. Alprostadil (PGE_1) can be injected directly into the corpus cavernosum or administered as a transurethral suppository to cause vasodilation and enhance tumescence.

(1) It relaxes trabecular smooth muscle, which allows blood flow to the lacunar spaces of the penis.

6. ***Glaucoma***
   a. **Latanoprost** ($PGF_{2\alpha}$ analogue) reduces intraocular pressure by increasing the uveoscleral outflow of aqueous humor.
7. ***Pulmonary hypertension***
   a. PGI_2 analogues (**epoprostenol**, **treprostinil**, and **iloprost**) are strong vasodilators of pulmonary and systemic vascular beds.

C. **Adverse effects.** Adverse effects of eicosanoids include local pain and irritation, bronchospasm, and GI disturbances, including nausea, vomiting, cramping, and diarrhea.

V. SALICYLATES AND NONSTEROIDAL ANTI-INFLAMMATORY DRUGS

A. Mechanism of action

1. NSAIDs are used to **suppress the symptoms of inflammation** and **relieve pain** (analgesic action) and **fever** (antipyretic action).
2. ***Anti-inflammatory effect***
   a. PGE_2 and PGI_2 are primarily involved with inflammation. They promote blood flow in the inflamed region, enhance edema formation, and enhance leukocyte infiltration.
   b. The anti-inflammatory effect of NSAIDs is due to the **inhibition of COX-1 and COX-2**. COX-2 plays an important role in the inflammatory process, although the effect of its inhibition on inflammation is not fully understood.
      (1) **Aspirin irreversibly inactivates** COX-1 and COX-2 by acetylation of a specific serine residue. This distinguishes it from **other NSAIDs**, which **reversibly inhibit** COX-1 and COX-2.
      (2) **COX-2 selective agents inhibit COX-2 more than COX-1**. They inhibit COX-2-mediated PGI_2 synthesis in the vascular endothelium.
         (a) Rationale for development: Inhibition of COX-2 would **reduce the inflammatory response and pain but not inhibit the cytoprotective action of prostaglandins** in the stomach. Unfortunately, this can cause an increased risk for serious cardiovascular thrombotic events.
   c. NSAIDs have no effect on LOX and therefore do not inhibit the production of leukotrienes.
3. ***Analgesic effect (decrease pain)***
   a. PGE_2 and PGI_2 are the most important prostaglandins involved in pain. They are hyperalgesic in the periphery and centrally. Inhibition of their synthesis is a primary mechanism of NSAID-mediated analgesia.
4. ***Antipyretic effect (decrease fever)***
   a. The antipyretic effect of NSAIDs is believed to be related to inhibition of production of prostaglandins induced by interleukin-1 (IL-1) and interleukin-6 (IL-6) in the hypothalamus and the "resetting" of the thermoregulatory system, leading to vasodilatation and increased heat loss.

B. Indications

1. NSAIDs are first-line drugs used to **arrest inflammation and the accompanying pain** of rheumatic and nonrheumatic diseases.
   a. They are used in **rheumatoid arthritis**, juvenile arthritis, **osteoarthritis**, psoriatic arthritis, **ankylosing spondylitis**, reactive arthritis (Reiter syndrome), **dysmenorrhea**, bursitis, and tendonitis.
      (1) NSAIDs suppress the signs of underlying inflammatory response but may not reverse or resolve the inflammatory process.
   b. Treatment of chronic inflammation requires higher doses than those used for analgesia and antipyresis; consequently, the incidence of adverse drug effects is increased.
   c. In some cases, anti-inflammatory effects may develop only after several weeks of treatment.
2. NSAIDs are used to **alleviate mild to moderate pain**.
   a. They are more effective for pain associated with integumental structures (pain of muscular and vascular origin, arthritis, and bursitis) than for pain associated with the viscera.
   b. They are less effective than opioids.

3. NSAIDs are used to **reduce elevated body temperature**. They have little effect on normal body temperature.
4. **Aspirin reduces** the **formation of thrombi**.
   a. At low doses, aspirin is more selective for COX-1.
   b. This inhibition occurs in the portal circulation in which acetylation of COX-1 results in decrease in TXA_2 synthesis and the effect of this inhibition lasts for the lifetime of the anucleate platelets.
   c. Low-dose aspirin has significantly greater antithrombotic activity than other NSAIDs and is useful in preventing or reducing the risk of myocardial infarction in patients with a history of myocardial infarction, angina, cardiac surgery, and cerebral or peripheral vascular disease.
   d. It is also used prophylactically to reduce recurrent transient ischemia, unstable angina, and the incidence of thrombosis after coronary artery bypass grafts.
5. Salicylic acid is used **topically** to treat **plantar warts**, **fungal infections**, and **corns**.
   a. It causes destruction of keratinocytes and dermal epithelia by the free acid.

C. Adverse effects

1. **Gastrointestinal events**
   a. GI problems are the most common adverse effects. These may include **nausea, vomiting**, diarrhea, constipation, **dyspepsia, epigastric pain**, bleeding, and **ulceration** of the stomach, duodenum, and small intestine.
      (1) Elderly patients and patients with a history of GI bleeding or peptic ulcer disease are at the greatest risk.
      (2) These effects are most likely due to a **decrease in the production and cytoprotective activity of prostaglandins**, as well as a direct chemical effect on gastric cells.
      (3) Substitution of enteric-coated or timed-release preparations, or the use of nonacetylated salicylates, may decrease gastric irritation.
2. **Hypersensitivity (intolerance)** (also known as aspirin or NSAID-exacerbated respiratory disease)
   a. Hypersensitivity is relatively **uncommon**, but can result in rash, bronchospasm, rhinitis, edema, or an anaphylactic reaction with shock, which may be life-threatening.
      (1) The incidence is highest in patients with asthma and nasal polyps.
      (2) **Cross-hypersensitivity** may exist between aspirin and other NSAIDs.
      (3) It is thought that inhibiting the COX pathway diverts arachidonic acid metabolites to the LOX pathway, leading to increased synthesis of cysteinyl leukotrienes (proinflammatory mediators that have an important role in the pathophysiology of asthma).
         (a) Leukotriene-modifying agents, such as a leukotriene-receptor antagonist (montelukast or zafirlukast), can help prevent exacerbations.
3. **Reye syndrome**
   a. Reye syndrome is an illness characterized by **vomiting**, **hepatic disturbances**, and **encephalopathy**.
   b. It occurs when **aspirin** or other **salicylates** are used to **control fever during viral infections** (influenza and chickenpox) in children and adolescents.
   c. **Acetaminophen** is recommended as a substitute for children with **fever of unknown etiology**.
4. **Renal impairment**
   a. NSAIDs may **reduce renal blood flow** and compromise existing renal function.
5. **Cardiovascular events**
   a. Although **aspirin has cardioprotective effects, other NSAIDs** can cause an increased risk of serious cardiovascular thrombotic events, such as **myocardial infarction** or **stroke**.
   b. Compared with other nonselective NSAIDs, **COX-2 selective inhibitors** have an **increased incidence of heart attack and stroke**.
      (1) One potential reason for the increased risk of serious (and potentially fatal) adverse cardiovascular thrombotic events: inhibition of COX-2-mediated production of the vasodilator, PGI_2, by endothelial cells, while not affecting the prothrombotic actions of COX-1 in platelets, increases the chance of blood clots.

6. **Prolonged bleeding time**
   a. **Platelet** adhesion and **aggregation** may be **decreased**. Patients on anticoagulant therapy or with coagulation disorders must be monitored closely.
   b. **Aspirin irreversibly** inhibits platelet COX-1 and COX-2 and, therefore, irreversibly **inhibits TXA_2 production**, suppressing platelet adhesion and aggregation.
7. **Sulfonamide allergy**
   a. **COX-2 selective inhibitors** contain the sulfonamide structure; therefore, caution must be used in those with a sulfa allergy.

D. Drug interactions

1. **Anticoagulants and antiplatelet agents**
   a. The antiplatelet properties of salicylates and NSAIDs in combination with other anticoagulant or antiplatelet agents may increase the risk of bleeding.
2. **Sulfonylureas**
   a. The **hypoglycemic action** of sulfonylureas may be **enhanced** when given with aspirin and certain NSAIDs due to displacement from their binding sites on serum albumin.
3. **Methotrexate**
   a. NSAIDs or salicylates should not be given in combination with methotrexate due to the risk of methotrexate toxicity, which may include **hematologic toxicity** (neutropenia, thrombocytopenia), **nephrotoxicity**, and **hepatotoxicity**.
   b. There are several potential mechanisms for this interaction, including decreased renal excretion of methotrexate.
4. **Alcohol**
   a. Patients should be advised that regularly consuming alcohol when taking NSAIDs or salicylates could increase the **bleeding risk**.
5. **Low-dose aspirin interaction with NSAIDs**
   a. Some nonselective NSAIDs may exhibit greater affinity than aspirin for the active site on the COX enzyme, limiting aspirin's irreversible inhibition of COX.
   b. COX-2 selective NSAIDs have less risk for this potential interaction.

E. Aspirin (acetylsalicylic acid) toxicity

1. Mechanism of toxicity
   a. Salicylate poisoning causes **uncoupling of oxidative phosphorylation** and disruption of normal cellular metabolism; it results in **excess production of lactic acid** and heat.
      (1) Central stimulation of the respiratory center results in hyperventilation, leading to respiratory alkalosis.
      (2) Metabolic acidosis follows, and an increased anion gap results from accumulation of lactate and exertion of bicarbonate.
2. Clinical presentation of **acute intoxication**
   a. Signs and symptoms may include **vomiting**, **hyperpnea**, **tinnitus**, and lethargy.
      (1) Salicylism is the occurrence of dizziness, vertigo, tinnitus, and similar effects that can occur with the use of anti-inflammatory doses of aspirin.
   b. In severe cases, patients may present with seizures, hyperthermia, and pulmonary edema.
   c. Arterial blood gas testing often shows a **mixed respiratory alkalosis and acidosis**.
3. Treatment may involve supportive care, enhanced elimination, and decontamination.

F. NSAID classification (Fig. 3.2)

1. Propionic acid derivatives
   a. **Ibuprofen**, **naproxen**, fenoprofen, flurbiprofen, and ketoprofen
2. Acetic acid derivatives
   a. Indomethacin, sulindac, ketorolac, etodolac, diclofenac, and aceclofenac.
   b. **Diclofenac** is a potent **anti-inflammatory** agent.
   c. **Ketorolac** is a **potent analgesic** and is used for the management of moderately severe acute pain that requires analgesia at the opioid level.

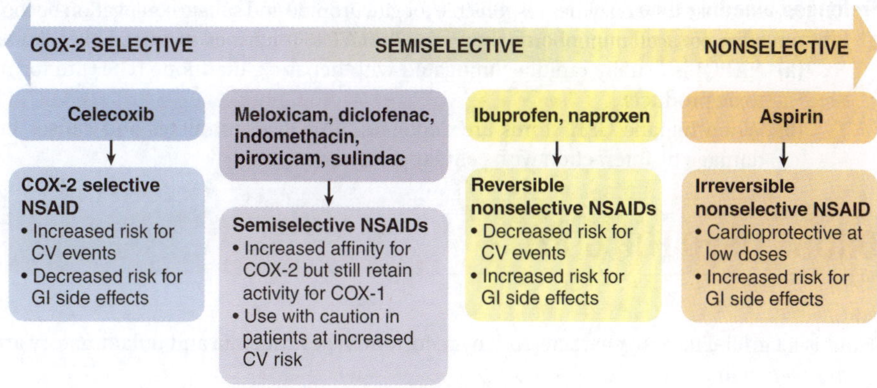

FIGURE 3.2. NSAID selectivity. COX, cyclooxygenase; CV, cardiovascular; GI, gastrointestinal; NSAID, nonsteroidal-anti-inflammatory drug.

(1) Due to the potential for **severe adverse effects**, it is indicated only for **short-term use** (use should not exceed 5 days).

d. **Flurbiprofen ophthalmic solution is used for inhibition of intraoperative miosis and reduction of postoperative inflammatory condition.**

3. Oxicam derivatives
   a. Piroxicam, meloxicam
4. Fenamate derivatives
   a. Mefenamic acid
   b. Used for the symptomatic relief of primary dysmenorrhea
5. Ketones
   a. Nabumetone.
   b. It is a non-acidic NSAID; it is a prodrug converted to an acidic metabolite which inhibits PG synthesis.
6. Sulfonanilide
   a. Nimesulide.
   b. Apart from inhibiting PG synthesis, it has additional actions which contribute to its anti-inflammatory and analgesic effects.
   c. It can cause hepatotoxicity, and it is banned for use in children younger than 12 years.
7. COX-2 selective agents
   a. **Celecoxib, etoricoxib, parecoxib**

G. Paracetamol (acetaminophen; *N*-acetyl-*p*-aminophenol)

1. ***Mechanism of action***
   a. Paracetamol is a **centrally acting analgesic and antipyretic** with **minimal anti-inflammatory** activity.
      (1) High concentrations of peroxides that occur at sites of inflammation reduce its COX inhibitory activity.
   b. It **reduces fever** through the inhibition of prostaglandin synthesis in the CNS and by inhibition of endogenous pyrogens in the **hypothalamus**.
2. ***Indications***
   a. It is used for the management of **mild to moderate pain** and for temporary **reduction of fever.**
3. ***Adverse effects***
   a. Paracetamol may cause a **mild increase in hepatic enzymes.**
   b. Overall, it is very well tolerated and has no clinically relevant effects on the cardiovascular and respiratory systems, platelets, and GI tract.
4. ***Toxicity***
   a. Severe liver damage can occur with overdose due to the accumulation of a minor toxic metabolite, *N*-acetyl-*p*-benzoquinone imine (**NAPQI**).

(1) At toxic doses, the enzymes responsible for glucuronide and sulfate conjugation become saturated; more acetaminophen is shunted to the CYP450 enzymes and metabolized to NAPQI.
  (a) NAPQI is usually rapidly conjugated with hepatic glutathione (GSH) to form nontoxic products.
  (b) When hepatic GSH stores are depleted, NAPQI accumulates and causes hepatic damage by interaction with cellular proteins.

VI. DRUGS USED FOR GOUT

A. Gout

1. Gout is a familial disease characterized by recurrent hyperuricemia and inflammatory arthritis with severe pain.
   a. It is caused by **deposits of uric acid** (the end product of purine metabolism) in joints, cartilage, and the kidney.
   b. Serum urate in excess of 6 mg/dL is associated with gout.
   c. Hyperuricemia can also occur during malignancies (leukemia, lymphoma) or due to certain medications (pyrazinamide, thiazide/loop diuretics, etc.).
2. Acute gout flares are treated with oral glucocorticoids or nonsalicylate NSAIDs, particularly **indomethacin**. In certain patients, **colchicine** may also be used.
3. Chronic gout is treated with a uricosuric agent, **probenecid**, which increases the elimination of uric acid. It can also be treated with **febuxostat** or **allopurinol**, which inhibit uric acid production. Drugs for chronic gout should not be initiated during an acute episode as their action may result in a fluctuation in the serum levels of urate, and thereby its precipitation in the joints/tissue, leading to acute gout flares.
4. Serious gout refractory to the above treatments can be treated with **rasburicase** and **pegloticase**, a recombinant uricase that is administered by infusion.

B. Colchicine

1. ***Mechanism of action.*** The mechanism of action of colchicine is unclear. It is an anti-inflammatory agent that **prevents polymerization of tubulin into microtubules.** It **interferes with migration of neutrophils** to sites associated with mediating gout symptoms.
2. ***Indications.*** Colchicine is used for the **relief of inflammation and pain in acute gouty arthritis**. It is most effective when taken within 24 hours of the acute gout flare.
3. ***Adverse effects*** include **GI distress** (nausea, vomiting, and diarrhea).
   a. Higher doses may result in hepatic impairment and blood dyscrasias.

C. Probenecid

1. ***Mechanism of action.*** Probenecid is an organic acid that **competitively inhibits** the **reabsorption of urate** at the **proximal renal tubule** (uric acid is predominantly reabsorbed at this site, in contrast to penicillin which is predominantly secreted). It increases urinary excretion of uric acid.
2. ***Indications.*** These agents are used for **chronic gout**, often in combination with colchicine.
3. ***Adverse effects.*** Increased urinary concentration of uric acid may result in the formation of urate stones (**urolithiasis**).
4. ***Drug interactions.*** Probenecid inhibits the excretion of other drugs that are actively secreted by renal tubules, including **penicillins**, cephalosporins, and methotrexate. Dose reduction of these drugs may be warranted. Salicylates may diminish the therapeutic effect of probenecid.

D. Allopurinol and febuxostat

1. ***Mechanism of action.*** These agents decrease uric acid production through **xanthine oxidase inhibition**. Xanthine oxidase is the enzyme responsible for the conversion of hypoxanthine to xanthine to uric acid (Fig. 3.3).
2. ***Indications.*** Both agents are used for the **chronic management** of **hyperuricemia** due to **gout**. Allopurinol is also approved for hyperuricemia due to cancer.
3. ***Adverse effects*** may include **skin rash**, **GI distress**, and increased liver enzymes. **Febuxostat** has an increased risk for **heart-related death** compared with allopurinol.

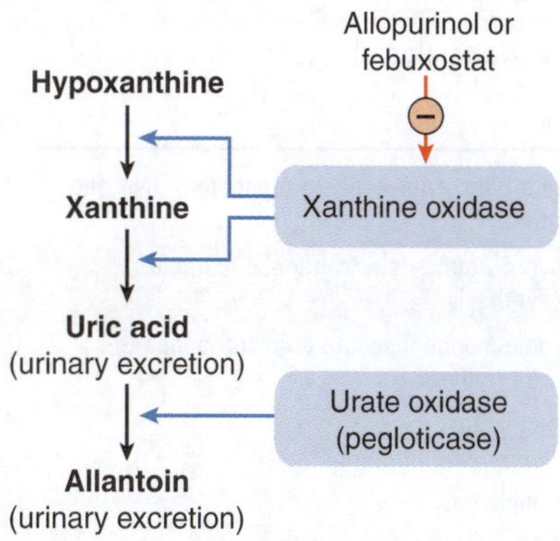

FIGURE 3.3. Mechanism of action of drugs used for gout.

E. Pegloticase

1. ***Mechanism of action.*** Uricase is an enzyme that **converts uric acid to the water-soluble allantoin** for renal excretion; it is absent in humans and high primates. Pegloticase is a pegylated, recombinant form of uricase (Fig. 3.3).
2. ***Indications.*** Pegloticase can reduce serum urate in a matter of hours. It is approved for use in patients with **gout** who have been **unresponsive to other drug therapies**.
3. ***Adverse effects.*** Pegloticase has the potential to cause serious side effects such as **anaphylaxis** and infusion reactions.
4. Rasburicase is also a recombinant uricase enzyme. It is approved for hyperuricemia associated with malignancy.

VII. ANTIRHEUMATOID AND IMMUNOSUPPRESSIVE DRUGS

A. Use of immunosuppressive agents

1. Immunosuppressive agents are used to treat syndromes or diseases that reflect **imbalances in the immune system**, including **rheumatoid arthritis**, **systemic lupus erythematosus**, inflammatory bowel disease, chronic active hepatitis, Goodpasture syndrome, autoimmune hemolytic anemia, and organ transplantation.
2. Many immunosuppressive agents used for the management of rheumatoid arthritis are considered disease-modifying antirheumatic drugs (DMARDs).
   a. These drugs decrease pain and inflammation but are also used to **reduce or prevent joint damage** and to **preserve the structure and function of the joints.**
   b. They are not designed for immediate symptom relief, as they may take **several weeks or months for full effect during which NSAIDs and/or glucocorticoids may be used for symptomatic relief.**
   c. Methotrexate (see Chapter 12) is the recommended initial drug for rheumatoid arthritis. Other drugs include sulfasalazine, hydroxychloroquine, leflunomide, or tumor necrosis factor (TNF) inhibitor.
3. Suppression of the immune system increases the risk of **opportunistic** viral, bacterial, and fungal **infections**, as well as increased risk of **malignancy**.

B. Conventional (nonbiologic) agents (Table 3.3)

1. **Azathioprine** (a derivative of mercaptopurine)
   a. ***Mechanism of action.*** The exact mechanism of azathioprine's immunosuppressive action is unknown.
      (1) It is a cytotoxic agent that **suppresses T-cell activity** to a greater degree than B-cell activity.
      (2) Its metabolites are **incorporated into replicating DNA to halt replication.**
      (3) They also **block pathways necessary for purine synthesis.**
      (4) It is metabolized to mercaptopurine, which is also immunosuppressive.

TABLE 3.3 Conventional (Nonbiologic) Agents

Drug	Mechanism	Adverse Effects
Azathioprine	Metabolites are incorporated into replicating DNA and halt replication	Nausea, vomiting, leukopenia
Leflunomide	Inhibits dihydroorotate dehydrogenase to inhibit pyrimidine synthesis	Gastrointestinal distress, neutropenia
Mycophenolate mofetil	Inhibits inosine monophosphate dehydrogenase to inhibit purine synthesis	Gastrointestinal distress, neutropenia
Cyclosporine	Calcineurin inhibitor	Nephrotoxicity, hypertension, gingival hyperplasia
Tacrolimus	Calcineurin inhibitor	Nephrotoxicity, hypertension
Sirolimus	Inhibits mTOR activity	Impaired wound healing, increased cholesterol, anemia

mTOR, mammalian target of rapamycin.

b. ***Indications*** include rejection prophylaxis for renal transplantation and rheumatoid arthritis. It is used off-label for other solid-organ transplants.

c. ***Adverse effects*** include nausea and vomiting and **leukopenia**.

d. ***Drug interactions.*** Azathioprine is metabolized to an inactive metabolite by **xanthine oxidase. Dose reduction** is necessary when azathioprine is administered with xanthine oxidase inhibitors such as **allopurinol** or **febuxostat**.

2. **Leflunomide** and **mycophenolate mofetil**

a. ***Mechanism of action.*** Both leflunomide and mycophenolate mofetil are prodrugs that inhibit T- and B-cell responses through the inhibition of nucleotide synthesis (Fig. 3.4).

(1) **Leflunomide inhibits dihydroorotate dehydrogenase** (DHODH), which inhibits **pyrimidine synthesis**.

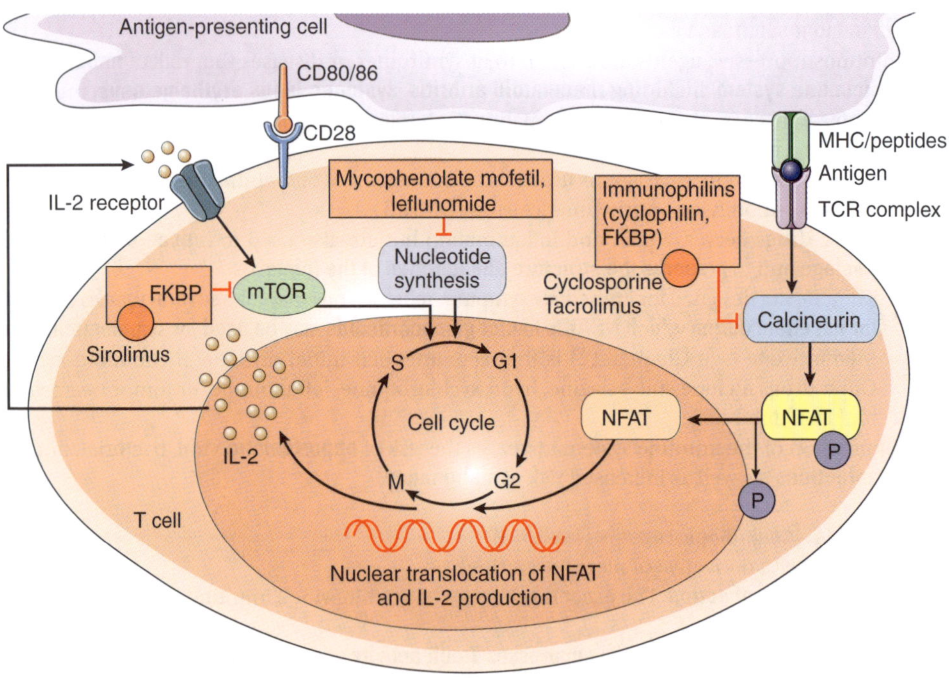

FIGURE 3.4. Mechanism of action of conventional (nonbiologic) agents. FKBP, FK binding protein; IL-2, interleukin-2; MHC, major histocompatibility complex; mTOR, mammalian (mechanistic) target of rapamycin; NFAT, nuclear factor of activated T cells; P, phosphate; TCR, T-cell receptor.

(2) **Mycophenolate mofetil inhibits inosine monophosphate dehydrogenase** (IMPDH) to inhibit **purine synthesis.**

b. ***Indications*** include rheumatoid arthritis for leflunomide and solid-organ transplant for mycophenolate mofetil.

a. ***Adverse effects*** include **GI distress, bone marrow suppression, increased susceptibility to infections**, and increased risk of secondary malignancies. Leflunomide can also cause **hepatotoxicity.**

3. **Cyclosporine** and **tacrolimus**

a. ***Mechanism of action.*** Both agents are **calcineurin inhibitors**; they bind to their respective immunophilins and inhibit the phosphatase action of calcineurin, which is then unable to dephosphorylate nuclear factor of activated T cells (NFAT) (Fig. 3.4).

(1) They prevent translocation of NFAT to the nucleus and inhibit production of interleukin-2 (IL-2) and IL-2-induced activation of resting T lymphocytes.

b. ***Indications*** include psoriasis, rheumatoid arthritis, solid-organ transplant, and graft-versus-host disease. Ophthalmic emulsions of cyclosporine can be used to increase tear production.

(1) Monitoring periodic trough levels is recommended during therapy.

c. ***Adverse effects*** may include **nephrotoxicity**, **hypertension**, headache, tremor, hirsutism, and hyperkalemia. Cyclosporine can also cause **gingival hyperplasia.**

d. ***Drug interactions.*** Both agents are major **substrates of CYP3A4** enzymes. Dose reductions are required when used in combination with strong CYP3A4 inhibitors.

4. **Sirolimus**

a. ***Mechanism of action.*** Sirolimus (also called rapamycin) **inhibits** mammalian target of rapamycin (**mTOR**), which is an important component of several signaling pathways (Fig. 3.4).

(1) Inhibition of mTOR interferes with protein biosynthesis and delays the G_1–S transition, which **blocks** the second phase of **T-cell activation**.

(2) B-cell differentiation is also inhibited.

b. ***Indications*** include rejection prophylaxis for renal transplantation. It is used off-label for other solid-organ transplants and graft-versus-host disease.

(1) Monitoring sirolimus levels in all patients is recommended.

c. ***Adverse effects*** include **anemia** and thrombocytopenia, **impaired wound healing**, increased risk of infection, and metabolic effects, including **increased cholesterol** and triglycerides.

C. Biologic agents (Table 3.4)

1. Biologic agents are genetically engineered proteins that target specific parts of the immune system to block immune response.

TABLE 3.4 Biologic Agents

Drug	Mechanism	Adverse Effects
Adalimumab	TNF inhibitors	In general, biologic agents are known to cause an increased risk of serious infections and malignancy
Infliximab		
Certolizumab		
Golimumab		
Etanercept		
Anakinra	IL-1-receptor antagonist	
Basiliximab	IL-2-receptor antagonist	
Tocilizumab	IL-6-receptor antagonist	
Abatacept	Selective T-cell costimulation blocker	
Antithymocyte globulin	Polyclonal antibody directed against T lymphocytes	
Natalizumab	Anti-integrin	
Rituximab	Anti-CD20	
Tofacitinib	Janus kinase inhibitor	

IL-1, interleukin-1; IL-2, interleukin-2; IL-6, interleukin-6.

2. **Infliximab**, **adalimumab**, **certolizumab**, **golimumab**, and **etanercept**
   a. ***TNF-α*** plays an important causative role in rheumatoid arthritis. It is responsible for inducing IL-1, IL-6, and other cytokines that further the disease.
   b. ***Mechanism of action.*** All agents interfere with endogenous TNF-α activity by **blocking TNF-α** and blocking its interaction with cell surface receptors. Most are monoclonal antibodies. Etanercept is a recombinant soluble TNF-receptor dimer.
   c. ***Indications*** for these agents include rheumatoid arthritis, plaque psoriasis, and many other autoimmune diseases.
   d. ***Adverse effects.*** Injection site infections are common. More serious adverse effects include an increased risk of **tuberculosis** and **lymphoma**.
3. **Anakinra**
   a. ***Mechanism of action.*** Anakinra is a human recombinant **IL-1-receptor antagonist**. It blocks the biologic activity of IL-1 by competitively inhibiting IL-1 binding to the IL-1 receptor to decrease the immune response in inflammatory diseases.
   b. ***Indications*** include rheumatoid arthritis.
   c. ***Adverse effects*** include injection site reactions and increased risk of **infections**.
4. **Abatacept**
   a. ***Mechanism of action.*** T-cell activation requires costimulation by an antigen-presenting cell. Abatacept **blocks the costimulatory signal**. It is a fusion protein consisting of a portion of human CTLA4 and a fragment of the Fc domain of human IgG1. Abatacept mimics endogenous CTLA4 and competes with CD28 for CD80 and CD86 binding. This prevents complete T-cell activation, reduces T-cell proliferation, and reduces plasma cytokine levels (Fig. 3.5).
   b. ***Indications.*** Abatacept is approved for use in rheumatoid arthritis.
   c. ***Adverse effects.*** The most common side effect with its use is **infection**.
5. **Tocilizumab**
   a. ***Mechanism of action.*** Tocilizumab is a **monoclonal antibody against the human IL-6 receptor**. IL-6 is a potent inflammatory cytokine involved in the pathogenesis of several autoimmune diseases including rheumatoid arthritis, multiple myeloma, and prostate cancer.
   b. ***Indications.*** Tocilizumab is approved for use in rheumatoid arthritis.
   c. ***Adverse effects*** may include increased **cholesterol, increased risk of serious infections, injection site reactions,** nasopharyngitis, and hypertension.

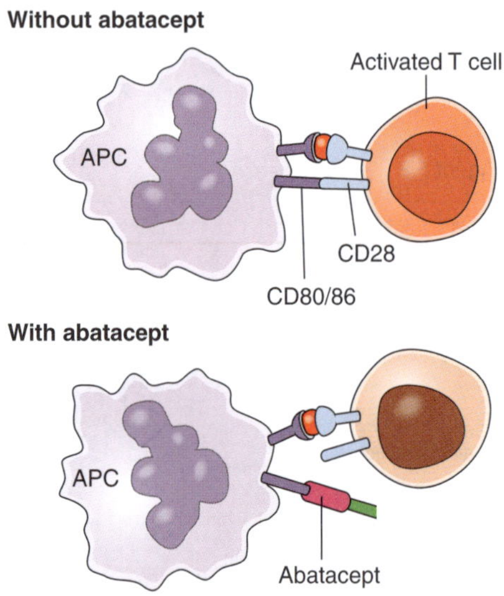

FIGURE 3.5. Mechanism of action of abatacept. APC, antigen-presenting cell.

6. **Tofacitinib**
   a. ***Mechanism of action.*** Tofacitinib selectively inhibits Janus kinases (JAK) and prevents the phosphorylation and activation of signal transducers and activators of transcription (STAT). It **interrupts the JAK–STAT signaling pathway** that normally influences cellular processes of hematopoiesis and immune cell function. It prevents cytokine- or growth factor–mediated gene expression and intracellular activity of immune cells.
   b. ***Indications.*** It is currently approved for rheumatoid arthritis and psoriatic arthritis.
   c. ***Adverse effects*** may include increased **cholesterol, increased risk of serious infections, injection site reactions**, nasopharyngitis, increased risk of lymphoma, and other malignancies.
7. **Rituximab**
   a. ***Mechanism of action.*** Rituximab is a **monoclonal antibody directed against CD20** on the surface of **B lymphocytes**. It binds to the surface of B cells and results in their destruction.
   b. ***Indications.*** It is currently approved for the management of rheumatoid arthritis and CD20-positive leukemia and lymphoma.
      (1) Rituximab, in combination with methotrexate, is approved for use in rheumatoid arthritis unresponsive to other therapies. It is also approved for treating refractory or large B-cell non-Hodgkin lymphoma.
   c. ***Adverse effects.*** Potentially severe adverse effects include **infusion reactions, mucocutaneous reactions**, and **hepatitis B reactivation**.
8. **Natalizumab**
   a. ***Mechanism of action.*** Natalizumab is a **monoclonal antibody against the α4 subunit of integrin** molecules. It prevents transmigration of leukocytes across the endothelium into the inflamed tissue.
   b. ***Indications*** include multiple sclerosis and Crohn disease.
   c. ***Adverse effects.*** It has been associated with the development of **progressive multifocal leukoencephalopathy** (PML), a neurologic disorder caused by an opportunistic viral infection that may lead to disability or death. Other adverse effects include increased risk of infections and depression.
9. **Antithymocyte globulin** (ATG)
   a. ***Mechanism of action.*** ATG is a purified immune globulin produced from hyperimmune serum of horses immunized with human thymocytes. It is involved with the **altered function or elimination of T lymphocytes**, resulting in decreased T-cell-mediated immune response. It can also directly promote the growth of hematopoietic stem cells.
   b. ***Indications.*** It is currently approved for aplastic anemia. It is also used for acute graft-versus-host disease.
   c. ***Adverse effects*** may include **serum sickness** and anaphylaxis.
      (1) Serum sickness is a type III hypersensitivity reaction due to administration of a foreign protein or serum. Symptoms may include fever, malaise, rash, arthralgias, and GI distress.
10. **Basiliximab**
   a. ***Mechanism of action.*** Basiliximab is a **monoclonal antibody that is an IL-2-receptor antagonist**. It inhibits IL-2-mediated activation of lymphocytes.
   b. ***Indications.*** It is used to prevent acute rejection in renal transplant.
   c. ***Adverse effects*** may include **hypertension**, GI distress, and increased risk of infection, including **urinary tract infections** and **viral infections**.

D. **Other immunosuppressive agents.** Other immunosuppressive agents are discussed in more detail in Chapter 8 on Drugs Acting on the Gastrointestinal Tract (sulfasalazine), Chapter 11 on Drugs Used in Treatment of Infectious Diseases (hydroxychloroquine), and Chapter 12 on Cancer Chemotherapy (methotrexate, cyclophosphamide, and thalidomide).

DRUG SUMMARY TABLE

Histamine H_1-Receptor Antagonists
Brompheniramine
Cetirizine
Chlorpheniramine
Clemastine
Cyproheptadine
Desloratadine
Dimenhydrinate
Diphenhydramine
Doxylamine
Fexofenadine
Levocetirizine
Loratadine
Meclizine
Promethazine

Histamine H_2-Receptor Antagonists
Cimetidine
Famotidine
Nizatidine
Ranitidine

Chromones
Cromolyn
Nedocromil

Ergots
Bromocriptine
Dihydroergotamine
Ergotamine
Methylergonovine

Serotonin-Receptor Agonists
Almotriptan
Buspirone
Eletriptan
Frovatriptan
Naratriptan
Rizatriptan
Trazodone
Sumatriptan
Zolmitriptan

Serotonin-Receptor Antagonists
Cyproheptadine
Dolasetron
Granisetron
Ondansetron
Palonosetron

Eicosanoids
Alprostadil
Carboprost tromethamine
Dinoprostone
Epoprostenol
Iloprost
Latanoprost
Misoprostol
Treprostinil

NSAIDs
Aspirin
Celecoxib
Diclofenac
Etodolac
Fenoprofen
Flurbiprofen
Ibuprofen
Indomethacin
Ketoprofen
Ketorolac
Meclofenamate
Mefenamic acid
Nabumetone
Naproxen
Piroxicam
Sulindac
Tolmetin

Nonopioid Analgesic
Paracetamol

Gold Salts
Auranofin
Gold sodium thiomalate

Antigout Drugs
Allopurinol
Colchicine
Febuxostat
Pegloticase
Probenecid

Immunosuppressive Drugs (including DMARDs and Biologic Agents)
Abatacept
Adalimumab
Anakinra
Antithymocyte globulin
Azathioprine
Basiliximab
Cyclophosphamide
Cyclosporine
Etanercept
Hydroxychloroquine
Infliximab
Methotrexate
Mycophenolate Mofetil
Mycophenolate Sodium
Sirolimus
Tacrolimus
Thalidomide

Review Test

Directions: Select the best answer for each question.

1. A 32-year-old man presents to his primary care physician with complaints of burning and watery eyes and constant sneezing. He experiences these symptoms each spring for about 1 month. The patient is a long-haul truck driver and is concerned about potential side effects of any new medications. Which of the following drugs would be most appropriate to treat this patient?

(A) Cimetidine
(B) Dimenhydrinate
(C) Fexofenadine
(D) Promethazine
(E) Scopolamine

2. A 30-year-old man is diagnosed with stage III testicular cancer. He undergoes a radical inguinal orchiectomy and followed by chemotherapy with etoposide and cisplatin. Which of the following medications would help manage chemotherapy-induced nausea and vomiting?

(A) Diphenhydramine
(B) Ondansetron
(C) Ranitidine
(D) Sumatriptan
(E) Buspirone

3. A 24-year-old woman has a history of migraine headaches with accompanying aura. During her last attack, ergotamine was much less effective; therefore, her neurologist uses an alternative to treat her current attack. Agonist activity at which of the following receptors would be the best target for the new treatment?

(A) α-Adrenoreceptors
(B) Histamine H_1
(C) Prostaglandin FP
(D) Serotonin 5-HT_{1B}
(E) Muscarinic M_3

4. A 79-year-old woman is admitted to the hospital with acute renal failure. She has a history of rheumatoid arthritis managed with methotrexate but stated that the pain in her hands was much worse over the last week; therefore, she took additional pain medication. Which of the following drugs is most likely responsible for the adverse renal effect?

(A) Paracetamol
(B) Colchicine
(C) Ibuprofen
(D) Prednisone
(E) Allopurinol

5. A neonate is diagnosed with an atrial septal defect of congenital origin. It will require surgical repair, and adequate systemic perfusion requires that the patency of the ductus arteriosus be maintained. Which of the following agents would be the best to accomplish this goal?

(A) Alprostadil
(B) Celecoxib
(C) Indomethacin
(D) Treprostinil
(E) Travoprost

6. A 65-year-old man presents to his primary care physician with complaints of severe pain and redness in his left big toe. Blood work revealed a uric acid level of 8.3 mg/dL (normal: 3.4–7 mg/dL). Few weeks after controlling the acute episode, his physician started him on a new medication for the chronic management of this condition. What is the mechanism of action of this new medication?

(A) Blocks the metabolism of xanthine to uric acid
(B) Catalyzes the oxidation of uric acid to xanthine
(C) Decreases the oxidation of allantoin to uric acid
(D) Inhibits the function of urate oxidase
(E) Stimulates the function of xanthine oxidase

7. A 35-year-old man presents to his doctor with complaints of epigastric pain. The patient has a history of a lower back injury in which his pain is managed with diclofenac. He is diagnosed with gastritis. Which of the following best explains the reason for the patient's symptoms?

(A) Inhibition of phospholipase A_2
(B) Inhibition of COX-1 production of PGE_2
(C) Inhibition of COX-2 production of PGI_2
(D) Inhibition of COX-2 production of TXA_2
(E) Inhibition of 5-lipoxygenase production of LTA_4

8. A 30-year-old primipara with no comorbidities has excessive bleeding following labor. She is administered an intramuscular injection of a drug which promptly controlled the bleeding. Which of the following drugs was likely administered?

(A) Almotriptan
(B) Bromocriptine
(C) Mefenamic acid
(D) Methylergometrine
(E) Prednisolone

9. A 35-year-old woman presents to her physician with a chief complaint of headaches and occasional vomiting for several months. She also complains of milky discharge from her breasts and a lack of menstruation for the last 3 months. Further testing reveals a large pituitary adenoma. Which is the mechanism of action for the medication that would treat this condition?

(A) 5-HT_3 antagonist
(B) α-Adrenoceptor agonist
(C) Dopamine agonist
(D) IL-1 antagonist
(E) H_1 antagonist

10. A 24-year-old woman, who is 42 weeks pregnant, is admitted to the hospital for induction of labor. A fetal heart monitor shows that the fetus is in no acute distress. Sterile examination reveals that she is minimally dilated without significant effacement. Due to an unfavorable cervix, she is given an agent for cervical ripening prior to oxytocin administration. What medication was most likely given?

(A) Carboprost
(B) Dinoprostone
(C) Epoprostenol
(D) Latanoprost
(E) Treprostinil

11. A 7-year-old girl is diagnosed with chickenpox, in which her symptoms included a red, itchy rash and fever. Two days later, she is taken to the emergency room due to persistent vomiting and mental status changes. Her blood work reveals elevated liver enzymes. Which of the following medications, when given at an appropriate dose, may cause this patient presentation?

(A) Paracetamol
(B) Aspirin
(C) Celecoxib
(D) Ibuprofen
(E) Naproxen

12. A 24-year-old man is admitted to the hospital after a kidney transplant. He is placed on appropriate immunosuppression to prevent rejection. About 48 hours after starting the new treatment regimen, the patient complains of a headache and tremors. His blood pressure is 140/82 mm Hg. What medication most likely caused this patient presentation?

(A) Azithromycin
(B) Cyclosporine
(C) Leflunomide
(D) Mycophenolate mofetil
(E) Sirolimus

13. A 42-year-old woman is started on a new medication for the management of rheumatoid arthritis. Her rheumatologist explains the possible adverse effects and schedules her return visit to assess lipid parameters 6 weeks following initiation. Which of the following medications was most likely prescribed?

(A) Anakinra
(B) Abatacept
(C) Etanercept
(D) Rituximab
(E) Tocilizumab

Answers and Explanations

1. **The answer is C.** Fexofenadine is a potent histamine H_1-receptor antagonist; its poor central nervous system (CNS) penetration reduces sedative effects. Dimenhydrinate and promethazine are first-generation H_1-receptor antagonists used for nausea and vomiting; adverse effects include sedation. Cimetidine is a histamine H_2-receptor antagonist. Scopolamine is an anticholinergic used for motion sickness; drowsiness is an adverse effect.
2. **The answer is B.** Ondansetron is a 5-HT_3-receptor antagonist approved for the prevention of chemotherapy-induced nausea and vomiting. Diphenhydramine, buspirone, sumatriptan, and ranitidine are not used for the management of nausea and vomiting.
3. **The answer is D.** The triptans are effective against acute migraine attacks; they act as agonists at serotonin 5-HT_{1B} and 5-HT_{1D} receptors. Agonists at α-adrenergic receptors, like epinephrine, cause vasoconstriction but are not effective for migraines. Antihistamines and agents that interfere with the prostaglandin FP receptor or muscarinic receptor would not be effective either.
4. **The answer is C.** NSAIDs, such as ibuprofen, are associated with renal toxicity. When taken with methotrexate, the risk of nephrotoxicity increases due to a drug–drug interaction. Prednisone is effective in alleviating the inflammation in rheumatoid arthritis but is not associated with adverse renal effects. Colchicine and allopurinol are used to treat gout, not rheumatoid arthritis.
5. **The answer is A.** E-series prostaglandins, such as alprostadil, are responsible for maintenance of the ductus. Inhibitors of prostaglandin biosynthesis, such as indomethacin and celecoxib, cause closure of the ductus. Treprostinil and travoprost are prostaglandin analogues used to treat pulmonary arterial hypertension and glaucoma, respectively.
6. **The answer is A.** The patient most likely has gout, which commonly presents with swelling, inflammation, and redness at the base of the great toe. High uric acid levels are also common. Allopurinol and febuxostat are xanthine oxidase inhibitors that prevent the metabolism of hypoxanthine and xanthine to uric acid. They can be used for the chronic management of gout.
7. **The answer is B.** Inhibition of COX-1 (by diclofenac) in gastric epithelial cells depresses mucosal cytoprotective prostaglandins, especially PGE_2. This can lead to GI symptoms, including gastritis or gastric ulcers. Inhibition of prostaglandin synthesis by COX-2 induced at sites of inflammation does not affect the action of the constitutively active housekeeping COX-1 isozyme found in the GI tract. Although diclofenac is considered a preferentially selective COX-2 inhibitor, peptic ulcer is still an important adverse effect. Diclofenac does not inhibit 5-lipoxgenase or phospholipase A_2.
8. **The answer is D.** Methylergometrine is a uterine-selective ergot used for the prevention or treatment of postpartum hemorrhage. Almotriptan is used to treat migraine. Bromocriptine is an ergot derivative used to treat hyperprolactinemia and acromegaly. Mefenamic acid, an NSAID used to treat dysmenorrhea, and prednisolone are not indicated for the treatment of postpartum hemorrhage.
9. **The answer is C.** Elevated prolactin secretion can induce galactorrhea, amenorrhea, and infertility in women. Dopaminergic agonists, such as bromocriptine and cabergoline, inhibit prolactin secretion. They can be used to treat hyperprolactinemia, as with pituitary adenomas, or for suppression of normal lactation.
10. **The answer is B.** Dinoprostone (PGE_2) reduces the collagen network within the cervix and is used for cervical ripening. Carboprost ($PGF_{2\alpha}$) stimulates uterine contractions similar to natural labor contractions and is currently approved for termination of pregnancy. Latanoprost (PGF_2 analogue) reduces intraocular pressure by increasing the outflow of aqueous humor and is used for glaucoma. Epoprostenol and treprostinil (PGI_2 analogues) are strong vasodilators used for pulmonary hypertension.

11. **The answer is B.** The patient has Reye syndrome, a condition characterized by hepatic encephalopathy and liver steatosis. Symptoms may include mental status changes and increased liver enzymes. It can occur in young children given aspirin during a febrile viral infection (such as chickenpox).

12. **The answer is B.** Calcineurin inhibitors, such as cyclosporine and tacrolimus, can cause headache, tremor, and hypertension. These adverse effects may be due to increased drug levels; therefore, decreasing the drug dose may help alleviate symptoms. The other medications listed do not generally cause this side effect profile.

13. **The answer is E.** Tocilizumab, an IL-6-receptor antagonist, is associated with increases in lipid parameters, including total cholesterol. Lipid parameters should be assessed about 4–8 weeks after initiation and about every 24 weeks thereafter.

Chapter 4

Drugs Acting on the Central Nervous System

Competencies Addressed: PH1.18–PH1.22

I. SEDATIVE–HYPNOTIC DRUGS

Sedatives are drugs which aim to reduce anxiety and are commonly used in various anxiety disorders. Hypnotics are drugs which induce or maintain sleep and hence are primarily used in insomnia.

A. Benzodiazepines

1. *General properties*

a. Benzodiazepines (BZs) offer significant advantages over barbiturates and hence have replaced them as sedative-hypnotics.

(1) BZs have a **great margin of safety.** They are safer and have fewer side effects. Abuse and dependence liability is less when compared with barbiturates.

(2) They exhibit a **ceiling effect,** whereas barbiturates exhibit a linear dose effect, which can progress from sedation to respiratory depression, coma, and death (Fig. 4.1).

b. Most BZs have qualitatively similar therapeutic actions but differ in their relative lipid solubility, biotransformation, and elimination half-life.

c. They are classified as short, intermediate, or long acting.

(1) Shorter-acting agents are generally more useful for insomnia because they cause less hangover on awakening. They can be used in patients with difficulty in onset of sleep.

(2) Longer-acting BZs are generally more useful for anxiety. They are also useful for chronic insomnia.

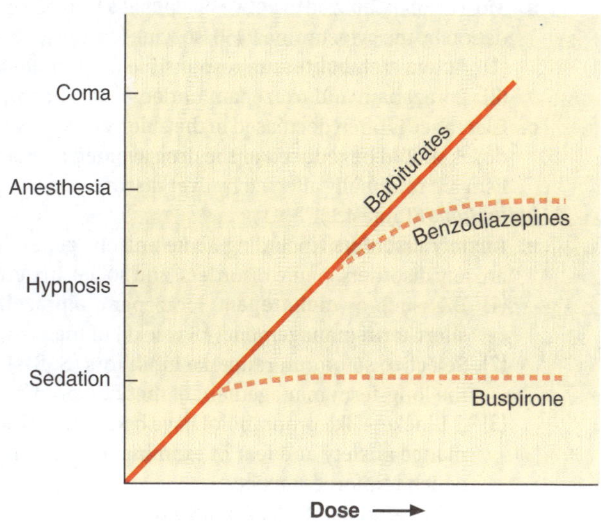

FIGURE 4.1. Theoretical dose–response relationships for sedative–hypnotic drugs and buspirone.

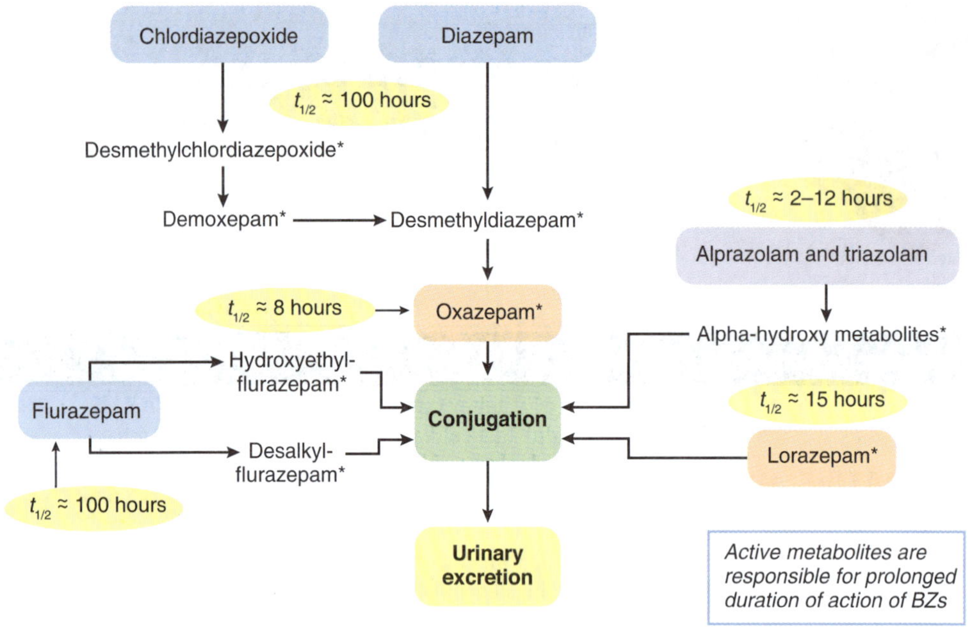

FIGURE 4.2. Biotransformation of benzodiazepines (BZs). Most BZs are metabolized by the liver to active compounds (except lorazepam, temazepam, oxazepam). (*) Active metabolite.

2. *Mechanism of action* (see Fig. 4.2)
- **a.** BZs are γ-aminobutyric acid ($GABA_A$)-receptor agonists. They bind to an alpha/gamma subunit interface on $GABA_A$-activated chloride channels.
  - **(1)** They **increase the frequency of $GABA_A$-receptor opening**.
    - **(a)** This results in increased chloride conductance and hyperpolarization, and leads to inhibition of synaptic transmission in the central nervous system (CNS), as well as inhibition of neuronal depolarization by excitatory neurotransmitters.
  - **(2)** These drugs have **no action in the absence of GABA** (only GABA facilitatory actions).
- **b.** The **alpha-1 subunit** mediates the **sedative, hypnotic, and amnesic** properties.
- **c.** The **alpha-2 subunit** mediates the **anxiolytic, myorelaxant**, and **anticonvulsant** properties.

3. *Pharmacologic properties*
- **a.** BZs that are **highly lipid soluble**, such as midazolam, triazolam, and diazepam, have a **more rapid onset** of action.
- **b.** Most are **metabolized to active compounds** by the liver through phase I hepatic microsomal oxidation by the cytochrome P450 isozyme (except lorazepam, temazepam, oxazepam) (Fig. 4.2).
  - **(1)** **Active metabolites** are responsible for **prolonged duration** of action of BZs.
  - **(2)** Lorazepam and oxazepam undergo extrahepatic conjugation.
- **c.** Clearance is often decreased in the elderly and in patients with liver disease. In these patients, doses should be reduced or the drug avoided altogether. Lorazepam and oxazepam metabolism are minimally affected by liver disease.

4. *Indications* (Table 4.1)
- **a.** **Anxiety disorders** (including acute anxiety, generalized anxiety disorder [GAD], situational anxiety disorders, panic disorders, and social anxiety disorder or social phobia)
  - **(1)** BZs such as **clonazepam**, lorazepam, **alprazolam**, and **diazepam** are effective for the short-term management (<6 weeks) of many anxiety disorders.
  - **(2)** Selective serotonin reuptake inhibitors (SSRIs) are now considered first-line agents for the long-term management of these disorders.
  - **(3)** β-Blockers like propranolol have been used in acute stressful conditions, such as performance anxiety and fear of examinations, as they cut down on sympathetic overactivity which reinforces anxiety.
  - **(4)** Other antianxiety drugs: Buspirone

TABLE 4.1 Classification and Indications of Benzodiazepines

Drug (Half-life)	Primary Indications
Ultrashort acting	
Remimazolam[a]	Short procedural sedation
Short acting ($t_{1/2}$ < 5 hours)	
Midazolam	Preanesthetic, procedural sedation
Triazolam	Sleep-onset insomnia
Intermediate acting ($t_{1/2}$ 5–24 hours)	
Alprazolam	Anxiety and panic disorders
Clonazepam	Myoclonic and absence seizures
Estazolam	Insomnia
Lorazepam	Anxiety, insomnia, status epilepticus, preanesthetic
Oxazepam	Anxiety, alcohol withdrawal syndrome
Temazepam	Sleep-onset and sleep maintenance insomnia
Long lasting ($t_{1/2}$ > 24 hours)	
Chlordiazepoxide[b,c]	Anxiety, alcohol withdrawal syndrome
Clorazepate[d]	Anxiety, focal (partial)-onset seizures
Diazepam[b,c]	Anxiety, preanesthetic, febrile seizures, alcohol withdrawal syndrome
Flurazepam	Insomnia
Prazepam[b,d]	Anxiety
Quazepam	Chronic insomnia

[a]Rapid onset, short duration of action due to rapid metabolism by a nonspecific tissue esterase.
[b]Converted to the long-acting, active metabolite.
[c]For withdrawal from ethanol and other sedative–hypnotics.
[d]Prodrug.

(a) Buspirone is a **non-BZ partial agonist at serotonin (5-HT1$_A$) receptors**, which selectively **relieves anxiety without the sedation**, hypnosis, general CNS depression, or drug abuse liability of the BZs (see Fig. 4.1).
  i. It has no other BZ-like activities.

(b) ***Indications.*** A week or more of administration may be required to achieve the therapeutic effects; therefore, it is **used primarily to treat GAD.**

(c) ***Adverse effects.*** Buspirone may cause **dizziness**, drowsiness, nervousness, dysphoria, tachycardia, or gastrointestinal (GI) distress.

5. ***Indications.*** A week or more of administration may be required to achieve the therapeutic effects; **therefore, it is used primarily to treat GAD.**
6. ***Adverse effects.*** Buspirone may cause **dizziness,** drowsiness, nervousness, dysphoria, tachycardia, or GI distress.
   a. **Insomnia**
      (1) **Temazepam**, flurazepam, and triazolam have a rapid onset and sufficient duration of action with minimal hangover.
   b. **Seizures**
      (1) BZs elevate the seizure threshold.
      (2) Intravenous (IV) **lorazepam** or **diazepam** may be used for the initial treatment of status epilepticus and drug- or toxin-induced seizures.
      (3) **Clonazepam and clobazam** can be used for myoclonic and absence seizures.
      (4) The development of tolerance precludes their long-term use.
   c. **Anesthesia and short medical or surgical procedures**
      (1) Shorter-acting BZs, such as **midazolam**, are preferred for their anxiolytic, **sedative**, and **amnestic actions** before and during surgery, endoscopy, or bronchoscopy.
      (2) **Ultrashort-acting remimazolam** has been recently approved for short procedural (less than half an hour) sedation.
   d. **Muscle relaxation**
      (1) **Diazepam** is used to treat spontaneous muscle spasms, spasms associated with endoscopy, and the spasticity of cerebral palsy.
   e. **Acute mania** of bipolar disorder (for the initial management of agitation)

f. Acute alcohol withdrawal

(1) Lorazepam, diazepam, and chlordiazepoxide are frequently used to reduce alcohol withdrawal symptoms, such as psychomotor agitation.

7. *Adverse effects and precautions*

a. Daytime drowsiness, sedation, and ataxia are common adverse effects.

(1) BZs may impair judgment and interfere with motor skills, particularly in the elderly leading to falls and fracture, and impair driving; abnormal sleep behaviors may occur.

b. These drugs may **depress respiration** at higher than hypnotic doses, an effect that can be exaggerated in patients with chronic obstructive pulmonary disease or obstructive sleep apnea.

c. Rebound insomnia may occur on discontinuation.

d. In the **elderly**, overuse of BZs is the most common cause of **reversible confusion** and amnesia.

e. BZs, particularly when given intravenously, like remimazolam, decrease blood pressure and heart rate in patients with impaired cardiovascular function.

f. Pregnancy: All BZs should be particularly avoided during the first trimester of pregnancy; they are associated with neonatal hypotonia and withdrawal; use of BZs during lactation should be avoided unless a compelling indication is present.

8. *Drug interactions*

a. BZs enhance CNS depression when taken in combination with other drugs that depress the CNS, most notably alcohol and opioids.

b. Drugs like erythromycin, clarithromycin, ritonavir, itraconazole, ketoconazole, nefazodone, and grapefruit juice are inhibitors of CYP3A4 and can affect the metabolism of BZs.

9. *Tolerance, abuse, and dependence*

a. Tolerance develops to the sedative, hypnotic, and anticonvulsant actions of BZs.

(1) **Cross-tolerance** occurs with other sedative-hypnotic agents, including **alcohol** and **barbiturates**.

b. Psychological and physical dependence can develop if high doses are given over a prolonged period.

c. Abrupt discontinuation may result in withdrawal symptoms, including confusion, anxiety, agitation, restlessness, insomnia, and seizures.

(1) Withdrawal occurs sooner and is more severe after abrupt discontinuation of shorter-acting BZs.

(2) Tapering the dose or substituting with longer-acting BZs, such as diazepam, can minimize withdrawal symptoms.

(3) If not treated appropriately, BZ withdrawal can be life threatening.

10. Overdosage of benzodiazepines

a. Clinical features: These include severe sedation, cognitive impairment, and ataxia, often accompanied by slurred speech, hypotension, and bradycardia. Respiratory depression needs to be promptly reversed. **The drug of choice is flumazenil 0.2 mg/min IV** till the patient regains consciousness. Activated charcoal administration is contraindicated due to the risk of aspiration owing to altered mental status.

B. Flumazenil

1. *Mechanism of action.* Flumazenil is a **competitive antagonist** at **BZ receptors**.

2. *Indications.* It is used to **prevent** or **reverse** the **CNS effects** from **BZ overdose**. It may also speed recovery from the effects of BZs used in anesthetic and diagnostic procedures.

a. It has a short duration of action, which often necessitates multiple dosing.

b. It will **not reverse** the **effects** of **barbiturates** or **alcohol**.

3. *Adverse effects.* Flumazenil may precipitate withdrawal, and can cause agitation and anxiety.

C. Barbiturates

1. *General properties*

a. Barbiturates have been largely replaced by BZs, non-BZ sedative-hypnotic agents, and the SSRIs for the treatment of anxiety and sleep disorders.

b. Use of barbiturates is limited due to **strong sedative** effects, rapid tolerance, drug interactions, abuse potential, and **lethality in overdose due to dose-related respiratory depression** with cerebral hypoxia (Fig. 4.1).

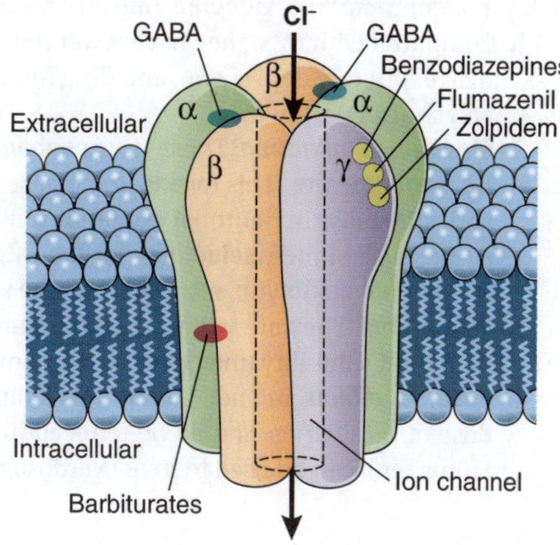

FIGURE 4.3. Representation of GABA receptor–chloride channel receptor complex. Binding of GABA to its receptor causes the closed chloride channel to open. Binding of benzodiazepines to its receptor allosterically enhances binding to GABA. This causes increased chloride conductance and further hyperpolarization of the cell, making it less excitable. Barbiturates, benzodiazepines, ethanol, and other sedative–hypnotic drugs act on the GABA receptor. GABA, γ-aminobutyric acid.

2. ***Mechanism of action*** (Fig. 4.3)
   a. Barbiturates interact with a binding site on the γ-aminobutyric acid **($GABA_A$)-receptor–chloride channel complex** that is separate from the BZ-binding site.
   b. At **low doses**, barbiturates **allosterically prolong the GABA-induced opening of chloride channels** and enhance GABA-inhibitory neurotransmission.
   c. At **higher doses**, these drugs have **GABA-mimetic** activity (they open chloride channels independently of GABA).
3. ***Indications*** (Table 4.2)
   a. Ultrashort-acting agents, such as thiopental, can be used for anesthesia induction and short-term maintenance.
   b. Long-acting agents, such as phenobarbital, can be used for the treatment of seizures, including status epilepticus.
4. ***Adverse effects and precautions***
   a. Barbiturates can cause sedation, tolerance, dependence, and respiratory depression.
   b. They may **increase porphyrin synthesis** by the induction of hepatic δ-aminolevulinic acid synthase, which can **precipitate** the symptoms of **acute intermittent porphyria**.
   c. Barbiturate overdosage: Treated with gastric lavage, supportive measures, alkaline diuresis, and hemodialysis; there is no specific antidote.
5. ***Drug interactions***
   a. With long-term use, barbiturates may **induce the synthesis of hepatic microsomal enzymes** and may increase the metabolism of numerous other drugs.
   b. They enhance CNS depression when taken in combination with other drugs that depress the CNS, most notably alcohol.

TABLE 4.2 Classification and Indications of Barbiturates

Drug and Classification	Indications
Ultrashort acting Thiopental Methohexital	Intravenous general anesthesia
Intermediate acting Amobarbital Pentobarbital Secobarbital	Preanesthetic medication and regional anesthesia; sedation and hypnosis (largely supplanted by benzodiazepines)
Long acting Phenobarbital Mephobarbital	Seizure disorders; withdrawal syndrome from sedative–hypnotics

D. Zolpidem, zopiclone, zaleplon, and eszopiclone (also known as "Z" drugs)

1. Compared with BZs, they have fewer reports of dependency, abuse potential, rebound insomnia, respiratory depression, and drug interactions (due to specific selectivity for alpha-1 subunit and shorter half-lives).
2. ***Mechanism of action.*** These drugs **enhance** the activity of **GABA** by acting at the α_1 subunit of **BZ_1-receptor site.** This results in increased chloride conductance, neuronal hyperpolarization, and a decrease in neuronal excitability, leading to sedative and hypnotic effects.
   a. Because of their **selectivity for the BZ_1**-receptor site over the BZ_2-receptor site, they **exhibit minimal anxiolytic**, myorelaxant, and anticonvulsant properties.
3. ***Indications.*** They are widely used for **short-term treatment of insomnia**. Due to their relatively high lipid solubility, they have a rapid onset of action.
4. ***Adverse effects*** include modest **daytime sedation**, headache, dizziness and GI upset. The dose of these drugs should be reduced in the elderly and in patients with hepatic impairment. Flumazenil can be used to treat overdosage by these drugs.

E. Melatonin

1. Principal hormone of pineal gland involved in synchronizing sleep with the body's circadian rhythm
2. Used for treatment of jetlag and sleep disturbances in shift workers

F. Ramelteon

1. ***Mechanism of action.*** It is a selective agonist at **melatonin MT1 and MT2 receptors** that are involved in the promotion of sleep and that maintain the normal circadian rhythm.
2. ***Indication.*** Ramelteon is prescribed for patients who have difficulty falling asleep.
3. ***Adverse effects*** include dizziness and fatigue.
4. It is devoid of rebound insomnia and dependence.

G. Suvorexant/daridorexant

1. These are orexin receptor antagonists (block binding of wake-promoting neuropeptides orexin A and orexin B to receptors OX1R and OX2R), and are indicated for the treatment of insomnia, characterized by difficulties with sleep onset and/or sleep maintenance.
2. **Adverse effects** include daytime sedation, impaired motor co-ordination, including impaired driving, complex sleep behaviors, worsening of depression, and suicidal ideation.
3. **Contraindicated** in patients with narcolepsy.

II. ANTIPSYCHOTIC (NEUROLEPTIC) DRUGS

A. Introduction

1. Antipsychotic drugs are used in the management of schizophrenia and other disorders with psychotic features.
   a. Patients with **schizophrenia** often experience disorders of perception, thinking, speech, and emotion.
      (1) **Positive symptoms** include **hallucinations**, delusions, and disorganized thoughts and behavior.
      (2) **Negative symptoms** include decreased expressiveness, **apathy**, **flat affect**, and lack of energy.
      (3) Other symptoms may include cognitive impairment and anxiety.
2. Although schizophrenia cannot be cured, antipsychotic drugs may **ameliorate the symptoms**.
3. Antipsychotic drugs may be classified as either **typical** or **atypical** agents.

B. Dopaminergic neural pathways

1. **Nigrostriatal pathway**
   a. This pathway is involved in the coordination of **voluntary (purposeful) movement**.
   b. **Blockade** of the dopamine **(DA) D_2 receptors** in this pathway is responsible for **extrapyramidal symptoms** (EPS).

2. **Mesolimbic and mesocortical pathways**
   a. These pathways are most closely related to **behavior** and **psychosis** (regulation of affect, reinforcement, and cognitive function).
   b. Research suggests that an excessive activation of the DA mesolimbic pathway is related to positive symptoms, while negative and cognitive symptoms might be caused by mesocortical dysfunction.
3. **Tuberoinfundibular pathway**
   a. DA released by these neurons physiologically **inhibits prolactin secretion** from the anterior pituitary.

C. Mechanism of action

1. **Typical** antipsychotic drugs are **D_2-receptor antagonists** in the mesolimbic pathway.
   a. Binding affinity is very strongly correlated with clinical antipsychotic and extrapyramidal effects.
      (1) They help **alleviate the positive symptoms** of schizophrenia but do not alleviate negative symptoms.
2. **Atypical** antipsychotic drugs are **5-HT_2-receptor antagonists**. They are **also D_2-receptor antagonists** but have less potent D_2 antagonism compared with typical antipsychotic agents.
   a. They **alleviate both positive and negative symptoms.**
   b. Compared with typical agents, they have limited extrapyramidal side effects.

D. Specific agents

1. ***Typical antipsychotics***
   a. **High-potency** drugs include **trifluoperazine, fluphenazine haloperidol, and trifluperidol.**
      (1) Compared with the low-potency agents, they have a higher affinity for the DA receptor and are more likely to cause **extrapyramidal reactions.**
      (2) **Haloperidol** is a preferred drug for acute schizophrenia, Tourette syndrome, and Huntington disease.
      (3) **Penfluridol** is a longer-acting congener preferred for chronic cases of schizophrenia.
   b. **Low-potency** drugs include **thioridazine** and **chlorpromazine.**
      (1) Compared with the high-potency agents, they have more **autonomic effects** due to increased **anticholinergic** and **antiadrenergic** activities.
      (2) They are less likely to produce acute extrapyramidal reactions and more likely to produce **sedation** and **postural hypotension.**
2. ***Atypical antipsychotics***
   a. ***Atypical antipsychotic agents*** include **clozapine, olanzapine, quetiapine, ziprasidone, risperidone, amisulpride, zotepine,** and **aripiprazole.**
      (1) They have generally replaced the typical drugs for the **initial treatment** of first-episode patients.
      (2) **Clozapine** is reserved for **treatment-resistant** patients due to its adverse effect profile.
   b. **Newer atypical antipsychotics** include **brexpiprazole** (congener of aripiprazole, modulates serotonin (5-HT)–DA activity), **cariprazine** (DA D3/D2-receptor partial agonist with additional serotonergic/histaminergic actions), and **lumateperone** (presynaptic partial agonist/postsynaptic antagonist at D2 receptor/antagonist at 5-HT_{2A} receptors/glutamate modulator) approved for maintenance treatment of schizophrenia.

E. Indications

1. **Schizophrenia**
2. **Suicidal behavior in schizophrenia or schizoaffective disorder**
   a. Manic phase in bipolar disorder (clozapine is the only approved drug for these indications)
3. Schizoaffective disorders
4. Atypical psychotic disorders
5. Depression with psychotic manifestations
6. Tourette syndrome
7. Nausea or vomiting
   a. Antiemetic activity is due to the D_2-receptor blockade in the chemoreceptor trigger zone (CTZ) of the medulla.

b. Prochlorperazine is a typical antipsychotic but is approved only for the treatment of nausea and vomiting.

F. Adverse effects and contraindications (Tables 4.3 and 4.4)

Selection of a specific antipsychotic agent for therapeutic use is often based on its associated adverse effects rather than therapeutic efficacy. The adverse effects of antipsychotic agents are due to their antagonist actions at the DA and histamine receptors in the CNS and due to their antagonist actions at muscarinic cholinoceptors and α-adrenoceptors in the periphery.

1. *Extrapyramidal syndromes (EPS)*

a. The nigrostriatal pathway is involved in the coordination of voluntary movement. Blockade of the D_2 receptors in this pathway is responsible for EPS.

b. EPS is a major cause of **noncompliance.**

c. Extrapyramidal effects are **most likely to occur with high-potency typical antipsychotic drugs** that have a high affinity for D_2 receptors in the basal ganglia.

(1) They are unlikely to occur with most atypical antipsychotic drugs.

d. EPS include the following:

(1) **Acute muscular dystonia** (may occur during the first week of therapy)

TABLE 4.3 Potency and Adverse Effects of Typical Antipsychotic Drugs

Drugs	Oral Dose (mg)	Extrapyramidal Effects[a]	Autonomic Effects	Sedation
Conventional drugs				
Aliphatic phenothiazines				
Chlorpromazine	100	++	+++	+++
Triflupromazine	50	++	+++	+++
Piperidine phenothiazines				
Thioridazine[b]	100	+	+++	+++
Mesoridazine	50	+	+++	+++
Piperazine phenothiazines				
Trifluoperazine	10	+++	++	++
Fluphenazine[c]	5	+++	++	++
Butyrophenones				
Haloperidol	2	+++	+	
Other related drugs				
Molindone	20–200	+++	++	++
Loxapine	20–250	+++	++	++

[a]Excluding tardive dyskinesia.
[b]Cardiotoxicity.
[c]Esterification (enanthate or decanoate) results in depot form.

TABLE 4.4 Adverse Effects of Atypical Antipsychotic Drugs

Atypical Drugs	Extrapyramidal Effects[a]	Hypotensive Activity	Sedation	Weight Gain	Increased Prolactin
Aripiprazole	+/−	+	+/−	+/−	+/−
Clozapine[b]	+/−	++	+	+++	+/−
Olanzapine	+/−	+	++	+++	+/−
Quetiapine	+/−	++	++	++	+/−
Risperidone[c]	++	+	+	+	++
Ziprasidone[d]	+/−	+/−	+	+/−	+/−

[a]Excluding tardive dyskinesia.
[b]Agranulocytosis.
[c]Little extrapyramidal effects at low doses.
[d]QTc prolongation.

(a) Symptoms may present as **involuntary muscle contractions**, including spasms of the tongue, face, and neck (torticollis).

(b) More common in children younger than 10 years and in girls; resolves spontaneously; intramuscular promethazine/hydroxyzine can be used to treat the condition.

(2) **Akathisia** (may develop as early as the first month or two of treatment)

(a) Symptoms include **motor restlessness**, including a compelling urge to move or an inability to sit still.

(b) Central anticholinergics (benztropine) and BZs like clonazepam and diazepam can be used to treat; resistant cases can be treated with propranolol.

(c) May require dose reduction or changeover to an atypical antipsychotic drug.

(3) **Parkinsonian-like syndrome** (may develop from 5 days to weeks into treatment)

(a) Symptoms include **mask facies**, **resting tremor**, **cogwheel rigidity**, shuffling gate, and psychomotor retardation (bradykinesia).

(b) Treated with central anticholinergics (benztropine).

(4) **Rabbit syndrome:** Characterized by **perioral tremors** (occur after few years of therapy)

(a) Requires treatment with central anticholinergics

2. ***Tardive dyskinesia (TD)***

a. TD is a **hyperkinetic** movement disorder that may be **irreversible**.

b. It generally occurs after **chronic use of DA-receptor blocking agents**.

(1) It is more likely to occur in the elderly or in institutionalized patients who receive long-term, high-dose therapy.

(2) TD is much more likely with typical antipsychotic agents than with atypical agents.

c. Clinical manifestations may include **smacking of lips**, choreoathetoid movements of the tongue, facial grimacing, and **choreiform** or **athetoid movements**.

d. Discontinuation of drug therapy is critical.

3. ***Neuroleptic malignant syndrome (NMS)***

a. NMS is a rare but **life-threatening idiosyncratic reaction** to antipsychotic (neuroleptic) medications.

b. It is characterized by **autonomic instability, muscle rigidity**, diaphoresis, profound **hyperthermia**, and myoglobinemia.

c. Treatment may include discontinuing drug therapy and initiating supportive measures, including the use of **bromocriptine** to **overcome the DA-receptor blockade**, and the use of muscle relaxants such as diazepam or **dantrolene** to **reduce muscle rigidity**.

4. ***Endocrine and metabolic disturbances***

a. **Hyperprolactinemia** may occur due to D_2-receptor antagonist activity in the anterior pituitary (**tuberoinfundibular** pathway).

(1) In **women**, these disturbances include spontaneous or induced **galactorrhea, loss of libido**, and delayed ovulation and menstruation or amenorrhea.

(2) In **men**, these disturbances include **gynecomastia** and **impotence**.

(3) It is most common with typical agents and **risperidone** (an atypical agent).

b. **Weight gain** is likely with most typical antipsychotic agents and the atypical antipsychotic agents, **clozapine** and **olanzapine**.

c. **Hyperglycemia** and **dyslipidemia** have been reported for atypical agents.

(1) These drugs may exacerbate or precipitate **diabetes mellitus** or **hyperlipidemia**.

5. ***Histamine H_1-receptor blockade***

a. **Sedation** occurs due to central histamine-receptor blockade.

b. It is more likely to occur with low-potency antipsychotic agents and with the atypical agents like **quetiapine**.

6. ***α-Adrenoceptor blockade***

a. Blockade of α-adrenoceptors is more likely to occur with low-potency typical agents and atypical antipsychotic agents.

b. **Orthostatic hypotension** and possibly syncope can result from peripheral vasodilation; this effect may be severe and may result in reflex tachycardia.

c. Elderly patients and those with heart disease are more at risk.

d. This blockade may cause **impotence** and **inhibition of ejaculation** in men.

7. ***Muscarinic cholinoceptor blockade***
   a. Blockade of muscarinic cholinoceptors is more common with typical low-potency antipsychotic agents and with the atypical agent clozapine.
   b. It can produce atropine-like effects, resulting in **dry mouth**, constipation, **urinary retention**, tachycardia, and blurred vision. Confusion may also occur.
   c. Elderly patients are at an increased risk.
8. ***Seizures***
   a. Antipsychotic drugs can lower the seizure threshold and may lead to seizures or precipitate or unmask epilepsy.
   b. Among the first-generation antipsychotics, **chlorpromazine** appears to be associated with the greatest risk of seizures.
   c. Among the atypical antipsychotics, **clozapine** is thought to be most likely to cause convulsions.
9. ***Cardiac arrhythmias***
   a. Cardiac arrhythmias are more likely with **thioridazine** and **ziprasidone**, which can prolong the QT interval and lead to conduction block and sudden death.
10. ***Agranulocytosis***
   a. Clozapine has a small but significant risk of agranulocytosis (up to 3%); for this reason, it requires frequent monitoring of white blood cell counts and is not used as a first-line agent.

G. Drug interactions

1. Certain antipsychotic drugs produce additive anticholinergic effects with tricyclic antidepressants (TCAs), antiparkinsonian drugs, and other drugs with anticholinergic activity.
2. Smoking causes CYP1A2 induction and can decrease clozapine and olanzapine levels.
3. Antipsychotics have potentiated sedative effects in the presence of CNS depressants such as sedative–hypnotics, opioids, and antihistamines.

III. ANTIDEPRESSANT DRUGS

A. Therapeutic efficacy

1. All antidepressant drugs have a similar therapeutic efficacy, although individual patients may respond better to one drug than to another. Selection is often based on associated adverse effects.
2. Although the initial effects of antidepressants on monoamine transmission occur early, their **therapeutic effect occurs only after several weeks of drug administration** and is more closely associated with adaptive changes in neuronal receptors and second messenger activity (Table 4.5).
3. Adaptive desensitization of prejunctional norepinephrine (NE) and 5-HT autoreceptors may also be factors (Fig. 4.4).
4. Adaptive changes in neurotrophic factors such as **brain-derived neurotrophic factor (BDNF)** have also been implicated.

B. Selective serotonin reuptake inhibitors

1. ***Specific agents*** include **fluoxetine, fluvoxamine, sertraline, paroxetine, dapoxetine, citalopram**, and **escitalopram**.
2. Compared with TCAs, SSRIs cause minimal or no sedation, no cognitive and psychomotor impairment, and no anticholinergic and α-adrenergic blocking side effects (suitable for elderly); they do not precipitate seizures and do not cause arrhythmias.

TABLE 4.5 Time Frame of Physiologic Changes with Antidepressant Therapy

Time Frame	Physiologic Changes	Therapeutic Goals
Hours/days	Synaptic signaling, receptor regulation	Improvement in sleep and appetite
Weeks	Intracellular signaling, post-translational modification, gene expression	Improvement in other signs and symptoms of depression
Months/years	Neuroplasticity, neurogenesis	Prevention of recurrent affective episodes

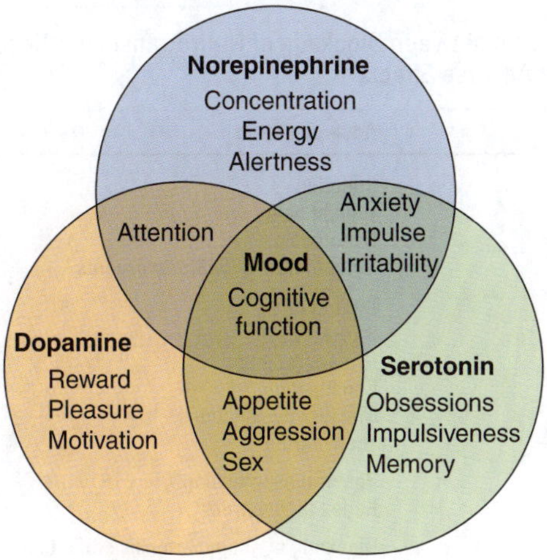

FIGURE 4.4. Monoamine activity.

3. ***Mechanism of action.*** SSRIs are selective inhibitors of 5-HT uptake. They allosterically inhibit the serotonin transporter (SERT) to potentiate the action of 5-HT (Fig. 4.5).
4. ***Indications*** include **major depressive disorder, anxiety disorders**, panic disorder, obsessive-compulsive disorder (OCD), post-traumatic stress disorder (PTSD), premenstrual dysphoric disorder (PMDD) (especially citalopram), premature ejaculation (especially dapoxetine), bulimia nervosa, and binge-eating disorder.
5. ***Adverse effects*** (Table 4.6)
   a. **GI distress** (nausea, diarrhea, heartburn) (generally transient)
   b. **Sexual dysfunction**
   c. Stimulation (often mild and transient)
      (1) Patients may experience agitation, anxiety, increased motor activity, insomnia, tremor, and excitement.
   d. **Weight gain** (especially paroxetine)
   e. **Epistaxis and ecchymosis**

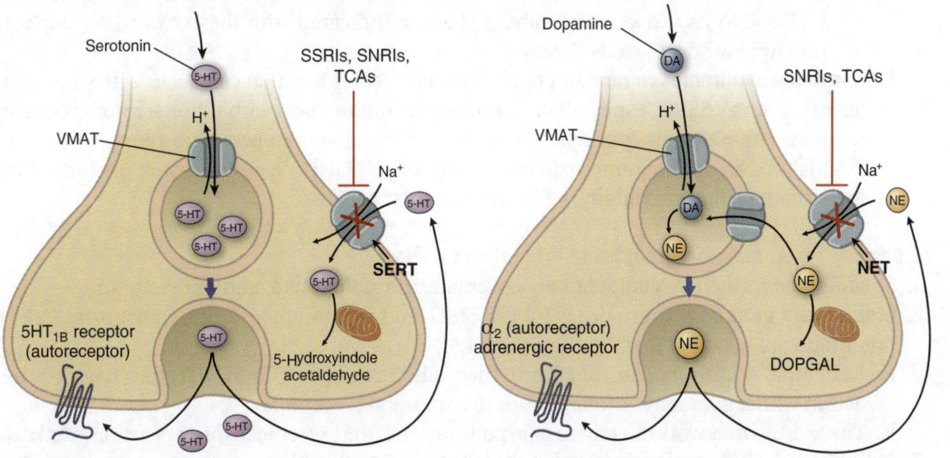

FIGURE 4.5. Mechanism of action of SSRIs, SNRIs, and TCAs. 5-HT, serotonin; DOPGAL, 3,4-dihydroxyphenyl-glycoaldehyde; NE, norepinephrine; NET, norepinephrine transporter; SERT, serotonin transporter; SNRI, selective serotonin–norepinephrine reuptake inhibitor; SSRI, selective serotonin reuptake inhibitor; TCA, tricyclic antidepressant; VMAT, vesicular monoamine transporter. Note: TCAs also block other receptors (H1, 5-HT2, a1, muscarinic). (Modified from Golan D. Principles of Pharmacology. 4th ed. Philadelphia, PA: Wolters Kluwer Health, 2016, Fig. 15.5.)

TABLE 4.6 Relationship between Blockade of Neurotransmitter Receptors and Antidepressant-Induced Adverse Effects

Receptor Subtype	Adverse Effects
Histamine H_1 receptors	Sedation Weight gain Hypotension Potentiation of CNS depressants
Muscarinic receptors	Dry mouth Blurred vision Urinary retention Constipation Memory dysfunction Tachycardia
α_1-Adrenoceptors	Postural hypotension Reflex tachycardia
α_2-Adrenoceptors	Blockade of antihypertensive effects of clonidine, α-methyldopa
Serotonin receptors	Ejaculatory dysfunction

CNS, central nervous system; 5-HT, serotonin.
Data from Charney DS, et al. Treatment of depression. In: Schatzberg AF, Nemeroff CB, eds. Textbook of Psychopharmacology. Washington, DC: American Psychiatric Press, 1995:578; Adapted from Richelson EJ. Side effects of old and new generation antidepressants: a pharmacologic framework. Clin Psychiatry 1991;9:13–19.

6. ***Precautions***
   - a. SSRIs (and all other antidepressants) may increase **suicidal ideation** for **children**, **adolescents**, and young adults.
   - b. **Discontinuation syndrome** may occur on abrupt discontinuation of SSRIs.
     - (1) Symptoms may include dizziness, nausea, headache, and fatigue.
     - (2) The drugs should be tapered on discontinuation to minimize symptoms.
     - (3) Paroxetine is the most likely to cause these symptoms.
     - (4) Fluoxetine has the longest half-life and is the least likely offender.
7. ***Drug interactions***
   - a. Fluoxetine and paroxetine are potent inhibitors of **CYP2D6** and **CYP3A4**; they can potentiate the actions of other drugs metabolized by the same enzymes such as clozapine, warfarin, TCAs, haloperidol, β-blockers, and carbamazepine.
     - (1) Tamoxifen, a medication used for the treatment of breast cancer, is metabolized via CYP2D6 to its active metabolite. It is contraindicated with these two SSRIs due to the potential for decreased efficacy.
   - b. **Serotonin syndrome** is a rare, but potentially fatal, condition that can occur with serotonergic agents, such as SSRIs, especially when used in combination with other serotonergic agents (triptans, tramadol, meperidine, linezolid, serotonin–norepinephrine reuptake inhibitors [SNRIs], TCAs, monoamine oxidase inhibitors [MAOIs]). Symptoms may include **tremor**, **hyperthermia**, **muscle rigidity**, and cardiovascular collapse.

C. Selective serotonin–norepinephrine reuptake inhibitors

1. ***Specific agents*** include **venlafaxine**, desvenlafaxine, **duloxetine**, and milnacipran.
2. ***Mechanism of action.*** These drugs inhibit SERT and the norepinephrine transporter (NET) to potentiate the action of 5-HT and NE (Fig. 4.5).
   - a. Individual drugs vary considerably in their inhibition of SERT and NET; they have less interaction with cholinergic, adrenergic, or histaminergic receptors.
   - b. These drugs may work directly on pain pathways, but the exact mechanism of action is unknown.
3. ***Indications*** include **major depressive disorder**, anxiety disorders, panic disorder, OCD, PTSD, PMDD, hot flashes, and **chronic pain disorders** such as fibromyalgia and diabetic neuropathy. Duloxetine is indicated in stress urinary incontinence in women as it increases the urethral tone.
4. ***Adverse effects*** (Table 4.6)
   - a. Adverse effects are similar to those with SSRIs.

b. Additional noradrenergic-related effects include **increased blood pressure** and heart rate, insomnia, and anxiety.
c. Duloxetine use is associated with rare hepatotoxicity.

5. ***Precautions*** are similar to those with SSRIs, including the risk of **discontinuation syndrome** and the risk of **suicidal ideation for children**, adolescents, and young adults.
6. ***Drug interactions***
   a. Duloxetine causes CYP2D6 inhibition. Caution must be taken when taken with CYP2D6 substrates, including tamoxifen.
   b. SNRIs carry the risk of serotonin syndrome when combined with other serotonergic agents (see Section III.B).

D. Tricyclic antidepressants

1. ***Specific agents*** include **amitriptyline**, desipramine, **imipramine**, **trimipramine, doxepin, clomipramine, dothiepin**, and **nortriptyline**.
2. ***Mechanism of action.*** These drugs inhibit SERT and NET to potentiate the action of 5-HT and NE (Fig. 4.5).
   a. Individual drugs vary considerably in their inhibition of SERT and NET.
   b. These drugs may work directly on pain pathways, but the exact mechanism of action is unknown.
   c. They also block α-adrenergic (α_1), histamine (H_1), and muscarinic (M_1) receptors, which accounts for many of their side effects.
3. ***Indications.*** Compared with SSRIs and SNRIs, these are now considered **second-line** drugs for the treatment of **depression**. TCAs like imipramine are used infrequently to suppress enuresis in children (older than 6 years) and adults. TCAs may be used for **neuropathic pain** conditions, attention-deficit/hyperactivity disorders in children, and prophylaxis of migraine (amitriptyline).
4. ***Adverse effects*** (Table 4.6)
   a. Adverse effects are similar to those with SSRIs and SNRIs.
   b. **Anticholinergic** effects may include constipation, **dry mouth**, **urinary retention**, and blurred vision. Confusion may also occur, especially in the elderly.
   c. **Antihistamine** effects may include **sedation** and **weight gain**.
   d. **α-Blocking properties** can cause **orthostatic hypotension**, which may lead to reflex tachycardia.
   e. TCAs can also have several other effects on the cardiovascular system, including tachycardia, conduction defects, and arrhythmias.
   f. Other side effects may include sexual dysfunction, diaphoresis, acute hepatitis, and tremor; seizures may be precipitated.
5. ***Precautions***
   a. Precautions are similar to those with SSRIs and SNRIs, including the risk of **discontinuation syndrome** and the risk of **suicidal ideation** for **children**, adolescents, and young adults.
   b. **Overdose** with TCAs can be very dangerous, in which as little as 10 times the daily dose could be fatal. Toxicity is usually due to **QT prolongation**, leading to arrhythmias. It can also lead to anticholinergic toxicity and **seizures**.
   c. **Treatment** of overdose includes supportive treatment with gastric lavage, respiratory support, fluid replacement, maintenance of blood pressure and body temperature, correction of acidosis with bicarbonate infusion, diazepam for convulsions, and propranolol/lidocaine for arrhythmias.
6. ***Drug interactions***
   a. TCAs may have additive effects with drugs that have anticholinergic and antihistamine properties.
   b. TCAs carry the risk of serotonin syndrome when combined with other serotonergic agents (see Section III.B).

E. Dopamine–norepinephrine reuptake inhibitor

1. ***Specific agent.*** Bupropion.
2. ***Mechanism of action.*** The mechanism for bupropion is not well understood. It may **increase the availability of NE and DA** via reuptake inhibition of NE trans-porter and DA transporter (DAT). It may also cause presynaptic release of NE and DA. It is also a **noncompetitive antagonist of nicotinic acetylcholine receptors** (nAChR) and may help bock the reinforcing effects of nicotine.

3. ***Indications*** include major depressive disorder, seasonal affective disorder, and **smoking cessation**. It does not cause sexual dysfunction and **may be used in patients with SSRI-induced sexual dysfunction**.
4. ***Adverse effects*** include noradrenergic-related effects such as tachycardia and insomnia. It also **lowers seizure threshold** and has a dose-related risk for seizures.
5. ***Precautions.*** Use is **contraindicated** in patients with **a history of seizures** or certain conditions with a high seizure risk such as patients with a history of **eating disorders**, including anorexia or bulimia; it is not suitable for anxiety disorders.
6. ***Drug interactions.*** Bupropion should not be given with MAOIs due to the increased risk of stimulant effects, including hypertension.

F. Monoamine oxidase inhibitors

1. ***Specific agents*** include nonselective inhibitors like **phenelzine**, tranylcypromine, isocarboxazid (less commonly used due to high toxicity and significant food and other drug interactions), monoamine oxidase (MAO)-A selective inhibitor like moclobemide (used in depression), and MAO-B selective inhibitor like selegiline (used in Parkinson disease [PD]).
2. ***Mechanism of action.*** MAOIs **inhibit** the mitochondrial enzyme, **MAO**. They **increase the 5-HT and NE available in the cytoplasm**, which leads to increased uptake and storage of 5-HT and NE in synaptic vesicles (Fig. 4.6).
   a. MAO inhibition continues for up to 3 weeks after their elimination from the body. There are two isoenzyme forms of MAO:
      (1) MAO-A: Involved in oxidative deamination of 5-HT and NE
      (2) MAO-B: Involved in deamination of phenylethylamine
3. ***Indications.*** Reversible inhibitors of MAO-A (RIMAs) are used rarely, usually only when other antidepressants have proved ineffective or for "atypical" depression; they are also used in social phobia.
4. ***Adverse effects*** include headache, insomnia, dizziness, nausea, constipation, and rarely liver damage.
5. ***Precautions*** are similar to those with other antidepressants, including the risk of **discontinuation syndrome** and the risk of **suicidal ideation** for **children**, adolescents, and young adults.
6. ***Drug interactions***
   a. MAOIs may cause **serotonin syndrome** in the presence of other serotonergic agents (see Section III.B).
      (1) Most antidepressants should be discontinued at least 2 weeks prior to starting a MAOI.
      (2) MAOIs should also be discontinued for at least 2 weeks before starting a serotonergic agent.
   b. They can cause **significant hypertension** when combined with other **sympathomimetic agents**, including pseudoephedrine, an over-the-counter (OTC) decongestant.

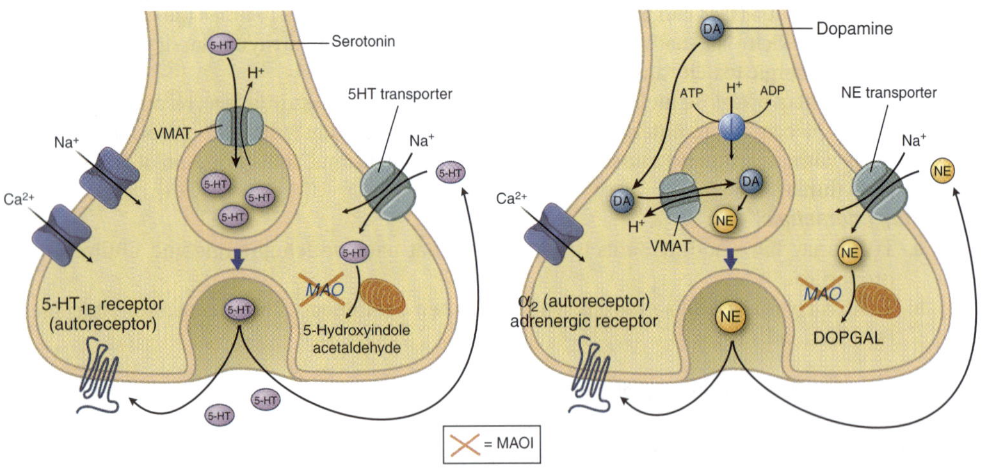

FIGURE 4.6. Mechanism of action of MAOIs. DOPGAL, 3,4-dihydroxyphenyl-glycoaldehyde; 5-HT, serotonin; MAO, monoamine oxidase; MAOI, monoamine oxidase inhibitor; NE, norepinephrine; VMAT, vesicular monoamine transporter. (Modified from Golan D. Principles of Pharmacology. 4th ed. Philadelphia, PA: Wolters Kluwer Health, 2016, Figs. 15.2 and 15.3.)

7. ***Food interactions.*** MAOIs prevent the breakdown of tyramine in the gut. Ingesting large amounts of **dietary tyramine** may cause **malignant hypertension**, **stroke**, or **myocardial infarction**.
   a. Patients should avoid consuming tyramine-containing foods, including aged cheese, beer, red wine, processed meats, and pickled or fermented food.

G. Serotonin ($5HT_2$)-receptor antagonists

1. ***Specific agents.*** **Trazodone** and nefazodone.
2. ***Mechanism of action.*** These drugs inhibit reuptake of 5-HT (at high doses) and act as $5HT_{2A}$-receptor antagonists. Both drugs also block the α_1-adrenergic receptor. Trazodone also blocks the H_1 receptor.
3. ***Indications.*** Both drugs can be used for the management of depression. **Trazodone** is often used for the management of **insomnia**.
4. ***Adverse effects***
   a. These drugs are **highly sedating**, particularly trazodone; they cause drowsiness and dizziness.
   b. These drugs may cause postural hypotension in the elderly.
   c. Sexual effects are limited, although **trazodone** may cause **priapism** in men.
   d. **Nefazodone** has been associated with a rare **hepatotoxicity** resulting in hepatic failure and death.
5. ***Precautions.*** Similar to other antidepressants, these agents increase the risk of **suicidal ideation** for **children**, adolescents, and young adults.
6. ***Drug interactions.*** Similar to many other antidepressants, they carry the risk of **serotonin syndrome** when combined with other serotonergic agents (see Section III.B).

H. Tetracyclic antidepressants

1. ***Specific agents.*** **Mirtazapine** and maprotiline.
2. ***Mechanism of action***
   a. **Mirtazapine** is an **antagonist at the presynaptic α_2-adrenergic receptor**, which results in increased release of NE and 5-HT. It is also a **potent antagonist of 5-HT_2 and 5-HT_3** receptors and H_1 receptors, and labeled as noradrenergic and specific serotonergic antidepressant (NaSSA); it is suitable for those with insomnia.
   b. Maprotiline's mechanism is similar to that of the TCAs, in which it inhibits NET and increases the synaptic concentration of NE. It has little effect on 5-HT reuptake.
3. ***Indications.*** Both agents can be used for the management of depression.
4. ***Adverse effects.*** Both drugs cause **sedation**. **Mirtazapine** can cause **increased appetite** and lead to **weight gain**; it is sometimes used for this purpose. Maprotiline can cause TCA-like side effects, including the potential for seizures or cardiotoxicity.

I. Atypical antidepressants

1. Agents include mianserin, tianeptine, amoxapine, and amineptine.
   a. **Mianserin** inhibits neither sNE nor 5-HT uptake; it blocks presynaptic alpha-2 receptors, thereby increasing their release; it is an antagonist at H_1, 5-HT_2, and 5-HT_{1c} receptors; it is less commonly used due to blood dyscrasias and liver damage.
   b. **Tianeptine** and **amineptine** increase 5-HT uptake, and are preferred in depression with anxiety.
   c. **Amoxapine** also has **DA-receptor antagonist** activity, in addition to inhibiting NE uptake; it carries the risk of **EPS**.

IV. LITHIUM (AND ANTICONVULSANTS USED TO TREAT BIPOLAR DISORDER)

A. Mechanism of action (see Fig. 1.1D)

1. The mechanism of action for lithium is unclear.
2. One hypothesis states that **lithium depletes inositol** in the CNS and dampens neurotransmission dependent on this second messenger.

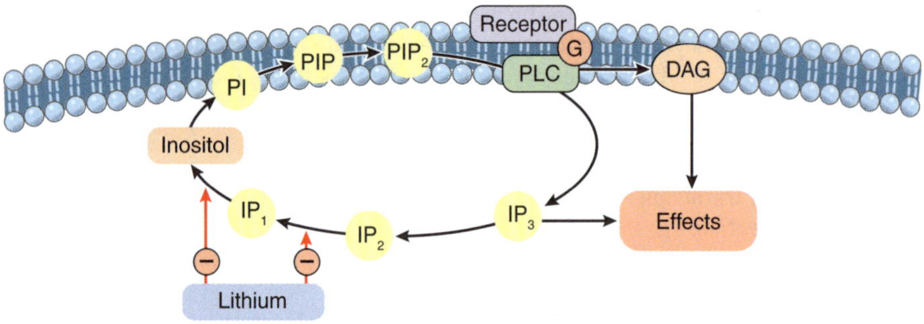

FIGURE 4.7. Mechanism of action of lithium. DAG, diacylglycerol; IP_1, inositol phosphate; IP_2, inositol 4,5-bisphosphate; IP_3, inositol 1,4,5-trisphosphate; PIP_2, phosphatidylinositol 4,5-bisphosphate; PLC, phospholipase C.

   a. Lithium inhibits inositol monophosphatase, thus decreasing inositol and, consequently, causing **decreased activity of the second messengers diacylglycerol and inositol 1,4,5-trisphosphate** (Fig. 4.7).
3. Another hypothesis states that it may have effects on protein kinase C, and subsequent neuroplastic alterations may be important to its therapeutic action.
4. Lithium's effects may also be due to the inhibition of glycogen synthase kinase-3 (GSK-3) activity with changes in energy metabolism and gene expression.
5. It also has reported effects on nerve conduction; on the release, synthesis, and action of biogenic amines; and on calcium metabolism.

B. Pharmacologic properties

1. The onset of the therapeutic effect takes 2–3 weeks.
2. It is **eliminated almost entirely by the kidney**; 80% is reabsorbed in the proximal renal tubule.
3. Lithium has a **low therapeutic index**; plasma levels must be monitored continuously.
   a. Levels should be maintained between 0.5 and 1.2 mmol/L.

C. Indications

1. ***Bipolar disorder (manic episodes and maintenance therapy)***
   a. Lithium normalizes mood in 70% of patients.
   b. Long-term treatment with lithium is associated with a reduced risk of suicide attempts and suicide deaths.
   c. Antipsychotic agents and BZs can be used in the initial stages of the disease to control acute agitation.

D. Adverse effects

1. The most common side effects with lithium include GI distress **(nausea, diarrhea), tremor**, edema, **weight gain** (may be due to sodium retention), and **cognitive impairment**.
   a. Nausea, tremor, and cognitive impairment are dose related and may decrease with dose reduction or dividing the daily dose to smaller amounts.
2. Lithium administration produces **polydipsia** and **polyuria (lithium-induced diabetes insipidus)**, which occurs as the kidney collecting tubule becomes unresponsive to antidiuretic hormone (reversible).
3. Long-term lithium therapy may cause renal impairment.
4. Lithium can **decrease thyroid function**, which is often reversible and nonprogressive.
   a. Some patients may develop **benign, reversible thyroid enlargement** (goiter) caused by reducing tyrosine iodination and the synthesis of thyroxine.
   b. It more rarely causes hypothyroidism.

E. Precautions and contraindications

1. Lithium is generally contraindicated during the first trimester of pregnancy due to possible risk of **fetal congenital abnormalities**, including cardiac anomalies (Ebstein anomaly).

2. Lithium is also contraindicated in patients with **sick sinus syndrome** due to increased depression of the sinus node.

F. Drug interactions

1. Diuretics by causing sodium loss promote proximal tubular reabsorption of sodium as well as lithium which can increase the plasma lithium levels.
2. **Lithium levels may increase** when given with **thiazide diuretics**, **nonsteroidal anti-inflammatory drugs** (except aspirin), angiotensin-converting enzyme inhibitors, and certain antibiotics such as tetracyclines and metronidazole.

G. Toxicity

1. Levels greater than 1.5 mmol/L may cause drowsiness, vomiting, diarrhea, ataxia, confusion, dizziness, and severe tremors.
2. Levels greater than 2.5 mmol/L may cause neurologic complications, clonic movements of the limbs, seizures, circulatory collapse, and coma.
3. Levels greater than 3.5 mmol/L are potentially lethal.
4. **Treatment of lithium toxicity:** No specific antidote; symptomatic treatment; excretion can be enhanced using osmotic diuretics and sodium bicarbonate infusion or hemodialysis.

H. The anticonvulsants **carbamazepine, valproic acid**, and **lamotrigine** have been used successfully for the management of bipolar disorder and are currently used extensively, either alone or as adjuncts to lithium therapy. These drugs may work through by promoting balance of GABA and glutamate activity. Atypical antipsychotics like **olanzapine, risperidone, aripiprazole**, and **quetiapine** with or without **BZs** are now preferred for control of acute mania. Severe cases might warrant the use of IM **olanzapine or haloperidol.**

V. DRUGS USED TO TREAT PARKINSON DISEASE

A. Parkinson disease

1. PD is a progressive neurodegenerative disease often characterized by **resting tremor**, **rigidity**, **bradykinesia**, **loss of postural reflexes**, and, occasionally, behavioral manifestations.
2. It occurs due to the **progressive degeneration of DA-producing neurons** in the substantia nigra pars compacta, which is thought to cause an imbalance in DA and acetylcholine (ACh) action on neurons of the corpus striatum.
   a. The net effect of the decreased DA activity (and relative increase in ACh activity) is a net loss of inhibitory regulation of the neuronal release of GABA.
   b. This leads to the characteristic movement disorders associated with PD.
3. Drugs that decrease DA activity, such as antipsychotics, may lead to a parkinsonian-like syndrome.

B. Therapeutic goal

1. Drugs are **used to increase DA activity** or **reduce ACh activity** in order to restore their balance in the corpus striatum.
   a. At this time, it is not possible to reverse the degenerative process.

C. Levodopa (L-dopa) and carbidopa

1. ***Mechanism of action***
   a. **Levodopa** circulates in the plasma and **crosses the blood–brain barrier (BBB)**, where it is **converted to DA (Fig. 4.8)**.
      (1) It interacts with postjunctional D_2 and D_3 receptors to activate inhibitory G proteins, inhibit adenylyl cyclase, and decrease cAMP levels (see Fig. 1.1C).
   b. **Carbidopa** is a **peripheral decarboxylase inhibitor** that inhibits the peripheral plasma breakdown of levodopa in the systemic circulation (before it crosses the BBB), thereby prolonging its plasma half-life, and reduces the dose of levodopa to **prevent its adverse effects like nausea, vomiting, cardiac complications, and "on–off effect"** (Fig. 4.8).

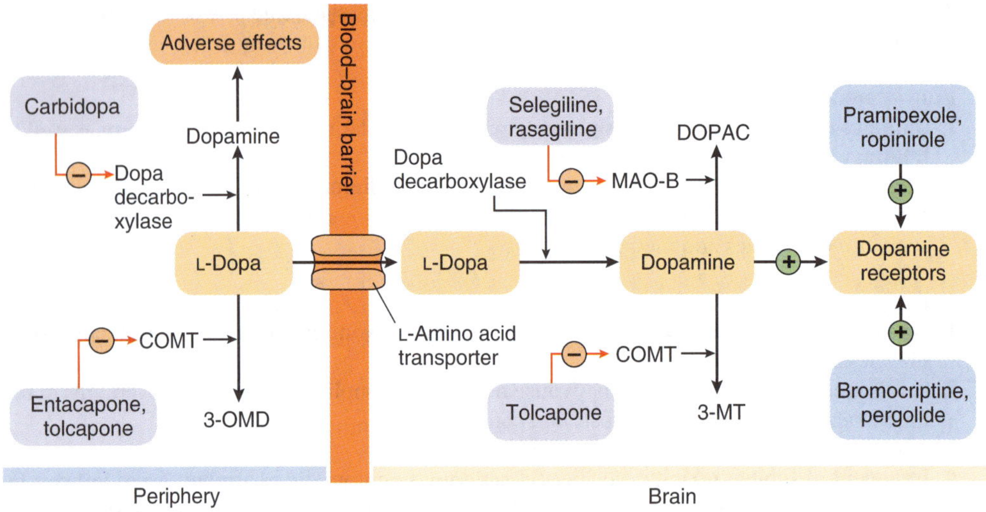

FIGURE 4.8. Mechanism of action for drugs used in Parkinson disease. 3-MT, 3-methoxytyramine; 3-OMD, 3-*ortho*-methyldopa; COMT, catechol-*O*-methyltransferase; DOPAC, dihydroxyphenylacetic acid; L-Dopa, levodopa; MAO, monoamine oxidase.

c. These drugs are administered in a fixed combination. They also prevent the interaction of levodopa with pyridoxine. However, involuntary movements and behavioral abnormalities, somnolence, and postural hypotension seen with levodopa may not be minimized.

2. *Therapeutic effects*

a. Clinical improvement, including major improvement in functional capacity and quality of life, occurs in 70% of patients after several weeks of treatment.

b. Tremor is more resistant to therapy. There is little effect on behavioral symptoms.

c. The **therapeutic effects of levodopa** begin to **diminish after 2–5 years**.

(1) It is believed that neuronal degeneration progresses to the extent that the remaining functional neurons are unable to process and store (as DA) enough exogenously administered L-dopa to compensate for the decreased endogenous DA levels.

3. *Adverse effects*

a. Gastrointestinal distress

(1) Nausea and vomiting may occur due to the direct effects of DA in the GI tract and CTZ. Tolerance to the emetic effect may develop.

(2) These effects are less frequent when administered with carbidopa.

b. Cardiovascular effects

(1) Tachycardia, or rarely atrial fibrillation, may occur due to increased circulating catecholamines.

(2) Postural hypotension is common and tends to diminish with continuing treatment.

c. Mydriasis and precipitation of an attack of acute glaucoma can develop.

d. Dyskinesias may occur in 80% of patients on long-term treatment.

(1) Dyskinesias include repetitive involuntary abnormal movements affecting the face, trunk, and limbs. They are the **major limiting factor** in therapy.

(2) Akinesia paradoxica, a sudden freezing of movement, may follow an episode of dyskinesia and is often precipitated by stress.

e. Akinesias (loss or impairment of the power of voluntary movement)

(1) End-of-dose akinesia

(a) Each dose of L-dopa improves mobility for a period of time but is followed by the rapid return of muscle rigidity and akinesia before the end of the dosing interval.

(2) "On-off" akinesia

(a) Off-periods of akinesia alternate over the course of a few hours with on-periods of improved mobility (but often marked dyskinesia).

f. **Behavioral effects** may include depression, anxiety, and insomnia.
(1) Occasionally, it may cause nightmares, visual hallucinations, and drug-induced psychoses characterized by paranoia and confusion.

4. ***Drug interactions***
a. **Antiemetic** or **antipsychotic drugs** that block DA receptors **reduce** the **therapeutic action** of levodopa.
b. Levodopa should not be used with **MAO-A inhibitors**. This combination can cause a severe hypertensive crisis.
c. Pyridoxine (vitamin B_6) enhances metabolism of levodopa and may prevent its therapeutic effect unless given with a peripheral decarboxylase inhibitor.

5. ***Contraindications***
a. The use of levodopa is **contraindicated in patients with psychosis and narrow-angle glaucoma.**

D. Dopamine-receptor agonists

1. ***Specific agents*** include bromocriptine, **pramipexole**, **ropinirole**, rotigotine, and apomorphine.
2. ***Mechanism of action.*** These agents **directly stimulate DA receptors** to stimulate DA activity on the nerves of the striatum and substantia nigra (Fig. 4.8).
3. ***Indications.*** These drugs are alternative first-line drugs or are given in combination with levodopa–carbidopa for optimal treatment.
4. ***Adverse effects***
a. Similar to levodopa, these drugs can cause **nausea and vomiting**, postural hypotension, and **dyskinesias**.
b. Behavioral manifestations, including **confusion** and **hallucinations**, are more common and severe than with levodopa.
5. ***Contraindications*** include history of **psychiatric illness** or recent **myocardial infarction.**
6. **Ropinirole** is also used in restless leg syndrome.

E. Amantadine

1. ***Mechanism of action.*** Amantadine is an antiviral drug that **increases the release of DA** in the CNS by an unknown mechanism; it also antagonizes *N*-methyl-D-aspartate (NMDA) glutamate receptors.
2. ***Indications.*** It may be useful in the **early stages** of PD or as **adjunct** therapy.
a. Benefits may disappear after a few weeks of treatment.
3. ***Adverse effects***
a. Headache, insomnia, hallucinations, anticholinergic effects, and peripheral edema may occur.
b. Long-term use may lead to **reversible discoloration of the skin** (livedo reticularis) or, more rarely, congestive heart failure.

F. Monoamine oxidase inhibitors

1. ***Specific agents*** include **selegiline** and **rasagiline.**
2. ***Mechanism of action.*** These agents are **selective irreversible MAO-B** inhibitors that **decrease DA metabolism** in the CNS and prolong its action (Fig. 4.8).
3. ***Indications.*** They may be used as initial therapy or as adjuncts to levodopa therapy.
4. **Adverse effects** may include nausea, headache, and postural hypotension; selegiline can cause insomnia and agitation.
5. ***Drug interactions.*** These drugs should be avoided by patients taking SSRIs, TCAs, and meperidine, because of the possibility of precipitating **serotonin syndrome.**

G. Catechol-*O*-methyltransferase inhibitors

1. ***Specific agents*** include **entacapone** and **tolcapone.**
2. ***Mechanism of action.*** These drugs **inhibit catechol-*O*-methyltransferase (COMT)**, thereby **reducing the peripheral metabolism of levodopa** (Fig. 4.8).
a. The decreased clearance of L-dopa increases its CNS bioavailability.
b. **Entacapone acts only in the periphery**. It decreases the metabolism of levodopa to make more available to the brain.
c. **Tolcapone** acts in the periphery and the brain. In the brain, it inhibits the degradation of DA.

3. ***Indications.*** These agents can lead to a more smooth response in patients receiving levodopa, including more prolonged "on time."
4. ***Adverse effects*** include GI distress, postural hypotension, sleep disturbances, and orange discoloration of the urine.
   a. **Entacapone** is preferred because tolcapone has been rarely associated with acute, fatal hepatic failure.

H. Anticholinergic drugs

1. ***Specific agents*** include **benztropine**, orphenadrine, and trihexyphenidyl.
2. ***Mechanism of action.*** These drugs **block muscarinic receptors** and **suppress overactivity of cholinergic interneurons** in the striatum; they have a somewhat greater ratio of CNS to peripheral activity.
3. ***Indications.*** They are frequently used in the initial stages of mild PD (often in combination with levodopa). They have a **significant effect on tremor and rigidity** but little effect on bradykinesia and postural reflexes
   a. Drug of choice in drug-induced parkinsonism
4. ***Adverse effects.*** These drugs are associated with occasional **restlessness**, sedation, **confusion**, mood changes, **dry mouth**, mydriasis, constipation, tachycardia, and arrhythmias.
5. ***Contraindications.*** They are contraindicated in patients with **prostatic hypertrophy**, obstructive GI disease (e.g., paralytic ileus), and **narrow-angle glaucoma**.

VI. DRUGS USED TO TREAT ALZHEIMER DISEASE

A. Alzheimer disease

1. Alzheimer disease (AD) is a neurodegenerative disorder characterized by **accumulation of β-amyloid plaques**, formation of neurofibrillary tangles, and loss of cortical neurons.
2. It causes **memory loss** and is the most common cause of **dementia**.
   a. Cognitive deficits occur due to cholinergic deficiency in the cortex and basal forebrain.
3. Although available treatment can ameliorate some symptoms of the illness, there is no cure or treatment that will slow disease progression.

B. Acetylcholinesterase inhibitors (see Chapter 2)

1. ***Specific agents*** include **donepezil, rivastigmine**, and **galantamine**.
2. ***Mechanism of action.*** These agents reversibly **inhibit** centrally active **acetylcholinesterase**, the enzyme responsible for hydrolysis of ACh.
   a. This results in **increased concentrations of ACh** available for synaptic transmission in the CNS.
3. ***Adverse effects*** include **GI distress** (nausea, diarrhea), weight loss, and **sleep disturbances** (insomnia, vivid dreams). Bradycardia and hypotension may occur due to enhanced vagal tone.

C. NMDA-receptor antagonist

1. ***Specific agent.*** Memantine.
2. ***Mechanism of action.*** Glutamate may worsen AD by overstimulating glutamate receptors, leading to excitotoxicity and neuronal cell death. Memantine is an uncompetitive **antagonist of the NMDA glutamate receptors**.
3. ***Indications.*** Memantine is commonly added to cholinesterase inhibitor therapy when patients reach a moderate stage of AD or for patients who do not tolerate cholinesterase inhibitors.
4. ***Adverse effects.*** The most common side effects are **dizziness, constipation, headache, and drowsiness**. It has fewer side effects than cholinesterase inhibitors.

VII. ANTIEPILEPTIC DRUGS

A. Drug treatment of seizures

1. **Epilepsy** is a neurologic disorder associated with **abnormal electrical activity** of the **brain**. It is characterized by recurrent episodes of sensory disturbances, loss of consciousness, and recurrent seizures.

2. An ideal antiepileptic drug (AED) should be effective against multiple types of seizures, have a low toxicity profile, and have favorable pharmacokinetic parameters.
3. AEDs are effective, to some degree, for about 80% of patients. Lifelong treatment may be necessary.
   a. **Lack of compliance** is responsible for many treatment failures.
4. It may take weeks to establish adequate drug plasma levels and to determine the adequacy of therapeutic improvement. AEDs are **most effective** and have the **least adverse effects** when they are used as **monotherapy**.
   a. Addition of a second drug to the therapeutic regimen should be gradual, as should discontinuance of the initial drug before the substitution of an alternative drug, because seizures may occur on withdrawal.
5. AEDs should not be stopped during pregnancy as it may predispose to status epilepticus in the mother and seizures might cause birth defects in the fetus due to anoxic injury; minimum required dose should be maintained; teratogenic drugs like valproate should be replaced; prophylactic folic acid supplementation in later trimesters and vitamin K supplementation in the last month of pregnancy should be followed to minimize neural tubal defects and neonatal hemorrhagic disorders.

B. Mechanism of action

1. ***Sodium channel blockade***
   a. **Phenytoin, carbamazepine, oxcarbazepine, eslicarbazepine, valproic acid, lamotrigine, topiramate, cenobamate, lacosamide, rufinamide**, and **zonisamide** block sodium channels and inhibit the generation of action potentials. Their effect is related to their selective binding and prolongation of the inactivated state of the sodium channel (use dependence). They also decrease neurotransmission by actions on prejunctional neurons.
2. ***Calcium channel blockade***
   a. **Ethosuximide, valproic acid, zonisamide, gabapentin**, and **pregabalin** reduce the low-threshold T-type Ca^{2+} current that provides the pacemaker activity in the thalamus.
3. ***GABA channel potentiation***
   a. **Barbiturates** (e.g., phenobarbital) and **BZs** (e.g., diazepam, lorazepam, clonazepam) facilitate $GABA_A$-mediated inhibition of neuronal activity.
   b. **Tiagabine** inhibits a GABA transporter (GAT-1) in neurons and glia prolonging the action of the neurotransmitter.
   c. **Vigabatrin** inhibits GABA-transaminase, which degrades GABA and thereby prolongs the action of GABA.
   d. **Gabapentin and pregabalin** enhance GABA release.
   e. **Felbamate, topiramate**, and **valproic acid** may also facilitate the inhibitory actions of GABA.
4. **Inhibition of excitatory glutamate neurotransmission**
   a. **Phenytoin, phenobarbitone, lamotrigine, and levetiracetam** inhibit glutamate release; **felbamate, topiramate, and valproic acid block glutamate NMDA** receptors; perampanel antagonizes AMPA-type glutamate receptor noncompetitively.
5. ***Other mechanisms***
   a. Mechanism of **levetiracetam/brivaracetam** is unknown; however, it may inhibit calcium channels and facilitate GABA inhibitory transmission by binding selectively to a synaptic vesicular protein "Sv_2A."

C. Indications: drug of choice based on specific type of seizure

1. ***Partial (focal) epilepsy***
   a. **Simple.** Localized discharge; consciousness unaltered.
   b. **Complex.** Localized discharge that becomes widespread; accompanied by loss of consciousness.
   c. In both cases, first-line agents include **lamotrigine, levetiracetam, oxcarbazepine, carbamazepine, and lacosamide.**
2. ***Primary (idiopathic) generalized epilepsy***
   a. **Tonic–clonic (grand mal)**. Dramatic bilateral movements with either clonic jerking of the extremities or tonic rigidity of the entire body; accompanied by loss of consciousness.
      (1) For primary generalized tonic–clonic seizures, first-line agents include **lamotrigine, levetiracetam, valproic acid, topiramate**, and **zonisamide**.

b. **Absence** (petit mal). Sudden onset of altered consciousness that lasts 10–45 seconds, with up to hundreds of seizures per day; begins in childhood or adolescence.
   (1) For absence epilepsy without motor seizures, first-line agents include **ethosuximide** and **valproic acid**.
   (2) For absence epilepsy with generalized tonic–clinic seizures, the first-line agent is valproic acid.

c. **Myoclonic** syndromes. Lightning-like jerks of one or more extremities occurring singly or in bursts of up to a hundred; accompanied by alteration of consciousness.
   (1) For myoclonic seizures, the first-line agents are **valproic acid** and **levetiracetam**.
   (2) For myoclonic seizures with absence or generalized tonic–clonic seizures, the first-line agents include valproic acid, lamotrigine, and levetiracetam.

3. ***Secondary generalized epilepsy***
   a. First-line agents include **valproic acid**, **lamotrigine**, and **levetiracetam**.
4. **Status epilepticus** is a prolonged seizure (>20 minutes) of any of the types previously described. The most common is life-threatening generalized tonic–clonic status epilepticus.
   a. BZs, such as **lorazepam** or **diazepam**, are the first-line treatment.
   b. Treatment with a non-BZ AED is also recommended to prevent recurrence (even if convulsions have stopped). Fosphenytoin or valproic acid is commonly used.
5. Female of childbearing age with either genetic generalized epilepsy or focal epilepsy: **Lamotrigine, and levetiracetam** have minimal or no elevated risk for structural malformations, fetal growth restriction, and/or adverse neurodevelopmental effects when compared with drugs like valproate; however, various factors should be considered to provide the optimum balance between effective seizure control in the mother and minimal side effects versus risk to the developing fetus.
6. **Other rare causes of seizures:** Addition of **cannabidiol/rufinamide** has been tried for the treatment of seizures resistant to conventional drugs especially those associated with Lennox-Gastaut syndrome, Dravet syndrome, or tuberous sclerosis complex.

D. Other commonly used indications

1. **Carbamazepine** is a drug of choice to treat **trigeminal neuralgia**; it is also used to treat bipolar affective disorder.
2. **Valproic acid** is also used to treat **bipolar** affective disorder and is used for **migraine prophylaxis**.
3. **Topiramate** is also used for **migraine prophylaxis**.
4. **Gabapentin** and **pregabalin** are used to treat **postherpetic neuralgia** and **diabetic peripheral neuropathy**. Pregabalin is used to treat fibromyalgia.

E. Pharmacologic properties

1. Many AEDs are eliminated primarily by hepatic metabolism through microsomal cytochrome P450 enzymes.
2. **Carbamazepine** induces microsomal enzymes and **increases its own hepatic clearance** (autoinduction).
   a. Gradual dosage adjustment is required early in therapy.
3. **Phenytoin**
   a. Phenytoin is 90% bound to plasma proteins.
      (1) Hypoalbuminemia may result in a decrease in total but not free plasma phenytoin (increasing the dose may result in toxicity).
   b. Phenytoin metabolism is nonlinear; elimination kinetics shift from first order to zero order at moderate- to high-dose levels.
   c. A steep dose–response and **low therapeutic index** require that **phenytoin** plasma levels be carefully monitored.

F. Adverse effects (Table 4.7)

1. Most AEDs are associated with neurotoxic side effects that may include **somnolence**, **dizziness**, **fatigue**, **ataxia**, **vision problems**, difficulty concentrating, and **cognitive dysfunction**.
2. **Phenytoin** may cause **hirsutism** (in women), **gingival hyperplasia**, and facial coarsening.
3. **Valproic acid** and **carbamazepine** are associated with **weight gain**.

TABLE 4.7 Adverse Effects and Other Considerations for Antiepileptic Drugs

Drug	Adverse Effects	Other Considerations
Sodium channel blockers		
Carbamazepine	Diplopia, ataxia, cognitive dysfunction, hepatotoxicity, SIADH, blood dyscrasias, SJS, TEN	CYP P450 enzyme inducer; teratogenicity
Lacosamide	Dizziness, nausea, nasopharyngitis, diplopia	Few drug interactions
Lamotrigine	Rash, ataxia, SJS, TEN	Decreases efficacy of oral contraceptives; must be titrated slowly
Oxcarbazepine	Diplopia, ataxia, hyponatremia, agranulocytosis, SJS, TEN	Teratogenicity
Phenytoin	Ataxia, nystagmus, confusion, gingival hyperplasia, hirsutism, blood dyscrasias, SJS, TEN	CYP P450 enzyme inducer; high protein binding; teratogenicity Prodrug fosphenytoin has largely replaced phenytoin for IV use
Topiramate	Sedation, decreased cognition, speech or language problems, nephrolithiasis, weight loss, acute myopia, and secondary angle glaucoma	Also modulates GABA and glutamate release; decreases efficacy of oral contraceptives
Valproic acid	GI distress, hepatotoxicity, pancreatitis, alopecia, tremor, weight gain	Multiple mechanisms of action; CYP P450 enzyme inhibitor; highly protein bound, teratogenicity
Zonisamide	Sedation, dizziness, confusion, SJS, TEN	May also affect calcium channels
Cenobamate	Somnolence, dizziness, headache, fatigue, and diplopia; DRESS	Advised not to drive or operate heavy machinery
Rufinamide	Somnolence and vomiting; DRESS	Avoided in patients with short QT syndrome
Calcium channel blockers		
Ethosuximide	GI distress, ataxia, somnolence, headache, behavioral changes	Few drug interactions
Gabapentin	Peripheral edema, weight gain, ataxia, dizziness, sedation	Few drug interactions
Pregabalin	Peripheral edema, weight gain, ataxia, dizziness, sedation	Often considered more effective than gabapentin
GABA channel potentiation		
Barbiturates	Sedation, tolerance, dependence	CYP P450 enzyme inducer
Benzodiazepines	Sedation, tolerance, dependence	Many agents are metabolized by the liver to active metabolites
Tiagabine	Confusion, dizziness, GI distress, unexplained sudden death	High protein binding
Vigabatrin	Cognitive dysfunction, permanent visual loss	Weak CYP P450 enzyme inducer
Glutamate receptor inhibitor		
Felbamate	Sedation, dizziness, aplastic anemia, hepatic failure	May also facilitate inhibitory actions of GABA; not recommended for first-line therapy
Perampanel	Dizziness, somnolence, headache, fatigue, irritability, gait disturbance, serious neuropsychiatric effects, including alteration of mood and aggression, falls, nausea, and weight gain	Potential for abuse
Other mechanisms		
Levetiracetam/ brivaracetam	Sedation, headache, psychiatric symptoms (anxiety, irritability)	Brivaracetam may increase the plasma concentrations of phenytoin and the active (10,11-epoxide) metabolite of carbamazepine via inhibition of epoxide hydroxylase

DRESS, drug rash with eosinophilia and systemic symptoms; GABA, γ-aminobutyric acid; GI, gastrointestinal; IV, intraventricular; SIADH, syndrome of inappropriate antidiuretic hormone secretion; SJS, Stevens–Johnson syndrome; TEN, toxic epidermal necrolysis.

4. Valproic acid can cause a fine tremor at high doses.
5. Severe side effects
   a. **Carbamazepine** and **oxcarbazepine** are associated with **idiosyncratic blood dyscrasias** and severe rashes.

b. **Phenytoin is associated with fetal malformation** (fetal hydantoin syndrome), which includes growth retardation, microencephaly, and craniofacial abnormalities (e.g., cleft palate). It is possibly due to an epoxide metabolite of phenytoin. It can also cause idiosyncratic reactions requiring drug discontinuance (e.g., exfoliative dermatitis; blood dyscrasias, including agranulocytosis).
c. **Valproic acid** is associated with idiosyncratic **hepatotoxicity**. It may be fatal in infants and in patients using multiple anticonvulsants. It can also cause **fetal malformations**, including spina bifida, orofacial, and cardiovascular anomalies.
d. Many AEDs have **teratogenic potential**. This may call for the reduction or termination of therapy during pregnancy or before planned pregnancy. However, maternal seizures also present a significant risk to the fetus.

G. Drug interactions

1. **Carbamazepine**, oxcarbamazepine, **phenytoin**, and barbiturates **induce cytochrome P450 enzymes** and can decrease the serum concentration of many drugs, such as antipsychotics, oral contraceptives, and many antimicrobial drugs.
2. **Valproic acid** and felbamate are **cytochrome P450 enzyme inhibitors** that can increase the serum concentration of different drugs.
3. Free (unbound) phenytoin levels can increase when administered with drugs that compete for binding, such as carbamazepine or valproic acid.

VIII. GENERAL ANESTHETICS

A. Overview of general anesthetics

1. **General anesthesia** is characterized by a **loss of consciousness**, analgesia, **amnesia**, **skeletal muscle relaxation**, and inhibition of autonomic and sensory reflexes.
2. **Balanced anesthesia**
   a. Balanced anesthesia refers to a combination of drugs used to take advantage of individual drug properties while attempting to minimize their adverse actions.
   b. In addition to inhaled anesthetics and neuromuscular junction (NMJ)-blocking drugs, other drugs are administered preoperatively, intraoperatively, and postoperatively to ensure smooth induction, analgesia, sedation, and recovery (e.g., BZs, opioids).
3. **Stages of anesthesia.** The stages of anesthesia identify the progression of physical signs that indicate the depth of anesthesia. Newer, more potent agents progress through these stages rapidly, and, therefore, they are often obscured.
   a. **Stage I. Analgesia and amnesia (impaired consciousness)**
   b. **Stage II.** Excitation
   c. **Stage III. Surgical anesthesia (loss of consciousness)**
   d. **Stage IV.** Medullary depression
      (1) Respiratory and cardiovascular depression requires mechanical and pharmacologic support.

B. Mechanisms of action

1. Inhalation and IV anesthetic agents interact with **discrete protein-binding sites in nerve endings to activate ligand-gated ion channels**. These channels include the following:
   a. **$GABA_A$-receptor–chloride channels**
      (1) Most anesthetic agents directly and indirectly facilitate a GABA-mediated increase in chloride conductance to hyperpolarize and inhibit neuronal membrane activity.
   b. **Ligand-gated potassium channels**
      (1) Anesthetic agents increase potassium conductance to hyperpolarize and inhibit neuronal membrane activity.
   c. **NMDA receptors**
      (1) Certain anesthetics (e.g., nitrous oxide, ketamine) inhibit excitatory glutamate-gated ion channels.

TABLE 4.8 Properties of Inhalation Anesthetics

Anesthetic	Blood: Gas Partition Coefficient (λ)	Oil–Gas Partition Coefficient	Minimum Alveolar Concentration (MAC) (%)
Nitrous oxide	0.47	1.4	>100
Halothane	2.3	224	0.75
Enflurane	1.8	95	1.7
Isoflurane	1.5	98	1.4
Desflurane	0.42	19	2.0

C. Inhaled anesthetics (Table 4.8)

1. Classification of inhaled anesthetics
   a. ***Volatile anesthetics*** (easily vaporized liquids) (halogenated hydrocarbons)
      (1) **Isoflurane**, desflurane, sevoflurane, **halothane**, and enflurane
   b. ***Gaseous anesthetics***
      (1) **Nitrous oxide**
2. ***Pharmacokinetics of inhaled anesthetics***
   a. Inhaled anesthetics are administered as gases.
   b. Concentrations of halogenated inhalation anesthetics that produce good skeletal muscle relaxation generally produce unacceptable dose-related cardiovascular depression.
      (1) For this reason, NMJ-blocking drugs are commonly used for surgical muscle relaxation.
      (2) They are often administered with nitrous oxide, which decreases the extent of cardiovascular and respiratory depression at equivalent anesthetic depths.
   c. **Solubility**
      (1) The rate at which the partial pressure of an inhalation anesthetic reaches equilibrium between various tissues (CNS) and inspired air depends primarily on the solubility of the drug in blood.
      (2) The relative solubility of an inhalation anesthetic in blood relative to air is defined by its blood–gas partition coefficient, λ, which is directly related to the pharmacokinetics of an anesthetic (see Table 4.8):

$$\lambda = \frac{[\text{anesthetic}] \text{ in blood}}{[\text{anesthetic}] \text{ in gas}}$$

         (a) Drugs with a **low blood:gas partition coefficient (nitrous oxide) equilibrate more rapidly** than those with a higher blood solubility (halothane).
            i. Induction is slower with more soluble anesthetic drugs.
   d. **Inspired gas partial pressure**
      (1) **Anesthetic effect** occurs more **rapidly** with drugs that have a **high** partial pressure.
   e. **Pulmonary blood flow**
      (1) The gas partial pressure rises at a slower rate with higher pulmonary blood flows (speed for onset of anesthesia is reduced).
         (a) **Induction** of anesthesia is **faster** with **low pulmonary blood flows**.
   f. **Ventilation**
      (1) The **greater** the **ventilation**, the more **rapid rise** in **alveolar** and **blood partial pressure** of the drug is.
         (a) This leads to a more rapid induction of anesthesia.
   g. The rate of recovery is quicker when agents with low blood:gas partition coefficients (low solubility) are used.
3. ***Potency***
   a. **The minimum alveolar concentration (MAC)** is a relative term defined as the **concentration** of an inhalation agent in the alveoli that results in **immobility in 50% of patients** when exposed to a noxious stimulus, such as a surgical incision (after allowing sufficient time for agent to reach steady state).

(1) It is the effective dose $(ED)_{50}$ for absence of movement in response to surgical pain.
(2) Inhalant anesthetics have a steep dose–response relationship.

b. The **lower the MAC** value, the **more potent** the agent is.
(1) For example, isoflurane has a MAC of 1.2, indicating that immobility can be achieved at a relatively low concentration (compared with nitrous oxide that has an MAC of more than 100).

c. Increasing age, pregnancy, hypothermia, and hypotension will decrease MAC.

d. It decreases in the presence of adjuvant drugs such as other general anesthetics, opioids, sedative-hypnotics, or other CNS depressants.

e. MAC is independent of gender and weight.

4. ***Effects on organ function***

a. ***CNS effects***
(1) Inhaled anesthetics decrease the brain metabolic rate.
(2) They reduce vascular resistance and can increase cerebral blood flow.
(3) **High concentrations** of volatile anesthetic agents are **not recommended** in patients with or at risk for **increased intracranial pressure** (head injury, brain tumor).

b. **Cardiovascular effects**
(1) Most inhalation anesthetics **depress mean arterial pressure**, especially halothane and enflurane.
(2) Isoflurane, desflurane, and sevoflurane cause peripheral vasodilation.
(a) They preserve cardiac output better than halothane and enflurane.
(3) Nitrous oxide depresses myocardial function, although this may be offset by its activation of the sympathetic nervous system.
(4) Halothane sensitizes the heart to catecholamines, which may result in arrhythmias.

c. **Respiratory effects**
(1) Most inhaled anesthetics are **bronchodilators**.
(a) Desflurane is a pulmonary irritant and can cause bronchospasm.
(2) Nitrous oxide has the smallest effect on respiration.

5. ***Toxicity of inhaled anesthetics***

a. **Malignant hyperthermia** is a rare, but life-threatening, condition that may occur when anesthetics are used with neuromuscular blockers, like succinylcholine.
(1) Symptoms include **muscle spasm**, **hyperthermia**, **hypertension**, tachycardia, and electrolyte abnormalities.
(2) Treatment includes **dantrolene**, a muscle relaxant that blocks calcium, and supportive care.
(3) In susceptible individuals, the ryanodine receptor in skeletal muscle is abnormal, which interferes with calcium regulation in the muscle.

6. ***Other effects of commonly used inhalation anesthetics***

a. Inhalation anesthetics, except nitrous oxide, relax uterine muscle, an advantage during certain obstetrical procedures.

b. **Nitrous oxide does not have skeletal muscle relaxant properties and lacks sufficient potency to produce surgical anesthesia.**
(1) It is often **used in combination with other inhalation anesthetics** to increase their rate of uptake and to add to their analgesic activity while reducing their adverse effects.

D. Intravenous anesthetics and adjunct agents

1. Preoperative sedation and induction of general anesthesia often includes IV drug administration.

2. **Propofol**

a. Propofol has **rapid sedation, rapid onset**, and a **short duration of anesthesia**.

b. It produces no analgesia and has **minimal postoperative nausea and vomiting**.

c. ***Adverse effects*** include pain at injection site and systemic hypotension from decreased systemic vascular resistance. Since propofol is formulated within a 10% fat emulsion, hypertriglyceridemia is an expected side effect.

d. **Fospropofol** is a water-soluble **prodrug** of propofol that does not cause pain at the site of injection. However, paresthesia is an adverse effect.

3. **Barbiturates. Thiopental** and methohexital

a. Thiopental is highly lipid soluble. It results in a smooth, pleasant, and rapid induction (~20 seconds) and **minimal postoperative nausea and vomiting**, although there may be a "hangover."

b. It has a short duration of action (5–10 minutes) due to redistribution from highly vascular tissue, particularly brain tissue, to less vascular tissue such as muscle and adipose tissue.
c. The action of thiopental in the CNS is similar to that of inhalation anesthetics; it can produce profound respiratory and cardiovascular depression.
d. Thiopental has no analgesic or muscle relaxant properties.
e. Thiopental is an absolute contraindication for patients with acute intermediate porphyria or variegate porphyria.

4. Benzodiazepines

a. **Midazolam** may be used preoperatively for sedation and to reduce anxiety.
   (1) It is used intraoperatively with other drugs as part of balanced anesthesia.
   (2) It is used as a sole agent for surgical and diagnostic procedures that do not require analgesia (endoscopy, cardiac catheterization).
   (3) Lorazepam and diazepam may also be used for these purposes.
b. Midazolam produces clinically useful anterograde amnesia.
c. Midazolam has a more rapid onset and shorter elimination time than diazepam and lorazepam and produces less cardiovascular depression.
d. The actions of the BZs can be reversed with flumazenil.

5. Opioids. Fentanyl, sufentanil, and **remifentanil**

a. Opioids are administered preoperatively as adjuncts to inhalation and IV anesthetic to reduce pain.
b. **Remifentanil** has a rapid onset of action and a short duration of action due to metabolism by nonspecific esterases in the blood and certain tissues.
c. **Fentanyl**, at high doses, is used to achieve general anesthesia during cardiac surgery when circulatory stability is important.
   (1) It may be combined with muscle relaxants and nitrous oxide or very small doses of inhalation anesthetic.
d. Opioids increase the risk of preoperative and postoperative nausea and vomiting.

6. Etomidate

a. Etomidate is a nonbarbiturate anesthetic used as an alternative to propofol and thiopental for rapid-onset, short-duration anesthesia.
b. Unlike thiopental, it causes **minimal cardiorespiratory depression**, which is **useful** for the treatment of patients with **hemodynamic instability**.
c. Etomidate has no analgesic effect.
d. ***Adverse effects*** include pain at injection site, unpredictable and often severe myoclonus during induction of hypnosis, suppression of adrenocortical function (with continuous use), and postoperative nausea and vomiting.

7. Ketamine

a. Ketamine produces a **dissociative anesthesia**, an effect in which patients feel dissociated from their surroundings. It also causes analgesia and amnesia, with or without loss of consciousness.
b. This drug is thought to **block the effects of glutamic acid at NMDA receptors**.
c. It also has good bronchodilator activity.
d. Ketamine is a potent **cardiovascular stimulant**; it is **useful** for patients in **cardiogenic** or **septic shock**.
e. At low doses, it is used in infants and children (trauma, minor surgical and diagnostic procedures, changing dressings).
f. ***Adverse effects*** include distortions of reality, **terrifying dreams**, and **delirium**, particularly in adults.

8. Other agents given in conjunction with general anesthetics

a. **Dexmedetomidine**, a selective α_2-adrenoceptor agonist, is used for **sedation** for procedures or for intensive care unit sedation.
b. Neuromuscular blocking agents and antiemetics may also be used with general anesthetics.

9. Preanesthetic medication: Using specific drugs such as diazepam/lorazepam as sedative-antianxiety drugs, analgesics like morphine or pethidine, anticholinergics like glycopyrrolate, H_2 blockers/proton pump inhibitors to prevent aspiration pneumonia, as well as antiemetics like domperidone/metoclopramide/ondansetron before anesthesia can help make the experience safer and less unpleasant.

IX. OPIOID ANALGESICS AND ANTAGONISTS

A. Mechanism of action

1. Opioids such as morphine are believed to mimic the effects of endogenous opioid peptides by interaction with one or more receptors (μ, δ, κ) (Table 4.9).
   a. Interaction with **μ-receptors** contributes to supraspinal and spinal **analgesia**, **respiratory depression**, **sedation**, **euphoria**, **decreased GI transit**, and **physical dependence**.
   b. Interaction with **δ-receptors** also contributes to supraspinal and spinal **analgesia**.
   c. The significance of interaction with **κ-receptors** is unclear, but it may contribute to analgesia and also **psychotomimetic effects** (**dysphoria**) of some opioids.
   d. Some opioids are agonists at all opioid receptors, whereas others are partial agonists–antagonists at the opioid receptors.
2. Opioids produce **analgesia** by one or more of the following actions (Fig. 4.9).
   a. All opioids activate inhibitory guanine nucleotide-binding proteins (G_i) (see Fig. 1.1C).
      (1) Activate the **presynaptic** opioid receptor
         (a) They **inhibit adenylyl cyclase activity**, resulting in a reduction in intracellular cAMP and decreased protein phosphorylation.
         (b) They close voltage-dependent calcium channels to **inhibit release of excitatory neurotransmitters**, such as glutamate and substance P.
      (2) Activate **postsynaptic** opioid receptor
         (a) Opioids **promote the opening of potassium channels**, which hyperpolarizes the neuronal membrane and inhibits postsynaptic neurons.
   b. Opioids **raise the threshold to pain** by **interrupting pain transmission through ascending pathways** and activating the descending inhibitory pathways in the CNS. They also raise the pain threshold by action on peripheral sensory neurons.
   c. Opioids can **decrease emotional reactivity to pain** through actions in the limbic areas of the CNS. They dissociate the perception of pain from the sensation.

B. Indications of opioids

1. Analgesia

   a. Opioids are used for the management of moderate to severe pain, including postoperative pain, cancer pain, ischemic pain in myocardial infarction, and pain due to injury, burns, or trauma.

TABLE 4.9 Opioid Receptor Binding Affinity

Strong μ-receptor agonists	Fentanyl Hydromorphone Meperidine Methadone Morphine Oxymorphone
Mild-to-moderate μ-receptor agonists	Codeine Hydrocodone Oxycodone
Mixed receptor actions	Buprenorphine ■ Partial agonist at μ-receptor ■ Weak antagonist at κ-receptor Butorphanol ■ Agonist at κ-receptor ■ Partial agonist at μ-receptor Nalbuphine ■ Agonist at κ-receptor ■ Partial antagonist at μ-receptor Pentazocine ■ Agonist at κ-receptor ■ Partial agonist at μ-receptor

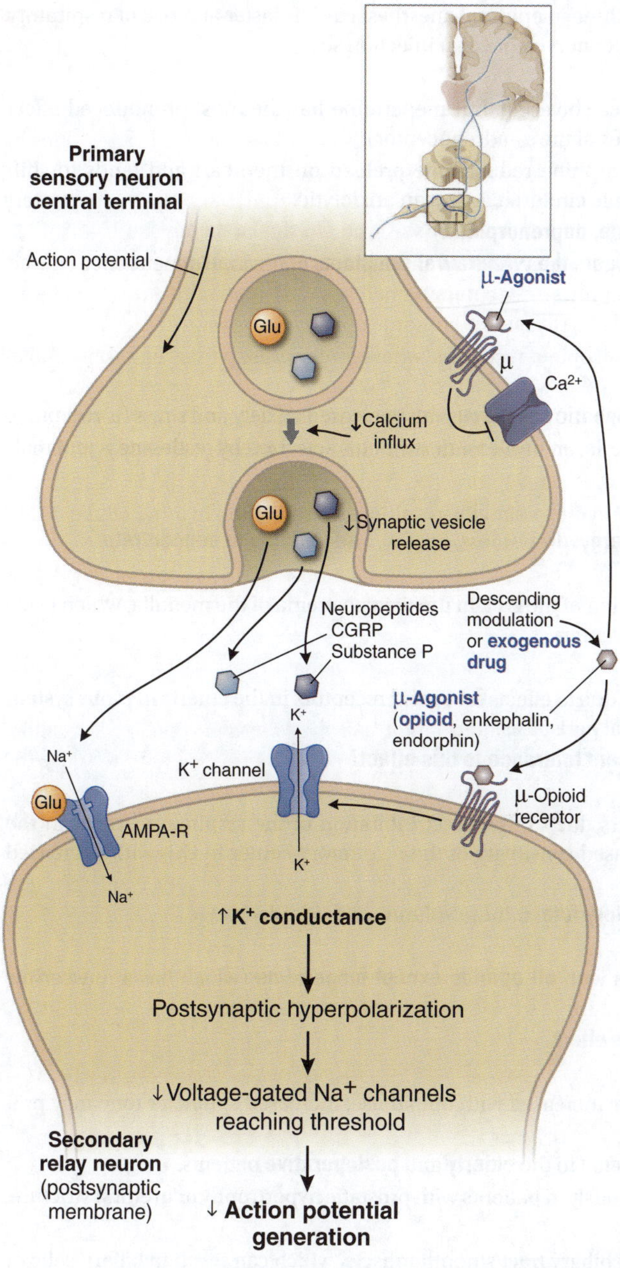

FIGURE 4.9. Mechanism of action of opioids. AMPA-R, alpha-amino-3-hydroxy-5-methyl-4-isoxazolepropionic acid receptor (glutamate-gated cation channels); CGRP, calcitonin gene–related peptide; Glu, glutamate. (Modified from Golan D. Principles of Pharmacology. 4th ed. Philadelphia, PA: Wolters Kluwer Health, 2016, Fig. 18.8.)

(1) The lowest effective dose of immediate-release opioids should be given, and no greater quantity should be prescribed than needed for the expected duration of pain severe enough to require opioids.

(2) Patient-controlled analgesia with fentanyl or transdermal patches can be used for chronic terminal illness as palliative therapy.

2. Diarrhea (diphenoxylate and loperamide)

3. Cough (codeine)

a. Opioids directly depress the cough center in the medulla.

4. Anesthesia

a. Opioids can be used before anesthesia and surgery due to their sedative, anxiolytic, and analgesic properties.

b. They can be used as an adjunct to anesthetic agents.

c. Fentanyl is preferred to morphine in epidural anesthesia as it is faster and risk of respiratory depression is less due to greater nerve uptake at injection site.

5. **Shivering (meperidine)**
   a. All opioid agonists can reduce shivering, but meperidine has the most pronounced effect (through its action on subtypes of the α_2-adrenoceptor).
6. Acute pulmonary edema: IV morphine reduces the preload on the heart and tends to shift blood from pulmonary to systemic circuit; it is also an anxiolytic.
7. **Physical dependence (methadone, buprenorphine)**
   a. Some opioids are used to **mitigate the withdrawal symptoms** of physical dependence caused by other opioids, including heroin.

C. Adverse effects of opioids

1. **Mood changes**
   a. Most patients experience a **euphoric sensation** with decreased anxiety and stress (μ-receptor).
   b. Some may experience dysphoria, an unpleasant state characterized by restlessness and malaise (κ-receptor).
2. **Somnolence**
   a. Patients may experience **lethargy**, drowsiness, apathy, and **inability to concentrate**.
3. **Nausea and vomiting**
   a. Opioids cause direct stimulation of the CTZ in the area postrema of the medulla, which leads to activation of the vomiting center.
4. **Constipation**
   a. This effect most likely occurs due to effects on opioid receptors in the enteric nervous system leading to decreased intestinal peristalsis.
   b. There is **no clinically significant tolerance to this effect**.
5. **Respiratory depression**
   a. Respiratory depression occurs due to the direct inhibition of the respiratory center in the brainstem and due to decreased sensitivity of the respiratory center to CO_2 with decreased hypoxic drive.
   b. It leads to **decreased respiratory rate**, minute volume, and tidal exchange.
6. **Miosis** (pinpoint pupils)
   a. Pupillary constriction occurs with **all opioids except meperidine** (which has a muscarinic blocking action).
   b. **No tolerance develops to this effect.**
7. **Urine retention**
   a. Ureteral and bladder tone are increased with opioid use; increased sphincter tone may precipitate urinary retention.
   b. This effect may be **more common** in the **elderly** and **postoperative** patients.
   c. Opioids should be used cautiously in patients with prostatic hypertrophy or urethral stricture.
8. **Pain from biliary spasm**
   a. Opioids cause contraction of biliary tract smooth muscle, which can result in biliary colic or spasm (except meperidine).
9. **Itching** and **flushing** (due to histamine release)

D. Tolerance

1. Tolerance occurs due to a direct neuronal effect of opioids in the CNS (cellular tolerance).
2. It occurs gradually with repeated administration; a **larger opioid dose is necessary to produce the same initial effect**.
   a. It begins with the first dose of an opioid but may not become clinically evident until after 2–3 weeks of frequent opioid administration.
3. A high degree of tolerance may develop to the analgesic, sedating, and respiratory depressant effects of opioid agonists. It does not develop to miosis and constipation.
4. Tolerance can be conferred from one opioid agonist to others (cross-tolerance).

E. Physical dependence

1. Physical dependence occurs with the development of tolerance to opioids and is similarly associated with changes in cellular signaling pathways.
2. It occurs with chronic therapy, in which **abrupt cessation of treatment results in a withdrawal syndrome.**
   a. Withdrawal may also be precipitated by administration of an opioid antagonist such as naloxone.
3. Symptoms of opioid withdrawal may include **lacrimation, rhinorrhea, yawning,** chills, **piloerection** (gooseflesh), muscle aches, **diarrhea**, anxiety, and **irritability**.
   a. Physical symptoms are often due to **autonomic hyperexcitability**.
   b. Administration of an opioid suppresses withdrawal symptoms almost immediately.
   c. The use of alpha-2-agonists, such as clonidine or lofexidine, can help with withdrawal symptoms by reducing the release of NE and decreasing sympathetic tone.

F. Psychological dependence and compulsive drug use (addiction)

1. The euphoria and other pleasurable activities produced by opioid analgesics can result in the development of addiction.
2. Addiction is a medical disorder of the brain reward pathways that is characterized by individuals' drug-seeking behavior and pathologic pursuit of reward.
   a. Addiction to opioids (and many other drugs of abuse) is due to the **increased release of DA in the nucleus accumbens** (Fig. 4.10).
   b. Cravings result in repeated relapse to opioid use, even in the presence of powerful consequences and strong motivation.
   c. It often leads to significant emotional and behavioral problems and has significant social manifestations, including problems at work and home.

G. Precautions and contraindications

1. Opioids are **contraindicated** if there is a **preexisting decrease in respiratory reserve** (e.g., emphysema) or excessive respiratory secretions (e.g., obstructive lung disease).
2. They are relatively contraindicated in patients with head injuries.
   a. Increased PCO_2 may cause cerebrovascular dilation, resulting in increased blood flow and increased intracranial pressure.
   b. Increased chances of respiratory depression.
   c. Assessment of head injury is difficult due to vomiting and miosis.
3. Opioids should be used cautiously during pregnancy because they may prolong labor and cause fetal dependence.
4. Infants and elderly are more susceptible to their respiratory depressant actions; elderly are also more prone to urinary retention.
5. They should be used in caution with patients with preexisting liver, kidney, and thyroid disorders.

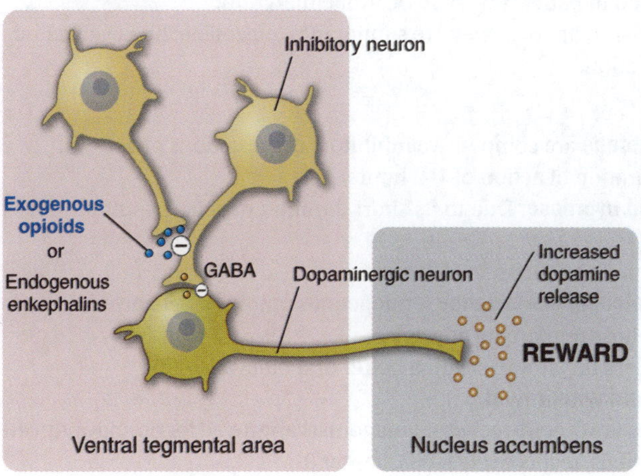

FIGURE 4.10. Opioid reward pathway. GABA, γ-aminobutyric acid. (Modified from Golan D. Principles of Pharmacology. 4th ed. Philadelphia, PA: Wolters Kluwer Health, 2016, Fig. 18.7.)

H. Drug interactions

1. **Drugs that depress the CNS** can add to or potentiate the respiratory depression caused by opioids (e.g., sedative–hypnotic agents).
   a. Concomitant use of BZs and opioids may lead to profound sedation, respiratory depression, coma, and death.
2. **Antipsychotic and antidepressant agents** with sedative activity potentiate the sedation produced by opioids.
3. Meperidine and tramadol may lead to serotonin syndrome when combined with other serotonergic agents.

I. Special considerations with specific agents

1. Morphine is the gold standard. In most cases, the 24-hour morphine equivalent dose is used to compare strengths of different opioid regimens, as well as to calculate equianalgesic doses for various preparations.
2. **Codeine** is **metabolized** by **CYP2D6** to **morphine**.
   a. Caution must be used in **CYP2D6 ultrarapid metabolizers**, since they may have extensive conversion to morphine and **increased opioid-mediated effects**.
   b. Can cause constipation, hence used in diarrhea.
3. **Fentanyl** and other synthetic subtypes may cause **severe truncal rigidity** when administered rapidly at a high dose.
4. **Meperidine** can cause CNS excitation (tremors, delirium, hyperreflexia), tachycardia, and **seizures**, at high doses, due to formation of a metabolite, normeperidine; it is less effective as a cough suppressant; miosis, urinary retention, and constipation are less prominent; it can cause anticholinergic side effects.
5. **Tramadol** is a weak opioid μ-receptor agonist that **also blocks reuptake of 5-HT and NE**. It may have special use for neuropathic pain.
   a. Its actions are only partially reversed by naloxone.
   b. Tramadol and tapentadol are associated with an increased risk of seizures and are contraindicated in patients with epilepsy.
6. **Methadone** is a **long-acting** opioid that is associated with a **less severe withdrawal** syndrome than morphine; it is often substituted for other opioids as a treatment for physical dependence. It is also used for maintenance therapy of the heroin-dependent patients.
7. **Buprenorphine** is a partial agonist at opioid μ-receptors and antagonist at κ-receptors. Due to its **slow dissociation** from **μ-receptors** and **long duration of action**, it is used in the treatment of opioid dependence, including those addicted to heroin.
   a. **Since it is a partial agonist, it can precipitate withdrawal if administered to patients already receiving a full opioid agonist.**
8. **Pentazocine** is a weak μ-antagonist and κ-agonist; it generally causes less sedation, biliary spasm, constipation, and respiratory depression. However, it causes tachycardia and hypertension and hence should be avoided in patients with myocardial infarction.
9. **Butorphanol and nalbuphine** are κ-analgesics; they are similar to pentazocine; however, nalbuphine is safe in myocardial infarction.

J. Opioid antagonists

1. **Naloxone, naltrexone, and nalmefene** are competitive inhibitors of the actions of opioids.
2. **Naloxone** has a relative short duration of action of 1–2 hours.
   a. It is used to treat **acute opioid overdose**. Due to its short duration of action, multiple doses may need to be administered.
3. **Naltrexone** has a longer duration of action, up to 48 hours.
   a. It is approved for **opioid and alcohol dependence** (endogenous opioids are involved in modulating the expression of alcohol's reinforcing effects).
4. Nalmefene is longer acting and less hepatotoxic with a better oral bioavailability.
5. These drugs will **precipitate opioid withdrawal**.
6. Methylnaltrexone and alvimopan are opioid-receptor antagonists approved for opioid-induced constipation and postoperative ileus, respectively (see Chapter 8).

K. Antidiarrheal agents (see Chapter 8)

1. **Diphenoxylate/atropine** and **loperamide** are indicated for the treatment of diarrhea.
   a. Atropine is added to diphenoxylate to discourage abuse.
2. They have **minimal dependence liability** or other centrally mediated opioid-like effects at therapeutic doses.
   a. Insolubility of diphenoxylate limits its absorption across the GI tract.
   b. Loperamide does not cross the BBB.

L. Antitussive agents (see Chapter 9)

1. **Dextromethorphan** is an OTC cough medication that is structurally related to codeine.
   a. It decreases the sensitivity of cough receptors and interrupts cough impulse transmission by depressing the medullary cough center.
   b. It has **little or no analgesic or addictive properties at therapeutic doses.**

X. DRUGS OF ABUSE (TABLE 4.10)

A. Definitions

1. Substance abuse disorder or addiction is defined as a maladaptive pattern of substance use that leads to significant impairment or distress.
   a. Individuals often continue to use the substance despite significant problems, including loss of control, health problems, disability, and failure to meet responsibilities at school, home, or work.
2. **Tolerance** is the **decreased intensity of a response to a drug following its continued administration**; a larger dose is necessary to produce the same effect.
   a. **Metabolic tolerance** (pharmacokinetic tolerance). The rate of drug elimination increases with long-term use from stimulation of its own metabolism.
   b. **Cellular tolerance** (pharmacodynamic tolerance). Biochemical adaptation or homeostatic adjustment of cells to the continued presence of a drug.
   c. **Cross-tolerance**. Tolerance to one drug confers at least partial tolerance to other drugs in the same drug class.
   d. Tolerance is often associated with the development of physical dependence.
3. **Sensitization (inverse tolerance)** occurs when repeated administration of a drug results in a greater effect with a given dose.
   a. A lower dose is required to achieve the same effect.
4. **Dependence** refers to the **biologic need to continue** to take a drug.
   a. **Physical dependence.** A latent hyperexcitability that is revealed when administration of a drug of abuse is discontinued after its long-term use (abstinent withdrawal). Continued drug use is necessary to avoid the withdrawal syndrome.
      (1) Withdrawal symptoms are often opposite to the short-term effects of the abused drug.
      (2) Withdrawal can occur due to abstinence from the substance or may be precipitated following the administration of an antagonist.
         (a) The severity of the withdrawal syndrome is directly related to the dose of the drug, how long it is used, and its rate of elimination.
         (b) Precipitated withdrawal has a more explosive onset and a shorter duration of action than withdrawal due to abstinence.
      (3) **Neonatal abstinence syndrome** (NAS) is caused when a baby withdraws from certain substances that he or she is exposed to in the womb before birth (often opioids).
   b. **Psychological dependence (addiction)** is defined as an overwhelming compulsive need to take a drug (**drug-seeking behavior**) to maintain a sense of well-being.
      (1) It is likely related to increased **DA activity** in the **nucleus accumbens**.
   c. **Cross-dependence** is defined as the ability of one drug to substitute for another pharmacologically similar drug to maintain a dependent state or to prevent withdrawal (e.g., diazepam for ethanol; methadone for heroin).

TABLE 4.10 Actions and Effects for Drugs of Abuse

Class	Examples	Actions	Effects
Alcohol	Ethanol	NMDA-receptor antagonist GABA-receptor modulator	Intoxication, sedation, memory loss
Barbiturates	Phenobarbital	GABA-receptor agonist and modulator	Sedation, respiratory depression
Benzodiazepines	Diazepam Lorazepam	GABA-receptor modulator	Sedation, respiratory depression
Cannabinoids	Marijuana	CB-receptor agonist	Giddiness, hunger
Inhalants	Toluene, nitrous oxide	Not known (may affect GABA or glutamate receptor)	Dizziness, intoxication
Nicotine	Cigarettes Chewing tobacco	Nicotinic ACh-receptor agonist	Alertness, muscle relaxation
Opioids	Heroin Oxycodone	μ-Receptor agonist	Euphoria, respiratory depression, sedation
Phencyclidine	PCP	NMDA-receptor antagonist	Hallucinations, aggressive behavior
Phenylethylamines	Ecstasy (MDMA)	Increases release of serotonin, dopamine, and norepinephrine	Wakefulness, emotional warmth, intimacy
Psychedelic agents	LSD Psilocybin	Partial agonist at 5-HT_2 receptor	Hallucinations, flashbacks
Psychostimulants	Amphetamine Cocaine	Dopamine and norepinephrine reuptake inhibitor	Euphoria, alertness, hypertension

5-HT, serotonin; ACh, acetylcholine; CB, cannabinoid; GABA, γ-aminobutyric acid; LSD, lysergic acid diethylamide; MDMA, methylenedioxymethamphetamine; NMDA, *N*-methyl-D-aspartate.

5. The degree of tolerance and physical dependence varies considerably among different classes of drugs.

B. General CNS depressants

1. Ethanol

a. ***Mechanism of action.*** The precise mechanism of action for ethanol in the CNS is unknown. It has a direct effect on $GABA_A$ receptors to acutely **enhance the inhibitory action of GABA** in the CNS. It also has an **inhibitory effect on glutamate activation** of NMDA receptors in the CNS.

b. ***Pharmacologic properties***

(1) Ethanol is rapidly absorbed from the stomach and small intestine and is rapidly distributed in total body water. Absorption is delayed by food.

(2) It is **oxidized** at low plasma concentrations **to acetaldehyde** by the liver cytosolic enzyme **alcohol dehydrogenase** (ADH), with the generation of reduced nicotinamide adenine dinucleotide (NADH) (Fig. 4.11).

(a) Excess NADH production may contribute to the metabolic disorders that are associated with chronic alcoholism, as well as lactic acidosis and hypoglycemia due to acute alcohol toxicity.

(b) Acetaldehyde is further oxidized by mitochondrial **aldehyde dehydrogenase to acetate**, which is further metabolized to CO_2 and H_2O (Fig. 4.11).

(3) The rate of oxidation often follows **zero-order kinetics** (due to a functional saturation of ADH), which is independent of time and drug concentration.

c. ***Acute effects***

(1) General **CNS depression**

(a) At **low-to-moderate levels** in nontolerant individuals (50–100 mg/dL), inhibition of inhibitory CNS pathways (disinhibition) occurs, resulting in **decreased anxiety**

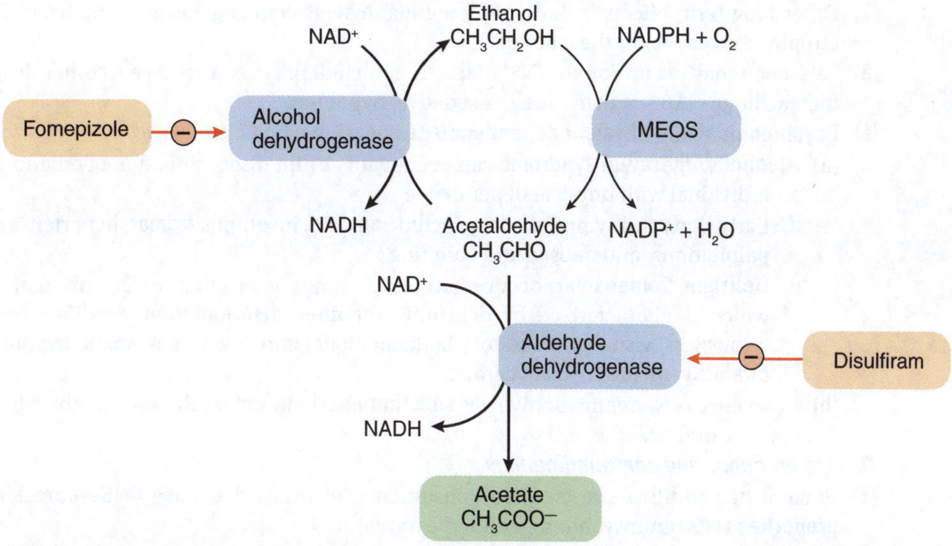

FIGURE 4.11. Metabolism of ethanol. MEOS, microsomal ethanol oxidizing system; NADH, nicotinamide adenine dinucleotide; $NADP^+$, nicotinamide adenine dinucleotide phosphate.

and **disinhibited behavior** with slurred speech, ataxia, and impaired judgment (drunkenness).

(b) At **moderate-to-toxic levels** (100–300 mg/dL), a dose-dependent general inhibition of the CNS occurs with increasing **sedation** and **respiratory depression** and **decreasing mental acuity** and motor function.

(c) At **toxic levels** (>300 mg/dL), CNS depression can result in **coma**, profound respiratory depression, and death.

(2) Other effects may include depressed myocardial contractility, vasodilation, diuresis, and GI effects (increased salivation, decreased GI motility, and nausea and vomiting).

(a) Hypothermia, due to vasodilation, can occur and may be significant in cases of severe overdose or in cold environments.

d. *Long-term effects*

(1) Liver disease is manifested by a progression from reversible fatty liver to alcohol hepatitis and to irreversible cirrhosis and liver failure.

(a) It is the most common adverse effect of long-term ethanol consumption.

(b) Other contributing factors to liver disease may include reduced glutathione as a free radical scavenger, damage to mitochondria, and malnutrition.

(2) Peripheral neuropathy with paresthesias of the hands and feet.

(3) Wernicke encephalopathy with ataxia, confusion, abnormal eye movements, and **Korsakoff psychosis** with impairment of memory that is often irreversible (**Wernicke–Korsakoff syndrome**).

(a) This is associated with **thiamine deficiency** secondary to malnutrition.

(4) Pancreatitis and **gastritis** may occur with chronic alcohol use.

(5) Heart disease

(a) Cardiomyopathy may develop due to ethanol-induced membrane disruption with decreased mitochondrial activity, among other effects.

(b) Arrhythmias (and seizures) may develop during "binge" drinking or during the ethanol withdrawal syndrome.

(c) Hypertension may occur, which may be reversible.

(6) Fetal alcohol spectrum disorder

(a) This disorder results from maternal abuse of ethanol during pregnancy.

(b) It is characterized by **growth abnormalities, microcephaly, poorly developed coordination**, and **underdevelopment of the midface region**.

i. Severe cases may lead to mental retardation and congenital heart abnormalities.

(7) Other long-term effects include mild anemia, hypoglycemia, gynecomastia, testicular atrophy, and cancer of the GI tract.

(8) **Tolerance** may occur due to CNS adaptation, including cross-tolerance to other drugs that facilitate GABA activity, such as sedative–hypnotics.

(9) **Psychological** and **physical dependence** can develop with chronic use.

(a) **Alcohol withdrawal syndrome** can occur with abrupt discontinuation of ethanol in an individual with physical dependence.

i. Early signs and symptoms may include **anxiety**, insomnia, **tremor**, hypertension, palpitations, and nausea and vomiting.

ii. **Delirium tremens** can occur about 48–96 hours after ethanol discontinuation, which is characterized by delirium (**agitation**, **disorientation**, modified consciousness, visual and auditory hallucinations) and **severe autonomic hyperexcitability**, including tachycardia.

(b) In severe cases, treatment involves **substituting** a **long-acting BZ**, such as chlordiazepoxide or diazepam.

e. ***Drug interactions and contraindications***

(1) Ethanol has additive effects when consumed with drugs that have **CNS-depressing properties** (BZs, antipsychotics, antidepressants).

(2) **Acute ethanol** use **decreases** the **metabolism** and augments the effects of many drugs because of its inhibitory effects on liver microsomal enzymes.

(3) **Long-term** ethanol use may **induce CYP P450 enzymes** and decrease drug effects due to increased metabolism (phenytoin, warfarin, barbiturates).

(4) Ethanol use is contraindicated during pregnancy and in patients with ulcers, liver disease, and seizure disorders.

f. ***Management of ethanol abuse***

(1) **Disulfiram inhibits aldehyde dehydrogenase**, resulting in the accumulation of toxic levels of acetaldehyde (Fig. 4.11).

(a) It discourages drinking by causing an **unpleasant physiologic reaction when alcohol is consumed**.

(b) Effects include **nausea**, vomiting, **flushing**, headache, and hypotension.

(c) Other drugs with disulfiram-like activity include metronidazole, sulfonylureas, and some cephalosporins.

(2) Naltrexone is an orally effective opioid-receptor antagonist that reduces craving for ethanol and reduces the rate of relapse of alcoholism.

(3) Acamprosate acts as a competitive inhibitor at the NMDA glutamate receptor.

(a) It reduces the incidence of relapse and prolongs abstinence from ethanol.

(4) Other drugs which have been tried include topiramate, baclofen, gabapentin, nalmefene, and ondansetron.

2. **Methanol (wood alcohol)**

a. Methanol can be found in windshield washing fluid and commercial solvents.

b. It is **metabolized to formaldehyde** by **ADH**, which is then oxidized to formic acid, a toxic metabolite, by aldehyde dehydrogenase.

c. Poisoning can lead to **visual disturbances**, including blurred vision and what patients describe as "being in a snowstorm." Other effects include bradycardia, acidosis, coma, and seizures.

d. Treatment of methanol toxicity includes the administration of **fomepizole**, an inhibitor of ADH that reduces the rate of accumulation of formaldehyde (Fig. 4.12).

e. Ethanol (10% in water) administered by a nasogastric tube can also be administered as an alternative; it competes with methanol for ADH and can act as a specific antidote.

f. Bicarbonate infusion helps to prevent acidosis and hemodialysis if serum concentration of methanol exceeds 50 mg/dL; cofactor therapy to increase elimination with IV leucovorin or folic acid can also be tried.

3. **Ethylene glycol**

a. Ethylene glycol can be found in **antifreeze** formulations and industrial solvents.

b. Due to its sweet taste, animals and children may ingest it.

c. It can lead to the deposition of **oxalate crystals** in **renal tubules** and delayed renal insufficiency.

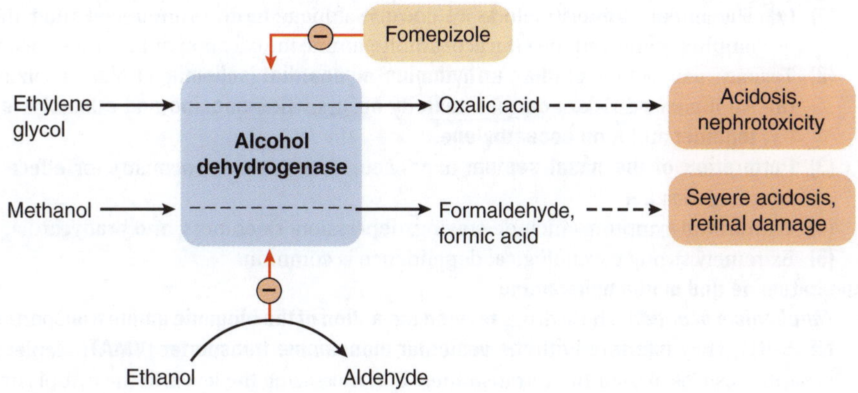

FIGURE 4.12. Metabolism of ethylene glycol and methanol.

d. Treatment of ethylene glycol toxicity includes the administration of **fomepizole** to reduce the accumulation of oxalate crystals (Fig. 4.12); ethanol is an alternative; cofactor therapy includes thiamine and pyridoxine supplementation.

4. **Gamma-hydroxybutyric acid (GHB)** is a **weak agonist at $GABA_B$ receptors.**

a. It can cause euphoria, enhanced sensory perceptions, a feeling of social closeness, and **amnesia**.

5. **Inhalants**

a. Inhalants contain volatile substances that have psychoactive properties when inhaled. **Children** and **adolescents** often abuse them. They are usually not addictive, but short-term high leads to repetitive use.

b. Abused substances may include **spray paints**, markers, **glues**, cleaning fluids, and aerosol products. Abusers can sniff, snort, or spray fumes into their nose or mouth (known as **bagging** or **huffing**).

c. ***Specific agents*** include volatile hydrocarbons, **nitrous oxide**, and nitrites.

d. ***Mechanism of action.*** Although the exact mechanism is unknown, they are thought to act as **CNS depressants** through actions at GABA or glutamate receptors. They are lipid soluble and are rapidly absorbed into the bloodstream.

(1) Nitrites produce their pleasurable effects by intense vasodilation that produces a sensation of heat and warmth.

e. ***Effects***

(1) CNS effects may include **slurred speech**, lack of coordination, **euphoria**, dizziness, and headache.

(2) Cardiac effects may include fatal arrhythmias.

(a) **Sudden sniffing death syndrome**, or **cardiovascular collapse**, may occur due to increased catecholamine release.

(3) Nitrates enhance sexual pleasure by dilating and relaxing blood vessels.

(4) Chronic exposure to the **aromatic hydrocarbons** (e.g., **benzene**, **toluene**) may result in **damage to several organ systems** and lead to bone marrow depression or liver or kidney damage.

C. CNS stimulants

1. **Cocaine**

a. ***Mechanism of action.*** **Cocaine inhibits the DAT** to decrease DA clearance from the synaptic cleft and cause an increased extracellular DA concentration (Fig. 4.13).

(1) It has similar effects on the NE and 5-HT terminals; however, reinforcing effects of cocaine correlate best with its effectiveness in blocking DAT.

b. ***Therapeutic uses***

(1) Cocaine is used as a **local anesthetic** for ear, nose, and throat surgery. It has inherent vasoconstrictor activity.

c. ***Effects***

(1) Acute exposure causes a sense of **euphoria** that includes a sense of well-being and optimism, increased **energy**, and **talkativeness**. It may also cause an **increase** in **heart rate** and **blood pressure** and a decreased appetite.

(a) The initial euphoric effects of cocaine appear more pronounced than those of amphetamine, but the effects of amphetamine intoxication outlast those of cocaine.

(2) Toxicity may include **cardiac arrhythmias**, **myocardial ischemia**, **stroke**, or seizures.

(a) An increased risk of **cardiac toxicity** occurs when **cocaine and ethanol are taken together** and **form cocaethylene**.

(3) **Perforation of the nasal septum** may occur due to the vasoconstrictor effects when snorting cocaine.

(4) Withdrawal symptoms include craving, depression, sleepiness, and bradycardia.

(5) Extremely strong psychological dependence is common.

2. Amphetamine and methamphetamine

a. ***Mechanism of action.*** These drugs **reverse the action of the biogenic amine transporters (DA, NE, 5-HT)**. They **interfere with the vesicular monoamine transporter (VMAT)**, depleting the synaptic vesicles of their neurotransmitters and increasing the levels in the cytoplasm. They also **reverse the action of the DAT and other biogenic amine transporters** to increase extracellular neurotransmitter concentrations (Fig. 4.13).

b. ***Effects*** **are similar to those caused by cocaine.**

(1) They cause increased alertness, **euphoria**, and confusion.

(2) Bruxism (**tooth grinding**) and skin flushing may occur.

(3) Long-term methamphetamine use may lead to **extreme weight loss**, severe **dental problems ("meth mouth")**, and skin sores caused by scratching.

(4) Higher doses can lead to increased blood pressure and heart rate and could potentially lead to hypertensive crisis, arrhythmias, and stroke.

(5) Unlike many other abused drugs, amphetamines are neurotoxic. Abusers may experience abnormal movements and psychotic episodes (paranoid psychosis).

(6) Extremely strong psychological dependence is common.

c. ***Therapeutic uses***

(1) **Methylphenidate** is an amphetamine congener used for **attention-deficit/hyperactivity disorder** and **narcolepsy**.

d. Atomoxetine is a selective NE reuptake inhibitor that is used to treat attention-deficit/hyperactivity disorder (ADHD) in children, adolescents, and adults. Since it is not a stimulant, it is considered a good alternative for patients with substance abuse problems or unable to tolerate the side effects of stimulants.

3. Methylenedioxymethamphetamine (MDMA, ecstasy)

a. ***Mechanism of action.*** MDMA increases the activity of DA, NE, and 5-HT. It differs from traditional amphetamines because it is structurally similar to 5-HT. For this reason, it causes increased release of 5-HT and inhibition of 5-HT reuptake.

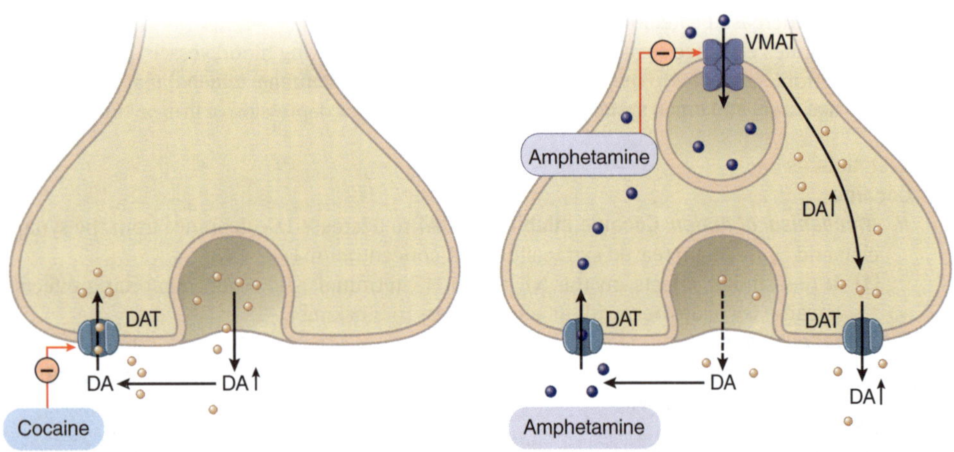

FIGURE 4.13. Mechanism of action of cocaine and amphetamine. DA, dopamine; DAT, dopamine transporter; VMAT, vesicular monoamine transporter.

b. *Effects*

(1) Acute effects include an **altered sense of time** and **pleasant sensory experiences** with enhanced perception. It increases feelings of **intimacy** and understanding.

(a) Increased 5-HT levels most likely account for the elevated mood, emotional closeness, and empathy felt by those who use ecstasy.

(2) Anxiety, insomnia, **dehydration**, hyperthermia, seizures, and serotonin syndrome can occur. These effects may occur hours, days, or weeks after use.

(3) Withdrawal is associated with long-term depression and aggression.

4. Nicotine is a constituent of tobacco, along with various gases and particulate matter.

a. *Mechanism of action.* Nicotine is an **agonist for** nAChR. It mimics the action of ACh at cholinergic nicotinic receptors of ganglia, in skeletal muscle, and in the CNS. It also activates the dopaminergic brain reward pathway.

b. *Pharmacologic properties*

(1) It is well absorbed from the lung after smoking and is rapidly distributed.

c. *Effects*

(1) It may cause nausea and vomiting in the early stages of smoking.

(2) Activity on the **central** nicotinic receptor may include **anxiolytic** effects, increased **arousal**, effects on psychomotor activity and cognitive function, and **suppressed appetite**.

(3) Activity on the **peripheral** nicotinic receptors may lead to **increased blood pressure** and **heart rate** and stimulate smooth muscle contraction.

(4) Smoking contributes to cancer of the lungs, oral cavity, bladder, and pancreas; obstructive lung disease; coronary artery disease; and peripheral vascular disease.

(5) Tolerance to the subjective effects of nicotine develops rapidly.

(6) It produces strong psychological dependence by increasing the activity of DA in the nucleus accumbens.

(7) The withdrawal-like syndrome indicative of physical dependence occurs within 24 hours and persists for weeks or months.

(a) Symptoms may include sleep disturbances, difficulty concentrating, irritability, impatience, restlessness, a dysphoric or depressed mood, decreased heart rate, and increased appetite or weight gain.

d. Smoking cessation

(1) The goal is to **reduce nicotine craving** and **inhibit the reinforcing effects** of nicotine.

(2) **Nicotine replacement therapy** contains small doses of nicotine to combat cravings and the urge to smoke.

(a) The amount of nicotine is decreased gradually over time until nicotine replacement is no longer needed.

(b) The nicotine dose is much lower than what a person would receive by smoking a cigarette (becoming addicted is rare).

(c) Options include gum, lozenges, patches, an oral inhaler, and nasal spray.

(3) **Varenicline** is a **partial nicotinic agonist** that prevents nicotine stimulation of mesolimbic DA system (and its association with nicotine addiction).

(a) It stimulates DA activity, but to a much smaller degree than nicotine does, resulting in **decreased craving and withdrawal symptoms.**

(b) ***Adverse effects*** may include insomnia and **abnormal dreams.**

(c) Use has been associated with **serious neuropsychiatric events**, including depression and suicidal ideation; risk versus benefit must be assessed.

(4) Bupropion is a weak inhibitor of DA and NE reuptake. The precise mechanism for smoking cessation is unclear, but it may act as an antagonist at nAChR function.

5. Modafinil is used to increase attention span in narcolepsy, sleep apnea syndrome, and shift-work disorder; it acts by inhibiting NE and DA uptake; it can also be used in cocaine withdrawal symptoms; it can cause headache, insomnia, confusion, dizziness, and personality disorders; armodafinil is a new long-acting congener.

6. Caffeine is used in combination with ergotamine for treatment of acute attacks of migraine; it is also used for apnea in premature infants.

D. Hallucinogens (psychotomimetics)

1. D-Lysergic acid diethylamide (LSD); also mescaline, psilocybin

a. ***Mechanism of action.*** LSD is a **psychedelic hallucinogen**. It acts at neuronal postjunctional **5-HT_{2A} receptors**.

b. ***Effects***

(1) It causes **altered consciousness**, euphoria, **increased sensory awareness** ("mind expansion"), **perceptual distortions**, and increased introspection.

(a) Trips can last up to 12 hours and lead to **depersonalization**, hallucinations, distorted time perception, shape and color distortion, and **mixed senses ("hear colors and see sound")**.

(b) A "bad trip" usually consists of severe anxiety, although at times it is marked by intense depression and suicidal thoughts.

(2) ***Effects*** are **unpredictable**.

(3) **Long-term effects** may include persistent psychosis, **flashbacks**, memory loss, anxiety, and depression.

c. The sympathomimetic activity of LSD includes pupillary dilation, increased blood pressure, and tachycardia. A high degree of tolerance to the behavioral effects of LSD develops rapidly.

d. Dependence and withdrawal do not occur with these drugs.

2. Phencyclidine (PCP, angel dust)

a. ***Mechanism of action.*** PCP is a **dissociative hallucinogen** that acts as an **antagonist at NMDA-type glutamate receptors**.

b. ***Effects***

(1) Low doses produce a state resembling ethanol intoxication.

(2) High doses cause euphoria, **hallucinations**, changed body image, and an increased sense of isolation and loneliness; it also impairs judgment, causes **paranoia/hostility**, and **increases aggressiveness**.

(a) Users may become severely disoriented, violent, or suicidal.

(b) They may experience an altered perception of pain and perception of the environment.

(3) High blood pressure, nystagmus, sweating, and tachycardia may occur.

(4) Chronic exposure may lead to long-lasting psychosis closely resembling schizophrenia.

(a) The agitated/psychotic state should be treated with a long-acting BZ.

(b) Prolonged psychotic behavior requires antipsychotic medication.

c. Ketamine is a general anesthetic primarily used in veterinary medicine that also causes dissociative effects (out-of-body experiences), similar to PCP.

d. Dextromethorphan, an OTC cough suppressant, may have these effects at high doses but is safe at recommended doses.

E. Marijuana (cannabis)

1. ***Mechanism of action.*** **Δ-9 tetrahydrocannabinol**, the active ingredient in marijuana, acts prejunctionally as an agonist to inhibit adenylyl cyclase through G-protein-linked cannabinoid receptors.

a. Through disinhibition of DA neurons, it inhibits the activity of GABA neurons in the ventral tegmentum area (VTA).

b. Cannabinol **CB_1 receptors**, which account for most CNS effects, are localized to cognitive and motor areas of the brain.

c. Cannabinol **CB_2 receptors** are found in the immune system among other peripheral organs.

d. **Anandamide and 2-arachidonoylglycerol** are naturally occurring ligands derived from arachidonic acid that act at prejunctional CB_1 receptors to inhibit the release of GABA and glutamate; their normal physiologic function is unclear.

2. Marijuana is mostly smoked but can be taken orally. It is very lipid soluble. The effects of smoking are immediate and last up to 2–3 hours.

3. ***Effects***

a. The **initial phase** of marijuana use (the "high") occurs within minutes and consists of **euphoria, uncontrolled laughter**, loss of sense of time, and increased introspection.

b. The **mellowing phase** occurs within 1–2 hours and includes **relaxation**, a dream-like state, sleepiness, and difficulty in concentration.

(1) Cognitive functions, including memory, reaction time, and coordination, are often impaired.

(2) At extremely high doses, acute psychosis with depersonalization has been observed.

c. The physiologic effects of marijuana include increased pulse rate and a characteristic reddening of the conjunctiva. It can also cause **increased appetite** and **dry mouth** and throat.

d. Tolerance to most effects develops after a few doses but disappears rapidly.

e. Heavy users may suffer from depression.

4. ***Therapeutic uses***

a. Therapeutic use of marijuana is controversial.

b. **Dronabinol** and **nabilone** are synthetic **Δ9-THC analogues** (see Chapter 8).

(1) Both are used as **antiemetic** therapy for chemotherapy-induced nausea and vomiting. Dronabinol is also used as an **appetite stimulant** for patients with acquired immune deficiency syndrome (AIDS).

DRUG SUMMARY TABLE

Sedative–Hypnotic Drugs
Barbiturates
Phenobarbitone
Benzodiazepines
Alprazolam
Clonazepam
Chlordiazepoxide
Diazepam
Flurazepam
Lorazepam
Midazolam
Nitrazepam
Oxazepam
Remimazolam
Temazepam
Triazolam
Nonbenzodiazepines
Eszopiclone
Zopiclone
Zaleplon
Zolpidem

Benzodiazepine Receptor Antagonist
Flumazenil

Melatonin Receptor Agonist
Ramelteon

Dual Orexin Receptor Antagonists
Daridorexant
Suvorexant

Antianxiety Drug
Buspirone

Antipsychotic Drugs
Typical
Chlorpromazine
Flupenthixol
Fluphenazine
Haloperidol
Loxapine
Perphenazine
Pimozide
Thioridazine
Thiothixene
Trifluoperazine
Trifluperidol
Triflupromazine
Atypical
Amisulpride
Aripiprazole
Asenapine
Clozapine
Olanzapine
Paliperidone
Quetiapine
Risperidone
Ziprasidone
Zotepine

Antidepressant Drugs
Selective serotonin reuptake inhibitors
Citalopram
Dapoxetine
Escitalopram
Fluoxetine
Fluvoxamine
Paroxetine
Sertraline
Serotonin–norepinephrine reuptake inhibitors
Desvenlafaxine
Duloxetine
Milnacipran
Venlafaxine
Tricyclic antidepressants
Amitriptyline
Clomipramine
Desipramine
Doxepin
Dothiepin
Imipramine
Nortriptyline
Protriptyline
Reboxetine
Trimipramine
Serotonin (5-HT$_2$) antagonists
Nefazodone
Trazodone
Dopamine–norepinephrine reuptake inhibitor
Bupropion
Atypical heterocyclic drugs
Amineptine
Amoxapine
Maprotiline
Mianserin
Mirtazapine
Tianeptine
Monoamine oxidase inhibitors
Moclobemide
Clorgyline

Drugs Used to Treat Bipolar Disorder
Carbamazepine
Lamotrigine
Lithium
Topiramate
Valproate

Antidiarrheal Agents
Difenoxin
Diphenoxylate
Loperamide

Antitussive Agent
Dextromethorphan

Drugs Used to Treat Parkinson Disease
Amantadine
Biperiden
Bromocriptine
Entacapone
Levodopa
Levodopa/carbidopa
Levodopa/benserazide
Orphenadrine
Pramipexole
Procyclidine
Rasagiline
Ropinirole
Selegiline
Tolcapone
Trihexyphenidyl

Drugs Used to Treat Alzheimer Disease
Donepezil
Galantamine
Memantine
Rivastigmine

Antiepileptic Drugs
Carbamazepine
Clonazepam
Clorazepate
Diazepam
Ethosuximide
Felbamate
Fosphenytoin
Gabapentin
Lacosamide
Lamotrigine
Levetiracetam
Lorazepam
Oxcarbazepine
Phenobarbital
Phenytoin
Pregabalin
Primidone
Rufinamide

(Continued)

Tiagabine
Topiramate
Vigabatrin
Zonisamide

Drugs Used for Alcohol Dependence
Acamprosate
Disulfiram
Naltrexone
Thiamine

Drugs Used for Methanol or Ethylene Glycol Toxicity
Ethanol
Fomepizole

Drugs Used for Nicotine Dependence
Bupropion
Nicotine replacement
Varenicline

General Anesthetics
Inhaled general anesthetics
Desflurane
Enflurane
Halothane
Isoflurane
Nitrous oxide
Sevoflurane

Intravenous general anesthetics
Etomidate
Ketamine
Methohexital
Midazolam
Propofol
Thiopentone

Adjunct agents
Dexmedetomidine
Fentanyl
Remifentanil
Sufentanil

Review Test

Directions: Select the best answer for each question.

1. A 42-year-old man is referred to a psychiatrist after telling his family physician that he often feels the need to drive back home to make sure that the garage door is shut. Over the past 6 months, he has started waking up 2 hours earlier to make it to work on time. Which of the following medications may help manage the patient's symptoms?

(A) Atomoxetine
(B) Bupropion
(C) Imipramine
(D) Sertraline
(E) Phenelzine

2. A 56-year-old man presents to his physician with persistent back pain due to an injury while making a delivery 3 months ago. The patient said that he often feels persistent numbness and tingling in his back, and the pain often travels down his leg. Which of the following medications may help manage the patient's symptoms?

(A) Duloxetine
(B) Fluoxetine
(C) Phenelzine
(D) Promethazine
(E) Trazodone

3. A 54-year-old woman presents to her physician with complaints of difficulty sleeping and decreased appetite. She no longer finds enjoyment in her hobbies, like embroidery and sewing, and often finds it difficult to start her day. Her doctor would like to start her on an antidepressant medication. The patient is currently on tamoxifen for breast cancer treatment and lisinopril for the management of high blood pressure. Which of the following antidepressants is contraindicated in this patient?

(A) Atomoxetine
(B) Escitalopram
(C) Fluoxetine
(D) Trazodone
(E) Venlafaxine

4. A 56-year-old man returns for a 6-month follow-up after starting sertraline for the treatment of depression. On questioning, he still has not returned to the activities he once enjoyed and is still not sleeping or eating well. The psychiatrist recommends increasing the dose of sertraline, but the patient reluctantly admits that he has not been taking it because he feels that it causes sexual dysfunction. Which of the following antidepressants should the physician consider prescribing to avoid this side effect?

(A) Bupropion
(B) Citalopram
(C) Duloxetine
(D) Imipramine
(E) Venlafaxine

5. A 36-year-old man presents to his physician with complaints of feeling down for the last 4 months. He says that he has experienced feelings of worthlessness almost daily, and although he always feels tired, he is never able to fall asleep. The patient also has concerns that his health is deteriorating. He currently smokes two packs of cigarettes per day and complains of a persistent hacking cough. He has tried nicotine patches with no success and wants to know whether there is a pill to try instead. What is the mechanism of action for an antidepressant that may also help with smoking cessation?

(A) Dopamine–norepinephrine reuptake inhibitor
(B) Monoamine oxidase inhibitor
(C) Selective serotonin reuptake inhibitor
(D) Serotonin–norepinephrine reuptake inhibitor
(E) Serotonin ($5HT_2$)-receptor antagonist

6. A 23-year-old man is brought to the emergency room after he is found walking the streets naked while proclaiming himself "the son of God." His urine toxicology screen is negative for illicit drugs or alcohol. During the interview with the on-call psychiatrist, the patient displays flight of ideas as he jumps from topic to topic. He is diagnosed with acute mania and started on a medication that inhibits inositol monophosphatase. Which of the following adverse effects is most likely associated with this medication?

(A) Hypertension
(B) Liver dysfunction
(C) Urinary retention
(D) Tremor
(E) Weight loss

7. A 63-year-old man returns to his oncologist's office for a routine visit 2 months after undergoing a partial colectomy for the treatment of colon cancer. He is currently on morphine for the management of pain and is concerned about adverse effects. Which of the following effects would most likely remain unchanged after starting morphine?

(A) Euphoria
(B) Miosis
(C) Nausea and vomiting
(D) Respiratory depression
(E) Sedation

8. A mother takes her 7-year-old girl to urgent care for a persistent cough that results in vomiting episodes after prolonged coughing spells. Further workup, including a throat culture, is negative. Which of the following medications could be used to manage her current symptoms?

(A) Dextromethorphan
(B) Diphenoxylate
(C) Loperamide
(D) Naloxone
(E) Tramadol

9. A 48-year-old woman is admitted for abdominal surgery due to a bowel obstruction. The surgeons prepare the patient for surgery and ask the nurse anesthetist whether the patient is ready for an incision. Which of the following signs should the nurse anesthetist look for to make sure that surgical anesthesia has been reached?

(A) Amnesia
(B) Analgesia
(C) Loss of consciousness
(D) Loss of eyelash reflex
(E) Respiratory depression

10. A 16-year-old boy visits his dentist for a routine checkup and is told that his wisdom teeth are severely impacted and should be removed. He is referred to an oral surgeon who uses an anesthetic with good analgesic and sedative properties but does not cause skeletal muscle relaxation. Which of the following anesthetic agents was used?

(A) Enflurane
(B) Halothane
(C) Isoflurane
(D) Nitrous oxide
(E) Thiopental

11. A 6-year-old boy is badly burned when his house catches on fire. He sustains full-thickness burns on approximately 40% of his body. Over the next few months, he requires multiple skin-grafting procedures and is given intravenous ketamine to help reduce pain associated with dressing changes. Which of the following adverse reactions should the healthcare team monitor for after administration?

(A) Distortion of reality and terrifying dreams
(B) Hyperthyroidism
(C) Malignant hyperthermia
(D) Myocardial infarction
(E) Respiratory distress

12. A 28-year-old woman with a history of alcoholism learns that she is pregnant after missing her last two menstrual periods. Over the course of her pregnancy, she misses many of her appointments and continues her normal heavy alcohol binges. Which of the following congenital abnormalities may affect the fetus?

(A) Abruptio placentae
(B) Cerebral palsy
(C) Fetal hemorrhage
(D) Microcephaly
(E) Spina bifida

13. A group of classmates bring a 16-year-old boy to the emergency room after he becomes agitated, hyperactive, and hypersexual at an all-night rave. The physician learns that the boy took several pills, which his friends thought were ecstasy. Which of the following describes the mechanism for this drug of abuse?

(A) Agonist at cannabinoid receptor
(B) Agonist at dopamine receptor
(C) Antagonist at the *N*-methyl-D-aspartate receptor
(D) Increases extracellular concentration of gamma-aminobutyric acid

(E) Increases extracellular concentration of serotonin

14. A 31-year-old man is transferred to the emergency room after complaining of chest pain and collapsing at a party. An electrocardiogram shows ventricular fibrillation. Physical examination reveals a perforated nasal septum. A close friend accompanying the patient thinks that he was using an illicit substance at the party. Which of the following drugs was the patient most likely abusing?

(A) Cocaine
(B) γ-Hydroxybutyric acid
(C) Lysergic acid diethylamide
(D) Marijuana
(E) Phencyclidine

Answers and Explanations

1. **The answer is D.** The patient most likely has obsessive–compulsive disorder (OCD). Selective serotonin reuptake inhibitors, such as sertraline, are used for the treatment of OCD. Atomoxetine, bupropion, imipramine, and phenelzine are not used for this indication.
2. **The answer is A.** Duloxetine, a SNRI, and some tricyclic antidepressants are used in the management of chronic pain. Promethazine is a dopamine receptor blocker used to treat nausea and vomiting. Trazodone is an atypical antidepressant that is highly sedating and may be used for depression or to help with sleep. Phenelzine is a MAOI, which is not indicated for the management of pain. Fluoxetine is a SSRI, which is not effective for pain management.
3. **The answer is C.** Fluoxetine, a SSRI, is a potent inhibitor of CYP2D6 and can potentiate the actions of other drugs metabolized by the same enzymes. Tamoxifen, a medication used for the treatment of breast cancer, is metabolized via CYP2D6 to its active metabolite. It is contraindicated with fluoxetine due to the potential for decreased efficacy. The other antidepressants do not have this drug interaction and can be given with tamoxifen therapy.
4. **The answer is A.** Sexual dysfunction is a common complaint with SSRIs (sertraline, citalopram), occurring in up to 40% of all patients, and a leading cause of noncompliance. It can similarly occur with SNRIs (duloxetine, venlafaxine) and TCAs (imipramine). Bupropion, a dopamine–norepinephrine reuptake inhibitor, does not cause sexual dysfunction and may be used in patients with SSRI-induced sexual dysfunction.
5. **The answer is A.** Bupropion, a dopamine–norepinephrine reuptake inhibitor, is an antidepressant that is useful as an aid in smoking cessation. The precise mechanism for smoking cessation is unclear, but it may act as an antagonist at nicotinic acetylcholine receptor function. The other agents do not affect nicotine receptors and are not indicated for smoking cessation.
6. **The answer is D.** Lithium use is associated with a fine tremor that can often be successfully managed with β-blockers. Lithium is associated with polydipsia and polyuria, not urinary retention. Likewise, it is also associated with weight gain. It does not cause hypertension or liver dysfunction.
7. **The answer is B.** Miosis (pinpoint pupils) occurs with all opioids except meperidine (which has a muscarinic blocking action). No tolerance develops to this effect. Additionally, tolerance does not develop to constipation. Patients will experience tolerance to other opioid effects, including euphoria, nausea, respiratory depression, and sedation.
8. **The answer is A.** Dextromethorphan is an opioid isomer available in over-the-counter cough remedies. It has no analgesic properties and limited abuse potential at recommended doses. Tramadol is a weak μ-opioid-receptor agonist, which also blocks serotonin and norepinephrine uptake and is used for neuropathic pain. Diphenoxylate is an opioid that, combined with atropine, is taken orally to treat diarrhea. Loperamide is an opioid that does not cross the blood-brain barrier and is also used for the treatment of diarrhea. Naloxone is an opioid antagonist used to reverse opioid overdose.
9. **The answer is D.** Loss of eyelash reflex and a pattern of respiration that is regular and deep are the most reliable indications of stage III, or surgical, anesthesia. Analgesia and amnesia are characteristics of stage I anesthesia, whereas the loss of consciousness is associated with stage II anesthesia. Stage IV anesthesia is an undesirable stage associated with respiratory and cardiovascular failure.
10. **The answer is D.** Nitrous oxide is an anesthetic gas that has good analgesic and sedative properties without the skeletal muscle–relaxing effects. It can be used along with other inhaled agents decreasing their concentrations and thus their side effects. Enflurane produces anesthesia, hypnosis, and muscle relaxation, as do the others, and is very pungent. Thiopental is a barbiturate

that is too short acting for this application. Halothane has a pleasant odor and produces a smooth and relatively rapid induction but decreases cardiac output and can result in an unpredictable hepatotoxicity. Isoflurane is associated with more rapid induction and recovery than halothane and may have some benefits in patients with ischemic heart disease.

11. **The answer is A.** Ketamine is a dissociative anesthetic related to phencyclidine (PCP) and is thought to block glutamic acid *N*-methyl-D-aspartate (NMDA) receptors. Its use is associated with distortions of reality, terrifying dreams, and delirium, more commonly in adults. Malignant hyperthermia may be associated with any of the inhaled anesthetics, such as halothane, in genetically prone individuals. Halothane and isoflurane sensitize the heart to catecholamines. Desflurane is especially irritating to airways, and enflurane can reduce cardiac output.

12. **The answer is D.** Fetal alcohol syndrome is a leading cause of congenital abnormalities, including microcephaly, growth retardation, and congenital heart defects. Abruptio placentae is more typical with maternal use of cocaine during pregnancy. Spina bifida is associated with valproic acid use during pregnancy. Fetal hemorrhage is a consequence of warfarin use during pregnancy. Cerebral palsy is caused by traumatic injury to the developing brain.

13. **The answer is E.** Ecstasy has preferential affinity for the serotonin reuptake transporter and increases the extracellular concentration of serotonin. Its use is often associated with "rave" parties. Phencyclidine (PCP) is an antagonist at the *N*-methyl-D-aspartate (NMDA) receptor, causing euphoria and hallucinations. Marijuana causes euphoria, uncontrollable laughter, loss of time perception, and increased introspection. It binds to the cannabinol CB_1 receptor. Benzodiazepines act on the GABA receptors. Amphetamines increase dopamine and norepinephrine levels.

14. **The answer is A.** Cocaine is cardiotoxic and can cause arrhythmias that can be life threatening. These effects are even more likely when alcohol is also consumed. Cocaine causes vasoconstriction, and snorting the drug causes necrosis and eventual perforation of the nasal septum. γ-Hydroxybutyric acid (GHB) is used as a "date rape" drug. Lysergic acid diethylamide (LSD) causes increased sensory awareness, perceptual distortions, and altered consciousness. Phencyclidine (PCP) can cause euphoria, hallucinations, an increased sense of isolation and loneliness, and increased aggression. Marijuana causes euphoria, laughter, a loss of time perception, and increased introspection.

Chapter 5

Drugs Acting on the Renal System

Competencies Addressed: PH1.24

I. DIURETICS

A. Introduction

1. ***Function.*** Diuretics **increase urine production** by acting on the kidney (Fig. 5.1). Most agents affect water balance indirectly by altering electrolyte reabsorption or secretion. Osmotic agents affect water balance directly.
2. ***Effects.*** **Natriuretic diuretics** produce diuresis, associated with **increased sodium (Na^+) excretion**, which results in a **concomitant loss of water** and a reduction in extracellular volume.
3. ***Indications.*** Diuretic agents are generally used for the management of edema, hypertension, congestive heart failure (CHF), and abnormalities in body fluid distribution.
4. ***Adverse effects.*** Diuretics can cause **electrolyte imbalances**, such as hypokalemia, hyponatremia, and hypochloremia, and disturbances in acid-base balance.

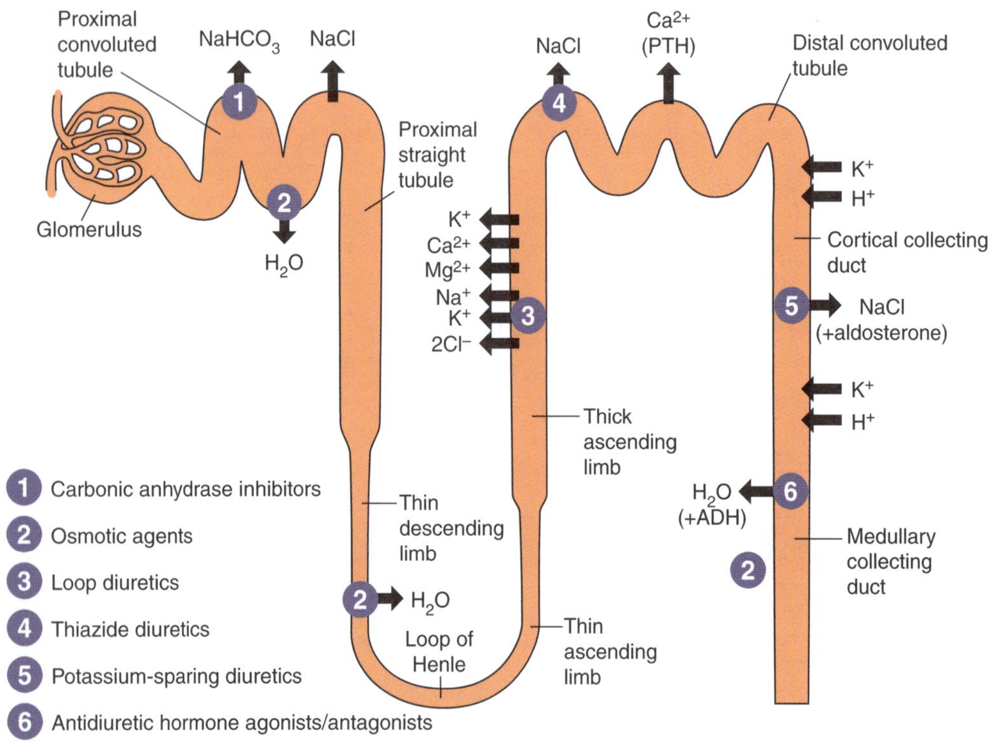

FIGURE 5.1. Sites of action of diuretic agents on the nephron.

B. Carbonic anhydrase inhibitors

1. ***Specific agents*** include **acetazolamide** and **methazolamide.**
2. ***Mechanism of action***
   a. Carbonic anhydrase (CA) is an enzyme predominately found in the **proximal convoluted tubule** of the nephron. It catalyzes the dehydration of H_2CO_3 to CO_2 at the luminal membrane and the rehydration of CO_2 to H_2CO_3 in the cytoplasm (Fig. 5.2).
   b. CA inhibitors cause **reversible inhibition of the CA** enzyme leading to reduced sodium and bicarbonate reabsorption and, therefore, **increased excretion of sodium, bicarbonate**, and water (Fig. 5.2).
3. ***Indications.*** CA inhibitors are rarely used as diuretics.
   a. These drugs are most useful in the treatment of **glaucoma**. They reduce aqueous humor production and, consequently, reduce ocular pressure.
   b. They may be used to produce **alkalinization of urine** to **enhance renal secretion of uric acid and cysteine.**
   c. They may be used for prophylaxis and treatment of **acute mountain sickness.**
   d. CA inhibitors are sometimes used as an adjuvant treatment for **epilepsy**, but the development of tolerance limits their use.
4. ***Adverse effects and contraindications***
   a. **Metabolic acidosis** may occur due to a reduction in bicarbonate stores. Urine alkalinity decreases the solubility of calcium (Ca^{2+}) salts and increases the risk for **renal calculi** formation (kidney stones). **Potassium (K^+) wasting** may be severe.
   b. Drowsiness and paresthesias are common following large doses.
   c. These agents are **sulfonamide derivatives**; therefore, precaution must be used in patients with a sulfa allergy.
   d. The use of these drugs is contraindicated in the presence of **hepatic cirrhosis.**

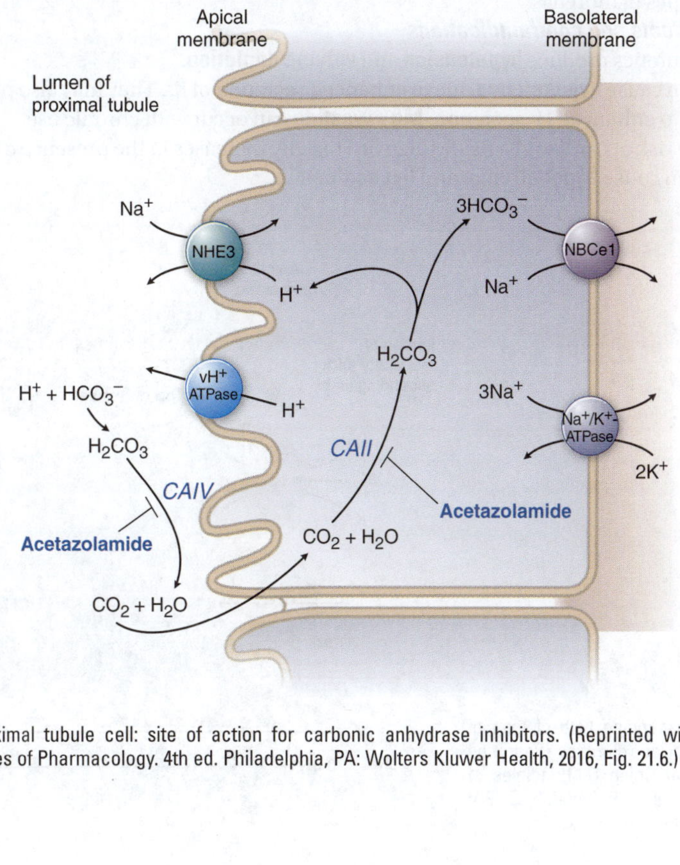

FIGURE 5.2. Proximal tubule cell: site of action for carbonic anhydrase inhibitors. (Reprinted with permission from Golan D. Principles of Pharmacology. 4th ed. Philadelphia, PA: Wolters Kluwer Health, 2016, Fig. 21.6.)

C. Loop diuretics

1. ***Specific agents*** include furosemide, bumetanide, torsemide, and ethacrynic acid.
2. ***Mechanism of action.*** Loop diuretics inhibit active sodium chloride (NaCl) reabsorption in the **thick ascending limb of the loop of Henle** by inhibiting the activity of the **$Na^+/K^+/2Cl^-$ symporter** (NKCC2) (Fig. 5.3). Diuresis occurs within 5 minutes of intravenous (IV) administration and within 30 minutes of oral administration.
   - **a.** Because of the high capacity for NaCl reabsorption in this segment, agents active at this site markedly increase water and electrolyte excretion and are referred to as **high-ceiling diuretics**.
   - **b.** They also reduce the lumen-positive potential (Fig. 5.3); therefore, magnesium (Mg^{2+}) and calcium (Ca^{2+}) excretion is increased.
   - **c.** They **block the kidney's ability to concentrate urine** by interfering with an important step in the production of a hypertonic medullary interstitium.
   - **d.** Loop diuretics cause increased renal prostaglandin production, which accounts for some of their activity. Nonsteroidal anti-inflammatory drugs (NSAIDs) can reduce the effectiveness of loop diuretics.
   - **e.** They increase systemic venous capacitance and decrease left ventricular filling pressure. This action is beneficial in patients with pulmonary edema and ensues before the diuretic action.
3. ***Indications***
   - **a.** Loop diuretics are used in the treatment of **CHF** by reducing **acute pulmonary edema** and edema refractory to other agents. When administered with thiazide diuretics, they have a synergistic effect.
   - **b.** These agents are used to treat **hypertension**, especially in individuals with **diminished renal function**. They reduce plasma volume and total peripheral resistance.
   - **c.** They may be used to treat acute **hypercalcemia** due to hyperparathyroidism or malignancy.
   - **d.** These drugs are often effective in producing diuresis in patients responding maximally to other types of diuretics.
4. ***Adverse effects and contraindications***
   - **a.** Loop diuretics produce **hypotension** and **volume depletion.**
   - **b.** They can cause **hypokalemia** due to enhanced secretion of K^+. They may also produce **alkalosis** due to enhanced H^+ secretion. **Mg^{2+} wasting** can occur with chronic use.
     - **(1)** The risk of cardiac glycoside (digoxin) toxicity increases in the presence of hypokalemia.
   - **c.** They can cause **hyponatremia** and **hypocalcemia**.

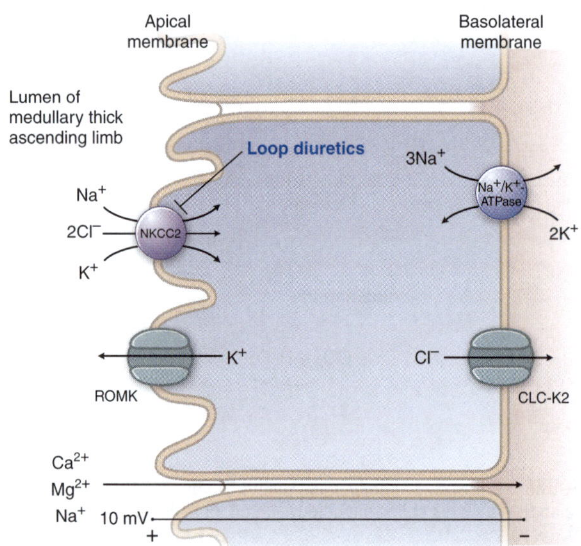

FIGURE 5.3. Thick ascending limb of loop of Henle: site of action for loop diuretics. (Reprinted with permission from Golan D. Principles of Pharmacology. 4th ed. Philadelphia, PA: Wolters Kluwer Health, 2016, Fig. 21.7.)

d. Loop diuretics can cause dose-related **ototoxicity**, more often in individuals with renal impairment.

(1) These effects are the most pronounced with ethacrynic acid.

(2) These agents should be administered cautiously in the presence of renal disease or with the use of other ototoxic agents, such as aminoglycosides.

e. They can cause **hyperglycemia, hyperlipidemia**, and **hyperuricemia**.

f. All loop diuretics, **except ethacrynic acid**, are **sulfonamides**; therefore, precaution must be used in patients with a sulfa allergy.

D. Thiazide and thiazide-like diuretics

1. *Specific agents*

a. True thiazides include **chlorothiazide** and **hydrochlorothiazide**. Chlorothiazide is the only thiazide available for parenteral use.

b. Thiazide-like drugs include **metolazone, chlorthalidone**, and **indapamide.**

(1) They have properties similar to those of thiazide diuretics but may be effective in the presence of renal impairment.

2. *Mechanism of action.* Thiazide diuretics inhibit active reabsorption of NaCl in the **distal convoluted tubule** by blocking the **Na^+–Cl^- cotransporter** (NCC) (Fig. 5.4). This results in the net excretion of sodium and an accompanying volume of water. Diuresis occurs within 1–2 hours.

a. They **decrease the diluting capacity of the nephron.**

b. These agents increase excretion of Na^+, Cl^-, K^+, and, at high doses, bicarbonate (HCO_3^-). They also **reduce excretion of Ca^{2+}**.

3. *Indications*

a. Thiazide diuretics are the preferred class of diuretic for the treatment of **essential hypertension** when renal function is normal.

(1) They are often used in combination with other antihypertensive agents to enhance their blood pressure–lowering effects.

(2) They reduce plasma volume and total peripheral resistance.

b. These agents reduce the formation of new calcium stones in **idiopathic hypercalciuria**. Thiazide diuretics may be useful in patients with **nephrogenic diabetes insipidus** that is not responsive to antidiuretic hormone (ADH).

c. They are often used in combination with a potassium-sparing diuretic to manage edema associated with renal dysfunction, hepatic cirrhosis, heart failure, and hormonal imbalances.

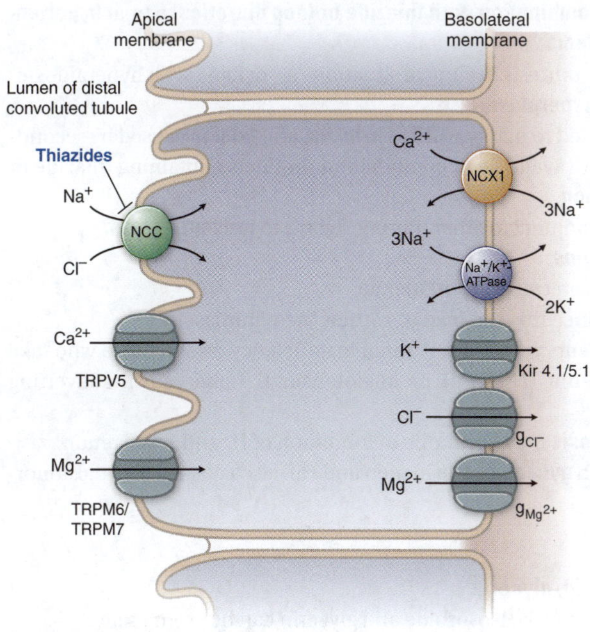

FIGURE 5.4. Distal convoluted tubule: site of action for thiazide and thiazide-like diuretics. (Reprinted with permission from Golan D. Principles of Pharmacology. 4th ed. Philadelphia, PA: Wolters Kluwer Health, 2016, Fig. 21.8.)

4. ***Adverse effects and contraindications***
   a. Thiazide diuretics produce electrolyte imbalances such as **hypokalemia**, **hyponatremia**, and **hypercalcemia**. Potassium supplementation may be required.
   b. The risk of cardiac glycoside (digoxin) toxicity increases in the presence of hypokalemia.
   c. These agents often **elevate serum urate**, presumably as a result of competition for the organic anion carriers (which also eliminate uric acid). Gout-like symptoms may appear.
   d. Thiazide diuretics can cause **hyperglycemia** (especially in patients with diabetes), **hypertriglyceridemia**, and **hypercholesterolemia**.
   e. These agents are **sulfonamide derivatives**; therefore, precaution must be used in patients with a sulfa allergy.

E. Potassium-sparing diuretics

1. ***Specific agents*** include **spironolactone**, **eplerenone**, **amiloride**, and **triamterene**.
2. ***Mechanism of action***
   a. Potassium-sparing diuretics reduce **Na^+ reabsorption** and **K^+ secretion** by antagonizing the effects of aldosterone in the collecting tubule.
   b. **Spironolactone** and **eplerenone inhibit the action of aldosterone** by competitively binding to the **mineralocorticoid receptor** and preventing subsequent cellular events that regulate K^+ and H^+ secretion and Na^+ reabsorption. An important action is a reduction in the biosynthesis of epithelial Na^+ channel (ENaC) in the principal cells of the collecting duct (Fig. 5.5).
      (1) These agents are active only when endogenous mineralocorticoid is present; the effects are enhanced when hormone levels are elevated.
      (2) **Eplerenone is highly selective** for the mineralocorticoid receptor.
      (3) **Spironolactone** binds to other nuclear receptors such as the **androgen** receptor or **progesterone** receptor. This may lead to additional side effects.
      (4) Therapeutic effects are achieved only after several days.
   c. **Amiloride** and **triamterene bind to and block the ENaC** and thereby decrease absorption of Na^+ and excretion of K^+ in the cortical collecting tubule, independent of the presence of mineralocorticoids (Fig. 5.5).
      (1) These drugs produce diuretic effects 2–4 hours after oral administration.
3. ***Indications***
   a. **Spironolactone** and **eplerenone** are not potent diuretics when used alone.
      (1) They are primarily used in **combination with thiazide or loop diuretics** to treat **hypertension**, **CHF**, and **refractory edema**.
      (2) They are also used to induce diuresis in clinical situations associated with hyperaldosteronism, such as in **adrenal hyperplasia**.
   b. **Amiloride and triamterene** are used to manage **CHF**, **cirrhosis**, and **edema** caused by secondary hyperaldosteronism. They are available in combination products containing thiazide or loop diuretics to treat **hypertension**.
   c. Often times, they are used as an adjunct to other diuretic agents to **prevent K^+ loss**.
4. ***Adverse effects and contraindications***
   a. All potassium-sparing diuretics can cause **hyperkalemia**.
      (1) Precaution must be taken since this can lead to cardiac arrhythmias.
      (2) The risk is increased in patients with chronic renal insufficiency and in those who take medications that inhibit renin (NSAIDs) or angiotensin II (angiotensin-converting enzyme inhibitors).
   b. **Hyperchloremic metabolic acidosis** may occur due to inhibition of H^+ and K^+ secretion.
   c. **Spironolactone** is associated with **gynecomastia** in men and can also cause menstrual abnormalities in women.

F. Osmotic diuretics

1. ***Specific agents.*** **Mannitol, isosorbide, glycerin**.
   a. Mannitol is administered intravenously. Isosorbide and glycerin can be given orally.

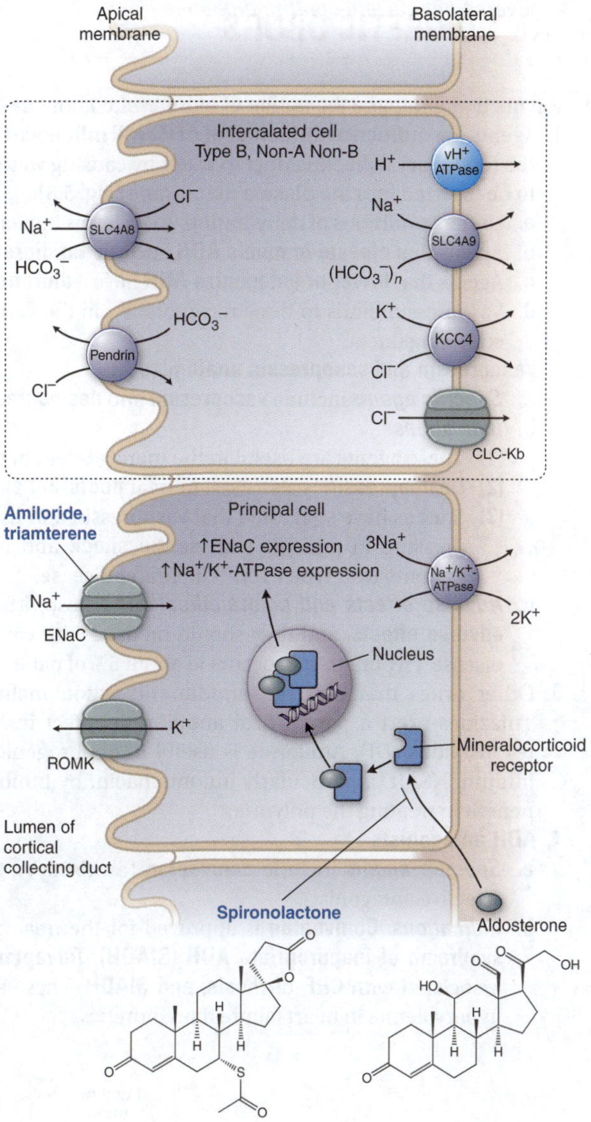

FIGURE 5.5. Cortical collecting duct: site of action for potassium-sparing diuretics. (Reprinted with permission from Golan D. Principles of Pharmacology. 4th ed. Philadelphia, PA: Wolters Kluwer Health, 2016, Fig 21.9.)

2. ***Mechanism of action***. Mannitol is **easily filtered** at the glomerulus but **poorly reabsorbed**. It increases the osmotic pressure of the glomerular filtrate, which **inhibits reabsorption of water and electrolytes** and increases urine output.
3. ***Indications***
   - **a.** Mannitol is commonly used to **reduce intracranial pressure** due to trauma and to **reduce intraocular pressure** prior to a surgical procedure.
   - **b.** It is used in **prophylaxis of acute renal failure** resulting from physical trauma or surgery. Even when filtration is reduced, sufficient mannitol usually enters the tubule to promote urine output.
4. ***Adverse effects and contraindications***
   - **a.** The osmotic forces that reduce intracellular volume ultimately **expand extracellular volume**; therefore, **precaution** must be taken in patients with **CHF** or **pulmonary congestion**.
   - **b.** The volume expansion may cause adverse effects such as headache and nausea.

II. ANTIDIURETIC DRUGS

A. Agents that influence the action of antidiuretic hormone (vasopressin)

1. Agents that influence the action of ADH will influence the permeability of the luminal surface of the medullary collecting duct to water by causing water-specific water channels (aquaporin II) to be inserted into the plasma membrane (Fig. 5.6).
   a. Under conditions of dehydration, ADH levels increase to conserve body water.
   b. Agents that **elevate or mimic ADH** have an **antidiuretic effect.**
   c. Agents that **lower or antagonize ADH** have a **diuretic effect.**
   d. Vasopressin binds to three receptors: $\mathbf{V_{1a}}$ in the vasculature, $\mathbf{V_{1b}}$ in the brain, and $\mathbf{V_2}$ in renal collecting ducts.
2. **Vasopressin and vasopressin analogues**
   a. ***Specific agents*** include **vasopressin** and **desmopressin (DDAVP)**.
   b. ***Indications***
      (1) These agents are useful in the management of **central diabetes insipidus**.
      (2) **Desmopressin** is also used to treat **nocturnal enuresis**.
      (3) Studies have suggested that vasopressin and its analogues are useful to maintain blood pressure in patients with **septic shock** and to increase **clotting factor VIII** in some patients with type I von Willebrand disease.
   c. ***Adverse effects and contraindications.*** These drugs can produce serious **cardiac-related adverse effects**, and they should be used with caution in individuals with coronary artery disease. Hyponatremia occurs in about 5% of patients.
3. Other drugs that exert an antidiuretic action include thiazides, amiloride, and NSAIDs. Thiazides exert a paradoxical antidiuretic effect in both pituitary and nephrogenic diabetes insipidus (DI). Amiloride is useful in nephrogenic DI, particularly when it is induced by lithium. NSAIDs, particularly indomethacin, by inhibiting renal prostaglandin synthesis can benefit in treating the polyuria.
4. **ADH antagonists**
   a. ***Specific agents*** include **conivaptan** (a mixed V_{1a} and V_2 antagonist) and **tolvaptan** (a V_2 selective antagonist).
   b. ***Indications.*** **Conivaptan** is approved for the treatment of **hypervolemic hyponatremia and syndrome of inappropriate ADH (SIADH). Tolvaptan** is approved for treating **hyponatremia** associated with **CHF, cirrhosis, and SIADH**. These agents may be more effective in treating hypervolemia in heart failure than diuretics.

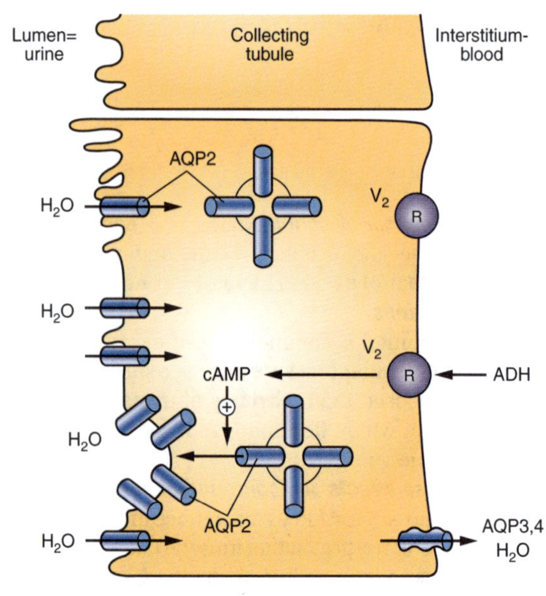

FIGURE 5.6. Medullary collecting duct: site of action for ADH agonists and antagonists.

c. ***Adverse effects*** may include nausea and xerostomia. Rapid correction of hyponatremia (>12 mEq/L/24 h) may cause **osmotic demyelination.**

(1) Symptoms of **osmotic demyelination** may include lethargy, confusion, behavioral disturbances, movement disorders, paresis, or seizures.

d. Nonreceptor antagonists of ADH action include **demeclocycline** and **lithium carbonate.** They may be useful in the treatment of **SIADH.**

(1) Adverse effects of demeclocycline

(a) It may cause photosensitivity.

(b) Dose-dependent nephrogenic diabetes insipidus is common with use (reversible on discontinuation).

(c) It may lead to tooth discoloration or tissue hyperpigmentation in children.

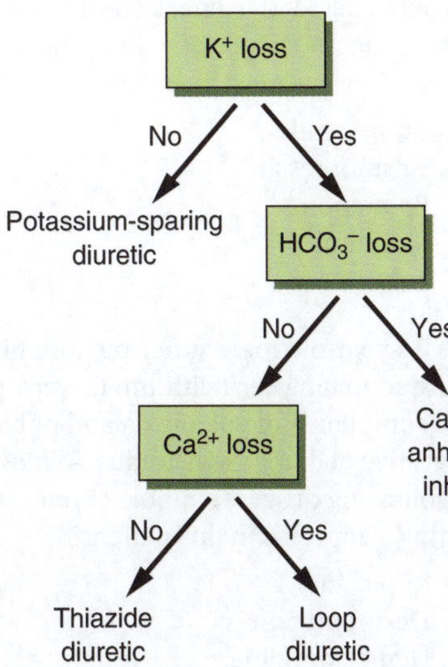

FIGURE 5.7. Identification of drug class based on plasma electrolyte changes.

DRUG SUMMARY TABLE

See Figure 5.7

Carbonic Anhydrase Inhibitors
Acetazolamide
Dichlorphenamide
Methazolamide

Loop Diuretics
Bumetanide
Ethacrynic acid
Furosemide
Torsemide

Thiazide Diuretics
Chlorothiazide
Hydrochlorothiazide

Thiazide-Like Diuretics
Chlorthalidone
Indapamide
Metolazone

Potassium-Sparing Diuretics
Amiloride
Eplerenone
Spironolactone
Triamterene

Osmotic Diuretics
Mannitol
Urea

Antidiuretic Hormone Agonists
Desmopressin
Vasopressin

Vasopressin Antagonists
Conivaptan
Demeclocycline
Lithium carbonate
Tolvaptan

Review Test

Directions: Select the best answer for each question.

1. A 35-year-old woman presents to her primary care office for her annual physical examination. She has no complaints. On examination, her blood pressure is slightly elevated at 145/85 mm Hg. She is physically fit and follows a healthy diet. Her doctor prescribes hydrochlorothiazide. What is the mechanism of action of this medication?

(A) Decreases net excretion of chloride, sodium, and potassium
(B) Increases excretion of calcium
(C) Inhibits reabsorption of sodium in the early distal convoluted tubule
(D) Inhibits reabsorption of sodium in the thick ascending limb of the loop of Henle
(E) Interferes with potassium secretion

2. A 7-year-old boy is brought to his pediatrician's office by his mother. He complains of sharp pain in his flanks, as well as dysuria and frequency. The doctor orders a 24-hour urine calcium test, and the results are abnormal. After additional workup, the child is diagnosed with idiopathic hypercalciuria and is started on a new medication. Which of the following medications was most likely prescribed?

(A) Acetazolamide
(B) Furosemide
(C) Hydrochlorothiazide
(D) Mannitol
(E) Spironolactone

3. A 45-year-old man with a history of hypertension treated with diuretic therapy presents to his doctor with complaints of a painful, swollen left big toe. Further testing reveals increased uric acid levels. Which of the following medications most likely caused this patient presentation?

(A) Acetazolamide
(B) Amiloride
(C) Hydrochlorothiazide
(D) Mannitol
(E) Spironolactone

4. A 63-year-old woman with euvolemic hyponatremia due to heart failure was started on a medication to help with the excretion of free water with minimal electrolyte loss. The physician decided to check labs frequently due to the concern for osmotic demyelination. What medication was most likely prescribed?

(A) Bumetanide
(B) Desmopressin
(C) Eplerenone
(D) Mannitol
(E) Tolvaptan

5. A 24-year-old male suffering from bipolar disorder on long-term lithium therapy presents with complaints of polydipsia and polyuria suggestive of diabetes insipidus. Which of the following drugs is suitable to relieve the presenting symptoms in this patient?

(A) Amiloride
(B) Desmopressin
(C) Demeclocycline
(D) Tolvaptan
(E) Terlipressin

6. An 87-year-old woman is admitted to the hospital and started on gentamicin for the treatment of an intra-abdominal infection. After 3 days of therapy, she complains of dizziness and tinnitus. The doctor is concerned about a drug interaction between the gentamicin and one of her medications used for swelling. Which of the following agents was the patient most likely taking?

(A) Torasemide
(B) Hydrochlorothiazide
(C) Mannitol
(D) Urea
(E) Spironolactone

7. A 54-year-old man develops congestive heart failure (CHF) after suffering his second myocardial infarction. His physician starts him on several new medications, including furosemide. At the follow-up examination, the patient is found to have hypokalemia. The addition of which medication may help resolve the hypokalemia and treat the CHF?

(A) Acetazolamide
(B) Allopurinol
(C) Ethacrynic acid
(D) Hydrochlorothiazide
(E) Spironolactone

8. A 60-year-old man presents to his family physician for his annual physical examination. On examination, the patient is found to be hypertensive. Laboratory results show low levels of potassium, high levels of aldosterone, and low levels of renin. The patient is diagnosed with Conn syndrome, or hyperaldosteronism. A computed tomographic (CT) scan of the abdomen reveals bilateral adrenal hyperplasia, which renders the patient inoperable; therefore, he is started on spironolactone. What is the mechanism of action of this agent?

(A) Blocks the mineralocorticoid receptor in the collecting tubule
(B) Increases cAMP for increased water permeability at the renal tubule
(C) Increases osmolarity of the glomerular filtrate to block tubular reabsorption of water
(D) Inhibits activity of the $Na^+/K^+/2Cl^-$ symporter in the thick ascending limb of the loop of Henle
(E) Inhibits carbonic anhydrase to blunt $NaHCO_3$ reabsorption in the proximal convoluted tubule

9. A 45-year-old woman with a long history of alcohol abuse presents to her physician for the treatment of cirrhosis-associated ascites. She is started on a new diuretic to improve the edema caused by cirrhosis. One month later, the patient returns for a checkup and her blood work shows the following results:

Na^+ 136 mEq/L (normal: 136–145 mEq/L)
Bicarbonate 23 mEq/L (normal: 22–28 mEq/L)
K^+ 5.2 mEq/L (normal: 3.5–5.0 mEq/L)
Ca^{2+} 9.9 mg/dL (normal: 8.5–10.5 mg/dL)
Uric acid 5.2 mg/dL (normal: 3.0–8.2 mg/dL)

Which of the following medications was most likely prescribed to the patient?

(A) Acetazolamide
(B) Amiloride
(C) Furosemide
(D) Hydrochlorothiazide
(E) Torsemide

10. A 57-year-old man develops progressive vision loss with a sensation of pressure behind his eyes. The ophthalmologist diagnoses the patient with glaucoma. To prevent further progression of the disease and to alleviate current symptoms, the physician starts the patient on acetazolamide therapy. What is the mechanism of action of this medication?

(A) Increases excretion of hydrogen
(B) Increases rate of formation of bicarbonate in the aqueous humor
(C) Increases uptake of sodium in the proximal tubule
(D) Inhibits carbonic anhydrase in all parts of the body
(E) Reduces reabsorption of bicarbonate

11. A 50-year-old man with mild hypertension presents to his physician with complaints of discomfort in his chest. He has slightly enlarged fat deposits in his breasts with prominent nipples. Which of the following medications most likely caused this patient presentation?

(A) Acetazolamide
(B) Amiloride
(C) Hydrochlorothiazide
(D) Metolazone
(E) Spironolactone

12. A patient has a history of anaphylaxis to trimethoprim/sulfamethoxazole. Which of the following diuretics, if required, can be prescribed to this patient?

(A) Acetazolamide
(B) Bumetanide
(C) Chlorthalidone
(D) Eplerenone
(E) Torsemide

Answers and Explanations

1. **The answer is C.** Thiazide diuretics inhibit active reabsorption of sodium chloride in the early distal convoluted tubule of the nephron by interfering with the Na/Cl cotransporter, resulting in net excretion of sodium and water. These agents increase net excretion of chloride, sodium, and potassium. They decrease excretion of calcium. Inhibiting reabsorption of sodium chloride in the thick ascending limb of the loop of Henle describes the mechanism of action of loop diuretics. Interfering with potassium secretion refers to the mechanism of action of potassium-sparing diuretics.
2. **The answer is C.** Thiazide diuretics, like hydrochlorothiazide, decrease excretion of calcium and thus can be used for idiopathic hypercalciuria. Loop diuretics, such as furosemide, stimulate tubular calcium excretion and can thus be used to treat hypercalcemia. Carbonic anhydrase inhibitors (acetazolamide), potassium-sparing diuretics (spironolactone), and osmotic diuretics (mannitol) do not have a significant impact on net calcium balance.
3. **The answer is C.** The patient is most likely experiencing a gout attack. Hydrochlorothiazide, a thiazide diuretic, can precipitate a gouty attack in predisposed individuals; this is because these agents increase serum uric acid as a result of competition for the organic acid carrier. Loop diuretics can also have this effect. The other agents listed do not have a significant impact on uric acid levels.
4. **The answer is E.** Tolvaptan, a vasopressin receptor antagonist, increases the excretion of free water without serum electrolyte loss to help with net fluid loss. It is indicated for hyponatremia, although caution must be used since rapid correction can potentially cause osmotic demyelination.
5. **The answer is A.** Desmopressin is not effective in nephrogenic diabetes insipidus. Similarly, terlipressin, which is mainly used for its vasoconstrictor action in bleeding esophageal varices, is not effective for this condition. Demeclocycline and tolvaptan are vasopressin antagonists, and, hence, are not useful in diabetes insipidus. Amiloride is used to treat lithium-induced diabetes insipidus. It is important to monitor the serum concentration of lithium as amiloride can increase renal reabsorption of lithium and predispose to toxicity.
6. **The answer is A.** Ototoxicity, as demonstrated by tinnitus and dizziness, is a potential adverse effect of loop diuretics. This effect is magnified when aminoglycoside antibiotics are added to the regimen. The other diuretic classes are not associated with ototoxicity.
7. **The answer is E.** Spironolactone is commonly added for the treatment of CHF since it counteracts the loss of potassium caused by the loop diuretics, such as furosemide. This agent is also effective in reducing the symptoms of refractory edema. Allopurinol is not used to treat CHF. Hydrochlorothiazide will exacerbate hypokalemia caused by the loop diuretics. Acetazolamide will not counteract hypokalemia. Ethacrynic acid is an example of another loop diuretic.
8. **The answer is A.** Spironolactone interferes with the action of the mineralocorticoid receptor and prevents cellular events that regulate potassium and hydrogen secretion and sodium reabsorption. It is an antagonist of mineralocorticoid receptors. It decreases the synthesis of sodium channels in the principal cells of the collecting ducts.
9. **The answer is B.** Amiloride, a potassium-sparing diuretic, can cause increased potassium levels. Hyperkalemia, a potentially life-threatening side effect, should be recognized as a possible result of amiloride use. The other agents are not potassium-sparing diuretics and are more likely to cause decreased potassium levels.
10. **The answer is D.** Acetazolamide belongs to a class of medications termed carbonic anhydrase inhibitors. These agents reduce bicarbonate reabsorption in the proximal tubule. They inhibit

carbonic anhydrase in all parts of the body, including the aqueous humor, which makes these agents very useful in the treatment of glaucoma. Acetazolamide inhibits excretion of hydrogen and concomitant sodium uptake.

11. **The answer is E.** Spironolactone antagonizes the action of the mineralocorticoid, progesterone, and androgen receptors. Inhibition of androgen receptors can lead to gynecomastia and breast tenderness, most often in men.

12. **The answer is D.** The best option for a patient with a severe allergy to sulfa is eplerenone. Diuretics that do not contain a sulfonamide group (such as amiloride, eplerenone, ethacrynic acid, spironolactone, and triamterene) are safe for patients with an allergy to sulfa. All other diuretics listed have the potential for cross-allergenicity (including anaphylaxis and skin rash) with sulfonamide-related compounds.

Chapter 6

Drugs Acting on the Cardiovascular System

Competencies Addressed: PH1.26–PH1.31

I. ANTIHYPERTENSIVE DRUGS

A. Principles of blood pressure regulation

1. **Blood pressure** is regulated by cardiac output, peripheral vascular resistance, and intravascular volume (controlled at the kidney).
2. **Baroreflexes adjust moment-to-moment blood pressure.** Carotid baroreceptors respond to stretch, and their activation inhibits sympathetic discharge.
3. The **renin–angiotensin system** provides tonic, longer-term regulation of blood pressure. Reduction in renal perfusion pressure results in increased reabsorption of salt and water. Decreased renal pressure stimulates **renin production** and leads to enhanced levels of **angiotensin II.** This agent, in turn, causes resistance vessels to constrict and stimulates aldosterone synthesis, which ultimately increases the absorption of sodium and water by the kidney.

B. Hypertension

The Joint National Committee (JNC) 8 guidelines define hypertension as systolic blood pressure (SBP) ≥140 mm Hg or diastolic blood pressure (DBP) ≥90 mm Hg, while the 2017 American College of Cardiology/American Heart Association (ACC/AHA) guidelines define it as SBP ≥130 mm Hg or DBP ≥80 mm Hg (Table 6.1).

C. Goal of therapy

1. The goal of the therapy is to **reduce elevated blood pressure**, which could ultimately lead to **end-organ damage, increased risk of stroke**, and **myocardial infarction (MI)** if left uncontrolled.
2. This goal is achieved through the use of various drug classes, and treatment often involves a **combination of agents** (Table 6.2).

TABLE 6.1 Classification of Hypertension

Category	Systolic Blood Pressure (mm Hg)	Diastolic Blood Pressure (mm Hg)
Optimal	<120	<80
Normal	120–129	80–84
High-normal	130–139	85–89
Grade 1 hypertension	140–159	90–99
Grade 2 hypertension	160–179	100–109
Grade 3 hypertension	≥180	≥110
Isolated systolic hypertension	≥140	<90
Isolated diastolic hypertension	<140	≥90

TABLE 6.2 Antihypertensive Drugs

Class	Drug	Adverse Effects	Indications
Diuretics			
Thiazide and thiazide-like diuretics	Chlorothiazide, hydrochlorothiazide, chlorthalidone, metolazone, indapamide	Hypokalemia, hyperuricemia, hyperglycemia	Monotherapy to treat moderate hypertension; in combination with other classes of drugs to treat severe hypertension
Loop diuretics	Furosemide, bumetanide, ethacrynic acid	Hypokalemia, hypomagnesemia, hyperuricemia, hypocalcemia, hypotension, volume depletion	Used in hypertension refractory to thiazide diuretics; used in the presence of azotemia
Potassium-sparing diuretics	Triamterene, spironolactone, amiloride	Hyperkalemia	Used in combination with a thiazide or loop diuretic to avoid potassium depletion
Peripheral sympatholytics			
β-Adrenergic antagonists	■ Nonselective (β_1 and β_2): Propranolol, timolol, nadolol, pindolol, penbutolol, carteolol ■ β_1-Selective: Acebutolol, atenolol, metoprolol	Fatigue, reduced exercise tolerance, bradycardia, masked hypoglycemia	Hypertension; may be combined with a diuretic for additive effects, or with a diuretic plus an α-adrenoceptor antagonist for resistant hypertension; also diminish cardiac oxygen demand
α_1- and β-adrenoceptor antagonists	Carvedilol, labetalol	Similar to other β-blockers; more likely to cause orthostatic hypotension and sexual dysfunction	May be useful in CHF
α_1-Adrenoceptor antagonists	Prazosin, terazosin, doxazosin	First-dose syncope, orthostatic hypotension	Monotherapy for mild-to-moderate hypertension; may be useful with a diuretic and a β-adrenoceptor antagonist
Inhibitors of renin–angiotensin			
Angiotensin-converting enzyme (ACE) inhibitors	Captopril, enalapril, lisinopril, ramipril, quinapril	Hyperkalemia, cough	Mild-to-severe hypertension
Angiotensin II receptor antagonists	Losartan potassium	Hyperkalemia, cough	Mild-to-severe hypertension
Renin inhibitor	Aliskiren	Hyperkalemia	Mild-to-severe hypertension
Calcium channel blockers	Nicardipine, nifedipine, felodipine	Peripheral edema	Hypertension
Central sympatholytics	Methyldopa, clonidine, guanabenz	Dry mouth, sedation, lethargy, depression	Chronic hypertension
Adrenergic neuronal blocking drugs	Guanadrel	Orthostatic hypotension; severe hypotension in presence of pheochromocytoma	Severe refractory hypertension
Vasodilators			
Arteriolar vasodilators	Hydralazine, minoxidil	Lupus-like syndrome may occur with hydralazine; minoxidil may cause severe volume retention	Hypertension refractory to β-blocker/thiazide diuretic combination
Arteriolar and venule vasodilator	Sodium nitroprusside	Excessive decrease in blood pressure may occur	Emergency situations in which rapid reduction in blood pressure is desired

CHF, congestive heart failure.

D. Principles of the renin–angiotensin system

1. Several parameters regulate the **release of renin** from the kidney cortex.
   a. Reduced arterial pressure, decreased sodium delivery to the cortex, increased sodium at the distal tubule, and stimulation of sympathetic activity all increase renin release.
2. Renin cleaves the protein angiotensinogen and releases angiotensin 1, receptor (AT1).
   a. AT1 is converted to angiotensin II by the activity of angiotensin-converting enzyme (ACE).
   b. Angiotensin II is a potent vasoconstrictor and stimulates the release of aldosterone, causing sodium and water retention.
3. Angiotensin II acts on several subtypes of angiotensin receptors.
   a. The pressor actions of angiotensin II are mediated by AT1 receptors.
4. Angiotensin II can also be produced locally in the myocardium, kidney, adrenals, or vessel walls by the action of chymases and cathepsins.
5. Drugs that interfere with the biosynthesis of angiotensin II (ACE inhibitors), or act as antagonists of angiotensin receptors (angiotensin receptor blockers [ARBs]), are indicated in all patients with left ventricular (LV) dysfunction, whether symptomatic or asymptomatic.
   a. Since AT1 is produced via pathways other than the ACE pathway, angiotensin II receptor antagonists may be more effective and specific in reducing angiotensin II actions.
   b. ACE inhibitors are becoming increasingly important in the treatment of congestive heart failure (CHF) and have been shown to prevent or slow the progression of heart failure in patients with ventricular dysfunction.
   c. Agents that inhibit **renin activity** are also useful for treating hypertension.

E. Diuretics (see Chapter 3)

1. Diuretics increase sodium excretion, lower blood volume, and reduce total peripheral resistance.
2. Thiazide diuretics, loop diuretics, and potassium-sparing diuretics can be used for the management of hypertension.
3. ***Thiazide diuretics***
   a. Thiazide diuretics are effective in lowering blood pressure 10–15 mm Hg.
   b. When administered alone, they are used for **mild or moderate hypertension**.
   c. They may be used in combination with sympatholytic agents or vasodilators in **severe hypertension**.
4. ***Loop diuretics*** are used in combination with sympatholytic agents and vasodilators for hypertension refractory to thiazide treatment.
5. ***Potassium-sparing diuretics*** are used to avoid potassium depletion, especially when administered with cardiac glycosides.

F. ACE inhibitors

1. ***Specific agents*** include benazepril, captopril, enalapril, fosinopril, lisinopril, moexipril, perindopril, quinapril, ramipril, trandolapril, and zofenopril.
2. ***Mechanism of action.*** ACE inhibitors inhibit the production of angiotensin II from AT1 by blocking the activity of ACE1; they do not inhibit ACE2. Blocking ACE1 also **reduces the breakdown of bradykinin, a potent vasodilator.**
   a. These agents **counteract** elevated peripheral vascular resistance and sodium and water retention resulting from angiotensin II and aldosterone.
      (1) They increase cardiac output, induce systemic arteriolar dilation (reduce afterload), **cause venodilation,** and **induce natriuresis,** thereby reducing preload.
      (2) They slow the progression of heart failure in patients with ventricular dysfunction. They prevent and reverse cardiac remodeling in heart failure and increase the LV ejection fraction in patients with heart failure with reduced ejection fraction (HFrEF).
3. ***Indications.*** ACE inhibitors are very useful in the treatment of **heart failure with reduced ejection fraction, reducing risk of recurrent post-MI, reducing the progression of renal disease in diabetic nephropathy**, and in treating **hypertension.** ACE inhibitors may be less effective in African Americans than in Caucasians.
4. ***Adverse effects***
   a. These agents have the potential to cause a dry, **nonproductive cough**, which resolves when therapy is discontinued (most likely due to increased bradykinin levels). Switching to an angiotensin II receptor blocker (ARB) can alleviate this.

b. **Angioedema** (life-threatening airway swelling and obstruction) is rare but can occur at any time, especially after the first dose (most likely due to increased bradykinin levels).

c. **Hyperkalemia** is also a common adverse effect due to reduced aldosterone levels.

d. **Modest reductions in glomerular filtration rate (GFR) and small increases in serum creatinine (SCr)** may occur with ACE inhibitors, particularly in patients with preexisting renal impairment or significant renal artery stenosis.

e. Hypotension and dizziness are also potential adverse effects, especially after the first dose, particularly in patients who are volume depleted or on diuretics.

f. Hypogeusia often described as metallic taste.

5. ***Contraindications***

a. **Bilateral renal artery stenosis**

(1) Normally, in bilateral renal artery stenosis, the increased levels of angiotensin II constrict the efferent arteriole in the kidney more than the afferent arteriole; this helps to maintain glomerular pressure in the kidney.

(2) ACE inhibitors block angiotensin II and prevent constriction of the efferent arteriole, leading to fall in glomerular pressure and filtration.

b. In addition, drugs that act on the renin–angiotensin system are **teratogenic** and should be discontinued in pregnancy.

G. Angiotensin II receptor blockers

1. ***Specific agents*** include azilsartan, candesartan, eprosartan, irbesartan, losartan, olmesartan, telmisartan, and valsartan.

2. ***Mechanism of action.*** These agents bind to the AT1 angiotensin II receptor and prevent angiotensin II from binding; this blocks the effects of angiotensin II, including aldosterone release and vasoconstriction.

a. AT1 receptors are coupled to the Gq protein and IP3 signal transduction pathway.

b. ARBs have similar effects to ACE inhibitors, including **reduced preload and afterload and decreased cardiac remodeling**.

c. Bradykinin levels are not increased since ARBs do not inhibit ACE.

3. ***Indications.*** ARBs have similar indications to ACE inhibitors; they are used for the management of **hypertension**, **heart failure**, and **post-MI**.

4. ***Adverse effects***

a. ARBs are more likely to cause **hypotension** than ACE inhibitors.

b. They can also cause **hyperkalemia**.

c. Since ARBs do not cause an increase in bradykinin levels, the incidence of **cough** and angioedema are less compared with ACE inhibitors ACE inhibitors.

5. ***Contraindications.*** Similar to ACE inhibitors, ARBs are also contraindicated in **bilateral renal artery stenosis** and **pregnancy**.

H. Renin inhibitors

1. ***Specific agent.*** Aliskiren.

2. ***Mechanism of action.*** This agent is a small molecule **direct inhibitor of renin**. It inhibits the conversion of angiotensinogen to AT1.

3. ***Indication.*** It is used for the management of **hypertension**.

4. ***Adverse effects*** may include diarrhea, angioedema, and hyperkalemia.

5. ***Contraindications.*** It should not be combined with ACE inhibitors or ARBs in patients with renal impairment or diabetes due to an increase in the risk of serious adverse effects. It is also teratogenic.

I. β-Adrenoceptor antagonists (β-blockers)

1. ***Specific agents*** include acebutolol, atenolol, carvedilol, esmolol, labetalol, metoprolol, pindolol, and propranolol.

2. ***Mechanism of action***

a. β-Adrenoceptor antagonists **block the response to β-stimulation** (from epinephrine and norepinephrine) in the heart; this results in **decreased heart rate**, **blood pressure**, and **myocar-**

dial contractility, resulting in **decreased myocardial oxygen requirements. They also inhibit renin secretion by the kidneys.**

(1) Some agents, such as **pindolol** and **propranolol**, are **nonselective** and affect both **β_1- and β_2-receptors.**

(a) These agents are **contraindicated in patients with asthma** due to the potential for bronchoconstriction from β_2 blockade (β_2-adrenoceptors promote bronchodilation).

(b) **Propranolol** also **decreases serum triiodothyronine** (T_3) concentrations via **inhibition of the 5′-monodeiodinase** that converts thyroxine (T_4) to T_3.

(2) **Cardioselective agents**, such as **atenolol** and **metoprolol**, are **β_1-selective.**

(a) These agents have less chance for bronchoconstriction and vasospasm.

(3) Agents such as **acebutolol** and **pindolol** have **intrinsic sympathomimetic activity (ISA).** They are partial agonists and provide low-level β-stimulation at rest but full β-receptor blockade at times of high sympathetic activity. Overall, they **cause less bradycardia** and may be useful in patients with diminished cardiac reserve or a tendency for bradycardia.

(4) **Labetalol** and **carvedilol** also have **α_1-adrenergic receptor blockade**, leading to **additional vasodilatory actions in the arteries**. They cause decreases in peripheral and coronary vascular resistance; this is especially useful in patients with CHF.

3. ***Indications***

a. β-Blockers have many indications. They are used in the management of hypertension, **angina** and **MI, arrhythmias (bisoprolol, propranolol, atenolol, carvedilol, metoprolol)**, and **heart failure (carvedilol, bisoprolol, nebivolol, metoprolol CR)**. As per the recent guidelines (JNC VIII report), their status has been shifted to that of add-on therapy in hypertension, particularly in patients with heart failure, post-MI, and angina.

4. ***Adverse effects***

a. β-Blockers may cause **decreased heart rate, blood pressure, contractility**, and **atrioventricular (AV) node conduction**.

b. Acute withdrawal can be dangerous and lead to exacerbation of ischemic symptoms, including angina or MI.

c. Nonselective agents may increase airway resistance and exacerbate peripheral artery disease (due to β_2-blockade).

d. β_2-Adrenoceptor blockade also decreases catecholamine-induced glycogenolysis.

e. Other noncardiac effects may include dizziness, drowsiness, and headache.

(1) Blockade of β-adrenoceptors in the central nervous system decreases sympathetic activity.

f. **β-Blockers may impair endurance exercise capacity, leading to fatigue.**

g. Some β-blockers also have unfavorable effects on lipid profile.

5. ***Contraindications***

a. β-Adrenoceptor antagonists are contraindicated in the presence of bradycardia and AV block.

J. Calcium channel blockers

1. ***Specific agents***

a. **Dihydropyridines** (DHPs) include **amlodipine, cilnidipine, felodipine, isradipine, nicardipine, nifedipine, and nimodipine**.

b. **Non-DHPs** include **diltiazem** and **verapamil**.

2. ***Mechanism of action.*** Calcium channel blockers (CCBs) produce a blockade of L-type (slow) calcium channels, which decreases contractile force and oxygen requirements. Agents cause **coronary vasodilation** and **relief of spasm**; they also **dilate peripheral vasculature** and **decrease cardiac afterload.**

a. The **DHPs** are **more specific for vascular smooth muscle**; since they can reduce systemic vascular resistance and arterial pressure, they are used for the management of hypertension. Systemic vasodilation leads to a reduced ventricular afterload and decreased oxygen demand.

b. The **non-DHPs affect cardiac myocytes and nodal tissue.** Verapamil is highly selective for the myocardium, whereas diltiazem has an intermediate selectivity, with both vasodilator and cardiac depressant actions.

(1) They can be used to **reduce oxygen demand** and **reverse coronary vasospasm** in angina.

(2) In addition, they have **antiarrhythmic effects**; they can **decrease conduction velocity**, prolong repolarization, and **decrease the firing rate of aberrant impulses** in the heart.

3. ***Indications***
   a. Since the **DHPs** are potent vasodilators with little effect on cardiac conduction and contractility, they are used for the treatment of **hypertension**. They can also be used for vasospastic (Prinzmetal) and chronic stable **angina.** They are used in peripheral vascular diseases like Raynaud syndrome too. Nimodipine is of value in ischemic cerebrovascular diseases.
   b. **Verapamil** and **diltiazem** are indicated for the treatment of **hypertension**, vasospastic (Prinzmetal) and chronic stable **angina**, and **cardiac arrhythmias.**
4. ***Adverse effects***
   a. DHPs may cause **flushing**, hypotension, headache, and **peripheral edema.** Few have the potential to cause reflex tachycardia and gingival hyperplasia.
   b. Non-DHPs may cause **bradycardia** and **decreased contractility exacerbating heart failure symptoms.** Caution must be used in patients with conduction defects. They can also cause **constipation.**
5. ***Drug interactions***
   a. Verapamil may produce AV block when used in combination with β-adrenoceptor antagonists.

K. α_1-Adrenoceptor antagonists (α_1-blockers)

1. ***Specific agents*** include **prazosin**, terazosin, and **doxazosin.**
2. ***Mechanism of action***
   a. α-Adrenoceptor antagonists **lower total peripheral resistance** by preventing stimulation (and consequent vasoconstriction) of α-receptors, which are located predominantly in resistance vessels of the skin, mucosa, intestine, and kidney.
      (1) They **reduce pressure by dilating resistance and conductance vessels.**
3. ***Indications.*** These drugs may be used in the treatment of **hypertension.** They are not often recommended for monotherapy and are usually administered with a diuretic and a β-adrenoceptor antagonist. The effectiveness of these drugs diminishes in some patients due to tolerance.
4. ***Adverse effects*** include **reflex tachycardia**, dizziness, and **orthostatic hypotension**, which can occur due to the loss of reflex vasoconstriction when standing. Nasal congestion may occur due to vasodilation in the nasal mucosa. Sexual dysfunction has also been reported.
5. Nonselective α-antagonists (phentolamine and phenoxybenzamine) can be used in combination with β-blockers for hypertensive emergencies associated with pheochromocytoma (a tumor of the adrenal gland that secretes large amounts of catecholamines).

L. α_2-Adrenergic agonists (centrally acting vasodilators)

1. ***Specific agents*** include methyldopa and **clonidine.**
2. ***Mechanism of action.*** These agents **stimulate α_2-receptors in the CNS** and **reduce sympathetic outflow**; they decrease heart rate and contractility, which reduces cardiac output. The reduced sympathetic outflow to the vasculature leads to **decreased total peripheral resistance.**
   a. Clonidine's hypotensive effect is also mediated by imidazoline receptors in the brainstem. Moxonidine and rilmenidine are second-generation imidazoline drugs with less toxicity compared with clonidine.
   b. Methyldopa is a prodrug, in which the false neurotransmitter, alpha-methylnorepinephrine, exerts the effects at the α_2-receptor. It also reduces adrenergic neurotransmission in the peripheral nervous system through its actions as a competitive inhibitor of DOPA decarboxylase (which converts DOPA to dopamine).
3. ***Indications*** may include **mild to moderate hypertension**; they are often used in combination with other agents, such as diuretics. Methyldopa is rarely used due to the potential for severe adverse effects, although it is a drug of choice in pregnancy. Imidazoline receptor ligands such as clonidine are also used in opioid withdrawal, chronic pain, Attention Deficit Hyperkinetic Disorder (ADHD), and smoking cessation.
4. ***Adverse effects*** may include drowsiness, dry mouth, and constipation. Sexual dysfunction may occur. Methyldopa may cause hepatotoxicity and autoimmune hemolytic anemia.
5. ***Precaution.*** Abrupt discontinuation of clonidine may lead to **rebound hypertension.**
6. Dexmedetomidine, a selective α_2-adrenoceptor agonist with anesthetic and sedative properties, is used for procedural and intensive care unit sedation.

M. Vasodilators

1. ***General mechanism of action***
   a. Vasodilators **reduce arterial resistance or increase venous capacitance**; the **net effect is a reduction in vascular pressure**.
   b. They relax smooth muscle and lower total peripheral resistance, thereby lowering blood pressure.
2. ***Mechanism and indications for specific agents***
   a. **Hydralazine**
      (1) Hydralazine reduces blood pressure directly by **relaxing arteriolar muscle.**
      (2) This drug is used for moderate to severe hypertension and may be used in hypertensive emergency in pregnancy.
      (3) It is often used in combination with β-blockers as it can elicit the **baroreceptor reflex** and cause **tachycardia**. In addition, it may be used with diuretic agents to reduce sodium retention.
      (4) Hydralazine may cause a **lupus-like syndrome**.
   b. **Minoxidil**
      (1) Minoxidil causes vasodilation by **directly relaxing arteriolar vessels**.
      (2) Similar to hydralazine, it also elicits the **baroreceptor reflex.**
      (3) It is used for symptomatic hypertension when other agents are not effective.
      (4) Minoxidil produces **hirsutism**; it is used to reduce hair loss.
   c. **Sodium nitroprusside**
      (1) This agent causes peripheral **vasodilation** by direct acting on both **venous and arteriolar smooth muscles**.
      (2) It is used in **hypertensive emergencies** because of its rapid action. On initial infusion, it may cause excessive vasodilation and hypotension. It may also be used in acute decompensated heart failure.
      (3) Sodium nitroprusside can be converted to cyanide and thiocyanate. The risk of **cyanide toxicity** is minimized by concomitant administration of sodium thiosulfate or hydroxocobalamin.
         (a) Cyanide toxicity may cause acidosis, tachycardia, mental status changes, and death.
      (4) In addition, it can cause a conversion of hemoglobin to methemoglobin and increase the risk for **methemoglobinemia**.

N. Other agents used for hypertension

1. **Fenoldopam** is a selective **agonist at dopamine DA_1 receptors** that increases renal blood flow while reducing blood pressure. It is used for the short-term management of severe hypertension, including **malignant hypertension**.

O. Agents used in pulmonary hypertension

1. **Endothelin receptor antagonists**
   a. ***Specific agents*** include ambrisentan and bosentan.
   b. ***Mechanism of action***
      (1) Plasma endothelin-1 is elevated in patients with pulmonary hypertension.
      (2) Ambrisentan is a selective endothelin A receptor antagonist.
      (3) Bosentan antagonizes both endothelin A and B receptors.
   c. ***Adverse effects*** include headache and peripheral edema.
   d. ***Contraindications.*** Both agents are likely to cause serious birth defects and should not be administered to pregnant women.
2. **Phosphodiesterase-5 inhibitors**
   a. ***Specific agents*** include **sildenafil** and **tadalafil**.
   b. ***Mechanism of action***
      (1) These agents specifically **inhibit phosphodiesterase type 5**, the class of enzymes that are responsible for the breakdown of cGMP.
      (2) The type 5 isoform is expressed in reproductive tissues and the lung.
      (3) Inhibition of the breakdown of cGMP **enhances the vasodilatory action of nitric oxide** in the corpus callosum and in the pulmonary vasculature.

c. ***Indications***
   (1) Sildenafil and tadalafil are approved for the management of **pulmonary hypertension**.
   (2) Sildenafil, tadalafil, and other phosphodiesterase-5 inhibitors, including vardenafil, are also used for the treatment of **erectile dysfunction**.

d. ***Adverse effects*** may include **headache**, **flushing**, and ocular disturbances. More serious adverse effects may include cardiovascular issues such as arrhythmias, heart block, cardiac arrest, stroke, and hypotension.

e. ***Drug interactions.*** They are **contraindicated in patients taking nitrates**, because of exacerbation of the cardiovascular effects. They should be used with caution in patients taking α_1-adrenoceptor antagonists due to the potential for hypotension.

3. The prostacyclin (PGI_2) analogue, epoprostenol, is also approved for the treatment of pulmonary hypertension.

P. Management of hypertensive emergency

1. It is a life-threatening condition associated with severely elevated blood pressure (SBP >180 mm Hg and DBP >120 mm Hg) and acute organ damage such as neurological, renal, or cardiac dysfunction requiring immediate reduction in the BP. Intravenous antihypertensives need to be given for hypertensive emergency tailored to the type of organ damage.
2. Hypertensive urgency is accompanied by no acute organ damage and can be managed by oral medications within 24–48 hours.
3. Intravenous drugs for hypertensive emergencies include clevidipine (an ultrashort-acting CCB), sodium nitroprusside (a potent vasodilator), nitroglycerine (a short-acting nitrate), enalaprilat (active form of the ACE inhibitor, enalapril), hydralazine (a vasodilator), labetalol (α- and β-blocker), esmolol (an ultrashort-acting β-blocker), and fenoldopam (a dopamine agonist). They prevent or minimize end-organ damage. A maximum BP reduction of 20%–25% within the first hour is recommended to prevent hypoperfusion of vital organs. This should be followed by a gradual decrease to 160/110–100 over the next 2–6 hours, with a further gradual reduction over the next 24–48 hours. Oral medications can be used after 6–12 hours of parenteral therapy.
4. Hypertensive urgency can be managed by amlodipine, verapamil (CCBs), moxonidine (an α_2-adrenergic agonist), urapidil (an α_1-blocker and 5-HT_{1A} agonist), and ACE inhibitors.

II. AGENTS USED TO TREAT CONGESTIVE HEART FAILURE

A. Overview

1. ***CHF*** results when the output of the heart is insufficient to supply adequate levels of oxygen for the body.
   a. **Impaired contractility** and **circulatory congestion** are components of failure.
      (1) The capacity to develop force during systole is compromised, and increased end-diastolic volume is required to achieve the same amount of work.
      (2) Heart rate, ventricular volume, and pressure are elevated, whereas stroke volume is diminished.
   b. Compensatory **elevation in angiotensin II** production results in **sodium retention** and **vasoconstriction** and increases both matrix formation and **remodeling**.
2. **Goals of pharmacologic treatment** (Fig. 6.1)
   a. Increase cardiac **contractility**.
   b. **Reduce preload** (LV filling pressure) and aortic impedance (systemic vascular resistance).
   c. Normalize heart rate and rhythm.
   d. Several agents that are used in the treatment of hypertension are also used for the management of CHF, including diuretics, ACE inhibitors, ARBs, and β-blockers (Fig. 6.2).
3. **Drugs used in heart failure also can be classified based on the ejection fraction:**
   a. HFrEF ≤40%: ACE inhibitors, ARBs, β-blockers, mineralocorticoid receptor antagonists, combination of valsartan with sacubitril (a neprilysin inhibitor), digoxin, SGLT2 inhibitors, diuretics.

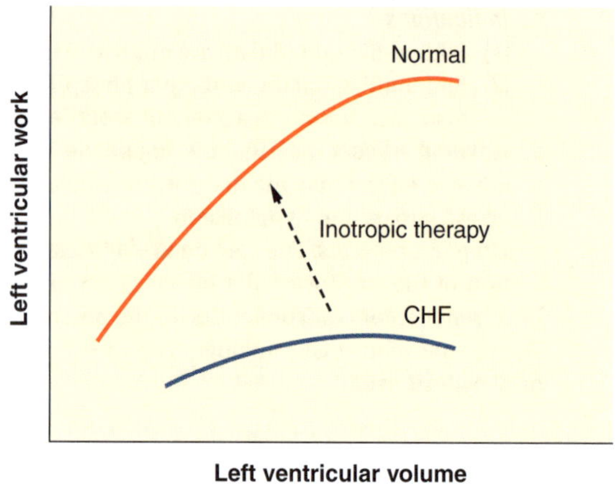

FIGURE 6.1. Pharmacologic goal in treating heart failure. CHF, congestive heart failure.

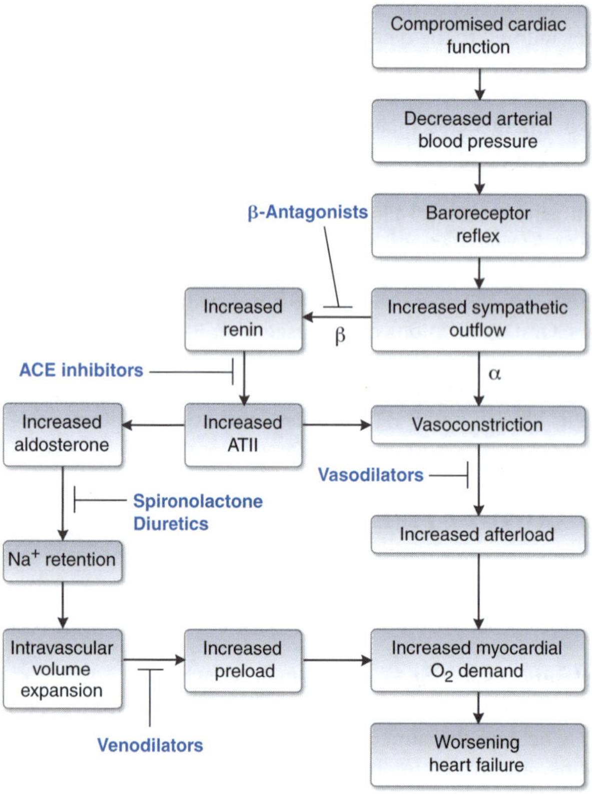

FIGURE 6.2. Pharmacologic treatment of heart failure. ACE, angiotensin-converting enzyme. (Reprinted with permission from Golan D. Principles of Pharmacology, 4th ed. Philadelphia, PA: Wolters Kluwer Health, 2016, Fig. 26.14.)

b. Heart failure with midrange ejection fraction (HFmrEF) 41%–49%: Patients may benefit with similar treatment as HErEF.

c. Heart failure with preserved ejection fraction (HFpEF) ≥50%: ACE inhibitors, ARBs, β-blockers, mineralocorticoid receptor antagonists, SGLT2 inhibitors.

B. Cardiac glycosides

1. *Specific agent.* Digoxin.

2. *Mechanism of action*

a. Digoxin **inhibits** the **sodium/potassium (Na^+/K^+)-ATPase pump in myocardial cells** leading to increased intracellular sodium (Na^+) and decreased intracellular potassium (K^+). The increased Na^+ leads to calcium (Ca^{2+}) influx via the sodium–calcium exchange pump, causing increased contractility (**positive inotropic effect**) (Fig. 6.3).

(1) Cardiac glycosides **increase stroke volume** and **enhance cardiac output**; blood volume, venous pressure, and end-diastolic volume decrease.

(2) **Improved circulation** reduces sympathetic activity and permits further improvement in cardiac function as a result of decreased systemic arterial resistance and venous tone.

b. In **supraventricular arrhythmias, digoxin enhances vagal tone.** It results in inhibition of the sinoatrial (SA) node and delayed conduction through the AV node. Overall, it **decreases heart rate and conduction velocity.**

3. ***Pharmacologic properties***

a. Digoxin has a **narrow therapeutic range**, and the dose must be individualized to maintain therapeutic effects and prevent adverse outcomes.

(1) Dosing levels for the treatment of CHF are generally lower than those required to decrease the ventricular response in atrial fibrillation.

b. It is **eliminated** by the kidneys.

4. ***Indications.*** Digoxin is used for the treatment of **CHF**. It is also used for supraventricular arrhythmias, including **atrial fibrillation** and atrial flutter.

5. ***Adverse effects and toxicity***

a. Digoxin may lead to cognitive dysfunction, **gastrointestinal distress** (anorexia, nausea, vomiting, diarrhea), and **visual disturbances**, including blurred vision or **yellow-green** disturbances (**halo effect**).

b. It may cause arrhythmias, including atrial tachycardias and AV block.

c. **Treatment of digoxin toxicity**

(1) The first manifestation of digoxin overdose is frequently fatigue or flu-like symptoms.

(2) **Potassium may help in alleviating arrhythmias.** Antiarrhythmic agents such as phenytoin and lidocaine may also be helpful in treating acute digoxin-induced arrhythmias.

6. **Antidigoxin antibodies** (digoxin immune FAB) and hemoperfusion are antidotes useful in acute toxicity.

7. ***Drug interactions***

a. **Loop and thiazide diuretics** cause **hypokalemia**, which may result in reduced competition for the Na/K-ATPase; this may **increase digoxin binding** and enhance its effects. The opposite is true for potassium-sparing diuretics.

b. Drugs that bind to digoxin, such as cholestyramine, may interfere with therapy.

c. Drugs that enhance hepatic metabolizing enzymes, such as phenobarbital, may lower the concentrations of the active drug.

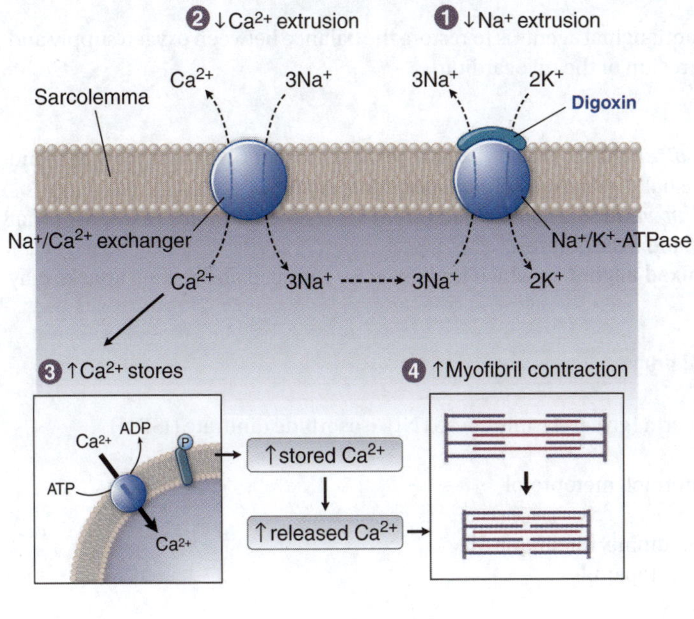

FIGURE 6.3. Mechanism of action for digoxin. (Reprinted with permission from Golan D. Principles of Pharmacology, 4th ed. Philadelphia, PA: Wolters Kluwer Health, 2016, Fig. 25.6.)

C. Phosphodiesterase-3 enzyme inhibitor

1. ***Specific agent.*** Milrinone.
2. ***Mechanism of action.*** This agent inhibits the phosphodiesterase enzyme type 3 in cardiac and vascular tissue; it causes an **increase in cyclic AMP** (cAMP), thereby activating calcium channels leading to **elevated intracellular Ca^{2+}** levels and **enhanced excitation contraction**. It reduces LV filling pressure and vascular resistance and **enhances cardiac output**.
3. ***Indication.*** It is used for short-term therapy in acute decompensated heart failure.
4. ***Adverse effects*** may include arrhythmias and hypotension.

D. Adrenergic agonist

1. ***Specific agent.*** Dobutamine.
2. ***Mechanism of action.*** Dobutamine is a synthetic catecholamine derivative that **increases contractility**; it acts primarily on **myocardial β_1-adrenoceptors** with lesser effects on β_2- and α-adrenoceptors. It **increases cAMP**-mediated phosphorylation and the activity of Ca^{2+} channels.
   a. Moderate doses of dobutamine hydrochloride do not increase heart rate.
   b. It does not activate dopamine receptors.
3. ***Indications***
   a. Dobutamine is used in **short-term therapy** in individuals with **severe chronic cardiac failure** and for inotropic support after a MI and cardiac surgery.
      (1) Since it does not substantially increase peripheral resistance, it is not useful in cardiac shock with severe hypotension.
   b. Combined infusion therapy with nitroprusside or nitroglycerin may improve cardiac performance in patients with advanced heart failure.
4. ***Adverse effects*** may include tachycardia and hypertension.
5. **Dopamine** stimulates both adrenergic and dopaminergic receptors.
   a. Lower doses stimulate dopaminergic activity and produce renal and mesenteric vasodilation.
   b. Intermediate doses stimulate dopaminergic and β_1-adrenergic activity to produce cardiac stimulation and renal vasodilation.
   c. High doses stimulate α-adrenergic receptors.

III. ANTIANGINAL AGENTS

A. Goal of therapy

1. The goal of therapy with antianginal agents is to restore the balance between oxygen supply and demand in the ischemic region of the myocardium.

B. Types of angina

1. ***Classic angina (angina of exercise, stable angina pectoris)*** occurs when oxygen demand exceeds oxygen supply, usually because of diminished coronary flow.
2. ***Vasospastic (Prinzmetal or variant) angina*** results from reversible coronary vasospasm that decreases oxygen supply and occurs at rest.
3. Some individuals have **mixed angina**, in which both exercise-induced and resting attacks may occur.

C. Classification of antianginal drugs

1. Nitrates
   a. Short acting: Nitroglycerin (glyceryl trinitrate [GTN]), isosorbide dinitrate (ISDN)
   b. Long acting: ISDN
2. β-blockers: Atenolol, bisoprolol, metoprolol
3. CCBs
   a. DHPs: Amlodipine, felodipine, nifedipine SR
   b. Non-DHPs: Diltiazem, verapamil

4. Others
   a. Ranolazine (a sodium channel blocker)
   b. Ivabradine (an I_f channel inhibitor)
   c. Nicorandil (a K^+ channel opener)
   d. Trimetazidine (a cytoprotective agent)

D. Nitrates

1. ***Specific agents*** include nitroglycerin (GTN), isosorbide mononitrate (ISMN), ISDN, and nitroprusside.
2. ***Mechanism of action***
   a. Nitrates relax vascular smooth muscle.
   b. They **activate guanylate cyclase** and increase cyclic guanine nucleotides. This activates cGMP-dependent kinases, ultimately leading to dephosphorylation of myosin light chain and **smooth muscle relaxation**.
   c. These drugs dilate all vessels.
      (1) **Peripheral venodilation decreases cardiac preload** and myocardial wall tension.
      (2) **Arterial dilation reduces afterload**.
      (3) Both actions lower oxygen demand by decreasing the workload of the heart.
   d. Redistribution of coronary blood flow to ischemic regions is increased in nitrate-treated patients.
   e. They ameliorate the symptoms of classic angina predominantly through the improvement of hemodynamics. Variant angina is relieved through the effects on coronary circulation.
3. ***Pharmacology***
   a. These drugs have a large first-pass effect due to the presence of high-capacity organic nitrate reductase in the liver, which inactivates drugs.
      (1) Nitrates have a $t_{1/2}$ of <10 minutes.
      (2) Sublingual administration avoids this effect.
   b. They form nitrosothiol in smooth muscle by reaction with glutathione.
      (1) The use of nitroglycerin for more than a few hours is associated with significant tolerance to the drug. This is thought to be due to depletion of enzymes responsible for bioactivation of the drug.
4. ***Indications for selected drugs***
   a. Nitroglycerin (GTN)
      (1) Sublingual administration is effective for **angina pectoris**, as it has a rapid onset and short duration of action.
      (2) Sustained-delivery systems are available and are used to maintain blood levels.
   b. ISMN and ISDN
      (1) These agents have a longer duration of action than nitroglycerin and are more effective for long-term management of coronary artery disease.
      (2) Both are indicated for the treatment and management of angina pectoris. Only ISDN is also used for the management of heart failure in combination with hydralazine.
      (3) ISMN is the active metabolite of ISDN; it has high bioavailability and a longer half-life than ISDN.
   c. Nitroprusside
      (1) This agent has a rapid onset of action; it is used intravenously for the management of acute hypertensive crises and for acute decompensated heart failure.
5. ***Adverse effects***
   a. These medications produce **vasodilation**, which can lead to several adverse effects, including **throbbing headache** (may be dose limiting), **flushing**, orthostatic hypotension, and reflex tachycardia.
   b. Cyanide toxicity and methemoglobinemia may occur with nitroprusside.
6. ***Drug interactions***
   a. Nitrates are **contraindicated with phosphodiesterase-5 inhibitors**, such as sildenafil and tadalafil, due to the potentiation of the vasodilatory effects of cGMP (Fig. 6.4).
      (1) This may lead to an increased risk of hypotensive effects and cardiovascular events.

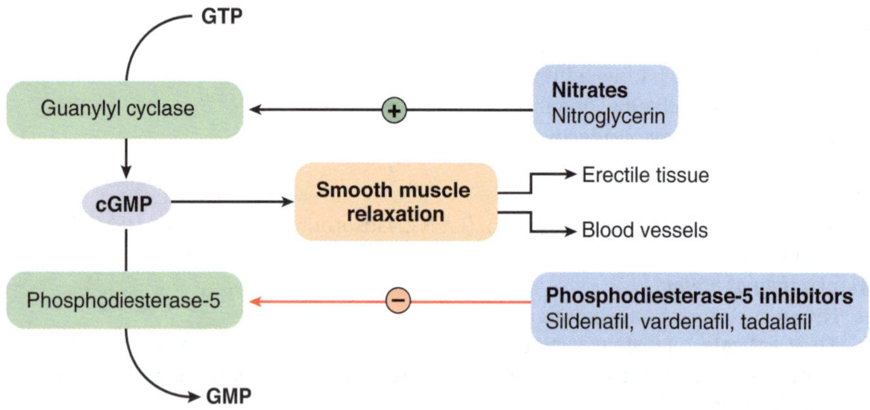

FIGURE 6.4. Drug interaction between nitrates and phosphodiesterase-5 inhibitors.

E. Dipyridamole

1. ***Mechanism of action***
   - **a.** Dipyridamole is a non-nitrate coronary vasodilator.
   - **b.** It inhibits the metabolism of adenosine deaminase and phosphodiesterase, leading to increased adenosine and cAMP.
   - **c.** It inhibits platelet aggregation and causes vasodilation.
   - **d.** It may also potentiate the effect of PGI_2 (prostacyclin) and PGD_2.
2. ***Indications***
   - **a.** The oral form may be used to decrease the risk of thrombosis in patients after artificial heart valve replacement (in combination with warfarin).
   - **b.** The intravenous version may be used as a diagnostic aid for coronary artery disease.
3. ***Adverse effects*** may include the worsening of angina, dizziness, and headache.

F. Ivabradine

1. **Mechanism of action.** It inhibits the funny electrical current (I_f channels) in the SA node leading to reduction in the heart rate without any effect on blood pressure and contractility of the heart (pure heart rate–lowering drug).
2. **Indications**
   - **a.** Stable angina pectoris intolerant to β-blockers
   - **b.** Chronic heart failure with reduced ejection fraction
3. **Adverse effects** include bradycardia and new-onset atrial fibrillation.

G. Ranolazine

1. **Mechanism of action.** It increases ATP production from glucose and improves myocardial functionality despite reduced oxygen supply.
2. **Indications.** Chronic stable angina improves exercise duration and reduces anginal attacks and consumption of nitroglycerin.
3. **Adverse effects.** These include dizziness, headache, and constipation.

H. Nicorandil

1. **Mechanism of action.** It acts by opening ATP-sensitive K^+ channels leading to vasodilation of arteries, veins, and coronary arteries. It is a vasodilator too (nitrate-like action).
2. **Indications.** It includes chronic stable angina.
3. **Adverse effects.** These include dizziness, headache, and ulceration of the skin and mucous membranes.
4. Pharmacotherapy of acute MI:
   - **a.** Relief of pain and anxiety
     - **(1)** Sublingual GTN 0.5 mg is given initially; if the pain is not relieved, administer IV GTN.
     - **(2)** Opioid analgesics: Morphine, pethidine.

b. Antiplatelet therapy: Aspirin 325 mg or $P2Y_{12}$ inhibitors such as clopidogrel, prasugrel, ticagrelor.
c. Fibrinolytic therapy
  (1) Greatest benefit occurs if administered within 3 hours (50% reduction in mortality). Mortality reduction of 10% can be achieved up to 10 hours after onset.
  (2) Fibrin-specific fibrinolytics include alteplase, reteplase, and tenecteplase to hasten myocardial reperfusion.
d. Anticoagulants to be continued till revascularization: Low-molecular-weight heparins such as enoxaparin or fondaparinux are preferred over unfractionated heparin.
e. Oxygenation: Lacks benefit in nonhypoxic patients.
f. β-Adrenergic blockers
  (1) Reduce heart rate, BP, and oxygen demand of the heart
  (2) Metoprolol, bisoprolol, carvedilol
g. Prevention of cardiac remodeling and subsequent CHF: ACE inhibitors/ARBs/spironolactone.
h. Stabilization of atherosclerotic plaque: Statins like atorvastatin.
i. Lifestyle modifications: Diet, exercise, smoking cessation, weight management.

IV. ANTIARRHYTHMIC DRUGS

A. Causes of arrhythmias

1. Arrhythmias may occur due to improper impulse generation and conduction.
  a. These manifest as abnormalities of rate or regularity or as disturbances in the normal sequence of activation of atria and ventricles.
2. Altered automaticity can arise from the following:
  a. Sinus node (sinus tachycardia and bradycardia)
    (1) Increased vagal activity can impair nodal pacemaker cells by elevating K^+ conductance, leading to hyperpolarization.
    (2) Increased sympathetic activity increases the rate of phase 4 depolarization.
    (3) Intrinsic disease can produce faulty pacemaker activity **(sick sinus syndrome)**.
  b. Ectopic foci are areas within the conduction system that may, in the diseased state, develop high rates of intrinsic activity and function as pacemakers.
  c. Triggered automaticity results from delayed afterpolarizations that reach threshold and are capable of initiating an impulse.
3. Abnormal impulse conduction in conduction pathways
  a. Heart blocks may produce **bradyarrhythmias.**
  b. Reentry circus conduction may produce **tachyarrhythmias.**

B. Review of the cardiac action potential

1. Action potentials are determined by changes in membrane conductance from the movement of ions in and out of cells.
2. Atrial and ventricular myocytes (fast-response fibers)
  a. ***Phase 0—rapid depolarization***
    (1) Rapid sodium influx occurs through fast-open sodium channels.
  b. ***Phase 1—initial repolarization***
    (1) Transient potassium channels open to return cell to 0 mV.
  c. ***Phase 2—plateau phase***
    (1) Influx of calcium occurs through L-type calcium channels.
    (2) The efflux of potassium through delayed rectifier potassium channels allows for electrical balance.
  d. ***Phase 3—repolarization***
    (1) The potassium channels remain open and calcium channels close to return membrane potential to −90 mV.
  e. ***Phase 4—resting phase***
    (1) Sodium and calcium channels are open and potassium channels are closed to keep membrane potential stable at −90 mV.

3. **Pacemaker cell action potential (SA and AV nodes) (slow-response fibers)**
   a. ***Phase 0—depolarization***
      (1) L-type calcium channels open to continue slow depolarization.
   b. ***Phase 3—repolarization***
      (1) Delayed rectifier potassium channels open for potassium efflux.
   c. ***Phase 4—spontaneous depolarization***
      (1) Depolarizing currents called "funny currents" cause the membrane potential to spontaneously depolarize.
      (2) Slow sodium channels open. Increased calcium conductance and decreased potassium conductance also occur.
   d. *These cells have automaticity and undergo spontaneous depolarization (they do not require external stimulation to initiate action potentials).*

C. Goals of therapy

1. Therapy aims to restore normal pacemaker activity and modify impaired conduction that leads to arrhythmias (Table 6.3).
2. Sodium or calcium channel blockade, prolongation of effective refractory period, or blockade of sympathetic effects on the heart achieves therapeutic effects.
3. Most antiarrhythmic drugs are classified by the Vaughan Williams classification system. The class I–IV agents are used for the management of tachyarrhythmias.
   a. Class I drugs block sodium channels. They are further divided into subclasses.
   b. Class II drugs are β-blockers.
   c. Class III drugs are potassium channel blockers.
   d. Class IV drugs are the non-DHP CCBs.
4. Adenosine and digoxin are not classified under this system; they are also used for the treatment of tachyarrhythmias.
5. In addition, atropine, which is used for the treatment of bradyarrhythmias, is not classified under this system.

TABLE 6.3 Antiarrhythmic Drugs

Group	Drugs	Mechanism	Indications
Class IA	■ Quinidine ■ Procainamide ■ Disopyramide	Moderately block Na^+ channels and K^+ channels; prolong action potentials	Suppress ventricular arrhythmias
Class IB	■ Lidocaine ■ Mexiletine	Weakly block Na^+ channels; shorten action potentials	Suppress ventricular arrhythmias
Class IC	■ Flecainide ■ Propafenone	Strongly block Na^+	Treat severe ventricular tachyarrhythmias
Class II	■ Propranolol ■ Atenolol ■ Nadolol	Block β-adrenoceptors	Suppress ventricular arrhythmias
Class III	■ Amiodarone ■ Ibutilide	Block K^+ channels; prolong refractory period	Suppress ventricular arrhythmias
Class IV	■ Verapamil ■ Diltiazem	Block Ca^+ channel	Treat reentrant supraventricular tachycardia; suppress AV node conduction
Other	Adenosine	Slows conduction time through the AV node and interrupts reentry pathways	Treats paroxysmal atrial tachycardia, including Wolff–Parkinson–White syndrome
Other	Atropine	Muscarinic antagonist	Increases heart rate in bradycardia and heart block
Other	Digoxin	Inhibits AV node conduction and increases vagal tone	Treats atrial fibrillation

AV, atrioventricular.

D. Class IA drugs (sodium channel blockers)

1. ***Specific agents*** include **disopyramide**, **procainamide**, and **quinidine**.
2. ***Mechanism of action*** (Fig. 6.5A)
   a. Class IA drugs cause moderate **blockade of fast-acting sodium channels** (in the open conformation), causing a moderate reduction in the phase 0 slope.
   b. They also **block potassium channels**, causing prolonged repolarization.
   c. They increase the action potential duration and effective refractory period.
3. ***Indications.*** These agents can be used in the management of atrial flutter and fibrillation, as well as supraventricular and ventricular tachyarrhythmias.
4. ***Adverse effects***
   a. All agents have the ability to cause **QT prolongation and torsade de pointes**, due to their potassium channel blockade.
   b. **Procainamide** may cause **drug-induced lupus-like syndrome**. It is associated with a positive antinuclear antibody test, especially in slow acetylators. Patients may experience symptoms similar to lupus, including arthritis and arthralgia.
   c. **Quinidine** can produce a cluster of symptoms called **cinchonism**, in which patients may experience **tinnitus**, headache, dizziness, and **visual changes**. It can also cause **gastrointestinal distress**, including nausea and diarrhea. It may also induce thrombocytopenia, most probably as a result of platelet-destroying antibodies developed in response to the circulating protein–quinidine complexes.
   d. These agents, especially disopyramide, have **anticholinergic activity**. They may cause dry mouth, dry eyes, urinary retention, constipation, and blurred vision.
5. ***Drug interactions***
   a. Quinidine increases digoxin plasma levels and the risk of digoxin toxicity, especially in the presence of hypokalemia.
   b. Quinidine is a strong inhibitor of CYP2D6 and may increase serum concentrations of CYP2D6 substrates. It is also a substrate of CYP3A4.

E. Class IB drugs (sodium channel blockers)

1. ***Specific agents*** include **lidocaine** (intravenous) and **mexiletine** (oral).
2. ***Mechanism of action*** (Fig. 6.5A)
   a. Class IB drugs cause **mild blockade of fast-acting sodium channels** (in the inactive, open conformation), causing a slight reduction in the phase 0 slope.
   b. They **shorten the repolarization period**.
   c. **Unlike other class I agents, they reduce the action potential duration** and effective refractory period.
   d. These agents are more **selective for hypoxic, depolarized tissue**, such as the ischemic myocardium.
3. ***Indications.*** These agents are used for ventricular tachyarrhythmias, especially after a MI.
4. ***Adverse effects***
   a. They may cause central nervous system effects, including dizziness, insomnia, **tremor**, or seizures.
   b. They may also cause depression of the cardiovascular system, including the potential for hypotension, asystole, and shock.
   c. Gastrointestinal distress may occur.

F. Class IC drugs (sodium channel blockers)

1. ***Specific agents*** include **flecainide** and **propafenone**.
2. ***Mechanism of action*** (Fig. 6.5A)
   a. These agents cause a **marked blockade of the fast-acting sodium channels** (in the closed conformation); they produce a pronounced reduction in the phase 0 slope.
      (1) They have a slow kinetic profile (slow association and dissociation).
   b. They do not have an effect on repolarization, with minimal effect on action potential duration and no effect on effective refractory period.
   c. Propafenone also possesses β-adrenoceptor antagonist activity.
3. ***Indications.*** These agents are indicated only for life-threatening supraventricular tachyarrhythmias and ventricular tachyarrhythmias.

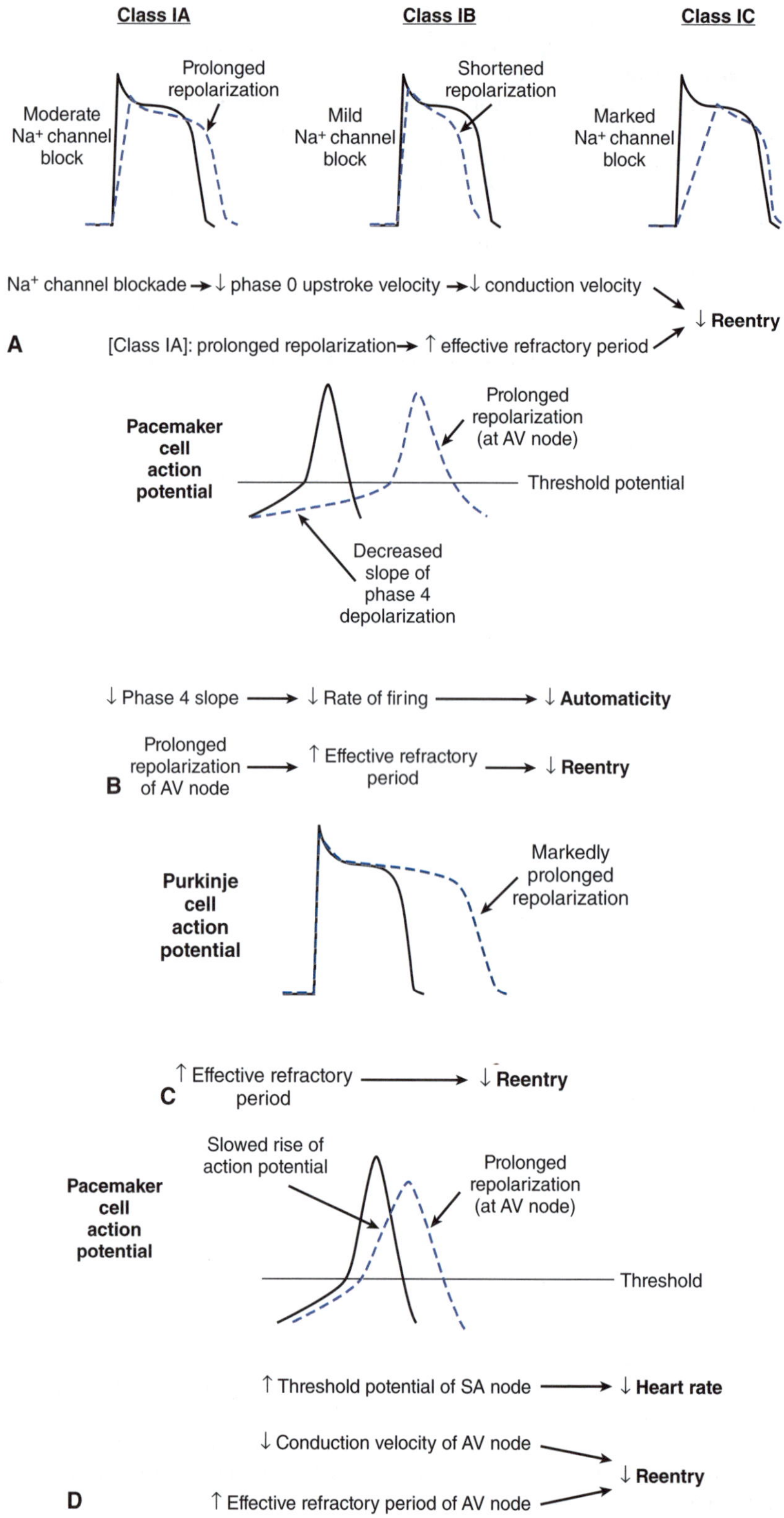

FIGURE 6.5. Effects of antiarrhythmic drugs on the action potential. **A.** Class I antiarrhythmic drugs (sodium channel blockers). **B.** Class II antiarrhythmic drugs (β-blockers). **C.** Class III antiarrhythmic drugs (potassium channel blockers). **D.** Class IV antiarrhythmic drugs (calcium channel blockers). AV, atrioventricular; SA, sinoatrial. (Reprinted with permission from Lilly L. Pathophysiology of Heart Disease, 6th ed. Philadelphia, PA: Wolters Kluwer Health, 2015, Figs. 17.12, 17.13, 17.14, and 17.15.)

4. ***Adverse effects***
   a. The use of these drugs is limited by their propensity to cause **proarrhythmic actions**. They are contraindicated post-MI and in ischemic heart disease.

G. Class II drugs (β-blockers)

1. ***Specific agents*** include acebutolol, atenolol, esmolol, and **metoprolol**.
2. ***Mechanism of action*** (Fig. 6.5B)
   a. β-Blockers block sympathetic activity at the β_1-adrenoceptors to **reduce heart rate (negative chronotropy), conduction velocity (negative dromotropy),** and **contractility (negative inotropy).**
      (1) They block adrenergic tone and decrease the slope of phase 4 repolarization.
      (2) They also caused prolonged repolarization at the AV node.
   b. They can increase action potential duration and the effective refractory period.
3. ***Indications*** include sinus tachycardia, atrial flutter and fibrillation, premature ventricular complexes (PVCs), and ventricular tachycardia.
4. ***Adverse effects*** may include hypotension, **bradycardia**, and the potential for heart block. Nonselective agents could cause bronchospasm.

H. Class III drugs (potassium channel blockers)

1. ***Specific agents*** include **amiodarone**, dronedarone, **sotalol**, **ibutilide**, and dofetilide.
2. ***Mechanism of action*** (Fig. 6.5C)
   a. These agents **inhibit potassium delayed rectifier currents**; they delay repolarization (phase 3) and prolong the action potential duration and effective refractory period.
   b. Sotalol also has class II actions.
   c. **Amiodarone and dronedarone have class I, II, III, and IV actions.**
3. ***Pharmacology***
   a. **Amiodarone** has a very **long half-life** (60–90 days).
      (1) The antiarrhythmic effects (and adverse effects) may last for months after the drug is discontinued.
   b. Dronedarone is structurally similar to amiodarone but lacks the iodine component.
4. ***Indications*** may include ventricular tachycardia (amiodarone, sotalol) and atrial fibrillation and flutter (amiodarone, dronedarone, sotalol, ibutilide, dofetilide).
5. ***Adverse effects***
   a. These agents have the potential to cause **QT prolongation and torsade de pointes** since they prolong repolarization and increase action potential duration.
   b. **Amiodarone** produces many dose-related and cumulative adverse effects, including the potential for **thyroid dysfunction** (due to iodine moiety), **liver dysfunction**, photosensitivity, corneal deposits, and **pulmonary fibrosis**.

I. Class IV drugs (calcium channel blockers)

1. ***Specific agents*** include the non-DHPs, **verapamil**, and **diltiazem**.
2. ***Mechanism of action*** (Fig. 6.5D)
   a. These agents **block the L-type calcium channels** in the myocardium during depolarization; their actions primarily occur in **nodal tissues** (SA and AV nodes).
   b. They decrease the conduction velocity and prolong repolarization at the AV node.
   c. They prolong the effective refractory period.
3. ***Indications.*** These agents can be used for the management of supraventricular tachycardia.
4. ***Adverse effects*** may include hypotension, **AV block**, and constipation.

J. Other drugs used for the treatment of tachyarrhythmias (sometimes referred to as class V agents)

1. **Adenosine**
   a. ***Mechanism of action***
      (1) Adenosine acts through specific **purinergic (P_1)** receptors.
      (2) It causes an increase in potassium efflux and decreases calcium influx.
      (3) This hyperpolarizes cardiac cells and decreases the calcium-dependent portion of the action potential.

(4) It slows conduction time through the AV node and interrupts reentry pathways through the AV node.

b. ***Pharmacology.*** It has a **very short duration of action**; the half-life is <10 seconds.

c. ***Indications***

(1) It is the drug of choice for the treatment of **paroxysmal supraventricular tachycardia**, including those associated with **Wolff–Parkinson–White** syndrome.

d. ***Adverse effects*** may include **chest discomfort**, **difficulty breathing**, dizziness, and **flushing**. Patients may experience an initial discomfort after administration, although it is **short lived** due to the short duration of action.

2. **Magnesium** decreases calcium influx and prevents early afterdepolarizations. It is used in the **management of torsade de pointes**.

3. **Digoxin** causes direct suppression of AV node conduction to increase effective refractory period and decrease conduction velocity. It **enhances vagal tone** and decreases the ventricular rate for the treatment of supraventricular arrhythmias.

K. Treatment of bradyarrhythmias

1. **Atropine**

a. ***Mechanism of action.*** Atropine **blocks the effects of acetylcholine**. It elevates sinus rate and AV nodal and SA conduction velocity and decreases the refractory period.

b. ***Indications.*** It is used to treat **bradyarrhythmias**, including symptomatic sinus bradycardia and AV block.

c. ***Adverse effects*** include dry mouth, mydriasis, and cycloplegia; it may induce arrhythmias.

2. **Isoproterenol**

a. ***Mechanism of action.*** Isoproterenol **stimulates β-adrenoceptors** and increases heart rate and contractility.

b. ***Indications.*** It is used to **maintain adequate heart rate** and cardiac output in patients with AV block.

c. ***Adverse effects*** include tachycardia, anginal attacks, headaches, dizziness, flushing, and tremors.

V. DRUGS THAT LOWER PLASMA LIPIDS

A. Overview

1. Dietary or pharmacologic reduction of elevated plasma cholesterol levels can reduce the risk of atherosclerosis and subsequent cardiovascular disease.

2. The association between cardiovascular disease and elevated plasma triglycerides is less dramatic, although **elevated triglycerides** can cause pancreatitis.

3. **Hyperlipoproteinemias**

a. **Cholesterol** is a nonpolar, poorly water-soluble substance.

(1) It is transported in the plasma in particles that have a hydrophobic core of cholesteryl esters and triglycerides surrounded by a coat of phospholipids, free cholesterol (nonesterified), and one or more apoproteins.

(2) These lipoprotein particles vary in the ratio of triglyceride to cholesteryl ester as well as in the type of apoprotein; they are identified as follows:

(a) **Very-low-density lipoprotein (VLDL)** particles

(b) **Low-density lipoprotein (LDL)** particles

(c) **Intermediate-density lipoprotein (IDL)** particles

(d) **High-density lipoprotein (HDL)** particles

b. Diseases of plasma lipids can be manifest as an elevation in triglycerides or as an elevation in cholesterol. In several of the complex or combined hyperlipoproteinemias, both **triglycerides and cholesterol can be elevated.**

B. Drugs useful in treating hyperlipidemias

1. **Inhibitors of cholesterol biosynthesis (statins)**

a. ***Specific agents*** include **lovastatin**, fluvastatin, **simvastatin**, **pravastatin**, **atorvastatin**, and **rosuvastatin**.

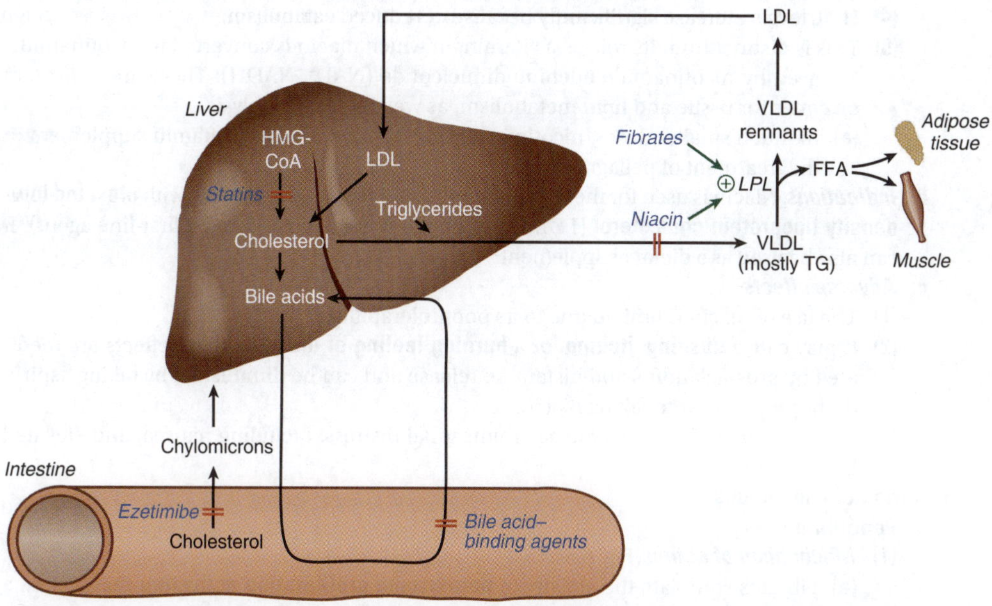

FIGURE 6.6. Sites of action for lipid-regulating drugs. CoA, coenzyme A; FFA, free fatty acids; HMG-CoA, 3-hydroxy-3-methylglutaryl coenzyme A; LDL, low-density lipoprotein; LPL, lipoprotein lipase; VLDL, very-low-density lipoprotein; TG, triglyceride. (Reprinted with permission from Lilly L. Pathophysiology of Heart Disease, 6th ed. Philadelphia, PA: Wolters Kluwer Health, 2015, Fig. 17.20.)

b. ***Mechanism of action*** (Fig. 6.6)

(1) These drugs function as competitive inhibitors of 3-hydroxy-3-methylglutaryl coenzyme A reductase **(HMG-CoA reductase)**, the rate-limiting enzyme in cholesterol biosynthesis.

(2) Reduced cholesterol synthesis results in a compensatory increase in the hepatic uptake of plasma cholesterol mediated by an increase in the number of LDL receptors.

(3) Drugs that inhibit cholesterol biosynthesis are quite effective at lowering LDL cholesterol and total cholesterol. They can **reduce total cholesterol** by as much as 30%–50% and LDL cholesterol by as much as 60%.

c. ***Indications***

(1) These agents can be used for the management of familial and nonfamilial **hypercholesterolemia**, including hyperlipidemia and mixed dyslipidemia. They can also be used for hypertriglyceridemia.

(2) They are used in the prevention of cardiovascular disease.

d. ***Adverse effects*** include **myopathy/rhabdomyolysis** (increased creatine phosphokinase [CPK]) and **elevations in aminotransferases**, with the potential for hepatotoxicity.

e. ***Drug interactions***

(1) Caution must be used with other drugs that increase the risk for skeletal muscle toxicity, such as daptomycin. The incidence of myopathy also increases with concomitant use of certain drugs like niacin and fenofibrates.

(2) Fewer drug interactions occur with pravastatin, fluvastatin, and rosuvastatin since they are not metabolized through CYP3A4.

2. Niacin (nicotinic acid) (vitamin B_3)

a. ***Mechanism of action*** (Fig. 6.6)

(1) Niacin can exert cholesterol- and triglyceride-lowering effects at high concentrations.

(2) Niacin reduces plasma VLDL by **inhibiting the synthesis and esterification of fatty acids in the liver and reducing lipolysis in adipose tissue**; it markedly decreases plasma triglyceride levels.

(3) As the substrate VLDL concentration is reduced, the concentrations of IDL and LDL also decrease, thereby reducing plasma cholesterol levels.

(4) HDL levels increase significantly because of reduced catabolism.

(5) This is distinct from its role as a vitamin, in which niacin is converted to nicotinamide, followed by nicotinamide adenine dinucleotide (NAD^+, NADH). These are important enzymes for tissue and lipid metabolism, as well as glycogenolysis.

(a) In much smaller doses, nicotinic acid can also be used as a vitamin supplement in the treatment of pellagra.

b. ***Indications.*** Niacin is used for the treatment of dyslipidemias, for patients with **elevated low-density lipoprotein cholesterol** (LDL-C) (although it is not considered a first-line agent). It can also be used as a dietary supplement.

c. ***Adverse effects***

(1) The use of niacin is limited due to its poor tolerability.

(2) It may cause **flushing**, **itching**, or a **burning feeling of the skin**; these effects are mediated by prostaglandins and histamine release and can be diminished by taking aspirin or ibuprofen prior to taking niacin.

(3) Other adverse effects include gastrointestinal distress, including nausea, and elevated liver enzymes.

3. Fibric acid analogues

a. Fenofibrate

(1) ***Mechanism of action*** (Fig. 6.6)

(a) Fibrates stimulate the activity of **peroxisome proliferating activating receptor** α, a class of nuclear receptor.

(b) Activation of these receptors alters the transcription of a number of genes involved in triglyceride metabolism, including lipoprotein lipase and apolipoprotein CIII.

(c) This **increases** the **peripheral catabolism of VLDL** and **chylomicrons**, resulting in a reduction in the plasma concentration of VLDL, most notably in triglycerides.

i. An increase in VLDL metabolism can raise LDL cholesterol, especially in patients with baseline hypertriglyceridemia.

(d) Fibrates **reduce hepatic synthesis of cholesterol**, which further reduces plasma triglycerides.

(2) ***Indications***

(a) Fenofibrate is indicated as an adjunct agent for the management of **hypertriglyceridemia**. It is also used to raise HDL.

(b) It is approved for the management of hypercholesterolemia or mixed hyperlipidemia, although it is not a first-line agent and should not be used in the absence of hypertriglyceridemia.

(3) ***Adverse effects and contraindications***

(a) A common adverse effect is elevated serum transaminases.

(b) Fenofibrate may also cause gastrointestinal distress, including dyspepsia.

(c) It can cause gallstones and myalgia.

(4) ***Drug interactions***

(a) Fenofibrate can **displace** other albumin-bound drugs, most notably the **sulfonylureas** and **warfarin**; this may increase their free fraction and augment their effects.

(b) It can increase the risk of myopathy when used with statins; therefore, close monitoring is recommended when used together.

b. Gemfibrozil

(1) ***Mechanism of action*** (Fig. 6.6)

(a) The mechanism of action for gemfibrozil is not clear.

(b) It decreases VLDL levels through **inhibition of lipolysis and decreases in hepatic fatty acid uptake**, as well as inhibition of hepatic secretion of VLDL.

(c) It also increases HDL cholesterol.

(d) It may be more effective in reducing triglycerides than fenofibrate.

(2) ***Indications.*** It is used for the management of **hypertriglyceridemia**.

(3) ***Adverse effects*** may include gastrointestinal distress, including dyspepsia, abdominal pain, and nausea.

(4) ***Drug interactions.*** It can increase the risk of myopathy when used with statins; therefore, close monitoring is recommended when used together.

4. Ezetimibe

a. ***Mechanism of action*** (Fig. 6.6)

(1) Ezetimibe **acts within the intestine** to reduce cholesterol absorption.

(a) Cholesterol is absorbed from the small intestine by a process that includes specific transporters including the **Niemann–Pick C1-like 1** (NPC1L1) protein, which is important for sterol absorption in the gut.

(b) Ezetimibe binds to and **inhibits the function of NPC1L1,** thereby reducing cholesterol absorption.

b. ***Indications.*** It is approved for **primary hyperlipidemia** and homozygous familial hypercholesterolemia.

c. ***Adverse effects*** may include fatigue, abdominal pain, and diarrhea.

5. Bile acid sequestrants

a. ***Specific agents*** include **cholestyramine, colestipol**, and colesevelam.

b. ***Mechanism of action*** (Fig. 6.6)

(1) Bile acid sequestrants are **positively charged molecules that bind to the negatively charged bile acids** in the intestines.

(a) They are hydrophilic, but they are not absorbed across the intestine.

(b) In the intestine, the resins bind bile salts and **prevent enterohepatic reutilization of bile acids.**

(c) In addition, they **impair the absorption of dietary cholesterol.**

c. ***Indications.*** Bile acid sequestrants are effective in **reducing plasma cholesterol** (10%–20%) in patients with some normal LDL receptors. This excludes patients who completely lack functional LDL receptors because of a genetic defect (homozygous familial hypercholesterolemia). They are usually reserved for second-line therapy or in combination with statins.

d. ***Adverse effects***

(1) Bile acid sequestrants produce **gastrointestinal distress**, including constipation, nausea, and abdominal discomfort. Colesevelam has fewer gastrointestinal side effects.

(2) Since they are not absorbed into the blood, they are unlikely to cause systemic effects.

e. ***Drug interactions***

(1) These agents interfere with the absorption of fat-soluble vitamins and anionic drugs, such as digoxin and warfarin.

DRUG SUMMARY TABLE

Diuretics	ACE Inhibitors	β-Adrenoceptor Antagonists (Also Class II Antiarrhythmic Drugs)
Loop diuretics	Benazepril	Acebutolol
Bumetanide	Captopril	Atenolol
Ethacrynic acid	Enalapril	Bisoprolol
Furosemide	Fosinopril	Carvedilol
Torsemide	Lisinopril	Esmolol
	Quinapril	Labetalol
Thiazide diuretics	Moexipril	Metoprolol
Chlorothiazide	Perindopril	Nadolol
Hydrochlorothiazide	Ramipril	Timolol
Methyclothiazide	Trandolapril	Penbutolol
		Pindolol
Thiazide-like diuretics	**Angiotensin Receptor Blockers**	Timolol
Chlorthalidone	Azilsartan	
Metolazone	Candesartan	**Calcium Channel Blockers (CCBs)**
Indapamide	Eprosartan	
	Irbesartan	***Dihydropyridines***
Potassium-sparing diuretics	Losartan	Amlodipine
Amiloride	Olmesartan	Isradipine
Eplerenone	Valsartan	Nicardipine
Spironolactone	Telmisartan	Nifedipine
Triamterene		Nisoldipine
	Renin Inhibitor	
	Aliskiren	

(Continued)

Nondihydropyridines (also class IV antiarrhythmic drugs)
Diltiazem
Verapamil

α_1-Adrenoceptor Antagonists (α_1-Blockers)
Doxazosin
Prazosin
Terazosin

α_2-Adrenergic Agonists (Centrally Acting Vasodilators)
Clonidine
Guanabenz acetate
Methyldopa

Vasodilators for Hypertension
Hydralazine
Minoxidil
Sodium nitroprusside

Other Agents for Hypertension
Fenoldopam

Endothelin Receptor Antagonists
Ambrisentan
Bosentan

Phosphodiesterase-5 Enzyme Inhibitors
Sildenafil
Tadalafil
Vardenafil

Cardiac Glycosides
Digoxin

Phosphodiesterase-3 Enzyme Inhibitor
Milrinone

Nonselective Adrenergic Agonist
Dobutamine

Antianginal Agents

Nitrates
Isosorbide dinitrate
Isosorbide mononitrate
Nitroglycerin
Nitroprusside

Non-nitrate coronary vasodilator
Dipyridamole

Antiarrhythmic Drugs

Class IA drugs
Disopyramide
Procainamide
Quinidine

Class IB drugs
Lidocaine
Mexiletine

Class IC drugs
Flecainide
Propafenone

Class III drugs
Amiodarone
Dofetilide
Dronedarone
Ibutilide
Sotalol

Inhibitors of Cholesterol Biosynthesis
Ezetimibe
Nicotinic acid

Statins
Atorvastatin
Fluvastatin
Lovastatin
Pitavastatin
Pravastatin
Rosuvastatin
Simvastatin

Fibric acid analogues
Fenofibrate
Gemfibrozil

Bile acid sequestrants
Cholestyramine
Colesevelam
Colestipol

Review Test

Directions: Select the best answer for each question.

1. A 62-year-old patient presents to the emergency room with complaints of palpitations and dizziness. An electrocardiogram was positive for QT prolongation (QTc = 0.61 second) and the physician is concerned about torsade de pointes. Two days prior, the patient started a new medication for the treatment of atrial fibrillation. Which of the following medications most likely caused this patient presentation?

(A) Diltiazem
(B) Lidocaine
(C) Mexiletine
(D) Quinidine
(E) Propafenone

2. A 59-year-old man presents to the emergency room with shortness of breath, chest tightness, and nausea. He is diagnosed with a non-ST-elevation myocardial infarction and started on appropriate therapy. Two hours later, the patient complains of palpitations and an electrocardiogram shows ventricular tachycardia. Which of the following medications is the most appropriate treatment for this arrhythmia?

(A) Atropine
(B) Digoxin
(C) Flecainide
(D) Lidocaine
(E) Quinidine

3. A 32-year-old woman presents to her family physician with complaints of tremors, anxiety, and heat intolerance. After further evaluation, she is diagnosed with hyperthyroidism. Which of the following medications may help decrease her symptoms?

(A) Amlodipine
(B) Digoxin
(C) Lisinopril
(D) Propranolol
(E) Verapamil

4. A 49-year-old woman presents to her primary care physician for the management of hypertension. Her past medical history is significant for severe asthma. Which of the following β-blockers would be most appropriate to use for this patient?

(A) Atenolol
(B) Nadolol
(C) Propranolol
(D) Sotalol
(E) Timolol

5. A 48-year-old man is taken to the emergency department by ambulance for a blood pressure of 220/170 mm Hg. He is diagnosed with hypertensive emergency and started on a nitroprusside infusion. Six hours later, the patient is confused. Further evaluation reveals lactic acidosis. What is the most likely cause of these symptoms?

(A) Accumulation of nitroprusside due to its long half-life
(B) Negative inotropic activity of nitroprusside
(C) Production of hydroxocobalamin from nitroprusside
(D) Production of thiocyanate from nitroprusside
(E) Renal precipitation of nitroprusside

6. A 76-year-old woman presents to her cardiologist with a 5-month history of dry cough. She denies any other symptoms. Her past medical history includes a myocardial infarction about 6 months prior, for which she was started on several new medications. Which of the following medications most likely caused this patient's cough?

(A) Digoxin
(B) Lisinopril
(C) Lovastatin
(D) Metoprolol
(E) Nitroglycerin

7. A 28-year-old woman presents to her cardiologist for the management of atrial fibrillation. The physician prescribes a new medication after several others were ineffective. A year later, the patient complains to her primary care physician about fever, myalgia, and rash. Laboratory tests reveal a positive antinuclear antibody (ANA) test. The doctor attributes her symptoms to a side effect of her antiarrhythmic medication. Which of the following medications caused these symptoms?

(A) Amiodarone
(B) Atenolol
(C) Hydralazine
(D) Procainamide
(E) Quinidine

8. A 51-year-old woman is admitted to the hospital with a diagnosis of paroxysmal supraventricular tachycardia associated with accessory bypass tracts. The physician attempts vagal maneuvers prior to pharmacologic treatment without success. The patient is treated with a medication by rapid intravenous infusion. Shortly after, she experiences chest discomfort, difficulty breathing, and flushing. Which of the following medications was administered?

(A) Adenosine
(B) Amiodarone
(C) Digoxin
(D) Diltiazem
(E) Quinidine

9. A 76-year-old man presents to his cardiologist for the management of congestive heart failure. He is started on a new medication and asked to follow up in 2 weeks. At his follow-up appointment, the patient complains of nausea and abdominal pain. His wife tells the doctor that he has been confused over the past couple of days and recently complained of vision changes. What is the mechanism of action for the medication that most likely caused this patient presentation?

(A) Blocks β_1-receptor activity
(B) Decreases vagal tone
(C) Inhibits angiotensin-converting enzyme
(D) Inhibits reabsorption of sodium in the loop of Henle
(E) Inhibits sodium/potassium-ATPase pump

10. A 67-year-old man is started on lidocaine for the management of a life-threatening ventricular arrhythmia after a myocardial infarction. Which change in the electrocardiogram will most likely occur after administration of this medication?

(A) Decreased PR interval
(B) Decreased QT interval
(C) Increased QRS interval
(D) Increased QT interval
(E) Increased PR interval

11. A 55-year-old woman is admitted to the surgical intensive care unit after a coronary artery bypass graft. She is given a dose of milrinone after developing hypotension, since her cardiac output, as measured by the Swan-Ganz catheter, is significantly lower than previous measurements. What is the mechanism of action for this medication?

(A) Activates cholinergic receptors
(B) Decreases cyclic AMP
(C) Decreases left ventricular filling pressure
(D) Decreases intracellular calcium
(E) Potentiates cardiac phosphodiesterase type 3

12. A 64-year-old man is admitted to the hospital after a right hemicolectomy for colon cancer. His past medical history is also significant for congestive heart failure. The day after the surgery, his blood pressure drops. Further evaluation leads to a diagnosis of cardiogenic shock, and he is started on dobutamine to maintain systemic perfusion and preserve end-organ performance. What is the mechanism of action for this medication?

(A) α_2-Receptor antagonist
(B) β_1-Receptor agonist
(C) β_2-Receptor antagonist
(D) Dopamine-receptor agonist
(E) Dopamine-receptor antagonist

13. An 85-year-old woman is admitted to the cardiovascular unit of the hospital due to arrhythmias. The electrocardiogram displays ventricular fibrillation, which is quickly converted to atrial fibrillation with rapid ventricular response. The physician orders amiodarone to manage the arrhythmia. The patient is worried about long-term effects of this medication. What may occur after long-term administration?

(A) Cinchonism
(B) Fracture
(C) Gingival hyperplasia
(D) Lupus
(E) Pulmonary fibrosis

14. A 56-year-old woman presents to her primary care physician with complaints of muscle pain, cramping, and weakness in her legs. Her symptoms started shortly after starting a new medication for the management of hyperlipidemia. Laboratory results are positive for an elevated serum creatine phosphokinase. After further discussion, the patient reveals that she consumes grapefruit juice on a daily basis. Which of the following drugs most likely caused this patient presentation?

(A) Daptomycin
(B) Ezetimibe
(C) Gemfibrozil
(D) Niacin
(E) Simvastatin

15. A 68-year-old man presents to his family physician with intermittent chest discomfort and occasional shortness of breath. After further evaluation, the symptoms are attributed to anginal pain and the patient is started on nitroglycerin. His past medical history is significant for hypertension and erectile dysfunction. Three days later, the patient is taken to the hospital by ambulance due to syncope and severe hypotension. He tells the doctor that his symptoms occurred shortly after intercourse. The doctor is concerned about a drug interaction with nitroglycerin. An interaction occurred with which drug may have caused these symptoms?

(A) Digoxin
(B) Milrinone
(C) Propranolol
(D) Sildenafil
(E) Verapamil

Answers and Explanations

1. **The answer is D.** Quinidine is a class IA antiarrhythmic that causes prolonged repolarization and is associated with QT interval prolongation and torsade de pointes arrhythmias. The other medications are not associated with QT prolongation. Diltiazem is a calcium channel blocker (class IV antiarrhythmic agent). Lidocaine and mexiletine are class IB antiarrhythmic agents, and propafenone is a class IC antiarrhythmic agent.
2. **The answer is D.** Lidocaine is a class IB antiarrhythmic agent that is selective for hypoxic tissue and is effective for the management of ventricular tachycardia associated with an acute myocardial infarction (MI). It does not slow conduction and has little effect on atrial function. Digoxin, quinidine, and atropine can induce tachyarrhythmias. Flecainide is contraindicated for the treatment of life-threatening ventricular tachyarrhythmias in patients without structural heart disease.
3. **The answer is D.** Hyperthyroidism may increase β-adrenoceptors. β-Adrenoceptor antagonists such as propranolol can decrease symptoms of hyperthyroidism, including palpitations, tachycardia, anxiety, tremor, and heat intolerance. In addition, propranolol slowly decreases serum triiodothyronine (T_3) concentrations via inhibition of the 5′-monodeiodinase that converts thyroxine (T_4) to T_3. The other medications will not help manage many of the symptoms associated with hyperthyroidism.
4. **The answer is A.** Atenolol is a β_1-selective agent, which is safer in patients with asthma. The other agents are nonselective (β_1/β_2). The sympathetic nerves in the bronchioles activate β_2-adrenoceptors, which promotes bronchodilation. Nonselective agents can cause β_2-blockade, which may lead to bronchoconstriction. For this reason, nonselective agents are contraindicated in patients with asthma or chronic obstructive pulmonary disease.
5. **The answer is D.** The toxicity of nitroprusside is caused by the release of cyanide and the accumulation of thiocyanate. Hydroxocobalamin is used to reduce the toxicity of nitroprusside through the formation of the less toxic cyanocobalamin.
6. **The answer is B.** Angiotensin-converting enzyme (ACE) inhibitors, such as lisinopril, commonly cause a dry nonproductive cough. It has been described in 5%–20% of patients treated with an ACE inhibitor and usually begins within 1–2 weeks of starting therapy. It typically resolves on treatment discontinuation. The other medications listed do not have this adverse effect.
7. **The answer is D.** Long-term use of procainamide can cause systemic drug-induced lupus, in which symptoms may include fever, rash, myalgia, and arthritis. A positive antinuclear antibody (ANA) test generally occurs in most patients on procainamide for more than 2 years. Although hydralazine can also cause drug-induced lupus, it is not used for the management of atrial fibrillation. The other medications do not cause drug-induced lupus.
8. **The answer is A.** Adenosine is the drug of choice for the treatment of paroxysmal supraventricular tachycardia, including those associated with Wolff–Parkinson–White syndrome. It has a very short duration of action; the half-life is <10 seconds. Adverse effects may include chest discomfort, difficulty breathing, dizziness, and flushing, although they are short lived due to the short duration of action.
9. **The answer is E.** Digoxin, a cardiac glycoside, has a narrow therapeutic index and must be monitored closely to prevent toxicity. Symptoms of acute toxicity may include gastrointestinal distress and mental status changes. Vision changes may also occur. For the treatment of heart failure, digoxin causes inhibition of the sodium/potassium-ATPase pump in myocardial cells, leading to an increase in intracellular sodium. This promotes calcium influx via the sodium–calcium exchange pump and causes increased contractility. For the treatment of arrhythmias, it increases vagal activity, resulting in inhibition of the sinoatrial (SA) node and delayed conduction through the atrioventricular (AV) node. It also decreases sympathetic tone.

10. **The answer is B.** Lidocaine is a class IB antiarrhythmic agent. It causes mild sodium channel block and shortens repolarization, leading to a decreased QT interval. Class IA drugs increase the QRS and QT intervals. Class IC drugs increase the QRS interval; they also increase the PR interval. In addition, class II and IV drugs increase the PR interval.

11. **The answer is C.** Milrinone reduces left ventricular filling pressure and thus enhances cardiac output. It inhibits cardiac phosphodiesterase type 3 and increases cyclic AMP (cAMP) and, therefore, intracellular calcium.

12. **The answer is B.** Dobutamine acts on β_1-receptors; it increases cyclic AMP (cAMP)–mediated phosphorylation and the activity of calcium channels. It does not act on dopamine receptors. It is also an agonist at β_2- and α_1-receptors.

13. **The answer is E.** Amiodarone is a class III antiarrhythmic agent that produces many dose-related and cumulative adverse effects, including the potential for thyroid dysfunction, liver dysfunction, photosensitivity, corneal deposits, and pulmonary fibrosis. Quinidine may cause cinchonism. Procainamide may cause drug-induced lupus.

14. **The answer is E.** A common adverse effect of statins, such as simvastatin, is muscle pain and cramping. Rhabdomyolysis secondary to myoglobinuria or myopathy may occur. This risk is increased with high doses and with concomitant use of strong CYP3A4 inhibitors, including grapefruit juice. Although cholesterol medications, such as fibrates and niacin, are unlikely to cause this patient presentation on their own, when used in combination with a statin, they may increase the risk for myopathy. Daptomycin can cause myopathy and elevated creatine kinase but is used for gram-positive infections, not high cholesterol.

15. **The answer is D.** Nitroglycerin stimulates cGMP production. Sildenafil, a phosphodiesterase (PDE)-5 inhibitor, prevents cGPM metabolism. Both drugs cause their vasodilatory effects through increased cGMP; when given together, they may cause a synergistic effect on blood pressure.

Chapter 7

Drugs Used in Anemia and Disorders of Hemostasis

Competencies Addressed: PH1.25, PH1.35

I. DRUGS USED IN THE TREATMENT OF ANEMIA

A. Iron

1. **Structure and storage of iron** (Fig. 7.1)
   a. Iron is an integral component of heme. About **70% of total body iron** is found in **hemoglobin**. Heme iron is also an essential component of **muscle myoglobin** and of several enzymes, including catalase, peroxidase, and cytochromes.
   b. Iron is **stored** in reticuloendothelial cells, hepatocytes, and intestinal cells as **ferritin** (a particle with a ferric hydroxide core and a surface layer of the protein apoferritin) and hemosiderin (aggregates of ferritin–apoferritin).
2. **Absorption and transport**
   a. Iron is primarily absorbed from the duodenum and upper part of the jejunum.
   b. Heme iron (found in animal products, e.g., meat, fish, poultry) is more readily absorbed across the intestine than inorganic non-heme iron (found in plant-based foods, e.g., green leafy vegetables, legumes, dry fruits).
   c. Inorganic iron in the **ferrous state (Fe^{2+})** is much **more readily absorbed** than that in the **ferric state (Fe^{3+})**.

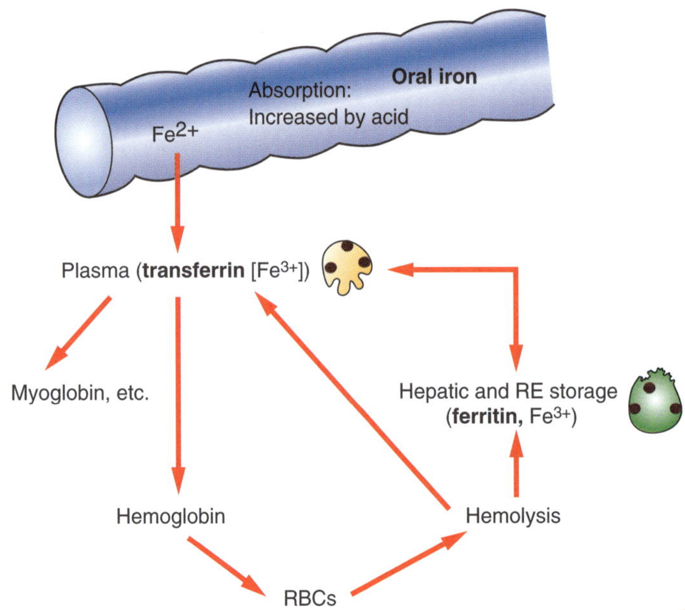

FIGURE 7.1. Absorption and circulation of iron within the body.

(1) Gastric acid and ascorbic acid promote the absorption of ferrous iron.

d. Iron is actively transported across the intestinal cell; it is then oxidized to ferric iron and stored as ferritin or transported to other tissues.

e. Iron is **transported** in the plasma bound to the glycoprotein **transferrin**.

(1) Specific cell surface receptors bind the transferrin–iron complex, and the iron is delivered to the recipient cell by endocytosis.

(2) Transferring saturation refers to the percentage of transferrin molecules saturated with iron (key marker in assessing iron status).

3. Regulation

a. Iron storage is regulated at the level of absorption.

(1) Except for menstruation and bleeding disorders, very little iron is lost from the body, and no mechanism exists for increasing excretion.

(2) **Hepcidin**, a peptide hormone synthesized in the liver, regulates intestinal iron absorption.

(3) **Mucosal block** induced by excessive iron suppresses intestinal iron absorption for a specific duration.

b. When plasma iron concentrations are **low**:

(1) The number of **transferrin receptors** is **increased** (facilitating cellular absorption).

(2) **Ferritin** synthesis is **decreased** (reducing tissue iron storage).

c. When iron stores are **high**:

(1) Intestinal **absorption** is **decreased**.

(2) Synthesis of **transferrin** is **decreased** (inhibiting additional cellular uptake).

(3) **Ferritin** synthesis is **increased**.

4. Causes of iron-deficiency anemia

a. **Bleeding** (~30 mg of iron is lost in a normal menstrual cycle)

b. Dietary deficiencies

c. Malabsorption syndromes (celiac disease, Whipple disease)

d. Increased iron demands (pregnancy, lactation)

5. Iron salt supplements

a. ***Oral agents (ferrous fumarate, ferrous gluconate, ferrous sulfate, polysaccharide iron complex, ferric maltol, carbonyl iron)***

(1) All are therapeutically equivalent and have similar adverse effects when doses are adjusted according to iron content.

(2) Approximately **25%** of orally administered iron is **absorbed**.

(3) Oral iron treatment may require **3–6 months to replenish body stores**.

(4) **Adverse effects**

(a) **Gastrointestinal (GI) distress** (**nausea**, cramps, flatulence, **constipation**, and **diarrhea**) is very common.

(b) Other effects include **black tarry stools** and a metallic taste.

(5) **Drug and food interactions**

(a) Medications that **reduce gastric acid** (antacids, histamine receptor blockers, and proton pump inhibitors [PPIs]) can **reduce iron absorption**.

(b) **Calcium**-containing food and beverages (coffee, tea, dairy products, soybeans) **may impair iron absorption**.

b. ***Parenteral agents (ferric carboxymaltose, ferric gluconate, ferumoxytol, iron isomaltoside, iron sucrose, and iron dextran)***

(1) Intravenous (IV) iron may be preferred over oral iron in patients with:

(a) Intolerable GI side effects of oral iron

(b) Iron absorption disorders caused by inflammatory bowel disease, gastric surgery, or hereditary absorption defects

(c) Severe anemic conditions (when rapid correction is desired)

(d) Renal failure–caused anemia treated with erythropoietin

(e) Unresolved ongoing bleeding that causes acceptable oral doses of iron therapy to be exceeded

(2) **Adverse and toxic effects**

(a) **Allergic or infusion reactions** may occur with IV administration, including urticaria, bronchospasm, and anaphylaxis.

i. Premedication may be given to those with a history of asthma or multiple drug allergies.

(b) **Iron sucrose and ferric gluconate** have been found to be effective and safe with a low risk of adverse effects.

(3) In acute iron toxicity, which is potentially fatal in children, **deferoxamine**, an iron-chelating agent, may be used. It **binds iron** and promotes excretion.

B. Vitamin B_{12}

1. ***Structure***
   a. **Vitamin B_{12}** is an essential **cofactor**, in which various groups are covalently linked to the cobalt atom, forming the cobalamins.
      (1) **Methylcobalamin** is a coenzyme essential for the production of methionine and *S*-adenosylmethionine from homocysteine and for the production of tetrahydrofolate from methyltetrahydrofolate.
      (2) **Deoxyadenosylcobalamin** participates in the mitochondrial reaction that produces succinyl-CoA from methylmalonyl-CoA.
         (a) Vitamin B_{12} deficiency leads to the production of abnormal fatty acids.
2. ***Transport and absorption***
   a. In the stomach, **dietary vitamin B_{12}** complexes with **intrinsic factor**, a peptide secreted by the parietal cells. The intrinsic factor–vitamin B_{12} complex is absorbed by active transport in the distal ileum.
   b. Vitamin B_{12} is transported in the plasma bound to the protein transcobalamin II and is taken up by and stored in hepatocytes.
3. ***Effects of B_{12} deficiency***
   a. Vitamin B_{12} is **essential** for **normal DNA synthesis** and **fatty acid metabolism.**
   b. Vitamin B_{12} is not synthesized by eukaryotic cells and is normally obtained from microbial synthesis.
   c. Loss of vitamin B_{12} from the body is very slow (2 μg/day); hepatic stores are sufficient for up to 5 years.
   d. A **deficiency** results in **impaired DNA replication**, which is most apparent in tissues that are actively dividing, such as the GI tract and erythroid precursors.
   e. The appearance of large **macrocytic (megaloblastic) red cells** in the blood is characteristic of this deficiency.
   f. Vitamin B_{12} deficiency can also result in **irreversible neurologic disorders.**
   g. Vitamin B_{12} (along with vitamin B_6 and folic acid) participates in the metabolism of homocysteine to cysteine. Elevations in homocysteine are associated with accelerated atherosclerosis.
4. ***Specific agents*** include **cyanocobalamin, hydroxocobalamin, and methylcobalamin.**
5. ***Pharmacologic properties***
   a. **Parenteral administration** of vitamin B_{12} is standard because the vast majority of situations requiring vitamin B_{12} replacement are due to **malabsorption**.
      (1) Uncorrectable malabsorption requires lifelong treatment.
      (2) Improvement in hemoglobin concentration is apparent in 7 days and normalizes in 1–2 months.
6. ***Indications***
   a. For the management of **pernicious anemia** (inadequate secretion of intrinsic factor with subsequent reduction in vitamin B_{12} absorption)
   b. After a partial or total **gastrectomy** (to mitigate loss of intrinsic factor synthesis)
   c. For vitamin B_{12} deficiency caused by **dysfunction** of the **distal ileum** with defective or absent absorption of the intrinsic factor–vitamin B_{12} complex
   d. For insufficient dietary intake of vitamin B_{12} (occasionally seen in strict vegetarians)
7. ***Adverse effects*** of vitamin B_{12} are uncommon, even at large doses.

C. Folic acid (vitamin B_9)

1. ***Structure***
   a. Folic acid is composed of three subunits: pteridine, *para*-aminobenzoic acid (PABA), and one to five glutamic acid residues.

2. ***Pharmacologic properties***
   a. Most folate is absorbed in the proximal portions of the small intestine and is transported to tissues bound to a plasma-binding protein.
   b. Folic acid requires **reduction by dihydrofolate reductase** to the **active metabolite methyltetrahydrofolate**.
   c. The cofactors of folic acid provide single carbon groups for transfer to various acceptors and are **essential for the biosynthesis of purines** and the pyrimidine deoxythymidylate.
   d. Catabolism and excretion of vitamin B_9 are more rapid than those of vitamin B_{12}; hepatic reserves are sufficient for only 1–3 months.
3. ***Effects of folic acid deficiency***
   a. A **deficiency** in folic acid results in **impaired DNA synthesis**; mitotically active tissues such as erythroid tissues are markedly affected.
4. ***Indications***
   a. Anemia due to folic acid deficiency is most often caused by dietary insufficiency or malabsorption and can be treated by oral folic acid supplementation.
   b. **Folic acid deficiency in pregnant women** is associated with an increased **risk of neural tube defects** in the fetus; therefore, supplementation is recommended.
   c. It may be used in cases of rapid cell turnover, such as hemolytic anemia.
   d. **Vitamin B_{12} deficiency should be ruled out before using folic acid** as the only treatment for anemia, especially since neurologic deficits of vitamin B_{12} deficiency may be irreversible. High-dose folic acid supplementation alone should not be used in megaloblastic anemia.
5. ***Adverse effects*** are **uncommon** with folic acid supplementation.

D. Pyridoxine (vitamin B_6)

1. Sideroblastic anemias are characterized by decreased hemoglobin synthesis and intracellular accumulation of iron in erythroid precursor cells.
   a. Iron is available but not incorporated into hemoglobin in a normal manner.
   b. Agents that antagonize or deplete pyridoxal phosphate can cause this type of anemia.
   c. Hereditary sideroblastic anemia is an X-linked trait.
2. **Pyridoxine (vitamin B_6)** can be used for the **management of sideroblastic anemia**, although it has **variable efficacy** with inherited forms of the disease.

E. Hydroxyurea

1. ***Mechanism of action (in sickle cell disease)***
   a. **Sickle cell disease** (SCD) refers to genetic disorders resulting from the presence of a **mutated** form of hemoglobin, **hemoglobin S** (HbS).
      (1) The mutated hemoglobin distorts the red blood cells (RBCs) into a crescent shape at low oxygen levels. The sickle-shaped cells are not flexible and many burst apart or stick to vessel walls causing a blockage or decreasing blood flow.
   b. **Hydroxyurea** increases the production of **fetal hemoglobin**, which makes **red cells resistant to sickling** and reduces the expression of adhesion molecules.
2. ***Indications***
   a. **Hydroxyurea** has been shown to reduce or prevent several complications due to SCD. It is effective in **reducing painful episodes** and the necessity of blood transfusions.
3. ***Adverse effects*** include GI distress and changes in the skin, hair, and nails. **Myelosuppression** is the major dose-limiting toxicity.

F. Drugs acting on erythroid precursor cells

1. Erythropoietin (EPO) is produced by the kidney. It is essential for normal reticulocyte production. Synthesis is stimulated by hypoxia.
2. Erythropoiesis-stimulating agents (ESAs)
   a. ***Specific agents*** include ***epoetin alfa*** and ***darbepoetin alfa***.
   b. ***Mechanism of action***
      (1) ESAs stimulate the **proliferation** and **differentiation** of **erythroid precursor cells** in the bone marrow.
      (2) They induce the **release of reticulocytes** from the bone marrow into the bloodstream, where they **mature to erythrocytes**.

(3) **Increased hemoglobin** and **hematocrit** levels follow the increased reticulocyte count.
(4) The action of ESAs **requires adequate stores of iron**.

c. ***Administration***
(1) Epoetin alfa has a shorter half-life and is administered subcutaneously (SubQ) three times a week, versus darbepoetin, which is administered weekly.

d. ***Indications***
(1) Both agents are approved for patients with anemia due to **chronic kidney disease** or anemia due to **chemotherapy** in patients with cancer.
(2) Epoetin alfa is also approved for anemia due to zidovudine in human immunodeficiency virus (HIV)–infected patients.
(3) In some situations, they may be used to reduce the need for transfusions.
(a) When a rapid increase in hematocrit is needed, RBC transfusions are effective in 1–3 hours, whereas ESAs may take 2–6 weeks.

e. ***Adverse effects*** may include **hypertension** and headache, most likely due to rapid expansion of blood volume. They can also cause **thrombosis**.

f. ***Precautions***
(1) The serum **hemoglobin** concentration of patients treated with an ESA should **not exceed 12 g/dL**.
(a) Hemoglobin levels above this target have been shown to increase the risk of **mortality** and **serious cardiovascular** and **thromboembolic events**, including myocardial infarction and stroke.
(2) ESAs may increase the risk for **tumor progression** or shorten overall survival in patients with breast, non–small cell lung, head and neck, lymphoid, and cervical cancers.
(3) The lowest dose of ESA necessary to prevent RBC transfusion should be used in order to prevent the severe adverse outcomes.

II. DRUGS ACTING ON MYELOID CELLS

A. Myeloid growth factors

1. Filgrastim, lenograstim, and pegfilgrastim (granulocyte colony-stimulating factor [G-CSF])

a. ***Mechanism of action***
(1) G-CSFs **stimulate bone marrow production, maturation**, and **activation** of **neutrophils** to increase their migration and cytotoxicity.
(2) They do not increase the number of basophils, eosinophils, or monocytes.

b. ***Administration***
(1) Pegfilgrastim is pegylated, giving it a longer half-life; it allows for one single SubQ dose compared with the daily administration required by filgrastim.

c. ***Indications***
(1) G-CSFs may be used **following** the administration of **chemotherapy** when **neutropenia** is **anticipated** ("primary prophylaxis").
(2) They may also be used during **retreatment after a previous cycle** of **chemotherapy** caused **neutropenic fever** ("secondary prophylaxis").
(3) G-CSFs are used to shorten the duration of chemotherapy-induced neutropenia after bone marrow transplantation.

d. ***Adverse effects*** may include cutaneous reactions, nausea, and **bone pain**.

2. Sargramostim (granulocyte–macrophage colony-stimulating factor [GM-CSF])

a. ***Mechanism of action***
(1) Sargramostim stimulates **proliferation**, differentiation, and **activity** of **neutrophils, eosinophils, monocytes,** and **macrophages**.

b. ***Indications***
(1) **Reduce** the **duration of neutropenia** and incidence of infection in patients receiving myelosuppressive chemotherapy or bone marrow transplantation
(2) **Mobilize peripheral blood progenitor cells** prior to collection
(3) For bone marrow graft failure

c. ***Adverse effects*** may include **bone pain**, fever, nausea, and rash.

3. **Romiplostim**

a. ***Mechanism of action***

(1) Romiplostim **binds to the thrombopoietin (TPO) receptor**. It produces a dose-dependent **increase in platelets**.

b. ***Indications.*** It is approved for **chronic immune thrombocytopenia** (ITP) in adults and children.

c. ***Route of administration:*** Subcutaneous injection.

d. ***Adverse reactions*** include headache and arthralgias. Risk of thromboembolic events is also reported.

III. DRUGS USED IN HEMOSTATIC DISORDERS

A. Parenteral anticoagulants

1. **Heparin (unfractionated heparin [UFH])**

a. ***Structure***

(1) Heparin is a large sulfated polysaccharide polymer that is isolated from porcine or bovine intestines.

(2) Each batch is a mixture of different-length polysaccharides, with an average molecular weight of 15,000–20,000 Da.

b. ***Mechanism of action*** (Fig. 7.2)

(1) Heparin potentiates the action of antithrombin III (ATIII). It **binds to ATIII** via a key pentasaccharide sequence and **irreversibly inactivates factor IIa (thrombin) and factor Xa**. It also inactivates coagulation factors IXa, XIa, and XIIa. By decreasing thrombin-mediated events in coagulation, including the conversion of fibrinogen to fibrin, fibrin-mediated clot formation is inhibited.

(a) It does not have anticoagulant activity on its own; binding to ATIII is required. It causes a conformational change, which converts ATIII from a slow to a rapid inhibitor of coagulation.

(b) Only one-third of molecules contain the pentasaccharide sequence needed to bind antithrombin.

(c) Anticoagulant activity is influenced by chain length (need 18 saccharides to bind thrombin).

(2) It provides anticoagulation immediately after administration. Its anticoagulant effects are reversible once it is cleared from the circulation (either by stopping the infusion or by administration of protamine sulfate).

(3) It cannot inhibit clot-bound factor IIa or Xa.

c. ***Indications***

(1) It provides preoperative prophylaxis against **deep vein thrombosis** (DVT) and reduces **pulmonary embolism** (PE) risk in patients with established thrombosis.

(2) It is used for the treatment of **acute coronary syndrome** (ACS), DVT, or PE.

(3) Heparin can be given to prevent stroke or systemic arterial embolism in patients with atrial fibrillation or mechanical or prosthetic heart valves.

(4) It prevents clotting in extracorporeal circulation devices (e.g., hemodialysis, cardiac surgeries).

d. ***Administration and monitoring***

(1) Heparin must be given by IV infusion or deep SubQ injection.

(a) Bioavailability is less with SubQ injection compared with that with IV.

(2) It is not injected intramuscularly (IM) due to the potential for hematoma.

(3) **Activated partial thromboplastin time (aPTT)** is commonly used to monitor heparin therapy. Achieving and maintaining a therapeutic level may be difficult. Few laboratories are transitioning to monitor actual heparin activity using anti-factor Xa analysis.

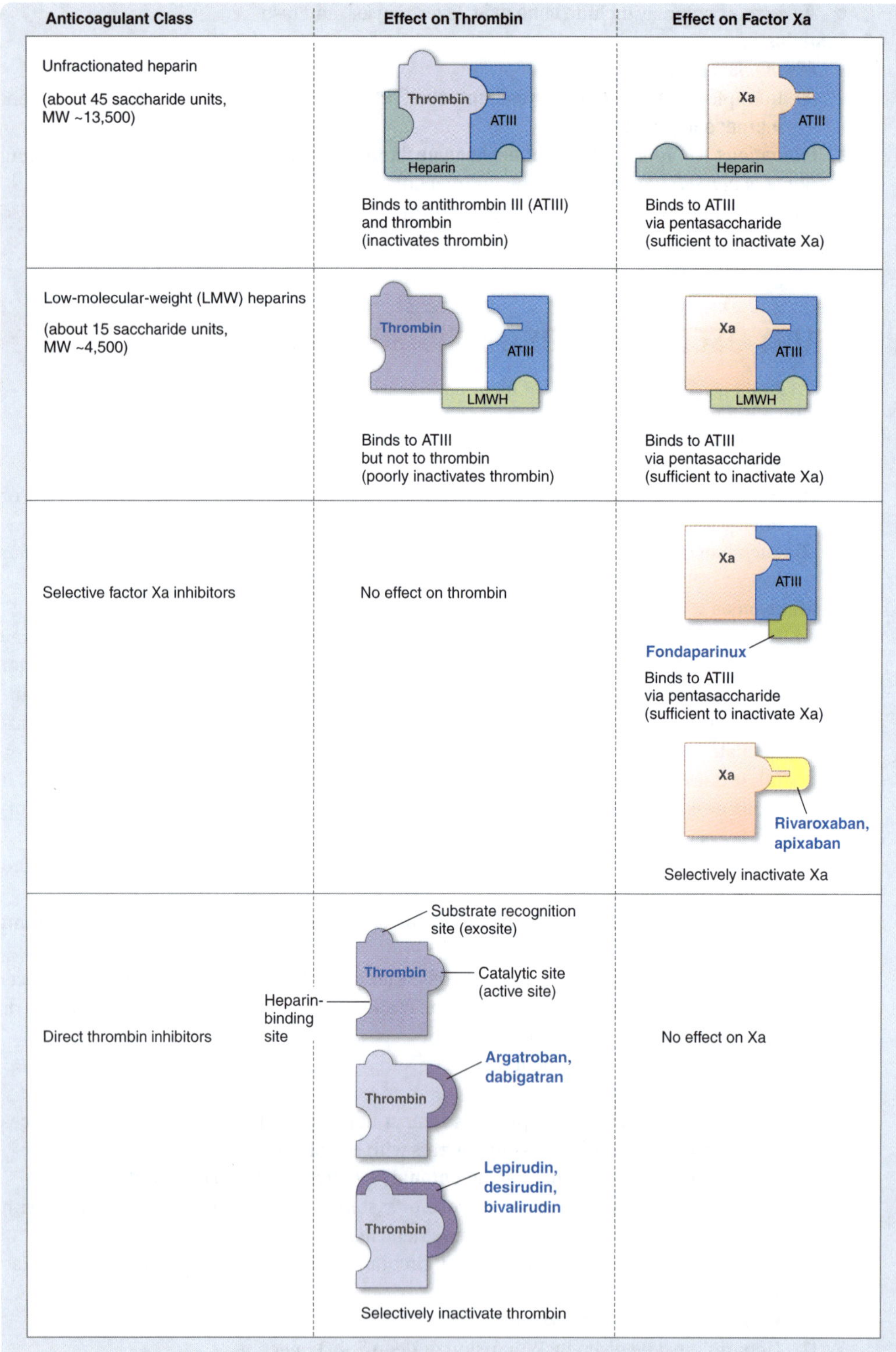

FIGURE 7.2. Mechanism of action for heparin, low-molecular-weight heparin, selective factor Xa inhibitors, and direct thrombin inhibitors. LMWH, low-molecular-weight heparin. (Reprinted with permission from Golan D. Principles of Pharmacology. 4th ed. Philadelphia, PA: Wolters Kluwer Health, 2016, Figure 23.15; Adapted from Lefkovits J, Topol EJ. Direct thrombin inhibitors in cardiovascular medicine. Circulation 1994;90:1522–1536, Figure 1.)

e. ***Adverse effects***

(1) **Bleeding** is a common and potentially dangerous adverse effect.

(a) **Protamine** sulfate can be given for **heparin reversal**.

i. Protamine is a positively charged alkaline protein. When given in the presence of heparin, which is strongly acidic and negatively charged, a salt is formed and stops the anticoagulant activity of heparin.

(2) Moderate thrombocytopenia may occur.

(3) Rarely, **heparin-induced thrombocytopenia (HIT)** can occur.

(a) HIT is a prothrombotic disorder caused by **antibodies to complexes of platelet factor 4** (PF4) and heparin.

(b) It is a potentially life-threatening complication in which the antibodies cause **thrombocytopenia** (by peripheral platelet consumption) and **thrombosis** (by platelet activation).

(4) Long-term use may be associated with osteoporosis.

f. ***Precautions and contraindications***

(1) Heparin is contraindicated in patients with active bleeding and in patients with hemophilia, thrombocytopenia, hypertension, or purpura.

(2) It should not be used before or after brain, spinal cord, or eye surgery.

(3) Extreme caution is advised in the treatment of pregnant women.

g. ***Drug interactions***

(1) Heparin should not be used in combination with other drugs that interfere with platelet aggregation.

2. **Low-molecular-weight heparin (LMWH)**

a. ***Specific agents*** include **enoxaparin, dalteparin, nadroparin, reviparin, and tinzaparin**.

b. ***Mechanism of action*** (Fig. 7.2)

(1) LMWH acts by **increasing ATIII-mediated inhibition** of the formation and activity of **factor Xa**. It has a **higher ratio of anti–factor Xa to anti–factor IIa activity**. Similar to UFH, it decreases thrombin-mediated events in coagulation, including the conversion of fibrinogen to fibrin; therefore, fibrin-mediated clot formation is inhibited.

(a) It does not have anticoagulant activity on its own; binding to ATIII is required. It causes a conformational change, which converts ATIII from a slow to a rapid inhibitor of coagulation.

c. ***Indications***

(1) Enoxaparin is approved for the management of **ACS** and for **DVT prophylaxis** and treatment.

(2) Dalteparin is approved for DVT prophylaxis, extended treatment of venous thromboembolism (VTE) for patients with cancer, and unstable angina.

d. ***Administration and monitoring***

(1) LMWH offers a **greater pharmacokinetic predictability** and **longer half-life** than UFH, which allows for once- or twice-a-day SubQ dosing without the need for aPTT monitoring. It has a **higher SubQ bioavailability** compared with UFH.

(2) Similar to UFH, it should not be given IM.

e. Adverse effects, precautions, contraindications, and drug interactions are similar to those of heparin.

(1) Protamine will only partially reverse the anticoagulant effect of LMWH.

3. **Indirect factor Xa inhibitor**

a. ***Specific agent.*** **Fondaparinux.**

b. ***Mechanism of action*** (Fig. 7.2)

(1) It causes **ATIII-mediated selective inhibition of factor Xa**, which interrupts the coagulation cascade and inhibits thrombin formation and thrombus development.

(a) It does not have anticoagulant activity on its own; binding to ATIII is required. It causes a conformational change, which converts ATIII from a slow to a rapid inhibitor of coagulation.

c. ***Indications***
   (1) Fondaparinux is approved for **prophylaxis of thrombus formation** in patients undergoing hip or knee surgery, treatment of **PE**, and **DVT**.
   (2) Off-label, it may be used for the management of HIT.

d. ***Administration and monitoring***
   (1) It has a long half-life, allowing for once-daily dosing by SubQ administration.

e. Adverse effects, precautions, contraindications, and drug interactions are similar to those of heparin.
   (1) Protamine will not reverse the activity of fondaparinux.

4. **Parenteral direct thrombin inhibitors (DTIs)**
   a. ***Specific agents*** include **bivalirudin**, desirudin, and **argatroban**.
   b. ***Mechanism of action*** (Fig. 7.2)
      (1) These agents directly **bind** to the active site of **thrombin** and inhibit its downstream effects without the need for a cofactor.
   c. ***Indications.*** They can be used in settlings like HIT and allergy to heparin. They have a relatively short half-life and hence are typically administered by IV infusion.
      (1) **Bivalirudin** is approved for **percutaneous coronary intervention** (PCI) and percutaneous transluminal coronary angioplasty, in conjunction with aspirin. It may also be **used in HIT**.
      (2) Desirudin is approved for DVT prophylaxis in patients undergoing hip replacement surgery.
      (3) **Argatroban** is approved for prophylaxis or treatment of thrombosis in adults with HIT. It can also be used for PCI in adults who have or are at risk for **HIT**.
   d. ***Adverse effects***
      (1) Like other anticoagulants, DTIs can cause bleeding. There is no available reversal agent.

B. Oral anticoagulants

1. **Direct factor Xa inhibitors**
   a. ***Specific agents*** include **rivaroxaban**, **apixaban**, edoxaban, and betrixaban.
   b. ***Mechanism of action.*** Similar to fondaparinux, these agents inhibit factor Xa in both the intrinsic and extrinsic coagulation pathways (Fig. 7.2).
   c. ***Indications***
      (1) Rivaroxaban is approved for the prevention of embolic stroke in patients with atrial fibrillation with nonvalvular heart disease, for the prevention of VTE following hip or knee surgery, and for the treatment of VTE.
      (2) Apixaban is approved for the prevention of stroke in nonvalvular atrial fibrillation, for the prevention of VTE following hip or knee surgery, and for the treatment and long-term prevention of VTE.
      (3) Edoxaban is approved for the prevention of stroke in nonvalvular atrial fibrillation and to treat VTE following treatment with UFH or LMWH.
      (4) Betrixaban is approved for prophylaxis of VTE in adults hospitalized for an acute medical illness who are at risk for thromboembolic complications due to moderate or severe restricted mobility or other risk factors.
   d. ***Administration and monitoring***
      (1) Compared with warfarin, these agents have a rapid onset of action and shorter half-lives.
      (2) They can be given as a fixed oral dose and do not require close monitoring of therapeutic effect.
   e. ***Adverse effects*** include bleeding. **Andexanet alfa** is a catalytically inactive form of factor Xa that acts as a "decoy" to bind and sequester the anticoagulant. It was approved for **reverse anticoagulation** for apixaban and rivaroxaban.
   f. ***Precautions and contraindications*** are similar to those of other anticoagulants.
   g. ***Drug interactions***
      (1) Drugs that inhibit CYP3A4 enzymes can increase the effect of **rivaroxaban** and **apixaban**.

2. Oral direct thrombin inhibitor

a. ***Specific agent.*** **Dabigatran.**

b. ***Mechanism of action.*** This agent is an oral DTI. Similar to the parenteral DTIs, it **inhibits both free and fibrin-bound thrombin,** therefore inhibiting coagulation. Inhibition is reversible (Fig. 7.2).

(1) It prevents cleavage of fibrinogen to fibrin; prevents and activates factors V, VIII, XI, and XIII; and inhibits thrombin-induced platelet aggregation.

c. ***Indications.*** It is approved for **prophylaxis and treatment of DVT and PE.** It can also be used to reduce the risk of stroke and systemic embolism in patients with nonvalvular atrial fibrillation.

d. ***Adverse effects.*** The primary side effect of dabigatran is **bleeding. Idarucizumab** is a humanized monoclonal antibody Fab fragment that binds to dabigatran to **reverse** its anticoagulant effect.

e. ***Precautions and contraindications*** are similar to those of other anticoagulants. It should be used in with caution in renal impairment, as it can lead to prolonged clearance.

3. Warfarin

a. ***Mechanism of action***

(1) Vitamin K is required for the synthesis of several clotting factors in the liver.

(2) Warfarin is a **vitamin K antagonist.** It blocks the regeneration of vitamin K epoxide, thus **inhibiting synthesis** of the vitamin K–dependent clotting factors **II, VII, IX, and X,** as well as the **anticoagulant proteins C and S.**

(a) The clotting factors require carboxylation of a glutamate residue to become activated. Carboxylation requires the reduced form of vitamin K, but **warfarin inhibits the enzyme vitamin K epoxide reductase.**

(3) Clotting factors produced before warfarin therapy decline in concentration as a function of factor half-life.

(a) **Factor VII** has the **shortest** half-life of 4–6 hours. **Factor II** has the **longest** half-life ranging from 42 to 72 hours. Similar to factor VII, **protein C** also has a **short**-half life.

(b) Warfarin **initially decreases protein C levels (an anticoagulant)** faster than the coagulation factors. This may create a **transient hypercoagulable state.**

(c) It does not affect established thrombi.

b. ***Indications***

(1) Warfarin is used for the **prevention and treatment of VTE and pulmonary thromboembolism,** as well as embolic complications due to **atrial fibrillation** or cardiac valve replacement.

(2) It may also be used as an adjunct to reduce systemic embolism, such as a recurrent myocardial infarction or stroke, after a MI.

c. ***Administration and monitoring***

(1) Due to the **initial potential of a hypercoagulable state, bridging therapy** with UFH or LMWH may be used to **achieve immediate anticoagulation.**

(a) Overlapping therapy is often used for 5–7 days (to ensure that warfarin has adequately depleted the clotting factors).

(2) The **international normalized ratio (INR),** a standardized measurement of the prothrombin time (PT), is used to monitor warfarin therapy.

(a) Warfarin must be monitored regularly since it has a **narrow therapeutic range.** Levels can be affected by numerous drug or food interactions, as well as different disease states, such as hepatic dysfunction.

d. ***Adverse effects***

(1) **Bleeding** is a common and potentially dangerous adverse effect.

(a) In some cases of bleeding, **phytonadione (vitamin K)**) and **fresh frozen plasma** can be given to **reverse** warfarin's anticoagulant effect.

e. ***Precautions and contraindications***

(1) Many of the precautions and contraindications are similar to those of UFH and LMWH.

(2) In addition, warfarin is **contraindicated in pregnancy** since it can readily cross the placenta and cause hemorrhage in the fetus.

f. ***Drug interactions***

(1) Drugs that **inhibit CYP2C9** (amiodarone, fluconazole, and trimethoprim–sulfamethoxazole) and **CYP3A4** (clarithromycin and ketoconazole) may **increase INR** and increase the risk of **bleeding.**

(2) Drugs that **induce CYP2C9** (rifampin, carbamazepine, and phenobarbital) and **CYP3A4** (rifampin, carbamazepine, and phenytoin) can **decrease INR** and **decrease efficacy** of warfarin therapy.

(3) Aspirin and salicylates increase warfarin action by inhibiting platelet function and displacement of warfarin from plasma-binding sites.

(4) Certain antibiotics can decrease microbial vitamin K production in the intestine (inhibit microbes responsible for production of vitamin K precursors).

(a) This may result in hypoprothrombinemia, even without warfarin.

(5) Oral contraceptives decrease the effectiveness of warfarin by increasing plasma clotting factors and decreasing ATIII.

g. ***Food interactions***

(1) Vitamin K–containing foods, such as **green leafy vegetables** like spinach, can decrease the efficacy of warfarin. A balanced diet with consistent vitamin K intake is essential.

(2) Acute ingestion of **alcohol** can inhibit CYP2C9 and increase INR. Chronic ingestion may induce CYP2C9 and decrease INR.

C. Hemostatic agents

1. Vitamin K_1 (phytonadione)

a. Vitamin K_1 is found in certain foods and is available for oral or parenteral use. It is required for posttranslational modification of clotting factors II, VII, IX, and X.

b. Administration of vitamin K to **newborns** reduces the incidence of **hypoprothrombinemia**, which is especially common in premature infants.

c. IV administration is typical for patients with dietary deficiencies and for replenishment of normal levels reduced by antimicrobial therapy or surgery.

d. It is effective in reversing **bleeding episodes induced by warfarin**.

2. Plasma protein preparations include the following:

a. ***Specific agents***

(1) Lyophilized factor VIII concentrate and recombinant factor VIII

(2) Cryoprecipitate (plasma protein fraction obtained from whole blood)

(3) Concentrates of plasma (variable amounts of factors II, IX, X, and VII)

(4) Lyophilized factor IX concentrates, recombinant factor IX

(5) Recombinant factor VIIa

(6) Recombinant thrombin

(7) Antithrombin

(8) Anti-inhibitor coagulant complex—activated clotting factor

b. ***Indications***

(1) **Hemophilia A** (classic hemophilia, due to a deficiency in factor VIII).

(2) **Hemophilia B** (Christmas disease, due to a deficiency in factor IX).

(3) Hereditary ATIII deficiency.

(4) In some cases, human plasma can be lifesaving (trauma, massive transfusion, disseminated intravascular coagulation).

3. **Desmopressin acetate** increases **factor VIII** synthesis and can be used before minor surgery in patients with **mild hemophilia A**.

4. Inhibitors of fibrinolysis

a. **Aminocaproic acid** is a synthetic agent similar in structure to lysine. It competitively inhibits plasminogen activation (Fig. 7.3).

(1) It is used as an adjunct in the treatment of hemophilia, for postsurgical bleeding, and in patients with hyperfibrinolysis.

(2) **Tranexamic acid** is a more potent analogue of aminocaproic acid.

D. Antithrombotics (antiplatelet medications)

1. Aspirin (see Chapter 6)

a. ***Mechanism of action.*** Low doses of aspirin (81 mg) produce a clinically relevant antiplatelet effect through **irreversible inhibition of cyclooxygenase-1** (COX-1), which is required for the production of thromboxane A2 (promoter of platelet aggregation) (Fig. 7.4).

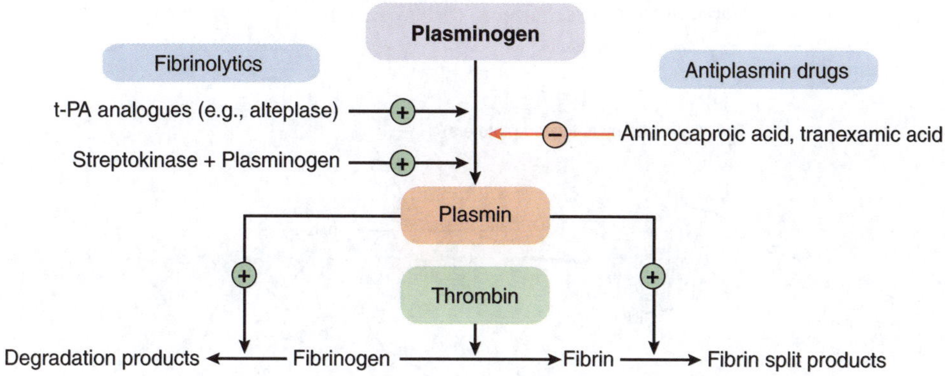

FIGURE 7.3. Mechanism of action for fibrinolytic and antifibrinolytic agents. t-PA, tissue plasminogen activator.

(1) Irreversible inhibition means that its **antiplatelet effect lasts for the life span of platelet** (7–10 days). The recovery of platelet function is usually 2–3 days.

(2) Higher doses (>325 mg) will also inhibit cyclooxygenase-2 (COX-2) and block prostaglandin synthesis for its analgesic and antipyretic effects.

(3) Other nonsteroidal anti-inflammatory drugs (NSAIDs) do not have comparable antithrombotic activity.

b. ***Indications.*** It has many indications, including coronary artery disease, ACS, stroke, VTE prevention, revascularization procedures, and stent placement.

c. ***Adverse effects.*** Its major adverse effect is **bleeding**, most commonly in the GI tract.

2. Dipyridamole

a. ***Mechanism of action.*** Dipyridamole promotes **vasodilation** and **inhibition of platelet aggregation**. It **inhibits phosphodiesterase (PDE)** breakdown of cyclic adenosine monophosphate (cAMP) and inhibits adenosine reuptake. Both increase cAMP, which inhibits platelet activation and aggregation (Fig. 7.4).

b. ***Indications***

(1) It is used with warfarin to decrease thrombosis in patients after artificial heart valve replacement.

(2) With aspirin, it is used to reduce the risk of stroke in patients who have had transient ischemia of the brain or complete ischemic stroke due to thrombosis.

c. ***Adverse effects*** may include abdominal distress, headache, and dizziness. Similar to other antiplatelet medications, it can increase the risk of bleeding. Dipyridamole is linked to **coronary steal phenomenon** in which it diverts blood flow away from the ischemic area to the nonischemic area due to vasodilatation.

d. **Cilostazol** is also a PDE inhibitor that increases cAMP and leads to platelet inhibition and vasodilation. It is used for the management of intermittent claudication.

3. $P2Y_{12}$-receptor inhibitors

a. ***Specific agents*** include **clopidogrel,** prasugrel, and **ticagrelor**, which are available as oral medications, and ***cangrelor***, which is available for IV therapy.

b. ***Mechanism of action*** (Fig. 7.4)

(1) The $P2Y_{12}$ receptors are located on the surface of platelets. Adenosine diphosphate (ADP) acts as an agonist on the $P2Y_{12}$ receptor, which inhibits adenylyl cyclase and allows for platelet activation.

(2) These agents **bind to the ADP $P2Y_{12}$ receptor on the platelet surface**, which prevents ADP-mediated activation of the GPIIb/IIIa-receptor complex, thereby **reducing platelet aggregation**.

c. ***Indications***

(1) Clopidogrel is approved to reduce the rate of MI and stroke in patients with ACS and in patients with a recent MI, recent stroke, or peripheral arterial disease. It is used off-label to prevent coronary stent thrombosis.

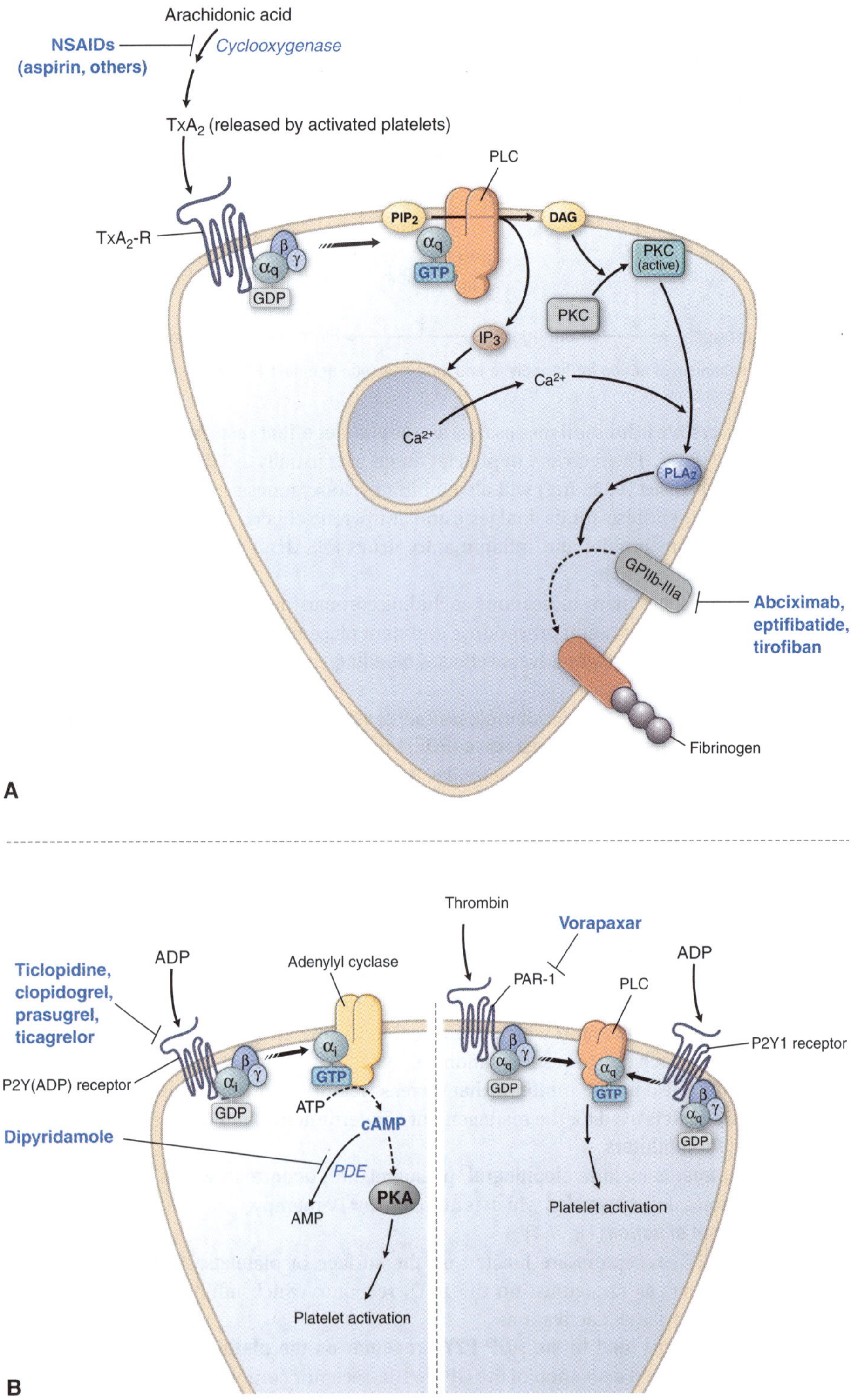

FIGURE 7.4. Mechanism of action for antiplatelet agents. NSAID, nonsteroidal anti-inflammatory drug. (Reprinted with permission from Golan D. Principles of Pharmacology. 4th ed. Philadelphia, PA: Wolters Kluwer Health, 2016, Figure 23.13.)

(2) Ticagrelor is approved to reduce MI and stroke in patients with ACS or a history of MI. It also reduces the rate of stent thrombosis in patients who have been stented for the treatment of ACS.

(3) Prasugrel is approved for ACS managed with PCI. Cangrelor is also used for PCI.

d. ***Adverse effects***

(1) These agents can increase the risk of **bleeding** and **hemorrhage**.

e. ***Drug interactions***

(1) **Clopidogrel** is a **prodrug**, and its effectiveness is dependent on its conversion to an active metabolite by the cytochrome P450 **CYP2C19 enzyme**.

(a) **PPIs**, like pantoprazole, **inhibit the CYP2C19** enzyme and **may prevent metabolism** of clopidogrel **to its active metabolite**.

(b) CYP2C19-poor metabolizers may also have decreased clopidogrel effectiveness.

4. GPIIb/IIIa inhibitors

a. ***Specific agents*** include **abciximab**, eptifibatide, and tirofiban.

b. ***Mechanism of action*** (Fig. 7.4)

(1) The abundant platelet glycoprotein GPIIb/IIIa plays a critical role in platelet aggregation. GPIIb/IIIa is an integrin that, when activated, binds to fibrinogen. There are two GPIIb/IIIa-binding sites on a fibrinogen molecule, thus permitting fibrinogen-mediated platelet aggregation.

(2) **Abciximab** is the Fab fragment of a chimeric monoclonal antibody that contains human and mouse IgG components. It **binds to GPIIb/IIIa and blocks fibrinogen binding**. It also binds to the vitronectin receptor.

(3) **Eptifibatide** is a small synthetic peptide that **competes for fibrinogen** binding to GPIIb/IIIa. **Tirofiban** is a peptide mimetic of low molecular weight that binds to the GPIIb/IIIa receptor.

(a) Both agents **inhibit ligand binding to the IIb/IIIa receptor** by their occupancy of the receptor but do not block the vitronectin receptor.

c. ***Administration.*** Due to their short half-lives, they are given by a continuous IV infusion.

d. ***Indications.*** These drugs have been approved for use in patients undergoing **PCI**, for unstable angina, and for post-MI. Use has decreased with newer antiplatelet agents.

e. ***Adverse effects.*** The most common adverse effect is **bleeding**, especially if used in combination with heparin.

5. Thrombin receptor antagonist

a. ***Specific agent.*** **Vorapaxar.**

b. ***Mechanism of action*** (Fig. 7.4)

(1) Vorapaxar is an antagonist of the protease-activated receptor-1 (PAR-1) that is expressed on platelets. It inhibits thrombin-induced platelet aggregation.

c. ***Indications.*** It is indicated in conjunction with aspirin or clopidogrel to reduce cardiovascular events in those with a history of MI or with peripheral artery disease.

d. ***Adverse effects*** include bleeding.

e. ***Precautions and contraindications***

(1) Due to the very long half-life, vorapaxar is effectively irreversible, in which inhibition of platelet aggregation may last up to 4 weeks after discontinuation.

(2) Due to its high risk for bleeding, use is contraindicated in patients with a history of stroke, transient ischemic attack (TIA), intracranial hemorrhage, or with active pathological bleeding.

E. Thrombolytics (fibrinolytic drugs)

1. Tissue plasminogen activator (tPA)

a. ***Specific agents*** include **alteplase, reteplase, saruplase,** and **tenecteplase**.

b. ***Mechanism of action*** (Fig. 7.3)

(1) tPA is an endogenous protease that causes local fibrinolysis by binding to fibrin in a thrombus and converting plasminogen to plasmin.

(2) These drugs **rapidly lyse thrombi** by **catalyzing** the **formation** of the protease **plasmin** from its precursor, plasminogen.

c. ***Pharmacological properties***

(1) Alteplase is a recombinant human protein produced in cultured cells.

(2) Tenecteplase and reteplase are genetically engineered form of human tPA that has a longer half-life, higher specificity for fibrin, and greater resistance to plasminogen activator inhibitor-1 than native tPA.

(a) The increase in half-life permits administration as a bolus rather than by continuous infusion.

d. ***Indications***

(1) Thrombolytics are used in patients with **acute arterial thrombosis** including acute myocardial infarction (AMI) and **stroke**.

(a) The use of thrombolytics has reduced morbidity and mortality associated with acute MI and ischemic stroke.

(b) Outcomes following its use are **improved if administration occurs promptly after the event** (within 3–6 hours).

(2) tPA has also been used in the treatment of PE and for DVT.

e. ***Adverse effects***

(1) The most common adverse effect of all thrombolytics is **bleeding**. Tranexamic acid and epsilon-aminocaproic acid (EACA) may be considered for correction of coagulopathy.

(a) Bleeding sites include both internal (intracranial, retroperitoneal, GI, genitourinary, respiratory) and superficial (venous cutdowns, arterial punctures, sites of recent surgical intervention) sites.

DRUG SUMMARY TABLE

Drugs Used for Anemia
Cyanocobalamin (vitamin B_{12})
Darbepoetin alfa
Epoetin alfa
Ferric carboxymaltose
Ferric gluconate
Ferrous fumarate
Ferrous gluconate
Ferrous sulfate
Ferumoxytol
Folic acid
Hydroxocobalamin
Hydroxyurea
Iron sucrose
Iron dextran
Polysaccharide iron complex
Pyridoxine (vitamin B_6)

Myeloid Growth Stimulators
Filgrastim
Pegfilgrastim
Romiplostim
Sargramostim

Anticoagulants
Argatroban
Apixaban
Betrixaban
Bivalirudin
Dabigatran
Dalteparin
Desirudin
Edoxaban
Enoxaparin
Fondaparinux
Heparin
Rivaroxaban
Warfarin

Anticoagulant Reversal Agents
Andexanet alfa
Idarucizumab
Phytonadione
Protamine sulfate

Hemostatic Agents
Desmopressin acetate
Factor VIIa
Factor VIII
Factor IX
Prothrombin complex concentrate
Phytonadione (vitamin K_1)
Prothrombin complex concentrate, activated, from human plasma
Thrombin

Antifibrinolytics
Aminocaproic acid
Tranexamic acid

Antithrombotics
Abciximab
Anagrelide
Aspirin
Cilostazol
Clopidogrel
Dipyridamole
Eptifibatide
Prasugrel
Ticagrelor
Tirofiban
Vorapaxar

Thrombolytics
Alteplase
Reteplase
Tenecteplase

Review Test

Directions: Select the best answer for each question.

1. A 48-year-old woman is admitted to the hospital with complaints of fatigue and dark tarry stools. One hour after admission, she begins vomiting what looks like coffee grounds. Laboratory results reveal an INR of 8.1. She has a history of deep vein thrombosis, for which she is taking warfarin. Which of the following would be the most appropriate treatment for this patient?

(A) Andexanet alfa
(B) Desmopressin
(C) Idarucizumab
(D) Phytonadione
(E) Protamine

2. A 66-year-old man presents to his oncologist with complaints of shortness of breath, especially with physical activity, such as climbing stairs. He also complains of constant fatigue. An electrocardiogram appears normal, but his hematocrit level is 8.1. He is currently being treated with chemotherapy for stage IV lung cancer. Which of the following drugs may be used to manage this patient's symptoms?

(A) Epoetin alfa
(B) Ferrous sulfate
(C) Filgrastim
(D) Pyridoxine
(E) Romiplostim

3. A 56-year-old woman presents to her physician with complaints of a temporary loss of peripheral vision, loss of coordination, and dizziness 2 days prior. She is still having trouble with coordination. Her family history reveals that her mother had a stroke at the age of 61 years. At this point in time, which of the following medications would be the best prophylactic regimen for this patient?

(A) Abciximab
(B) Aminocaproic acid
(C) Clopidogrel
(D) Enoxaparin
(E) Reteplase

4. A 53-year-old woman is brought to the emergency room by her husband, approximately 1 hour after complaining of constant abdominal pain, nausea, and shortness of breath. Further testing, including an electrocardiogram and cardiac enzyme tests, leads to a diagnosis of a moderate myocardial infarction due to occlusion of the left descending coronary artery. Which of the following would be the best course of treatment for this patient?

(A) Alteplase
(B) Darbepoetin alfa
(C) Fondaparinux
(D) Phytonadione
(E) Rivaroxaban

5. A 28-year-old woman presents to her obstetrician for her first prenatal appointment. She is 8 weeks pregnant. After an ultrasound and other routine testing, her physician gives her paperwork that covers the do's and don'ts for a safer pregnancy, including folic acid supplementation. If the patient disregards the recommendations for folic acid supplementation, what is the risk to the fetus?

(A) Cleft palate
(B) Congenital heart disease
(C) Down syndrome
(D) Neural tube defects
(E) Phenylketonuria

6. A 65-year-old man presents to his nephrologist for the management of end-stage renal disease. His glomerular filtration capacity is low enough to require dialysis. In addition to dialysis, his nephrologist also prescribes weekly injections of epoetin alfa. What is the mechanism for which this agent will help the patient?

(A) Decrease the release of reticulocytes from the bone marrow
(B) Decrease differentiation of reticulocytes in the bone marrow
(C) Decrease the amount of iron stored in the body
(D) Increase mitochondrial reactions that produce succinyl-CoA
(E) Increase proliferation of erythroid precursor cells in the bone marrow

7. A 37-year-old woman presents to her family physician for a routine appointment. Her past medical history is positive for heartburn, hypertension, iron-deficiency anemia, and migraines. Her medications include pantoprazole, lisinopril, hydrochlorothiazide, propranolol, sumatriptan, and ferrous gluconate. The patient complains of fatigue and light-headedness. Laboratory tests reveal low hemoglobin and ferritin levels. Her physician is worried about other drugs impairing iron absorption. Which of the patient's medications may be causing this drug interaction?

(A) Calcium carbonate
(B) Hydrochlorothiazide
(C) Lisinopril
(D) Propranolol
(E) Sumatriptan

8. A 78-year-old man presents to his hematologist for the management of pernicious anemia. His doctor prescribes a medication to prevent the development of irreversible neurologic disorders. His hemoglobin levels improve after 1 week of therapy. Which of the following medications was prescribed?

(A) Cyanocobalamin
(B) Factor VIII
(C) Ferrous sulfate
(D) Hydroxyurea
(E) Pyridoxine

9. A 56-year-old man presents to the emergency room with redness and swelling in his right calf. An ultrasound is positive for deep venous thrombosis. The patient is admitted to the hospital and started on warfarin therapy. The doctor also starts heparin to achieve immediate anticoagulation. Initial decreases in which of the following levels make heparin administration necessary?

(A) Factor II
(B) Factor VII
(C) Factor X
(D) Protein C
(E) Protein S

10. A 29-year-old man presents to the emergency department with the chief complaint of severe pain in his arms and legs. He has a history of sickle cell anemia, but due to insurance issues, he ran out of his medication that is supposed to prevent painful episodes and the necessity of blood transfusions. Which of the following medications was the patient supposed to take?

(A) Clopidogrel
(B) Cyanocobalamin
(C) Darbepoetin alfa
(D) Deferoxamine
(E) Hydroxyurea

11. A 74-year-old woman presents to the infusion center for her next cycle of chemotherapy for advanced lung cancer. After her previous treatment, she was admitted to the hospital with febrile neutropenia, in which she was treated with vancomycin for *Staphylococcus aureus* bacteremia. To prevent similar complications with this cycle, which medication should be given?

(A) Epoetin alfa
(B) Filgrastim
(C) Hydroxyurea
(D) Leucovorin
(E) Phytonadione

12. A 55-year-old woman undergoes an open cholecystectomy. She is admitted for postoperative observation and started on subcutaneous heparin treatment to prevent formation of deep venous thrombosis, a major risk factor for pulmonary embolism. How does heparin prevent these potential complications?

(A) Increases activity of antithrombin III
(B) Increases activity of factors II and X
(C) Increases conversion of fibrinogen to fibrin
(D) Inhibits clot-bound factors IX and XII
(E) Inhibits clot-bound lipoproteins

13. A 63-year-old man presents to his cardiologist for the management of atrial fibrillation. To reduce his risk of stroke, his physician starts him on a new anticoagulant. The patient is counseled to avoid drinking alcohol and to be consistent with his intake of green leafy vegetables. He is asked to return to the clinic in 1 week to monitor his international normalized ratio (INR). What is the mechanism of action for the anticoagulant that the patient was prescribed?

(A) Antithrombin III activator
(B) Direct thrombin inhibitor
(C) $P2Y_{12}$-receptor inhibitor
(D) Phosphodiesterase inhibitor
(E) Vitamin K antagonist

14. A 75-year-old man is brought to the emergency department by ambulance after being found on the floor by his wife. She tells the physician that his medical history includes two prior strokes, for which he takes clopidogrel. The patient is also on several other medications for the management of gastroesophageal reflux disease, hypertension, and hypercholesterolemia. After reviewing the patient's medication record, the physician is concerned that a drug interaction with clopidogrel may have caused this patient's symptoms. Which of the following medications is the physician concerned about?

(A) Atorvastatin
(B) Enalapril
(C) Losartan
(D) Omega-3 fatty acids
(E) Pantoprazole

15. A 60-year-old man who is a known case of hypertension and type 2 diabetes mellitus presents to the emergency department with acute onset of shortness of breath and pleuritic chest pain. Pulmonary angiogram confirms the diagnosis of acute pulmonary embolism. He is hemodynamically stable with BP of 136/88 mm Hg and pulse rate of 95 beats/min. There is no evidence of bleeding or active peptic under disease. The emergency physician initiates therapy with enoxaparin. Which of the following statements is correct?

(A) Enoxaparin is more efficacious than unfractionated heparin in pulmonary embolism.
(B) Enoxaparin has a quicker onset of action compared with unfractionated heparin.
(C) Enoxaparin is short-acting which allows termination of action if bleeding occurs.
(D) Enoxaparin can be given orally and hence is convenient for the patient.
(E) Enoxaparin is less likely to cause heparin-induced thrombocytopenia than unfractionated heparin.

Answers and Explanations

1. **The answer is D.** Phytonadione (vitamin K) can be used to reverse the effects of warfarin, a vitamin K antagonist. Vitamin K promotes liver synthesis of clotting factors (II, VII, IX, X). The other agents are not used to reverse the effects of warfarin. Andexanet alfa is approved to reverse anticoagulation due to apixaban and rivaroxaban. Idarucizumab binds to dabigatran to reverse its anticoagulant effect. Protamine is used to reverse the effects of heparin. Desmopressin can be used for hemophilia.
2. **The answer is A.** Epoetin alfa stimulates the production of erythrocytes, which are frequently diminished as a consequence of anticancer therapy. It will help correct the patient's hemoglobin level. Filgrastim is used to stimulate bone marrow production following the administration of chemotherapy to increase neutrophils and help prevent infection. Although it is given to patients with cancer undergoing chemotherapy, it would not manage his symptoms of fatigue. In some cases, pyridoxine (vitamin B_6) can be used to manage sideroblastic anemia. Romiplostim is used to increase platelets in patients with chronic immune thrombocytopenia.
3. **The answer is C.** The patient has symptoms consistent with a stroke or transient ischemic attack (TIA). Prophylactic antiplatelet therapy should be instituted once the diagnosis is confirmed. Clopidogrel is a $P2Y_{12}$-receptor inhibitor approved to prevent stroke in patients with a history of recent stroke. Although enoxaparin can be used for outpatient therapy, it is not used for this indication. Reteplase is a thrombolytic agent that may be used within hours of a thrombotic stroke, but not 2 days after a possible TIA. Aminocaproic acid is used as an adjunct for the treatment of hemophilia or for postsurgical bleeding. Abciximab is used for patients undergoing PCI or for unstable angina.
4. **The answer is A.** Thrombolytics such as the recombinant tissue plasminogen activator (tPA) alteplase reduce morbidity and mortality if used shortly after an acute myocardial infarction (AMI). They rapidly lyse thrombi by catalyzing the formation of the protease plasmin from its precursor, plasminogen. Darbepoetin alfa is an erythropoiesis-stimulating agent used to increase reticulocyte production. Fondaparinux and rivaroxaban are factor XA inhibitors used for DVT prophylaxis. Phytonadione is vitamin K, which is not used for this indication.
5. **The answer is D.** Folic acid supplementation has been shown to decrease the incidence of neural tube defects. The neural tube is the part of the embryo from which a baby's spine and brain develop. Folic acid supplementation helps prevent serious birth defects of the spinal cord (such as spina bifida) and the brain (such as anencephaly). Since these effects can occur at very early stages of pregnancy, women should begin taking folic acid before trying to conceive, whenever possible.
6. **The answer is E.** Epoetin alfa increases the rate of proliferation and differentiation of erythroid precursor cells in the bone marrow. It increases the release of reticulocytes. It also increases hemoglobin synthesis. The action of erythropoietin requires adequate iron stores, but it does not specifically decrease iron stores. Participation in the mitochondrial reaction that produces succinyl-CoA refers to the mechanism of action of one of the natural cobalamins, deoxyadenosylcobalamin.
7. **The answer is A.** Calcium carbonate is an antacid commonly used to manage mild heartburn symptoms. Calcium may impair iron absorption; therefore, it is important to monitor for decreased therapeutic effects of oral iron preparations when antacids like calcium carbonate are coadministered. The other medications listed will not affect iron absorption.
8. **The answer is A.** Cyanocobalamin, or vitamin B_{12}, is used for the management of pernicious anemia (inadequate secretion of intrinsic factor with subsequent reduction in vitamin B_{12} absorption). Ferrous sulfate is used for iron-deficiency anemia. Pyridoxine (vitamin B_6) can be used for the management of sideroblastic anemia. Hydroxyurea is used for sickle cell anemia.

9. **The answer is D.** Clotting factors produced before warfarin therapy decline in concentration as a function of factor half-life. Factor VII has the shortest half-life of 4–6 hours. Factor II has the longest half-life ranging from 42 to 72 hours. Similar to factor VII, protein C also has a short half-life. Warfarin initially decreases protein C levels (an anticoagulant) faster than the coagulation factors. This may create a transient hypercoagulable state. Heparin is required for anticoagulation due to the initial hypercoagulable state produced by warfarin therapy.
10. **The answer is E.** Hydroxyurea increases the production of fetal hemoglobin and has been shown to be effective in reducing painful episodes of sickle crisis. Darbepoetin alfa stimulates the proliferation and differentiation of erythroid precursor cells in the bone marrow in patients with anemia. Although it is used to decrease the necessity of transfusions in patients with chronic kidney disease or undergoing chemotherapy, it is not indicated for sickle cell anemia. Deferoxamine, cyanocobalamin (vitamin B_{12}), and clopidogrel are not used for these indications.
11. **The answer is B.** Filgrastim is a G-CSF used to stimulate bone marrow production, maturation, and activation of neutrophils to increase their migration and cytotoxicity. It can be used as secondary prophylaxis, after a previous cycle of chemotherapy caused neutropenic fever ("secondary prophylaxis"). The other medications are not used for this indication.
12. **The answer is A.** Heparin increases the activity of antithrombin by 1,000-fold. It binds to antithrombin III via a key pentasaccharide sequence and irreversibly inactivates factor IIa (thrombin) and factor Xa. It also inactivates coagulation factors IXa, XIa, and XIIa. By decreasing thrombin-mediated events in coagulation, including the conversion of fibrinogen to fibrin, fibrin-mediated clot formation is inhibited. It cannot inhibit clot-bound factor IIa or Xa.
13. **The answer is E.** The patient was most likely prescribed warfarin, which is a vitamin K antagonist. The international normalized ratio (INR), a standardized measurement of the prothrombin time (PT), is used to monitor warfarin therapy. Warfarin must be monitored regularly since it has a narrow therapeutic index. Vitamin K–containing foods, such as green leafy vegetables like spinach, can decrease the efficacy of warfarin. Acute alcohol ingestion can also affect warfarin levels.
14. **The answer is E.** The patient most likely had another stroke due to the decreased effectiveness of clopidogrel. Clopidogrel is a prodrug, and its effectiveness is dependent on its conversion to an active metabolite by the CYP2C19 enzyme. Proton pump inhibitors, like pantoprazole, inhibit the CYP2C19 enzyme and may prevent metabolism of clopidogrel to its active metabolite, therefore decreasing its effectiveness. The other medications do not interact with clopidogrel.
15. **The answer is E.** Enoxaparin is equally efficacious compared with unfractionated heparin in pulmonary embolism. Their efficacy is comparable. Both enoxaparin and UFH have a quicker onset of action. Enoxaparin is long-acting than UFH. It is given subcutaneously and not orally. Enoxaparin is less likely to cause heparin-induced thrombocytopenia than unfractionated heparin.

Chapter

8 Drugs Acting on the Pulmonary System

Competencies Addressed: PH1.32, PH1.33

I. INTRODUCTION TO PULMONARY DISORDERS

A. Asthma

1. ***Asthma is characterized by acute episodes of bronchoconstriction caused by underlying airway inflammation***.
   a. A hallmark of asthma is bronchial hyperreactivity to numerous kinds of endogenous or exogenous stimuli.
   b. In asthmatic patients, the response to various stimuli is amplified by persistent inflammation.
2. Early-phase response. ***Antigenic stimuli trigger the release of mediators*** (leukotrienes, histamine, PGD_2, and many others) that cause a bronchospastic response, with **smooth muscle contraction**, **mucus secretion**, and **recruitment of inflammatory cells**, such as eosinophils, neutrophils, and macrophages.
3. Late-phase response (may occur within hours or days). It is an inflammatory response in which the levels of histamine and other mediators released from inflammatory cells rise again and may induce bronchospasm. Eventually, fibrin and collagen deposition and tissue destruction occur. Smooth muscle hypertrophy occurs in chronic asthma.
4. Nonantigenic stimuli (cool air, exercise, and nonoxidizing pollutants) can trigger nonspecific bronchoconstriction after early phase sensitization.
5. The **methacholine challenge test** can be used in the diagnosis of asthma.
   a. Methacholine is a muscarinic cholinergic agonist.
   b. Nonasthmatic patients have a low-level response to methacholine, whereas asthmatic patients have hyperresponsiveness (exaggerated bronchoconstriction).

B. Chronic obstructive pulmonary disease

1. **Chronic bronchitis**
   a. Chronic bronchitis is characterized by **pulmonary obstruction** caused by excessive production of **mucus** due to hyperplasia and hyperfunctioning of mucus-secreting goblet cells; this causes a chronic (>2 months) cough.
   b. Smoking or environmental irritants often induce chronic bronchitis.
2. **Emphysema**
   a. Emphysema is a type of chronic obstructive pulmonary disease (COPD) characterized by **irreversible loss of alveoli** due to destruction of cell walls. This decreases the surface area available for gas exchange.

II. AGENTS USED TO TREAT ASTHMA AND OTHER BRONCHIAL DISORDERS

A. Categories of pharmacologic agents

1. Pharmacologic agents used to treat asthma are often divided into two broad categories.
   a. **Quick-relief medications (rescue medications; relievers)** are taken **as needed** for rapid, short-term relief of symptoms.
      (1) Examples include short-acting β_2-agonists and inhalational anticholinergics.
   b. **Long-term control medications (controllers)** are taken regularly to **control chronic symptoms** and prevent asthma attacks.
      (1) Examples include long-acting β_2-agonists, inhaled corticosteroids, leukotriene-receptor antagonists, and mast cell stabilizers.

B. Adrenergic agonists

1. ***Mechanism of action***
   a. Adrenergic agonists **stimulate β_2-adrenoceptors**, causing an increase in cyclic adenosine monophosphate (cAMP) levels, which leads to **relaxation of bronchial smooth muscle** (Fig. 8.1).
2. ***Short-acting β_2-adrenoceptor agonists (SABAs)***
   a. ***Specific agents*** include **salbutamol**, **levosalbutamol**, **terbutaline**, and **orciprenaline**.
      (1) These agents have **enhanced β_2-receptor selectivity** and are preferred because they produce **less cardiac stimulation** (except orciprenaline, which is relatively less selective).
      (2) They are generally administered by inhalation, in which their onset of action is 1–5 minutes.
   b. ***Indications.*** They are used for **quick relief of acute asthma symptoms**, such as shortness of breath, wheezing, and chest tightness.
   c. SABAs are prescribed for as-needed use and **should not be used routinely**.
      (1) Escalating use may be a sign that asthma is inadequately controlled.
      (2) Long-term use of these agents for the treatment of chronic asthma is associated with diminished control, perhaps due to β-receptor downregulation.
3. ***Long-acting β_2-adrenoceptor agonists (LABAs)***
   a. ***Specific agents*** include **salmeterol**, **formoterol**, and vilanterol (ultralong-acting).
      (1) These agents are administered as inhalants but have a slower onset of action and a longer duration of action than the short-acting preparations.
         (a) They have very lipophilic side chains that slow diffusion out of the airway.
   b. ***Indications.*** LABAs are **used in combination with inhaled glucocorticoids** for patients with moderate to severe asthma.

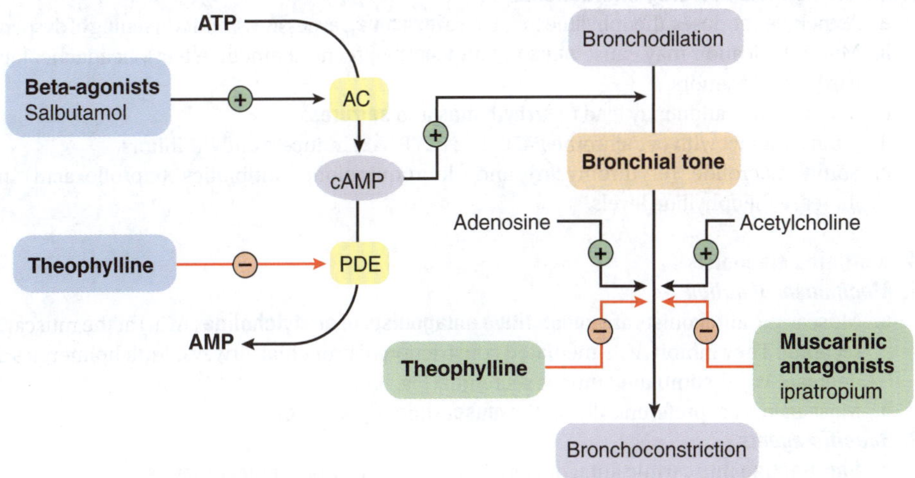

FIGURE 8.1. Mechanism of action for β_2-agonists, muscarinic antagonists, and methylxanthines. AC, adenylyl cyclase; cAMP, cyclic AMP; PDE, phosphodiesterase.

(1) They should never be prescribed as monotherapy.
(2) They are very effective for **long-term control of asthma** but should **not be used to treat an acute attack.**

c. Salbutamol and terbutaline can be administered orally for long-term control.

4. ***Adverse effects***
   a. The adverse effects of adrenergic agonists are based on receptor occupancy.
   b. They are minimized by inhalant delivery directly to the airways.
      (1) The most common adverse effect is skeletal muscle **tremor.**
      (2) **Increased heart rate and palpitations** may occur, especially with nonselective agents like metaproterenol.
      (3) β_2-Adrenoreceptor agonists may **decrease serum potassium levels.**

C. Methylxanthines

1. ***Specific agents*** include **theophylline, doxofylline, and aminophylline.**
2. ***Mechanism of action*** (Fig. 8.1)
   a. **Theophylline inhibits phosphodiesterase (PDE) enzymes** (mostly phosphodiesterase type 3 [PDE3] and phosphodiesterase type 4 [PDE4]); this prevents degradation of cAMP, leading to **bronchial smooth muscle relaxation.**
   b. It is also an **adenosine-receptor antagonist.**
      (1) Adenosine causes bronchoconstriction and promotes the release of histamine from mast cells.
   c. It may enhance calcium uptake through adenosine-mediated channels, leading to an increased force of contraction of diaphragmatic muscles.
3. ***Pharmacologic properties***
   a. Theophylline has a **narrow therapeutic index**; blood levels should be monitored to prevent drug intoxication. The therapeutic range is 5–15 mg/L.
   b. Clearance of theophylline has wide variability and is affected by diet, drugs, and liver function.
   c. It is metabolized in the liver and excreted by the kidney.
4. ***Indications***
   a. Theophylline can be used as **add-on therapy** when inhaled corticosteroids and/or β-adrenoceptor agonists inadequately control asthma symptoms.
   b. It may be used treat chronic bronchitis and emphysema.
      (1) Doxofylline is another oral methylxanthine claimed to produce lesser adverse drug reactions.
      (2) Aminophylline, a parenteral methylxanthine, has been used to treat severe acute asthma, although a favorable risk–benefit ratio has not been demonstrated.
   c. Caffeine, another methylxanthine, may be used to treat apnea in preterm infants (based on stimulation of the central respiratory center).
5. ***Adverse effects and drug interactions***
   a. At therapeutic doses, theophylline may cause **insomnia**, restlessness, and worsening of dyspepsia.
   b. Mild intoxication may cause **nausea and vomiting** (central emetic effect), headache, tachycardia, and tremors.
   c. Severe intoxication may lead to **arrhythmias** and **seizures.**
   d. It may interact with cytochrome P450-1A2 (CYP1A2) inducers and inhibitors.
   e. Some macrolide (erythromycin) and fluoroquinolone antibiotics (ciprofloxacin) may increase theophylline levels.

D. Muscarinic antagonists

1. ***Mechanism of action***
   a. Muscarinic antagonists are **competitive antagonists of acetylcholine** (ACh) at the muscarinic receptor. They inhibit ACh-mediated constriction of bronchial airways. Anticholinergics also decrease vagal-stimulated mucus secretion (Fig. 8.1).
   b. Most agents act preferentially on the **muscarinic M_3 receptor.**
2. ***Specific agents***
   a. **Short-acting** muscarinic antagonists (SAMA) include **ipratropium bromide.**
   b. **Long-acting** muscarinic antagonists (LAMA) include **tiotropium**, umeclidinium, and glycopyrronium.

3. ***Indications***
   a. All agents can be used for the **maintenance of COPD**.
   b. **Ipratropium** can be used for **acute asthma exacerbations**.
   c. **Tiotropium** can be used for **asthma maintenance** therapy.
4. ***Adverse effects***
   a. These agents are **given by inhalation. Systemic absorption is low**, although some absorption from the lung can occur.
   b. Ipratropium bromide and tiotropium are **quaternary ammonium compounds**; therefore, they are **poorly absorbed** and **do not cross the blood–brain barrier**.
      (1) For this reason, these agents have fewer adverse effects.
   c. **Dry mouth** and abnormal taste may occur. Urinary retention may be seen in elderly patients.

E. Glucocorticoids

1. ***Mechanism of action*** (Fig. 8.2)
   a. Glucocorticoids **bind to intracellular glucocorticoid receptors.** They form a steroid–receptor complex, which translocates to the nucleus and binds to glucocorticoid response elements in DNA.
      (1) This **alters the transcription of several genes**, including those coding for the β_2-adrenergic receptor and anti-inflammatory proteins.
   b. They can **reduce the number of inflammatory cells** and **decrease vascular permeability** and **mucus production.**
      (1) While they do not directly affect contractile function of the airway smooth muscle, they can produce a significant increase in airway diameter.
         (a) This effect is most likely from attenuating prostaglandin and leukotriene syntheses via annexin 1a and inhibiting the immune response, including production of cytokines and chemoattractants.
2. ***Specific agents*** include **beclomethasone, triamcinolone acetate, budesonide**, flunisolide, **fluticasone propionate, and ciclesonide.**
   a. Glucocorticoids are available as oral, parenteral, and inhaled agents.

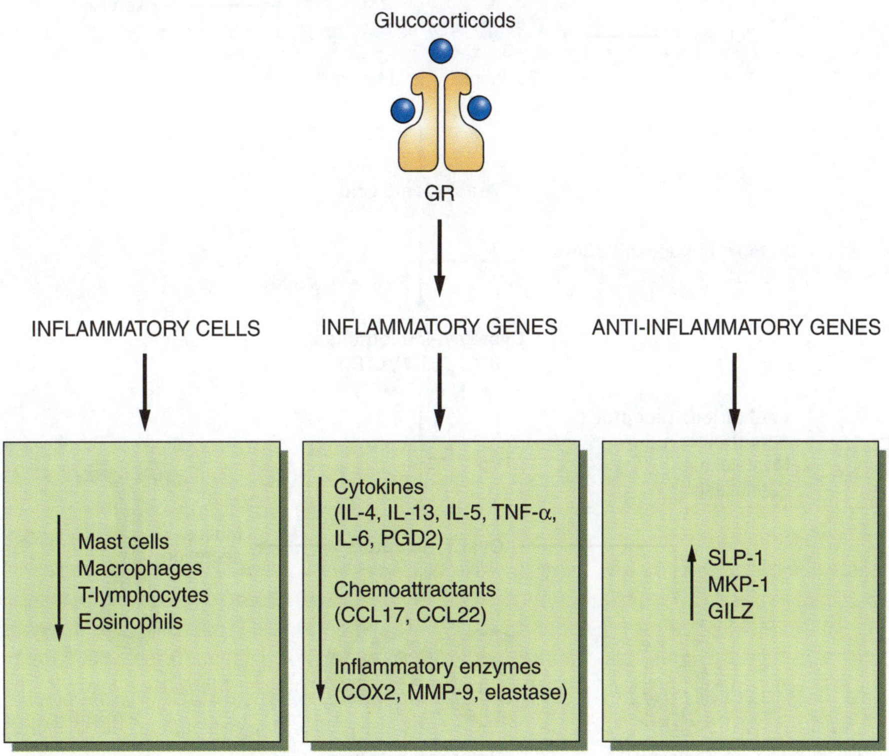

FIGURE 8.2. Effects of glucocorticoids in asthma. GILZ, glucocorticoid-induced leucine zipper; MKP-1, MAP kinase phosphatase; SLP-1, secretory leukoprotease inhibitor 1.

3. ***Indications***
   a. These are **first-line agents for the treatment of persistent asthma**.
      (1) Inhaled glucocorticoids may be recommended for the initial treatment of asthma, with additional agents added as needed.
      (2) They are used prophylactically rather than to reverse an acute attack.
      (3) Because of their systemic adverse effects, **oral glucocorticoids** (see Chapter 10) are usually reserved for patients with severe persistent asthma.
   b. Inhaled glucocorticoids are poorly effective in COPD.
4. ***Adverse effects***
   a. Systemic effects are decreased when administered by inhalation.
   b. Common adverse effects of inhaled glucocorticoids include hoarseness of voice and **oral candidiasis.** Patients should rinse their mouth with water (without swallowing) after each use to prevent oral candidiasis.
   c. Serious adverse effects of systemic glucocorticoids include adrenal suppression and osteoporosis. **Ciclesonide** is a prodrug with extensive first-pass metabolism; hence, it is less likely to cause the above-mentioned adverse effects.

F. Leukotriene pathway inhibitors

1. **Leukotriene-receptor antagonists**
   a. ***Specific agents*** include **zafirlukast, montelukast, and pranlukast.**
   b. ***Mechanism of action*** (Fig. 8.3)
      (1) Cysteinyl leukotrienes (CysLTs) are synthesized by eosinophils and mast cells, which are prominent in asthmatic inflammation. They are also released from the nasal mucosa following exposure to an allergen, leading to symptoms of allergic rhinitis.

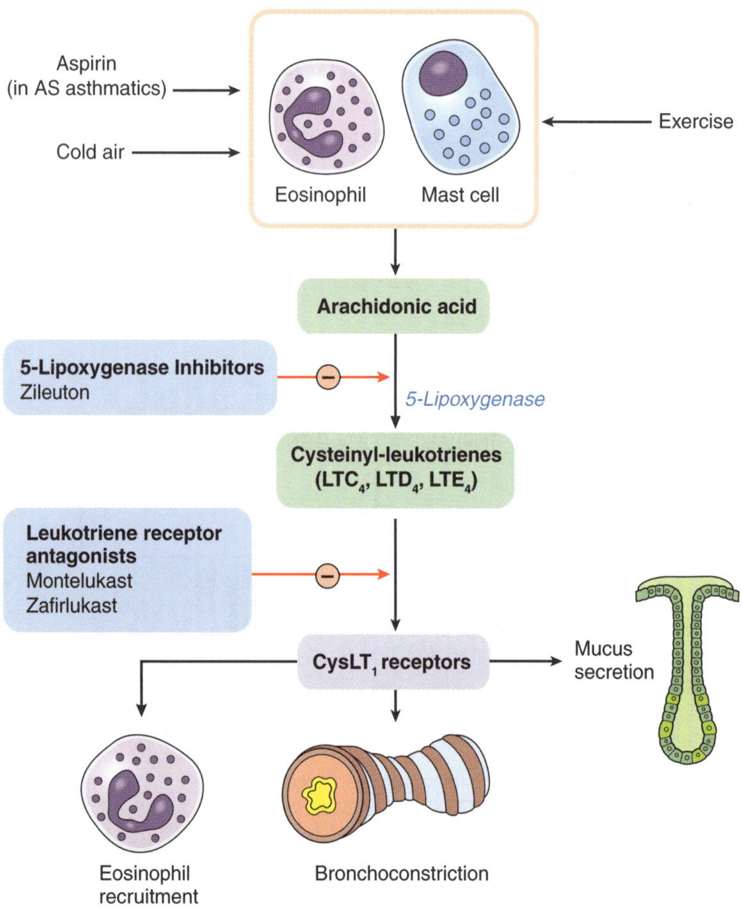

FIGURE 8.3. Mechanism of action of leukotriene pathway inhibitors.

(2) CysLTs include leukotriene C_4, D_4, and E_4 (LTC_4, LTD_4, LTE_4, respectively).

(3) Montelukast and zafirlukast are **CysLT type 1–receptor antagonists.**

(4) They **reduce airway edema, bronchoconstriction, and inflammatory cell infiltration.**

c. ***Indications.*** Montelukast and zafirlukast may be used for the prophylaxis and chronic treatment of asthma. Montelukast may also be used to relieve symptoms associated with allergic rhinitis. Both are administered orally.

d. ***Adverse effects*** of zafirlukast include headache and elevation in liver enzymes.

e. ***Drug interaction.*** Zafirlukast may increase the serum concentration of warfarin.

2. **5-Lipoxygenase inhibitor**

a. ***Specific agent.* Zileuton.**

b. ***Mechanism of action.*** Zileuton **inhibits 5-lipoxygenase**, the rate-limiting enzyme in leukotriene biosynthesis. Inhibiting leukotriene formation can help **decrease the inflammation, mucus secretion, and bronchoconstriction** associated with asthma (Fig. 8.3).

c. ***Indications.*** Zileuton is approved for the **prophylaxis and chronic treatment of asthma** in adults and children ≥12 years of age. It is administered orally.

d. ***Adverse effects.*** Zileuton can cause headaches. It also has the potential to cause **hepatotoxicity**; therefore, liver enzymes should be monitored; elderly women appear to be at the highest risk.

3. It is important to note that the leukotriene pathway is one of many responsible for the inflammatory symptoms associated with asthma. For this reason, **leukotriene pathway inhibitors are less effective than inhaled corticosteroids**, which affect several processes involved with inflammation.

G. Anti-IgE antibody

1. ***Specific agent.* Omalizumab.**

2. ***Mechanism of action.*** Omalizumab is a **monoclonal antibody that binds to human IgE's high-affinity Fc receptor, blocking the binding of IgE to mast cells**, basophils, and other cells associated with the allergic response (Fig. 8.4).

a. It also lowers free serum IgE concentrations by as much as 90%. Since it does not block the allergen–antibody reaction, it leads to a reduction in allergen concentrations.

b. These activities reduce both the early phase degranulation reaction of mast cells and the late-phase release of mediators.

3. ***Indications.*** Omalizumab is used as an adjunct treatment for **asthma** in patients older than 6 years whose asthma is **inadequately controlled with inhaled glucocorticoids and LABAs**, as well as in asthmatic patients with **allergies** (by allergy skin tests or in vitro measurements of allergen-specific IgE). It is administered by subcutaneous injection every 2–4 weeks.

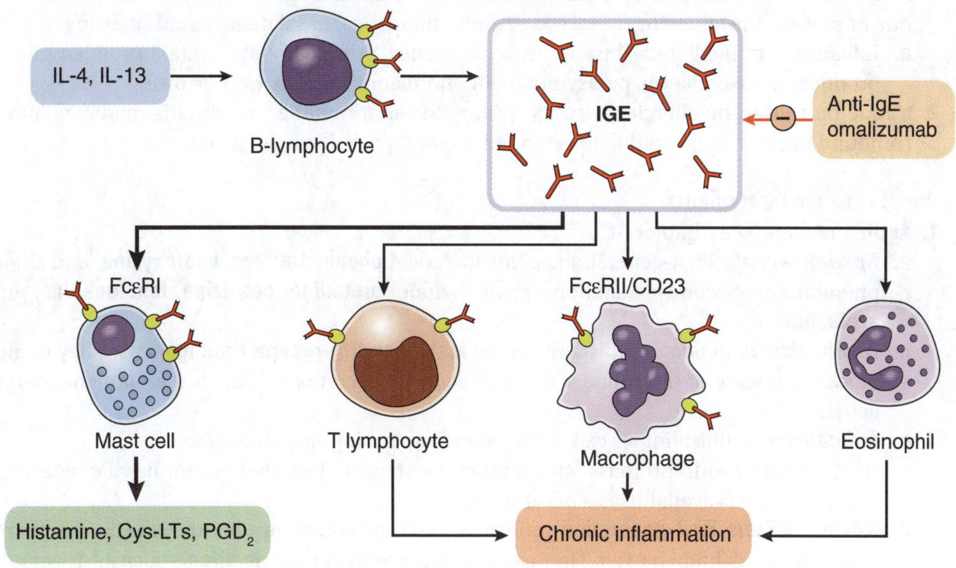

FIGURE 8.4. Mechanism of action for anti-IgE monoclonal antibodies.

4. ***Adverse effects*** include injection site reactions and arthralgia. It may also cause **anaphylaxis**; therefore, patients should be monitored after administration.
5. Newer monoclonal antibodies used for disease control in patients with severe eosinophilic asthma include the following:
   a. Anti-interleukin-5 antibody—mepolizumab, reslizumab.
   b. Anti-interleukin-4 antibody—dupilumab.
   c. Anti-interleukin-5 receptor antagonist—benralizumab.

   All these drugs are administered subcutaneously, except reslizumab which is intravenous. These are used as add-on medications when the inhalational corticosteroid–LABA combination produces inadequate response.

H. Chromones (see Chapter 6)

1. ***Specific agent.*** **Sodium cromoglycate (cromoglicic acid).**
2. ***Mechanism of action.*** Sodium cromoglycate is a **mast cell stabilizer.** It prevents the release of histamine and slow-reacting substance of anaphylaxis (SRS-A) from sensitized mast cells. It does not affect airway smooth muscle tone.
3. ***Indication.*** It can be given by nebulization for **chronic control of asthma**.
4. ***Adverse effects*** are rare but may include **dry mouth**, **throat irritation**, and **cough**.

I. Phosphodiesterase-4 enzyme inhibitor

1. ***Specific agent.*** **Roflumilast.**
2. ***Mechanism of action.*** Roflumilast is a PDE4 inhibitor; it leads to **increased cAMP levels and bronchodilation**. It may also have anti-inflammatory activity through inhibition of cytokine release and decreased neutrophils.
3. ***Indication.*** It is approved to **reduce the risk of COPD exacerbations**.
4. ***Adverse effects*** include nausea, diarrhea, and weight loss. It may be associated with neuropsychiatric reactions and should be used with caution in patients with a history of depression or suicidal thoughts and behavior.

III. DRUGS USED TO TREAT RHINITIS AND COUGH

A. Rhinitis

1. Rhinitis is inflammation and swelling of the mucous membrane of the nose, characterized by one or more of the following: nasal congestion, rhinorrhea, nasal itching, and sneezing.
   a. Inflammatory mediators (histamine, leukotrienes, prostaglandins, kinins) produce mucus production, vasodilation, parasympathetic stimulation, and airway narrowing.
2. It may be caused by allergies, viruses, vasomotor abnormalities, or rhinitis medicamentosa (rebound nasal congestion due to extended use of topical decongestants).

B. Agents used to treat rhinitis

1. **Antihistamines** (see Chapter 6)
   a. ***Specific agents.*** First-generation agents include **diphenhydramine**, **hydroxyzine**, and chlorpheniramine. Second-generation agents include **loratadine**, **cetirizine**, **fexofenadine**, and **azelastine**.
   b. ***Mechanism of action.*** Antihistamines are **histamine (H_1)-receptor antagonists**. They do not block the release of histamine. They also decrease secretions through their anticholinergic activity.
   c. ***Indications.*** Antihistamines can reduce sneezing, itching, and rhinorrhea.
      (1) Compared with intranasal glucocorticoids, they are less effective for nasal congestion. Azelastine is available as a nasal spray.
   d. ***Adverse effects.*** **First-generation** antihistamines cause **sedation** since they are lipophilic and cross the blood–brain barrier. They can also cause **anticholinergic effects** such as dry mouth and dry eyes. **Second-generation** agents **are less sedating**.

2. α-Adrenoceptor agonists

a. ***Specific agents.*** **Oxymetazoline** and **phenylephrine** are available as intranasal sprays. Phenylephrine and **pseudoephedrine** can be administered orally.

(1) While **intranasal** administration allows for rapid onset and has few systemic effects, it also has an increased risk for **rebound nasal congestion**.

(2) Oral administration allows for a longer duration of action but has an increased risk for systemic effects.

b. ***Mechanism of action.*** α-Adrenoceptor agonists reduce airway resistance by **constricting dilated arterioles in the nasal mucosa**.

c. ***Indication.*** They are used for the treatment of nasal congestion.

d. ***Adverse effects*** may include nervousness, tremor, insomnia, dizziness, and rhinitis medicamentosa (chronic mucosal inflammation due to prolonged use of topical vasoconstrictors, characterized by rebound congestion, tachyphylaxis, dependence, and eventual mucosal necrosis [atrophic rhinitis]). Use for more than 3 days is not recommended.

3. Inhaled corticosteroids

a. ***Specific agents*** include **beclomethasone**, budesonide, flunisolide, **fluticasone**, and **mometasone**.

b. ***Mechanism of action.*** Inhaled glucocorticoids exert their anti-inflammatory action through a wide range of effects on various inflammatory cells and mediators, including mast cells and histamine.

c. ***Indications.*** These agents are effective for the management of nasal congestion and maintenance therapy for allergic rhinitis. They require 1–2 weeks for full effect.

d. ***Adverse effects*** include **oral candidiasis**. Patients should rinse their mouth with water (without swallowing) after each use to prevent oral candidiasis.

4. Anticholinergics might be more effective in rhinitis, but the doses required produce systemic adverse effects.

a. **Ipratropium**, a poorly absorbed ACh antagonist administered by nasal spray, is approved for rhinorrhea associated with the common cold or with allergic or nonallergic seasonal rhinitis.

C. Cough

1. *Characteristics of cough*

a. **Cough is produced by the cough reflex, which is integrated in the cough center in the medulla.**

(1) The initial stimulus for cough probably arises in the bronchial mucosa, where irritation results in bronchoconstriction.

(2) Cough receptors, specialized stretch receptors in the trachea and bronchial tree, send vagal afferents to the cough center and trigger the cough reflex (Fig. 8.5).

(3) Cough can be productive or nonproductive. Expectorants and mucolytics are indicated in productive cough and antitussives in nonproductive cough. Use of antitussives in productive cough can exacerbate the respiratory infection by causing retention of secretions.

D. Agents used to treat cough

1. Antitussive agents

a. **Opioids. Codeine, pholcodine.**

(1) These agents decrease sensitivity of the central cough center to peripheral stimuli and decrease mucosal secretions.

(2) Antitussive actions occur at doses lower than those required for analgesia.

(3) These agents produce constipation, nausea, and respiratory depression.

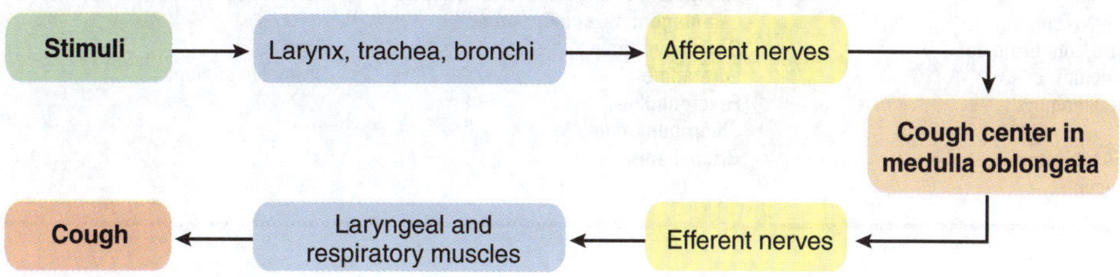

FIGURE 8.5. Mechanism of cough.

b. Noscapine, dextromethorphan. Noscapine is another opium alkaloid without any dependence liability. It does not have analgesic action.

(1) Dextromethorphan is the L-isomer of an opioid; it is active as an antitussive agent, but has less analgesic activity or addictive liability than codeine.

(2) Dextromethorphan is less constipating than **codeine**.

c. Benzonatate

(1) Benzonatate is a glycerol derivative chemically similar to procaine and other ester-type anesthetics.

(2) It reduces the activity of peripheral cough receptors and also appears to reduce the threshold of the central cough center.

d. Antihistaminics, such as chlorpheniramine and diphenhydramine, may relieve cough because of their sedative and anticholinergic properties.

2. Expectorants stimulate the production of watery, less-viscous mucus; they include **guaifenesin**.

a. Guaifenesin acts directly via the gastrointestinal tract to stimulate the vagal reflex.

b. Near-emetic doses of guaifenesin are required for beneficial effect; these doses are not attained in typical over-the-counter preparations.

c. Compounds such as potassium iodide, potassium citrate, and ammonium chloride also enhance bronchial secretions and are used as expectorants.

3. Mucolytics. Bromhexine, ambroxol, acetylcysteine, carbocysteine.

a. Bromhexine breaks down thick, tenacious sputum by releasing lysosomal enzymes which break down mucopolysaccharides.

b. Ambroxol is a metabolite of bromhexine with a similar action.

c. Acetylcysteine reduces the viscosity of mucus and sputum by **cleaving disulfide bonds**.

d. It is delivered as an inhalant and modestly reduces COPD exacerbation rates by roughly 30%. Oral formulation is also available.

e. Intravenous *N*-acetylcysteine is used as an antidote for acetaminophen toxicity (unrelated to its mucolytic activity).

f. Carbocysteine is a related drug which is orally administered.

DRUG SUMMARY TABLE

Short-Acting β_2-Adrenoceptor Agonists
Albuterol
Levalbuterol
Metaproterenol
Terbutaline

Long-Acting β_2-Adrenoceptor Agonists
Salmeterol
Formoterol
Terbutaline

Methylxanthines
Theophylline

Muscarinic Antagonists
Aclidinium
Glycopyrronium
Ipratropium bromide
Tiotropium
Umeclidinium

PDE4 Inhibitors
Roflumilast

Inhaled Glucocorticoids
Beclomethasone
Triamcinolone
Budesonide
Flunisolide
Fluticasone
Ciclesonide
Mometasone

Leukotriene Inhibitors
Zafirlukast
Montelukast
Zileuton

Anti-IgE Antibody
Omalizumab

Antihistamines (selected H_1-receptor antagonists, see Chapter 6)
Diphenhydramine
Loratadine
Fexofenadine
Chlorpheniramine
Brompheniramine

α-Adrenoceptor Agonists (selected, see Chapter 2)
Oxymetazoline
Phenylephrine
Pseudoephedrine

Antitussives
Codeine
Hydrocodone
Hydromorphone
Dextromethorphan
Benzonatate

Expectorants
Guaifenesin

Mucolytics
N-Acetylcysteine

Chromone
Cromolyn sodium

Review Test

Directions: Select the best answer for each question.

1. A 17-year-old male presents to the physician with complaints of a chronic cough that often increases with severity at different times throughout the day. His symptoms occur about twice a week and are beginning to interfere with his studies. Which of the following would be the most appropriate treatment for this patient?

(A) Budesonide
(B) Diphenhydramine
(C) Omalizumab
(D) Prednisone
(E) Theophylline

2. A 52-year-old woman presents to the emergency room with complaints of a severe asthma attack. A week prior, she was discharged from the hospital after being treated for a myocardial infarction. Her medications include daily low-dose aspirin. A diagnosis of drug hypersensitivity is made after further evaluation. What medication should be prescribed for the management of her drug hypersensitivity?

(A) Salbutamol
(B) Budesonide
(C) Ipratropium
(D) Theophylline
(E) Zafirlukast

3. A 20-year-old man presents to his primary care physician with complaints of worsening asthma. He is in college and participates in several intramural athletic programs, but in the last month, he has used his salbutamol inhaler at least 20 times following football practice. He has not been waking much at night. For the last 5 years, the patient has been well managed with inhaled glucocorticoids. Which of the following would be the best change in the treatment for this patient?

(A) Etanercept
(B) Salmeterol
(C) Sodium cromoglycate
(D) Triamcinolone
(E) Zileuton

4. A 62-year-old man presents to the emergency room with complaints of shortness of breath and light-headedness. Further workup reveals a tachyarrhythmia. The patient was recently started on moxifloxacin for the management of an upper respiratory infection, and the pharmacist is concerned that his symptoms are due to a drug interaction with his asthma medication. Which of the following medications was the patient most likely taking for the management of asthma?

(A) Salbutamol
(B) Budesonide
(C) Omalizumab
(D) Prednisone
(E) Theophylline

5. A 51-year-old woman is currently on theophylline for the management of chronic asthma. Which of the following statements correctly describes the action for this medication?

(A) Adenosine-receptor antagonist
(B) β-Receptor agonist
(C) Histamine-receptor agonist
(D) Muscarinic-receptor antagonist

6. A 24-year-old woman presents to the pharmacy to pick up a prescription for the management of her persistent cough. She was started on a medication that was supposed to decrease sensitivity of the central cough center to peripheral stimuli and decrease mucosal secretions. Which of the following medications was prescribed?

(A) Benzonatate
(B) Codeine
(C) Diphenhydramine
(D) Guaifenesin
(E) *N*-Acetylcysteine

7. A 74-year-old woman presents to her physician with complaints of urinary retention and dry mouth for the past 2 weeks. Recently, she was started on a new medication for the management of COPD. Which of the following medications most likely caused these symptoms?

(A) Budesonide
(B) Montelukast
(C) Salmeterol
(D) Theophylline
(E) Tiotropium

8. Which of the following monoclonal antibodies is not useful in the treatment of bronchial asthma

(A) Benralizumab
(B) Dupilumab
(C) Eculizumab
(D) Omalizumab
(E) Reslizumab

9. A 49-year-old man presents to his primary care physician with complaints of difficulty breathing. He has a 15-year history of smoking. Physical examination is positive for wheezing. Pulmonary function tests and lung diffusion studies are completed, and the patient is diagnosed with chronic obstructive pulmonary disease. He is prescribed tiotropium twice a day. Six months later, he returns to the clinic. Although he quit smoking, he has complaints of one episode of serious shortness of breath each day. Which of the following medications should be added to his treatment regimen?

(A) Beclomethasone
(B) Dexamethasone
(C) Roflumilast
(D) Omalizumab
(E) Zileuton

10. An adult female on low-dose fluticasone treatment for bronchial asthma complains of inadequate disease control for the past 6 weeks. An appropriate add-on drug in this case would be:

(A) Cromolyn sodium
(B) Formoterol
(C) Ipratropium
(D) Omalizumab
(E) Theophylline

Answers and Explanations

1. **The answer is A.** This is a fairly classical presentation of asthma, which should be confirmed with further pulmonary testing. Mild persistent asthma can be treated in several ways, but inhaled glucocorticoids, such as budesonide, are very effective. Oral prednisone has many side effects, especially in a young person. Omalizumab is for patients who are refractory to other treatments and those with allergies. Antihistamines such as diphenhydramine are poorly effective in asthma, and theophylline is only moderately effective.
2. **The answer is E.** The patient has drug hypersensitivity due to her recent history of aspirin. Aspirin's inhibition of cyclooxygenase most likely caused a shift of arachidonic acid metabolism to the leukotriene pathway, therefore leading to bronchoconstriction. Zafirlukast, a leukotriene-receptor antagonist, can help with the management of aspirin-induced asthma.
3. **The answer is B.** The patient's asthma is worsening, especially in response to exercise or increased allergen exposure, and the excess of short-acting β_2-agonists requires a change in medication. The best choice would be a long-acting β_2-agonist like salmeterol. Oral glucocorticoids, like triamcinolone, have many adverse effects, and sodium cromoglycate and zileuton are unlikely to be sufficiently efficacious in the worsening asthma. Etanercept is an anti-inflammatory used in rheumatoid arthritis.
4. **The answer is E.** Theophylline has a narrow therapeutic index; blood levels should be monitored to prevent drug intoxication. Clearance of theophylline has a wide variability and is affected by diet, drugs, and liver function. At therapeutic doses, theophylline may cause insomnia, restlessness, and worsening of dyspepsia. Severe intoxication may lead to arrhythmias and seizures. Fluoroquinolone antibiotics, such as moxifloxacin, can prolong QTc interval and precipitate serious arrhythmias in a patient receiving proarrhythmic drugs like theophylline.
5. **The answer is A.** Theophylline may have several mechanisms of action, but its adenosine-receptor antagonist activity and the inhibition of phosphodiesterase are best understood.
6. **The answer is B.** Opioids such as codeine decrease sensitivity of the central cough center to peripheral stimuli and decrease mucosal secretions. The antitussive actions occur at doses lower than those required for analgesia. Benzonatate reduces the activity of peripheral cough receptors. Guaifenesin is an expectorant that stimulates the production of watery, less-viscous mucus. *N*-Acetylcysteine is a mucolytic that reduces the viscosity of mucus and sputum by cleaving disulfide bonds. Diphenhydramine decreases mucosal secretions sue to its anticholinergic action but does not specifically inhibit the cough center.
7. **The answer is E.** Tiotropium is a muscarinic receptor antagonist. It is used for the maintenance of COPD. Although it is administered as an inhalation drug and systemic absorption is low, elderly patients may be at risk for adverse effects such as urinary retention and dry mouth, due to the anticholinergic activity. The other medications do not cause urinary retention or dry mouth.
8. **The answer is C.** Eculizumab is a monoclonal antibody directed against the complement protein and is used in the treatment of paroxysmal nocturnal hemoglobinuria. All other listed monoclonal antibodies are useful in asthma, particularly associated with elevated eosinophil counts (type 2 asthma).
9. **The answer is C.** Roflumilast is a fairly specific PDE4 inhibitor, useful to decrease exacerbations in patients with chronic obstructive pulmonary disease (COPD). Oral glucocorticoids such as dexamethasone, pose serious risks when used chronically and inhaled glucocorticoids, like beclomethasone, are not recommended in early stage COPD. Omalizumab and zileuton are ineffective in COPD.
10. **The answer is B.** When low-dose inhalational steroid alone is unable to adequately control the disease, addition of a long-acting beta-receptor agonist, such as formoterol, is recommended. Ipratropium is a short-acting muscarinic antagonist used to relieve acute attacks. The other drugs are not indicated at this stage of the disease.

Chapter 9

Drugs Acting on the Gastrointestinal Tract

Competencies Addressed: PH1.34

I. ANTIEMETICS

A. Pathophysiology of nausea and vomiting

1. Nausea and vomiting consists of three stages:
   a. Stage 1. **Nausea** is a subjective, unpleasant feeling of the need to vomit. It may be accompanied by tachycardia, diaphoresis, and salivation.
   b. Stage 2. **Retching**, or dry heaving, is the reverse movement of the stomach and esophagus without vomiting.
   c. Stage 3. **Vomiting** is the forceful expulsion of gastric contents due to powerful and sustained contractions of the muscles in the abdomen and thorax.
2. Vomiting occurs when the vomiting center (in the medulla) is stimulated.
   a. There are four important sources of afferent input to the vomiting center:
      (1) The **chemoreceptor trigger zone (CTZ)** (area postrema) is outside the blood–brain barrier (BBB). Drugs such as chemotherapy agents, opioids, and anesthetics stimulate the CTZ, as well as disease states such as uremia. It contains **dopamine (D_2)**, **serotonin (5-HT_3)**, opioid, and **neurokinin (NK_1)** receptors.
      (2) The **vestibular center** is important for sensory information about motion, equilibrium, and spatial orientation. It may play an important role in motion sickness. It is rich in **muscarinic (M_1)** and **histamine (H_1)** receptors.
      (3) The **vagal and spinal afferent nerves** from the **gastrointestinal (GI) tract** are rich in **5-HT_3** receptors. Irritation from chemotherapy, radiation therapy, distention, or acute infectious gastroenteritis can lead to release of mucosal serotonin and activation of these receptors; this stimulates vagal afferent input to the vomiting center and CTZ.
      (4) The **higher cortical centers** play a role in vomiting due to smell, sight, thought, or even **anticipatory vomiting** prior to chemotherapy.
   b. These afferent inputs will lead to activation of the vomiting center in the medulla, which has M_1, 5-HT_3, and H_1 receptors.

B. Antiemetics

1. **Muscarinic M_1-receptor antagonist**
   a. ***Specific agent.*** Scopolamine (hyoscine).
   b. ***Mechanism of action.*** It blocks the action of acetylcholine in the vestibular nuclei. **It reduces the excitability of labyrinthine receptors** and depresses conduction from the vestibular apparatus to the vomiting center.
   c. ***Indications.*** Scopolamine can be used for motion sickness and recovery from anesthesia and surgery.
   d. ***Administration.*** It is available as a transdermal patch programmed to deliver the medication over a 3-day period. When used postoperatively, the patch should be removed 24 hours after surgery.
   e. ***Adverse effects*** include drowsiness, dry mouth, and blurred vision.

2. **Histamine H_1-receptor antagonists**
   a. ***Specific agents*** include **meclizine** and **dimenhydrinate.**
   b. ***Mechanism of action.*** These agents act by inhibiting histamine and cholinergic pathways of the vestibular apparatus. They block the CTZ, diminish vestibular stimulation, and depress labyrinthine function through central anticholinergic activity.
   c. ***Indications.*** These agents are used to treat **motion sickness** and **vertigo**.
   d. ***Adverse effects.*** They cause varying degrees of sedation and dry mouth. They may also have other anticholinergic side effects.
3. **Dopamine receptor antagonists**
   a. ***Specific agents*** include **prochlorperazine, promethazine,** droperidol, metoclopramide, and domperidone.
   b. ***Mechanism of action.*** These agents **block dopaminergic** receptors in the brain, including the **CTZ**, and inhibit peripheral transmission to the vomiting center.
      (1) **Prochlorperazine** and **promethazine** also block **α_1-adrenoceptors** and have **anticholinergic** and **antihistaminic** activity.
      (2) **Metoclopramide** also blocks serotonin receptors in the CTZ. In addition, it enhances the response to acetylcholine of tissue in the upper GI tract causing **enhanced motility** and **accelerated gastric emptying**.
      (3) Domperidone blocks the D_2 receptors in the CTZ but does not penetrate the blood brain BBB unlike metoclopramide.
   c. ***Indications***
      (1) Promethazine is used to prevent and control nausea and vomiting associated with anesthesia and surgery, including postoperative nausea and vomiting (PONV). It is also approved for motion sickness.
      (2) Prochlorperazine is used for the management of severe nausea and vomiting.
      (3) Droperidol is approved for PONV.
      (4) **Metoclopramide** is used for the prevention of PONV and chemotherapy-induced nausea and vomiting (CINV). It is also indicated for **diabetic gastroparesis** and **gastroesophageal reflux**, due to its ability to stimulate gastric emptying.
   d. ***Adverse effects***
      (1) Adverse actions include anticholinergic effects such as drowsiness, dry mouth, and blurred vision (less pronounced with droperidol), **extrapyramidal effects and hyperprolactinemia** (due to dopamine D_2 receptor blockade in the nigrostriatal and tuberoinfundibular pathway, respectively), and orthostatic hypotension (due to α_1-receptor blockade). Domperidone, being devoid of the ability to cross the BBB, does not cause extrapyramidal effects or hyperprolactinemia. **Droperidol** use is associated with **QT prolongation** and **torsade de pointes.**
   e. ***Contraindications*** include **Parkinson disease**, because of the potential for extrapyramidal effects.
4. **Selective 5-HT_3-receptor antagonists**
   a. ***Specific agents*** include **ondansetron**, dolasetron, **granisetron**, and palonosetron.
   b. ***Mechanism of action.*** These agents **block** the effects of serotonin at **5-HT_3 receptors**, both peripherally on **vagal nerve** terminals and centrally in the **CTZ**.
   c. ***Indications.*** They are very effective for **CINV** and **PONV**. Some are also approved for radiation-induced nausea and vomiting (**RINV**). Palonosetron is a long-acting drug that is useful for the treatment of delayed CINV.
   d. ***Adverse effects*** may include headache and constipation.
5. **Cannabinoids**
   a. ***Specific agents*** include **dronabinol** and **nabilone.**
   b. ***Mechanism of action.*** Both are preparations of **Δ-9-tetrahydrocannabinol**, the active cannabinoid in marijuana. They act by inhibiting the vomiting center through **stimulation of a CB_1** subtype of cannabinoid receptors.
   c. ***Indications.*** Both agents may be used for **CINV**. Dronabinol is also approved for **anorexia** in patients with acquired immune deficiency syndrome (**AIDS**).
   d. ***Adverse effects*** include sedation, tachycardia, and hypotension.
6. **Benzodiazepines** (see Chapter 5)
   a. ***Specific agent.*** **Lorazepam.**

b. ***Mechanism of action.*** Lorazepam enhances the inhibitor effects of gamma-aminobutyric acid (**GABA**). The antiemetic mechanism is related to a combination of effects, including sedation, reduction in anxiety, and potential depression of the vomiting center.
c. ***Indications.*** It is used off-label as an adjunct with other agents for **CINV** or for **anticipatory nausea and vomiting** associated with chemotherapy.
d. ***Adverse effects*** may include sedation and amnesia.

7. **Neurokinin 1 (NK_1)-receptor antagonists**
   a. ***Specific agents*** include **aprepitant** and fosaprepitant (an intravenous prodrug of aprepitant).
   b. ***Mechanism of action.*** Aprepitant inhibits the **substance P/NK_1** receptor. It **augments the antiemetic activity of 5-HT_3-receptor antagonists** and **corticosteroids** to inhibit acute and delayed phases of chemotherapy-induced emesis.
   c. ***Indications.*** They are used for the management of **CINV, both acute and delayed**, usually in **combination with 5-HT_3 antagonists and corticosteroids.** Aprepitant is also approved for PONV.
   d. ***Adverse effects*** include fatigue. Aprepitant can also cause hiccups.
   e. ***Drug interactions.*** They are metabolized by CYP3A4 enzymes. They also moderately inhibit CYP3A4. Caution must be taken when used with other drugs that use the same pathway.

II. DRUGS USED TO MANAGE OBESITY

A. Sympathomimetic drugs

1. ***Specific agents*** include **phentermine**, phenylpropanolamine, and diethylpropion.
2. ***Adverse effects*** may include **tachycardia**, **hypertension**, insomnia, constipation, and nervousness. They have a high risk of **dependence**. None of these drugs are approved for use in India.

B. Lipase inhibitor

1. ***Specific agent.*** **Orlistat.**
2. ***Mechanism of action.*** Orlistat is a reversible **lipase inhibitor** of gastric and pancreatic lipases. It inactivates the enzymes, making them **unavailable to digest dietary fats**. Orlistat inhibits absorption of fats by approximately 30%.
3. ***Indications.*** It can be used for **weight loss** and obesity management in conjunction with a reduced-calorie and low-fat diet.
4. ***Adverse effects***
   a. The major side effects are GI related, including **oily rectal leakage** (fecal spotting), flatulence, and **diarrhea**.
   b. It **prevents absorption of fat-soluble vitamins** (A, D, E, K); therefore, supplementation may be necessary.
5. ***Contraindications***
   a. It should not be used in patients with **cholestasis** and **malabsorption syndromes**.

C. Glucagon-like peptide-1-receptor agonist

1. ***Specific agent.*** **Liraglutide.**
2. ***Mechanism of action.*** This agent is an analogue of human **glucagon-like peptide-1 (GLP-1)**. It increases **glucose-dependent insulin secretion**, decreases inappropriate glucagon secretion, increases β-cell growth/replication, **slows gastric emptying**, and decreases food intake.
3. ***Indications.*** It may be used for **chronic weight management**, in addition to reduced calorie intake and exercise. It is also indicated for the treatment of **type 2 diabetes.**
4. ***Adverse effects*** may include tachycardia, headache, and GI distress.

D. Serotonin agonist

1. ***Specific agent.*** **Lorcaserin.**
2. ***Mechanism of action.*** This is an **agonist** at serotonin **5-HT_{2C} receptors**. Downstream effects eventually result in satiety and decreased food intake.
3. ***Indications.*** It is used as an adjunct for **chronic weight management**, in addition to reduced calorie intake and exercise.
4. ***Adverse effects*** include headache and upper respiratory tract infections.

Serotonergic agents fenfluramine and dexfenfluramine can cause valvular defects and have thus been banned. Sibutramine, a serotonin–noradrenaline reuptake inhibitor, was associated with an increased risk of cardiovascular events and death, leading to its withdrawal from the market.

III. DRUGS USED TO INCREASE APPETITE

Megestrol is a **progestin** that stimulates appetite by antagonizing the metabolic effects of catabolic cytokines. It can be used for the treatment of **anorexia**, **cachexia**, or unexplained weight loss in patients with AIDS.

Dronabinol is a cannabinoid (CB_1)-receptor agonist that can also be used for anorexia in patients with AIDS.

Cyproheptadine is a 5-HT_{2a}-receptor antagonist with antihistaminic and anticholinergic action that has been used as an appetite stimulant in children.

Mirtazapine is an atypical antidepressant with appetite stimulant action which may be useful in underweight depressed patients.

IV. AGENTS USED FOR ACID PEPTIC DISEASES

A. Agents that neutralize acid (antacids)

1. ***General characteristics***
   a. Acid neutralization capacity of antacids is highly variable and depends on several factors including rate of dissolution (tablet vs. liquid), water solubility, rate of reaction with acid, and rate of gastric emptying.
2. ***Mechanism of action*** (Fig. 9.1)
   a. Antacids are weak bases that react with gastric hydrochloric acid (HCl) to form salt and water (H_2O). They rapidly reduce intragastric acidity.
   b. Example of reaction: $CaCO_3 + 2HCl \rightarrow CaCl_2 + H_2O + CO_2$.
3. ***Adverse effects and other characteristics for specific agents***
   a. **Sodium bicarbonate**
      (1) ***Adverse effects***
         (a) **Gastric distention** and **belching** may occur due to carbon dioxide.
         (b) Sodium chloride may cause **fluid retention**.
         (c) Some unreacted sodium bicarbonate is systemically absorbed and can cause **metabolic alkalosis**. It should not be used for long-term treatment.
      (2) ***Contraindications*** include hypertension, heart failure, and renal failure.
   b. **Calcium carbonate**
      (1) ***Adverse effects*** may include **nausea** and **belching**. Calcium carbonate is partially absorbed from the GI tract and may cause systemic effects like **metabolic alkalosis**. It should not be used for long-term treatment.
   c. **Magnesium hydroxide**
      (1) Magnesium hydroxide is not absorbed from the GI tract and therefore produces **no systemic effects**. This agent can be used for **long-term therapy**.
      (2) The most frequent adverse effect associated with magnesium hydroxide is **diarrhea**.
   d. **Aluminum hydroxide** may cause **constipation.**
   e. Many products have a **combination of magnesium hydroxide** and **aluminum hydroxide** to achieve a **counteracting balance** between each agent's adverse **effects on the bowel**.
   f. Sodium bicarbonate and calcium carbonate have the potential to cause milk-alkali syndrome, which is characterized by high blood calcium and metabolic alkalosis.

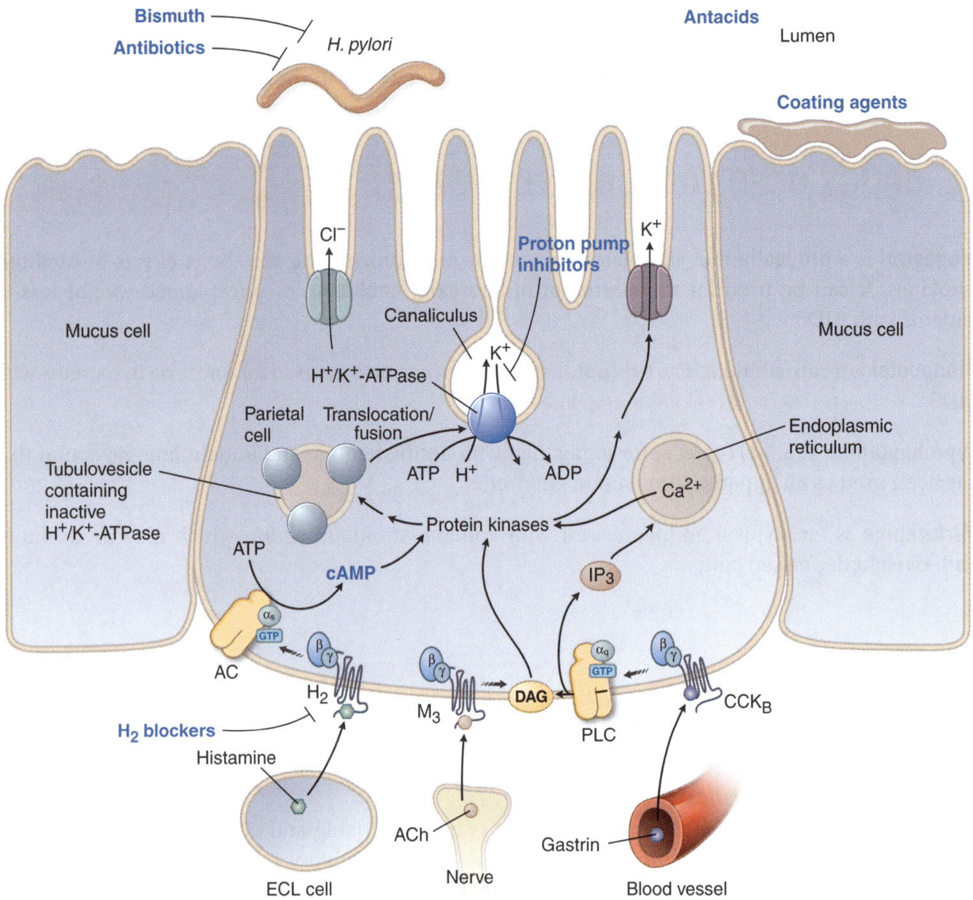

FIGURE 9.1. Mechanism of action for drugs used to manage gastric acidity. (Reprinted with permission from Golan D. Principles of Pharmacology. 4th ed. Philadelphia, PA: Wolters Kluwer Health, 2016, Fig. 47.4.)

4. ***Drug interactions.*** Antacids alter the bioavailability of many drugs:
   a. The **increase in gastric pH** produced by antacids decreases the absorption of acidic drugs and increases the absorption of basic drugs.
   b. The **metal ion** in some preparations can **chelate other drugs** (e.g., **digoxin** and **tetracycline)** and **prevent** their **absorption.**

B. Inhibitors of gastric acid production

1. Histamine H_2-receptor antagonists

a. ***Specific agents*** include **ranitidine**, **famotidine**, nizatidine, lafutidine, and cimetidine.

b. ***Mechanism of action*** (see Fig. 9.1)
   (1) The H_2-receptor antagonists act as **competitive inhibitors** of the histamine **H_2 receptor** on the parietal cell.
   (2) This results in a **decrease** in histamine-stimulated **gastric acid secretion.**
   (3) Although other agents such as gastrin and acetylcholine may induce acid secretion, **histamine** is the predominant final mediator that **stimulates parietal acid secretion.**
   (4) Famotidine binds tightly to the receptors and may have an inverse agonistic action. Lafutidine has additional gastroprotective effects.

c. ***Pharmacological properties***
   (1) These drugs are rapidly absorbed, and effects are observed within **a few minutes to hours.**
   (2) Although they are **less potent than proton pump inhibitors** (PPIs), they still suppress 24-hour gastric acid secretion by about 70%.

d. They predominantly inhibit **basal acid secretion**, which accounts for their efficacy in suppressing nocturnal acid secretion.

e. ***Indications*** include **peptic ulcer disease (PUD)**, **gastroesophageal reflux disease (GERD)**, stress-related gastritis (in intensive care settings), and non-ulcer-related dyspepsia.

f. ***Adverse effects***

(1) These agents are associated with **drowsiness**.

(2) Confusion may be seen with intravenous administration, especially in the elderly.

(3) **Cimetidine** is also an **androgen-receptor antagonist** and can induce galactorrhea, **gynecomastia**, and impotence.

g. ***Drug interactions***

(1) **Cimetidine** is a **cytochrome P-450 inhibitor.** It affects several pathways, including those catalyzed by CYP1A2, CYP2C9, CYP2D6, and CYP3A4.

(a) It can **increase the half-life** of drugs that are metabolized by this system, including **warfarin, theophylline, phenytoin,** and **benzodiazepines.**

2. Proton pump inhibitors

a. ***Specific agents*** include **omeprazole**, **lansoprazole**, dexlansoprazole, **esomeprazole**, **pantoprazole**, and rabeprazole.

b. ***Mechanism of action*** (see Fig. 9.1)

(1) They are covalent, **irreversible inhibitors** of the **H^+/K^+-ATPase pump** (proton pump) in parietal cells.

(2) As lipophilic weak bases, these agents are delayed-release **prodrugs** (to protect against their destruction by gastric acid) which get absorbed systemically and are activated in the acidic compartments of parietal cells.

(3) They are rapidly converted to an active cation, which forms a **covalent disulfide linkage to the H^+/K^+-ATPase proton pump**; this results in its inactivation, thereby blocking the transport of acid from the cell into the lumen.

c. ***Pharmacological properties***

(1) These agents **reduce** both **meal-stimulated** and **basal acid secretion.**

(2) Not all proton pumps are inhibited with the first dose; therefore, complete symptom relief may **take 3–4 days.**

(3) **Acid secretion resumes only after new pump molecules are synthesized** and inserted into the luminal membrane, providing a prolonged (up to 24- to 48-hour) suppression of acid secretion.

(4) Since they **block the final step in acid production**, PPIs are effective in acid suppression regardless of other stimulating factors.

(5) Their bioavailability is decreased significantly by food; ideally, they should be administered about 1 hour before a meal. This ensures that the optimal drug concentration in the blood coincides with the meal-induced activation of H^+/K^+-ATPase which results in maximal inhibition of the proton pumps.

d. ***Indications*** include GERD, PUD, Zollinger–Ellison syndrome, *Helicobacter pylori*–induced ulcers, and NSAID-induced ulcers. They are **more effective than H_2-antagonists.**

(1) PPIs are used in combination with antibiotics, and, in some cases, bismuth subsalicylate for the treatment of *H. pylori*–induced ulcers. Potential treatment regimens include the following:

(a) Quadruple therapy: Bismuth, metronidazole, tetracycline, and a PPI

(b) Triple therapy: Clarithromycin, amoxicillin, and a PPI

i. Typical regimen involves taking all the drugs twice daily for 2 weeks.

(c) Triple therapy: Clarithromycin, metronidazole, and a PPI

e. ***Adverse effects*** include nausea, abdominal pain, headache, and **hypomagnesemia**. PPIs may be associated with renal injury, and, on prolonged use, osteoporotic fractures.

f. ***Precautions*** include an increased risk for ***Clostridium difficile*–associated diarrhea**, especially in **hospitalized patients.**

(1) Reduced gastric acid might facilitate survival of these bacteria in the upper GI tract.

g. ***Drug interactions***

(1) Some PPIs, like pantoprazole, inhibit the CYP2C19 enzyme and may prevent metabolism of clopidogrel to its active metabolite, therefore decreasing its effectiveness.

(2) They may decrease the bioavailability of vitamin B_{12} and other drugs that require acidity for their GI absorption, such as digoxin and ketoconazole.

3. **Muscarinic antagonists**
   (1) **Specific agents** include pirenzepine, propantheline, and oxyphenonium.
   (2) Pirenzepine is M_1-selective muscarinic receptor antagonist which decreases gastric acid secretion.
   (3) Propantheline and oxyphenonium are nonselective antimuscarinics which also decrease GI motility.
   (4) These drugs are not commonly used due to their anticholinergic adverse effects and availability of better antiulcer drugs described above.

C. Agents that promote mucosal defense

1. **Sucralfate**
   a. ***Mechanism of action.*** Sucralfate is a complex salt of **sucrose sulfate** and **aluminum hydroxide**. It forms a **viscous gel** that binds to positively charged proteins and **adheres to gastric epithelial cells**, including areas of ulceration. It **protects** the surface of the stomach from **degradation by acid and pepsin.**
   b. ***Indications*** include **peptic ulcer** management (Fig. 9.1). Oral suspension is useful in chemotherapy-induced mucositis. Topical formulation can be used for bedsores, burns, and diabetic ulcers.
   c. ***Adverse effects*** may include **constipation** and nausea.
   d. ***Drug interactions.*** It may bind and impair absorption of certain medications, including quinolone antibiotics, phenytoin, and warfarin. Antacids decrease the polymerization of sucralfate to viscous gel consistency by raising the gastric pH >4 and hence decrease its effectiveness.
2. **Misoprostol**
   a. ***Mechanism of action.*** Misoprostol is an analogue of **prostaglandin E_1** that acts in the GI tract to **stimulate bicarbonate and mucus production**. It replaces the protective prostaglandins consumed with prostaglandin-inhibiting therapies, such as NSAIDs (see Fig. 9.1).
   b. ***Indication.*** It is used for the prevention of **NSAID-induced gastric ulcers**.
   c. ***Adverse effects*** may include diarrhea and abdominal pain.
   d. ***Precautions.*** It may cause **abortion**; therefore, it must be used with caution in women of childbearing age and is contraindicated in pregnant women.
3. **Colloidal bismuth subcitrate**
   a. **Mechanism of action.** In the acidic pH, it forms a protective coat over the ulcer base. It also has a cytoprotective effect and may directly inhibit *H. pylori*.
   b. **Indication.** It is used for the treatment of *H. pylori*–induced ulcers.
   c. **Adverse effects.** These include darkening of the tongue and black stools (temporary and harmless). (Also see **Antidiarrheal agents** below.)

V. DRUGS USED TO DISSOLVE GALLSTONES

A. Ursodiol

1. ***Mechanism of action.*** This drug's conjugated form **reduces hepatic synthesis and secretion of cholesterol into bile,** and its reabsorption by the intestine. It effectively **dissolves cholesterol gallstones**.
2. ***Indications.*** The capsules are used for the management of **noncalcified gallbladder stones** and for the prevention of gallstones in obese patients experiencing rapid weight loss. The tablets can be used for **primary biliary cirrhosis**. It requires administration for **months to reach full effect**.
3. ***Adverse effects*** may include diarrhea.

VI. DIGESTIVE ENZYME REPLACEMENTS

A. Pancrelipase

1. ***Mechanism of action.*** Pancrelipase (pancreatin) is a **digestive enzyme replacement** preparation of semipurified enzymes that contain various mixtures of lipase and proteolytic enzymes such as trypsin and amylase. The products dissolve in the duodenum and act locally to **break down fats, protein, and starch.**
2. ***Indications.*** It is used to treat **exocrine pancreatic insufficiency** associated with **cystic fibrosis** and **pancreatitis.**
3. ***Adverse effects*** are minimal, but may include occasional GI upset and hyperuricosuria.

VII. AGENTS THAT ACT ON THE LOWER GI TRACT

A. Agents used for constipation

1. **General characteristics**
   a. Laxatives (purgatives) act primarily on the large intestine to promote an **increase in the fluid** accumulated in the bowel, **decrease net absorption of fluid** from the bowel, or **alter bowel motility.** These actions facilitate the evacuation of fecal material.
   b. They should not be used chronically as they may induce "**laxative dependence.**"
   c. Many are contraindicated in bowel obstruction.
2. **Bulk-forming laxatives**
   a. ***Specific agents*** include **bran**, **psyllium**, methylcellulose, and polycarbophil.
   b. ***Mechanism of action.*** Bulk-forming laxatives absorb water in the intestine to form a bulky emollient gel, which promotes peristalsis and reduces transit time.
      (1) They produce laxation after 2–4 days; **adequate hydration** is required.
   c. ***Indications.*** These agents are the treatment of choice for **chronic constipation.**
   d. ***Adverse effects.*** They may cause abdominal cramps, bloating, and flatulence.
3. **Osmotic laxatives**
   a. ***Specific agents***
      (1) Salt-containing osmotic laxatives include **magnesium citrate**, magnesium hydroxide, and **sodium phosphate.**
      (2) Salt-free osmotic laxatives include **lactulose** and **polyethylene glycol (PEG) electrolyte solutions.**
   b. ***Mechanism of action.*** They **retain water** in the lumen by **osmosis.** They **distend** the **colon** and cause a reflex increase in **peristalsis** to promote bowel evacuation.
      (1) Onset of action typically occurs 3–6 hours after oral administration and 5–15 minutes after rectal administration.
      (2) They require adequate hydration for effect.
   c. ***Indications.*** These agents are used for both acute and chronic constipation.
      (1) PEG solutions may be used for bowel cleansing prior to rectal examination or surgery.
      (2) Lactulose can also be used for hepatic encephalopathy. Bacterial degradation of lactulose results in an acidic pH. This causes NH_3 to convert to NH_4^+, which is trapped in the colon for elimination, thereby reducing blood ammonia levels.
   d. ***Adverse effects***
      (1) Abdominal cramping, bloating, flatulence, and diarrhea may occur.
      (2) Sodium phosphate may cause hypernatremia and phosphatemia, especially in patients with renal dysfunction.
4. **Irritant (stimulant) laxatives (cathartics)**
   a. ***Specific agents*** include **bisacodyl** and **senna.**
   b. ***Mechanism of action.*** They have a number of poorly understood mechanisms. They **stimulate smooth muscle contractions** resulting from their irritant action on the bowel mucosa. Local bowel **inflammation also promotes accumulation of water and electrolytes.** The

increased luminal contents stimulate reflex peristalsis, and the irritant action stimulates peristalsis directly.

(1) The onset of action occurs in 6–12 hours.

(2) These agents require adequate hydration.

c. ***Indications.*** Both agents may be used for the temporary relief of occasional constipation. Bisacodyl is also approved for bowel cleansing prior to rectal examination or surgery.

d. ***Adverse effects*** may include abdominal cramps and electrolyte disturbances.

e. ***Precautions.*** Chronic use may result in **cathartic colon**, a condition of colonic distention, and development of laxative dependence.

5. **Stool softener**

a. ***Specific agent.*** **Docusate sodium.**

b. ***Mechanism of action***

(1) Docusate has a **detergent action** that facilitates the **mixing of water and fatty substances** to **increase luminal mass**.

(a) It is an anionic surfactant that reduces surface tension of the oil-water interface of stool, which results in enhanced incorporation of water and fat, allowing for stool softening.

(b) The onset of action is within 12–72 hours.

c. ***Indications.*** It is approved for occasional constipation with hard, dry stools. It may be used to **prevent straining** during defecation.

d. ***Adverse effects*** may include abnormal taste, abdominal cramping, and diarrhea.

e. ***Precaution.*** Prolonged or frequent use may result in dependence.

6. **Lubricating agent**

a. ***Specific agent.*** **Mineral oil.**

b. ***Mechanism of action.*** It **coats fecal contents** and thereby inhibits absorption of water; it softens and lubricates hard stools, allowing for easier passage of stool without irritating the mucosa.

c. ***Indications.*** It may be used for relief of occasional constipation. Rectal use may also help relieve fecal impaction.

d. ***Adverse effects*** may include abdominal cramps and **rectal discharge**.

e. ***Precautions and contraindications***

(1) Mineral oil **decreases the absorption of fat-soluble vitamins** (A, D, E, K).

(2) Aspiration of mineral oil may lead to **lipid pneumonitis.**

(a) For this reason, use is contraindicated in bedridden patients or those with difficulty swallowing.

7. **Opioid-receptor antagonists**

a. ***Specific agents*** include **methylnaltrexone** and alvimopan.

b. ***Mechanism of action.*** These agents **block opioid** binding at the **μ-receptor** in **peripheral tissues**, such as the **GI tract**. They inhibit the decreased GI motility and delay in GI transit time due to opioids.

(1) These agents **do not affect opioid analgesic effects**.

c. ***Indications.*** They are used for **opioid-induced constipation**. Alvimopan is approved only for postoperative ileus.

d. ***Adverse effects*** may include abdominal pain, flatulence, and nausea.

e. ***Precautions***

(1) **GI perforations** have been reported in patients with impaired structural integrity of the GI wall, such as PUD, diverticular disease, or infiltrative GI tract malignancies.

(2) They may be associated with opioid withdrawal symptoms, such as anxiety, chills, diarrhea, and yawning.

(3) Alvimopan has an increased incidence of myocardial infarction.

B. Antidiarrheal agents

1. **General characteristics**

a. Antidiarrheal agents may be used safely in patients with mild to moderate acute diarrhea.

b. They should not be used in patients with bloody diarrhea, high fever, or systemic toxicity due to the risk of worsening the underlying condition.

c. They should be discontinued in those whose diarrhea is worsening despite therapy.

2. **Opioid agonists**
   a. ***Specific agents*** include **loperamide, diphenoxylate plus atropine**, and difenoxin plus atropine.
   b. ***Mechanism of action.*** These agents act on the **opioid receptor** in circular and longitudinal **intestinal muscles**. They **inhibit peristalsis** and prolong transit time.
   c. ***Administration***
      (1) Difenoxin is the active metabolite of diphenoxylate.
      (2) At standard doses, they do not have analgesic properties, but at higher doses, they can cause central nervous system effects.
         (a) They are combined with small amounts of **atropine** to **discourage overdose** (due to potential for **anticholinergic side effects**).
            i. The anticholinergic properties of atropine may also contribute to the antidiarrheal action.
         (b) Prolonged use can lead to opioid dependence.
      (3) **Loperamide** does not cross the BBB. It has **no analgesic properties or potential for addiction**.
   d. ***Indications***
      (1) Diphenoxylate is approved for the adjunct management of diarrhea.
      (2) Difenoxin is used for the treatment of acute nonspecific diarrhea and acute exacerbations of chronic functional diarrhea.
      (3) Loperamide is used for chronic diarrhea associated with inflammatory bowel disease (IBD) in adults and acute nonspecific diarrhea and to reduce volume of ileostomy discharge. It may also be used for traveler's diarrhea.
   e. ***Adverse effects*** may include dizziness, drowsiness, and abdominal discomfort.
   f. ***Precautions.*** At high doses, they may cause severe constipation, paralytic ileus, or toxic megacolon. **Diphenoxylate should not be used in children younger than 13 years and loperamide in children younger than 4 years. Loperamide overdosage has been associated with serious adverse cardiac reactions in children as well as adults.**
3. **Racecadotril**
   a. **Mechanism of action.** It is a prodrug of thiorphan, which is an enkephalinase inhibitor. Thiorphan prevents the degradation of enkephalins in the GI tract. These enkephalins act via δ-opioid receptors, which help decrease the secretion of fluid and electrolytes into the GI lumen.
   b. **Indication.** It is used for the symptomatic treatment of acute diarrhea, including in children.
   c. **Adverse effects** may include hypersensitivity reaction/angioedema, skin reactions, tonsillitis, and headache.
   d. **Precautions.** Concomitant use with angiotensin-converting enzyme (ACE) inhibitors may increase the risk of angioedema. Unlike loperamide and diphenoxylate, which are antimotility antidiarrheals, racecadotril is an antisecretory drug that does not affect GI motility.
4. **Colloidal bismuth subcitrate (bismuth subsalicylate, bismuth subcitrate potassium)**
   a. ***Mechanism of action.*** It has **antisecretory** properties (due to salicylate moiety) and **antimicrobial** properties (due to bismuth) (see Fig. 9.1).
      (1) It may stimulate absorption of fluid and electrolytes across the intestinal wall.
      (2) It may inhibit synthesis of a prostaglandin responsible for intestinal inflammation and hypermotility.
      (3) It exhibits antimicrobial activity directly against bacterial and viral GI pathogens.
         (a) It **binds to toxins** produced by different microbes, such as *Escherichia coli.*
   b. ***Indications*** include diarrhea and dyspepsia. It is effective for the treatment and prophylaxis of **traveler's diarrhea**. It is also used for *H. pylori* eradication.
   c. ***Adverse effects*** include **fecal discoloration** (grayish black) and **tongue discoloration** (darkening). Tinnitus may also occur.
5. **Octreotide**
   a. ***Mechanism of action.*** Octreotide is an **analogue of somatostatin.** It decreases diarrhea by several mechanisms.
      (1) Octreotide acts directly on epithelial cells to **reduce the secretion** of a number of **pancreatic and GI hormones**, including **vasoactive intestinal polypeptide (VIP)**, serotonin, gastrin, secretin, and pancreatic polypeptide.

(2) It may also prolong intestinal transit time, promote intestinal absorption, and decrease secretion of fluids and electrolytes.

b. ***Indications***

(1) It is used in cases of **severe diarrhea** caused by **carcinoid syndrome** or by **excessive release of GI tract hormones,** including gastrin and VIP.

(2) It may be used off-label for the treatment of diarrhea caused by chemotherapy, graft-versus-host disease, short-gut syndrome, and dumping syndrome.

(3) It may be used in the treatment of neuroendocrine tumors of the GI tract.

c. ***Adverse effects*** may include mild GI distress and headache. It may cause the formation of gallstones due to alteration of fat absorption.

6. **Oral rehydration salt (ORS).** Oral rehydration is the mainstay of treatment in any form of diarrhea. Antidiarrheals are for symptomatic treatment only.

a. **Composition.** The low-osmolarity ORS used for oral rehydration consists of 2.6 g sodium chloride, 2.9 g trisodium citrate, 1.5 g potassium chloride, and 13.5 g anhydrous glucose, all dissolved in 1 L of water.

b. **Mechanism of action.** Oral rehydration relies on the fact that glucose-coupled sodium reabsorption in the intestine remains intact even in cases of severe diarrhea. Thus, glucose aids in sodium reabsorption; this along with chloride, potassium, and a buffer helps to replace the fluid lost in diarrhea.

c. **Indication.** It is used to treat mild to moderate dehydration. In cases of severe dehydration, ORS is administered along with IV fluids.

d. **Adverse effects.** Excess of sodium/glucose can result in edema, osmotic diarrhea, and nausea/vomiting.

7. **Zinc sulfate.** It is given along with ORS in children.

a. **Indication.** It is used to treat diarrhea in children.

b. **Mechanism of action.** Zinc reduces fluid secretion in the intestine, enhances immune response, and helps in intestinal epithelial regeneration. It decreases severity and duration of diarrhea and decreases recurrence.

c. **Adverse effects.** These include vomiting, regurgitation, abdominal pain, and dyspepsia.

C. Agent used for antiflatulence

1. Simethicone

a. ***Mechanism of action.*** Simethicone has the ability to collapse gas bubbles by forming a thin layer on their surface. It **alters the surface tension** of **gas and mucus bubbles** enabling them to **coalesce**, or form together. This **accelerates** the **passage of gas** through the GI tract through belching, passing of flatus, or increased absorption of gas into the bloodstream.

b. ***Indications.*** It is indicated for the management of **gas retention**, including the relief of pressure, **bloating**, fullness, and discomfort due to GI gas.

c. ***Adverse effects*** are minimal but may include mild diarrhea, nausea, and regurgitation.

D. Agents used in the treatment of irritable bowel syndrome

1. Antispasmodics (anticholinergic agents)

a. ***Specific agents*** include **dicyclomine** and **hyoscyamine**.

b. ***Mechanism of action.*** These agents **block the action of acetylcholine** in the **enteric plexus** and on smooth muscle to relieve symptoms of intestinal spasms.

c. ***Indications.*** They may be used for the management of irritable bowel syndrome (IBS) or other functional GI disorders.

d. ***Adverse effects*** may include dizziness, dry mouth, and blurred vision.

2. Serotonin (5-HT$_3$)-receptor antagonist

a. ***Specific agent.*** **Alosetron.**

b. ***Mechanism of action.*** Alosetron **blocks 5-HT$_3$ receptors** on **enteric neurons** in the GI tract to reduce pain, abdominal discomfort, urgency, and diarrhea.

c. ***Indication.*** It is approved for the treatment of **women** with **severe IBS** in whom **diarrhea** is the predominant symptom. Due to the risk of serious GI adverse reactions, it should be used only in women who have not responded to conventional therapy.

d. ***Adverse effects*** may include headache and constipation.

e. ***Precautions.*** Due to the risk for **ischemic colitis**, it should be discontinued immediately in patients who experience rectal bleeding, bloody diarrhea, or sudden worsening of abdominal pain (until further evaluation).

3. **Chloride channel activators**
   a. Type 2 chloride channels (ClC-2) help maintain fluid balance in the bowels.
      (1) Activation increases fluid in the bowel to help with the passage of stool.
   b. **Lubiprostone**
      (1) ***Mechanism of action.*** This agent **stimulates ClC-2** in the **small intestine**, thereby increasing intestinal fluid secretion and intestinal motility. It increases fluid in the bowels to help stool to pass.
      (2) ***Indications.*** It is approved for **IBS with constipation (females only)**, chronic idiopathic constipation, and opioid-induced constipation.
      (3) ***Adverse effects*** may include headache and nausea. **Dyspnea** may also occur, which is often described as chest tightness; it generally occurs shortly after taking the first dose and resolves within a few hours.
   c. **Linaclotide**
      (1) ***Mechanism of action.*** This agent **increases** cyclic guanosine monophosphate (**cGMP**) concentrations, which results in **chloride** and bicarbonate **secretion** into the **intestinal lumen**. Intestinal fluid increases, and GI transit time is decreased.
      (2) ***Indications.*** It is approved for IBS with constipation and chronic idiopathic constipation.
      (3) ***Adverse effects*** may include diarrhea, headache, and upper respiratory tract infections.
   d. Both agents are contraindicated with known or suspected bowel obstruction.

E. Agents used in inflammatory bowel disease

1. **General characteristics for IBD**
   a. IBD is a spectrum of chronic, idiopathic, and inflammatory intestinal conditions.
   b. It causes significant GI symptoms that may include diarrhea, abdominal pain, bleeding, anemia, and weight loss.
   c. IBD comprises two distinct disorders: ulcerative colitis and Crohn disease.
      (1) **Ulcerative colitis** is characterized by **confluent mucosal inflammation** of the colon starting at the **anal verge** and extending proximally.
      (2) **Crohn disease** is characterized by **transmural inflammation** of **any part** of the GI tract, but most commonly the area adjacent to the ileocecal valve.
         (a) The inflammation is not necessarily confluent; therefore, areas of inflammation may be in-between areas of relatively normal mucosa.
   d. Since the etiology and pathogenesis of these disorders remain unknown, medications are used to **dampen the generalized inflammatory response.**
      (1) Specific goals of pharmacotherapy include controlling acute exacerbations, maintaining remission, and treating specific complications, such as fistulas.
2. **5-Aminosalicylates (5-ASA)**
   a. ***Specific agents*** include sulfasalazine, olsalazine, balsalazide, and various forms of mesalamine.
   b. ***Mechanism of action***
      (1) The specific mechanism is unknown.
      (2) They may decrease inflammation by inhibiting cyclooxygenase and lipoxygenase to **decrease prostaglandin and leukotriene synthesis.**
      (3) They may **inhibit** the functions of **natural killer (NK) cells**, mucosal lymphocytes, and macrophages.
      (4) They may **scavenge oxygen-derived free radicals.**
   c. ***Formulations***
      (1) The effectiveness of therapy depends on achieving high drug concentration at the site of active disease.
      (2) They are believed to work **topically** (not systemically) in areas of diseased GI mucosa.
      (3) To **overcome the rapid absorption** of 5-ASA from the proximal small intestine, a number of formulations have been **designed to deliver it to various distal segments** of the small bowel or the colon, including delayed-release capsules and pH-dependent release.

d. ***Indications.*** These agents are most effective for the treatment of mild to moderate ulcerative colitis. They may also be used in Crohn disease.

e. ***Adverse effects*** are mainly related to the **sulfa moiety**. They may include headache, dyspepsia, and **skin rash**. Sulfasalazine may also cause oligospermia (reversible) and impair folate absorption.

3. In case of sulfasalazine, consisting of 5-ASA and sulfapyridine, the latter can get absorbed systemically. In case of rheumatoid arthritis, this systemically absorbed sulfapyridine has antirhuematoid effects.

4. Many other agents can be used for the management of IBD, including glucocorticoids, antimetabolites (azathioprine and methotrexate), and tumor necrosis factor (TNF) inhibitors (infliximab, adalimumab, certolizumab, and natalizumab). These agents are discussed in more detail in other chapters.

DRUG SUMMARY TABLE

Antiemetics
Benzodiazepine
Lorazepam
Cannabinoids
Dronabinol
Nabilone
Dopamine-receptor antagonists
Droperidol
Metoclopramide
Prochlorperazine
Promethazine
Histamine H_1-receptor antagonists
Dimenhydrinate
Diphenhydramine
Meclizine
Muscarinic M_1-receptor antagonist
Scopolamine
Neurokinin 1-receptor antagonists
Aprepitant
Fosaprepitant
Selective 5-HT_3-receptor antagonists
Dolasetron
Granisetron
Ondansetron
Palonosetron

Drugs Used to Manage Obesity
GLP-1-receptor agonist
Liraglutide
Lipase inhibitor
Orlistat
Serotonin agonist
Lorcaserin
Sympathomimetic drugs
Benzphetamine
Diethylpropion (generic only)
Phendimetrazine (generic only)
Phentermine
Drugs Used to Increase Appetite
Dronabinol
Megestrol

Agents Used to Neutralize or Inhibit Acid Production
Antacids
Calcium carbonate
Magnesium hydroxide
Magnesium hydroxide plus aluminum hydroxide
Sodium bicarbonate
Histamine H_2-receptor antagonists
Cimetidine
Famotidine
Nizatidine
Ranitidine
Proton pump inhibitors
Dexlansoprazole
Esomeprazole
Lansoprazole
Omeprazole
Pantoprazole
Rabeprazole

Mucosal Protective Agents
Misoprostol
Sucralfate

Agents Used for Constipation
Bulk-forming laxatives
Methylcellulose
Polycarbophil
Psyllium
Irritant (stimulant) laxatives (cathartics)
Bisacodyl
Senna
Lubricating agent
Mineral oil
Osmotic laxatives
Lactulose
Magnesium citrate
Magnesium hydroxide
Polyethylene glycol (PEG) electrolyte solution
Sodium phosphate
Opioid-receptor antagonists
Alvimopan
Methylnaltrexone
Naldemedine
Naloxegol
Stool softener
Docusate

Agents Used for Diarrhea and Flatulence
Bismuth subsalicylate
Difenoxin + atropine
Diphenoxylate + atropine
Loperamide
Octreotide
Simethicone

Agents for Inflammatory Bowel Disease (IBD)
5-Aminosalicylic acid derivatives
Sulfasalazine
Mesalamine
Olsalazine
Balsalazide
Antimetabolites
6-Mercaptopurine
Azathioprine
Methotrexate
Corticosteroids
Budesonide
Prednisolone
Methylprednisolone
Tumor necrosis factor (TNF) blocking agents
Adalimumab
Certolizumab
Infliximab
Natalizumab

Agents for Irritable Bowel Syndrome (IBS)
Antispasmodics (anticholinergic agents)
Dicyclomine
Hyoscyamine
Chloride channel activators
Linaclotide
Lubiprostone
Serotonin (5-HT_3)-receptor antagonist
Alosetron

Prokinetic agent
Metoclopramide

Drug Used to Dissolve Gallstones
Ursodiol

Digestive Enzyme Replacement
Pancrelipase

Review Test

Directions: Select the best answer for each question.

1. A 10-year-old girl is brought to the clinic with complaints of vomiting after eating at a food fest the previous day. She is prescribed an antiemetic to be taken for 3 days. Two days later, the child is brought again to the clinic due to acute spasm of the neck muscles. The antiemetic likely to have been prescribed to her is:

(A) Domperidone
(B) Dimenhydrinate
(C) Fosaprepitant
(D) Granisetron
(E) Metoclopramide

2. A 65-year-old woman presents to the infusion center for her first cycle of chemotherapy for stage III breast cancer. She is started on doxorubicin plus cyclophosphamide. The oncologist prescribes ondansetron and dexamethasone to prevent nausea and vomiting. In addition, he writes a prescription for a medication that will prevent delayed nausea and vomiting and augment the effect of the other antinausea medications. What medication was most likely prescribed?

(A) Aprepitant
(B) Dronabinol
(C) Lorazepam
(D) Meclizine
(E) Metoclopramide

3. A 57-year-old man presents to his physician with concerns about a history of motion sickness. He has plans to go on a cruise for his 25th wedding anniversary and does not want to be sick during his trip. The doctor writes a prescription for a medication to help prevent nausea and vomiting while on the cruise ship. What is the mechanism of action for the medication that was most likely prescribed?

(A) Cannabinoid (CB_1)-receptor agonist
(B) Dopamine (D_2)-receptor antagonist
(C) Muscarinic (M_1)-receptor antagonist
(D) Neurokinin (NK_1)-receptor antagonist
(E) Serotonin ($5\text{-}HT_3$)-receptor antagonist

4. A 53-year-old woman presents to her physician with complaints of bloody diarrhea and severe abdominal pain. She has a history of irritable bowel syndrome (IBS), in which diarrhea is the predominant symptom. Her doctor asks her to immediately discontinue the medication she takes for the management of IBS, until further testing is completed to rule out ischemic colitis. Which of the following medications was the patient most likely taking for IBS?

(A) Alosetron
(B) Dicyclomine
(C) Linaclotide
(D) Lubiprostone
(E) Simethicone

5. A 35-year-old woman presents to her family physician for her routine physical examination. The patient is obese, with a body mass index of 31 kg/m^2. She is currently on lisinopril for hypertension and atorvastatin for dyslipidemia. The patient tells the doctor that she is interested in taking an over-the-counter medication for weight loss but hesitant to start due to the side effects that may include rectal leakage, gas, and diarrhea. Which of the following medications is the patient interested in taking?

(A) Liraglutide
(B) Lorcaserin
(C) Megestrol
(D) Orlistat
(E) Phentermine

6. A 53-year-old man is started on daily clopidogrel following a peripheral artery percutaneous angioplasty. A month later, he develops frequent episodes of epigastric burning and pain which are not completely relieved with over-the-counter antacids. On visiting his physician, he is diagnosed to have gastritis. Which of the following medication use is discouraged in this patient?

(A) Famotidine
(B) Esomeprazole
(C) Pantoprazole
(D) Ranitidine
(E) Sucralfate

7. A young adult presents to his gastroenterologist for further evaluation of persistent burning stomach pain, heartburn, and nausea. In the past, he has been treated with ranitidine for peptic ulcer disease. His laboratory results are positive for elevated levels of gastrin. A colonoscopy reveals evidence of ulcers involving the jejunum. The patient is diagnosed with Zollinger–Ellison syndrome and started on a new medication that inhibits gastric acid production. What is the patient at risk for with the medication that was most likely prescribed?

(A) *C. difficile*–associated diarrhea
(B) Gastrointestinal perforation
(C) Ischemic colitis
(D) Lipid pneumonitis
(E) Milk-alkali syndrome

8. A 63-year-old woman is admitted to the hospital with complaints of early fullness after very small meals and vomiting undigested food. She has a long-standing history of poorly controlled diabetes. The physician is concerned about diabetic gastroparesis and starts her on an antinausea medication that will also help increase gastric motility. What medication was most likely started?

(A) Dimenhydrinate
(B) Droperidol
(C) Prochlorperazine
(D) Metoclopramide
(E) Ondansetron

9. A 3-year-old child with diarrhea developed paralytic ileus after being administered an antidiarrheal. The drug likely to have been prescribed is:

(A) Docusate sodium
(B) Octreotide
(C) Loperamide
(D) Racecadotril
(E) Zinc sulfate

10. A 33-year-old man presents to his primary care physician for a routine physical examination. The patient tells the doctor that he will be traveling to Mexico for a vacation the following month and is concerned about developing traveler's diarrhea. Which of the following agents can the physician recommend for prophylaxis against this condition?

(A) Bismuth subsalicylate
(B) Liraglutide
(C) Lorcaserin
(D) Octreotide
(E) Simethicone

11. A 45-year-old man presents to his infectious disease specialist for the management of acquired immune deficiency syndrome (AIDS). The patient complains of nausea and decreased appetite. The physician is concerned that the patient has lost about 6 kg over the past 2 months. Which of the following medications may help manage these symptoms?

(A) Dimenhydrinate
(B) Dronabinol
(C) Metoclopramide
(D) Ondansetron
(E) Phentermine

12. A 65-year-old man presents to his gastroenterologist with a 3-month history of watery diarrhea. Further testing reveals that the patient is hypokalemic with an absence of hydrochloric acid in his gastric secretions. He also has an elevated serum level of vasoactive intestinal peptide. The patient is diagnosed with a pancreatic islet cell tumor (VIPoma). Which agent would be most appropriate to treat the patient's symptoms?

(A) Bismuth subsalicylate
(B) Gastrin
(C) Glucagon
(D) Octreotide
(E) Sulfasalazine

Answers and Explanations

1. **The answer is E.** Metoclopramide is an antiemetic which blocks the D_2 receptors in the CTZ. The drug can also cross the blood–brain barrier and inhibit the dopamine receptors in the limbic system, resulting in extrapyramidal side effects such as acute dystonia. This is likely responsible for the acute spasm of the neck muscles in the given case. Although domperidone is also a D_2 blocker, it does not cross the blood–brain barrier. Dimenhydrinate, fosaprepitant, and granisetron are antiemetics which do not have any effect on the D_2 receptors.
2. **The answer is A.** Aprepitant is the first available substance P antagonist used for the prevention of both sudden and delayed chemotherapy-induced nausea and vomiting. It can be used synergistically with serotonin 5-HT_3 antagonists, such as ondansetron, and corticosteroids, such as dexamethasone. While the other drugs are used for the management of nausea and vomiting, they do not necessarily augment the effect of ondansetron and dexamethasone. In addition, except for palonosetron, they are not approved to help with delayed nausea and vomiting.
3. **The answer is C.** The patient was most likely prescribed scopolamine, a muscarinic (M_1)-receptor antagonist, which blocks the action of acetylcholine in the vestibular nuclei. The vestibular center is important for sensory information about motion, equilibrium, and spatial orientation. It may play an important role in motion sickness. Scopolamine reduces the excitability of labyrinthine receptors and depresses conduction from the vestibular apparatus to the vomiting center. It is approved for motion sickness. The other mechanisms are for drugs that help with nausea, but they do not act in the vestibular center and are not approved for motion sickness.
4. **The answer is A.** Alosetron, a 5-HT_3-receptor antagonist, has been shown to provide some relief of irritable bowel syndrome (IBS). It is approved for the treatment of women with severe IBS in whom diarrhea is the predominant symptom. Due to the risk for ischemic colitis, it should be discontinued immediately in patients who experience rectal bleeding, bloody diarrhea, or sudden worsening of abdominal pain (until further evaluation). Dicyclomine is an antispasmodic agent used in IBS. Lubiprostone and linaclotide are chloride channel activators used for IBS. Simethicone is used for flatulence. These agents do not carry the same risk for ischemic colitis.
5. **The answer is D.** The patient is interested in taking orlistat, a reversible lipase inhibitor of gastric and pancreatic lipases. Orlistat inactivates the enzymes, making them unavailable to digest dietary fats. It can be used for weight loss and obesity management in conjunction with a reduced-calorie and low-fat diet. The adverse effects are gastrointestinal related and may include oily rectal leakage, fecal spotting, flatulence, and diarrhea. Orlistat can also prevent absorption of fat-soluble vitamins (A, D, E, K); therefore, supplementation may be necessary. Liraglutide, lorcaserin, and phentermine are used for weight loss but do not have these adverse effects. Megestrol stimulates appetite.
6. **The answer is B.** The antiplatelet action of clopidogrel requires its conversion to the active form by CYP2C19 enzyme. Esomeprazole is a CYP2C19 inhibitor which can decrease the antiplatelet action by interfering with the activation of the prodrug. Pantoprazole, another proton pump inhibitor, does not have significant CYP2C19 inhibitory effect, and, hence, can be used with clopidogrel. Famotidine, ranitidine, and sucralfate do not have significant drug interactions with clopidogrel.
7. **The answer is A.** The patient was most likely started on a proton pump inhibitor (PPI). Compared with antacids and H_2 antagonists, PPIs are more potent acid suppressors. They are used for the treatment of Zollinger–Ellison syndrome. PPIs carry the risk for *C. difficile*–associated diarrhea. The other conditions are not likely with PPI therapy. Antacids, H_2 antagonists, and mucosal protective agents are not indicated for Zollinger–Ellison syndrome.

8. **The answer is D.** Poor gastric emptying is a manifestation of the neuropathy that accompanies long-standing diabetes. Metoclopramide is a prokinetic agent used in the treatment of diabetic gastroparesis. It is a dopamine-receptor antagonist used for nausea and vomiting but also enhances the response to acetylcholine of tissue in the upper GI tract, causing enhanced motility and accelerated gastric emptying. The other agents can help with the management of nausea and vomiting but do not enhance gastric motility.
9. **The answer is C.** Opioid receptor agonists, such as loperamide and diphenoxylate, have the risk of producing paralytic ileus and toxic megacolon, especially in children. In contrast, racecadotril, an enkephalinase inhibitor, is an antisecretory antidiarrheal with no effect on GI motility, making it suitable for children. Docusate, on the other hand, is a laxative and not used for treating diarrhea. Octreotide is an antisecretory drug useful to control diarrhea associated with carcinoid tumors. Zinc sulfate is used as an adjunct to oral rehydration therapy in children with diarrhea; it enhances fluid and electrolyte reabsorption and is not associated with paralytic ileus.
10. **The answer is A.** Bismuth subsalicylate is effective for both the treatment and the prophylaxis of traveler's diarrhea, most often due to *Escherichia coli*–contaminated water. Octreotide is used for severe diarrhea associated with carcinoid syndrome or excessive release of GI tract hormones. Liraglutide and lorcaserin are used for weight loss. Simethicone is used for flatulence.
11. **The answer is B.** Dronabinol contains Δ-9-tetrahydrocannabinol, the active cannabinoid in marijuana. It acts by inhibiting the vomiting center through stimulation of a CB_1 subtype of cannabinoid receptors. It may also enhance appetite by acting on these same receptors. It may help with the nausea and is also approved for anorexia in patients with acquired immune deficiency syndrome. Dimenhydrinate, metoclopramide, and ondansetron are also used for the management of nausea but would not help increase the patient's appetite. Phentermine is a sympathomimetic drug used for weight loss.
12. **The answer is D.** Octreotide is used in the treatment of endocrine tumors, such as gastrinomas, glucagonomas, and VIPomas, to help alleviate the diarrhea. Bismuth subsalicylate is used to treat traveler's diarrhea, and sulfasalazine is used treat such inflammatory bowel diseases as Crohn disease. Gastrin is a GI hormone.

Chapter 10

Drugs Acting on the Endocrine System

Competencies Addressed: PH1.24, PH1.36–PH1.41

I. HORMONE RECEPTORS

All known hormones, and drugs that mimic hormones, act via one of **two basic receptor systems:** membrane-associated receptors and intracellular receptors (see Chapter 1).

A. Membrane-associated receptors

1. Membrane-associated receptors bind **hydrophilic** hormones (which penetrate the plasma membrane poorly) outside the cell. Examples of hydrophilic hormones include insulin, adrenocorticotropic hormone (ACTH), and epinephrine.
2. Membrane-associated receptors transmit signals into the cell by a variety of second messenger mechanisms, including the following:
   a. Changes in cyclic adenosine monophosphate (cAMP) or cyclic guanosine monophosphate (cGMP) caused by changes in the activity of cyclases.
   b. Increased phosphoinositide turnover via increased phosphoinositide kinase activity.
   c. Changes in intracellular calcium (Ca^{2+}) by acting on intracellular stores or membrane Ca^{2+} channels.
   d. Changes in intracellular ions by action on specific channels. These include sodium (Na^+), Ca^{2+}, potassium (K^+), and chloride (Cl^-).
   e. Increased tyrosine phosphorylation on specific proteins by the action of tyrosine kinases.

B. Intracellular receptors

1. Intracellular receptors bind **hydrophobic** hormones (which penetrate the plasma membrane easily) inside the cell—either in the cytoplasm or in the nucleus. Examples of hydrophobic hormones include cortisol, retinol, and estrogen.
2. Intracellular receptors modulate the transcription rate of specific target genes to change the levels of cellular proteins.

II. THE HYPOTHALAMUS

A. Agents affecting growth hormone

1. Growth hormone–releasing hormone (GHRH)
   a. GHRH is produced by the hypothalamus within the arcuate nucleus.
   b. It binds to specific membrane GHRH receptors on pituitary somatotrophs and rapidly elevates serum growth hormone (GH; somatotropin) levels.
2. Somatotropin release-inhibiting hormone (somatostatin [SST])
   a. SST peptides are produced in the hypothalamus, pancreatic D cells, and other areas of the gastrointestinal (GI) tract.
   b. SST binds to SST receptors in the plasma membrane of target tissues.

c. SST **inhibits** many functions throughout the body, including the following:

(1) The release of **GH** and **thyroid-stimulating hormone** (TSH) from the pituitary

(2) The release of **glucagon** and **insulin** from the pancreas

(3) The secretion of a number of gut peptides, including **vasoactive intestinal polypeptide** (VIP), and **gastrin**

(4) The secretion of vasodilator hormones, especially within the gut

(5) The growth and proliferation of many cell types

3. SST analogues

a. Octreotide (see Chapter 8)

(1) ***Mechanism of action.*** Octreotide mimics natural **SST.** It has several different effects, including the following:

(a) Inhibition of serotonin release.

(b) Inhibition of secretion of gastrin, VIP, insulin, glucagon, secretin, motilin, and pancreatic polypeptide.

(c) Decreased secretion of TSH.

(d) Suppression of luteinizing hormone (LH) response to gonadotropin-releasing hormone (GnRH).

(e) Decreased GH and insulin-like growth factor-1 (IGF-1).

(f) Decreased splanchnic blood flow.

(g) In some cases, it is more potent than endogenous SST; for example, it provides more potent inhibition of GH, glucagon, and insulin.

(2) ***Indications***

(a) It is used to treat **acromegaly**.

(b) It is also used for the management of severe **diarrhea** associated with hypersecretory states such as VIP-secreting tumors **(VIPomas)** and chemotherapy-induced diarrhea.

(c) **Variceal/upper GI bleeding** and hepatorenal syndrome reduce splanchnic blood flow and portal pressure without any systemic hemodynamic effects.

(d) In **peptide receptor radionuclide therapy (PRRT)**, specific membrane SST receptors that are overexpressed in neuroendocrine neoplasms and their metastases are targeted.

(e) Other indications include gastrinomas, glucagonomas, TSH-secreting adenomas, prevention of exacerbation of chronic pancreatitis, and chylothorax in neonates.

(3) ***Adverse effects*** may include **nausea**, cramps, and increased **gallstone** formation. It may also cause hyperglycemia.

b. Lanreotide

(1) ***Mechanism of action***. Lanreotide is a **long-acting SST analogue**. Similar to SST and octreotide, it inhibits many endocrine, neuroendocrine, and exocrine functions. It causes decreased GH secretion and IGF-1 levels.

(2) ***Indications***

(a) It is approved for the long-term treatment of **acromegaly** in patients with suboptimal response to surgery or radiotherapy.

(b) It is also used for the treatment of carcinoid treatment and gastroenteropancreatic neuroendocrine tumors.

(3) ***Adverse effects*** may include bradycardia, hypertension, and GI distress, including abdominal pain, nausea, and diarrhea.

c. Pasireotide

(1) ***Mechanism of action.*** Pasireotide is a **subcutaneous long-acting SST analogue** with high affinity for SST receptor subtypes. It inhibits the secretion of GH, IGF-1, and ACTH.

(2) ***Indications***

(a) Acromegaly

(b) Cushing disease

(3) ***Adverse effects*** include hyperglycemia which requires monitoring. Few cases of QT prolongation have been reported.

B. Gonadotropin-releasing hormone agonists (see Chapter 12)

1. Endogenous GnRH is secreted from the preoptic area of the hypothalamus. It binds to specific receptors on pituitary gonadotrophs.
2. ***Specific agents*** include **leuprolide**, triptorelin, **goserelin**, nafarelin, and histrelin.
3. ***Mechanism of action*** (Fig. 10.1)
   a. GnRH agonists modulate the function of the hypothalamic–pituitary–gonadal axis.
   b. Short-term or **pulsatile administration increases** the synthesis and release of both **LH** and **follicle-stimulating hormone (FSH).**
   c. **Chronic administration inhibits** the release of both **LH** and **FSH** by causing a reduction in the number of GnRH receptors.
      (1) This leads to a subsequent **decrease** in levels of **testosterone**, **dihydrotestosterone**, and **estrogen**.
      (2) The use of these agents results in **castration levels of testosterone** in men and **postmenopausal levels of estrogen** in women.
4. ***Indications***
   a. Chronic administration (decreased LH and FSH) is useful in the treatment of **hormone-dependent hyperplasia and cancer**, including prostate cancer, breast cancer, endometriosis, and fibroids.
      (1) All agents are used in the management of **advanced prostate cancer.**
      (2) Goserelin can be used for the management of advanced breast cancer.
      (3) Leuprolide, nafarelin, and goserelin are indicated for endometriosis; leuprolide is also approved for the treatment of uterine fibroids.
   b. Pulsatile administration (increased LH and FSH) is used for **infertility** treatment.
   c. Leuprolide, triptorelin, nafarelin, and histrelin can be used for central precocious puberty.
5. ***Adverse effects*** may include **hot flashes**, **gynecomastia**, sexual dysfunction, and **decreased bone mineral density**. Ovarian hyperstimulation syndrome (OHSS) has been reported when used in infertility treatment. The long-term use of GnRH analogues can lead to hypoestrogenic symptoms in women and hypogonadism in men. Both men and women may experience loss of bone mineral density resulting in osteoporosis and risk of fractures.
6. ***Precautions***
   a. **Tumor flare** may occur in the **first few weeks** of treatment, due to initial increases in testosterone (in men with prostate cancer) and estrogen (in women with breast cancer). This presents as **worsening of disease symptoms**.

C. Gonadotropin-releasing hormone antagonists (see Chapter 12)

1. ***Specific agents*** include peptide antagonists such as **cetrorelix, ganirelix, degarelix**, and **abarelix** (injected subcutaneously), and nonpeptide antagonists like **elagolix and relugolix** (given orally).
2. ***Mechanism of action***. These agents **block the GnRH receptors** and **decrease** the release of **LH** and **FSH**.
   a. For their use in ovarian stimulation, delaying the LH surge prevents ovulation until the follicles are of adequate size.
   b. For their use in prostate cancer, they result in rapid androgen deprivation by decreasing testosterone production and levels.
      (1) Unlike the GnRH agonists, these agents do not cause a surge of testosterone or estradiol on initiation of therapy.
3. ***Indications***
   a. Cetrorelix and ganirelix are used for **controlled ovarian stimulation** in conjunction with gonadotropins.
   b. Degarelix and abarelix are used for the treatment of **advanced prostate cancer**.
   c. Ganirelix is used primarily in assisted reproduction technology for the prevention of premature LH surges during ovarian stimulation.
   d. Elagolix has been approved for managing **endometriosis** and **uterine fibroids**. Relugolix is a novel therapeutic option for **prostatic cancer**.
4. ***Adverse effects***
   a. Degarelix may cause **hot flashes** and increased transaminases. Cetrorelix and ganirelix may cause headache.

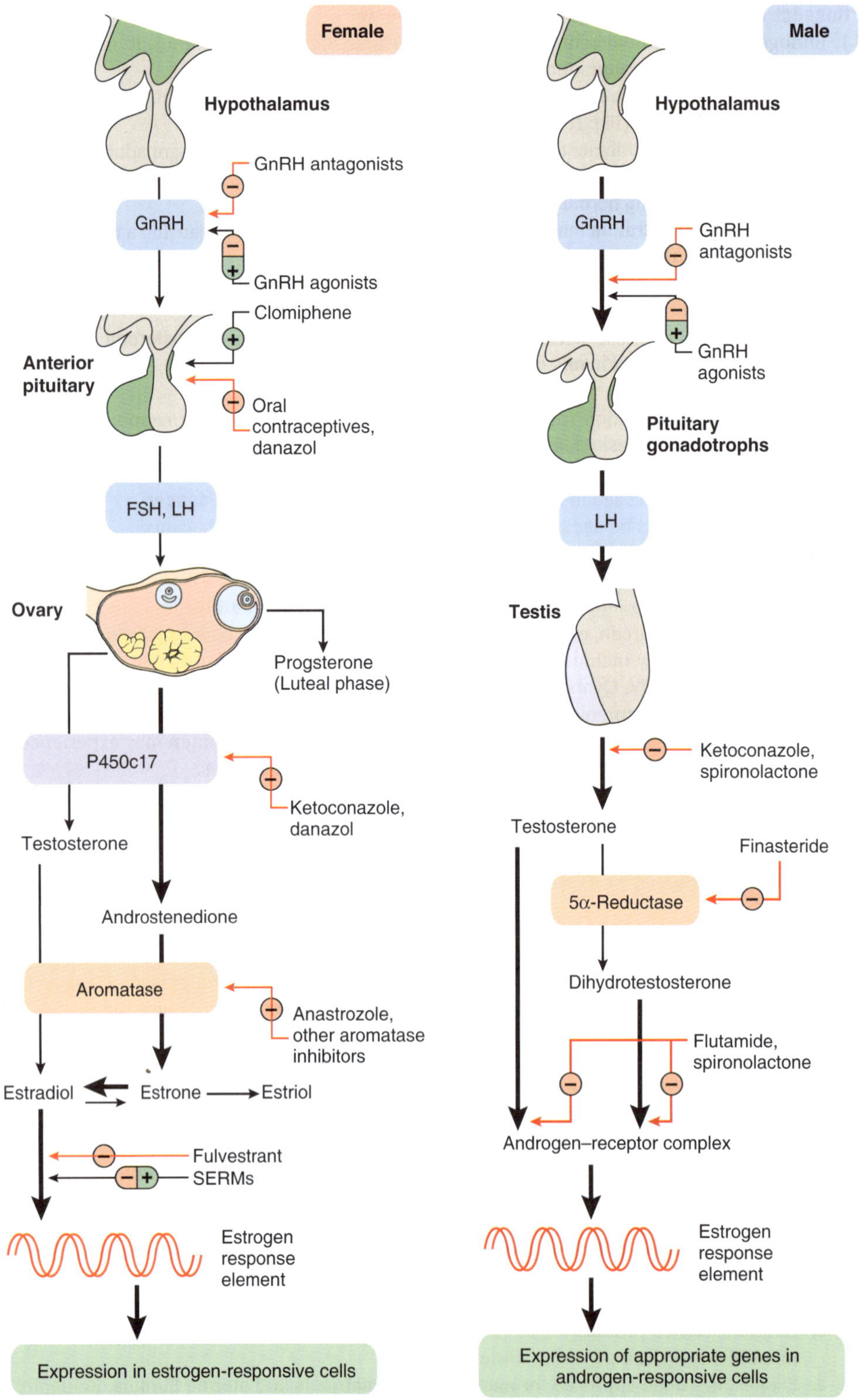

FIGURE 10.1. The hypothalamic–pituitary axis. The pituitary releases trophic hormones such as follicle-stimulating hormone (*FSH*) and luteinizing hormone (*LH*) in response to releasing hormones produced in the hypothalamus. It also releases adrenocorticotropic hormone (*ACTH*), which is not shown in this figure. The trophic hormones act on peripheral organs such as the ovary or testis to increase the production of gonadal steroids. Gonadal steroids in turn exert negative feedback on the hypothalamus and pituitary. GnRH, gonadotropin-releasing hormone; SERM, selective estrogen receptor modulator.

D. Prolactin-releasing factor and prolactin-inhibiting factor

1. Prolactin-releasing factor (PRF)

a. Various hormones stimulate prolactin secretion, including thyrotropin-releasing hormone (TRH), testosterone, estrogen, and VIP.

b. ***Dopamine antagonists*** and other drugs that reduce dopaminergic activity cause an **increase in prolactin secretion**, including the following:

(1) Antipsychotics (e.g., chlorpromazine, haloperidol)

(2) Antidepressants (e.g., imipramine)

c. ***Indications.*** Drugs that promote prolactin secretion are used for the treatment of lactation failure.

2. Prolactin-inhibiting factor (PIF)

a. ***Dopamine agonists inhibit prolactin*** secretion.

(1) Bromocriptine activates dopamine (D_2) receptors in the **tuberoinfundibular pathway**, which **inhibits pituitary prolactin secretion.**

(2) Cabergoline is a potent D_2 agonist with greater D_2 selectivity. It is more effective in reducing hyperprolactinemia than bromocriptine.

b. ***Indications***

(1) Inhibition of prolactin secretion in **amenorrhea**, **galactorrhea**, and prolactin-secreting tumors.

(2) Correction of female **infertility** secondary to hyperprolactinemia.

(3) Bromocriptine can be used for the treatment of Parkinson disease.

E. Corticotropin-releasing hormone

1. Corticotropin-releasing hormone (CRH) stimulates ACTH synthesis and release in pituitary corticotrophs.

2. Corticorelin is an analogue of human CRH. It is used diagnostically to discriminate between pituitary and ectopic sources of ACTH production and to differentiate between hypothalamic–hypophyseal and primary adrenal disease.

F. Thyrotropin-releasing hormone. TRH stimulates the secretion of TSH from the pituitary and induces prolactin secretion.

III. THE ANTERIOR PITUITARY

A. Growth hormone agonists and antagonists

1. GH is important for the **growth of skeletal muscle, linear bones, and organs.**

2. It has both direct and indirect actions mediated by the synthesis and release of IGF-1 from the liver and the kidney.

a. Direct actions of GH include antagonism of the action of insulin, stimulation of triglyceride hydrolysis in adipose tissue, increased hepatic glucose output, positive calcium balance, renal reabsorption of sodium and potassium, and production of somatomedins or IGFs in the liver and other tissues.

b. Indirect actions of GH mediated by IGF-1 include longitudinal growth of bones and growth of soft tissue, increased amino acid transport, DNA and RNA synthesis, proliferation of many tissues, and increased protein synthesis and positive nitrogen balance.

3. Recombinant human growth hormone

a. ***Specific agent.*** **Somatropin.**

b. ***Mechanism of action.*** Somatropin binds to dimeric GH receptors leading to transcription and translation of GH-dependent proteins, including IGF-1.

c. ***Indications***

(1) It is used for the treatment of **growth failure in pediatric patients**, including the following:

(a) Replacement therapy in children with GH deficiency

(b) Short stature associated with Turner syndrome

(c) Prader–Willi syndrome

(d) Chronic renal failure

(2) Other approved uses include long-term replacement of **GH deficiency** in adults, treatment of **cachexia** in patients with acquired immune deficiency syndrome (AIDS) wasting, and short bowel syndrome.

d. ***Adverse effects and contraindications***

(1) Edema, metabolic disturbances, and injection site reactions have been reported with GH treatment.

(2) Administration is contraindicated in obese patients, patients with closed epiphyses without GH deficiency, and patients with neoplastic disease.

4. GH-receptor antagonist

a. ***Specific agent.*** **Pegvisomant.**

b. ***Mechanism of action.*** Pegvisomant is a recombinant GH that selectively binds to GH receptors and **blocks the binding of endogenous GH**; this leads to decreased concentrations of GF-1 and other GH-responsive proteins.

c. ***Indication.*** It is used for the treatment of **acromegaly** subcutaneously.

d. ***Adverse effects*** may include headache, injection site reactions, and reversible elevation of liver enzymes.

B. Gonadotropins

1. ***LH and FSH***

a. ***Structure***

(1) LH and FSH are glycoproteins found in the anterior pituitary.

(2) **LH, FSH, and TSH are all composed of an identical α subunit**, with a β subunit unique to each hormone.

b. ***Actions and pharmacologic properties*** (Fig. 10.1)

(1) The activity of LH and FSH is mediated by specific membrane receptors that cause an increase in intracellular cAMP.

(2) In **women**

(a) LH increases **estrogen production** in the ovary and is required for **progesterone production** by the corpus luteum after ovulation.

(b) FSH is required for normal development and **maturation of the ovarian follicles.**

(3) In **men**

(a) LH induces **testosterone production** by the interstitial Leydig cells of the testis.

(b) FSH acts on the testis to stimulate **spermatogenesis** and the synthesis of androgen-binding protein.

c. ***Specific agents***

(1) **Urofollitropin** (purified human FSH)

(2) **Follitropin alfa** or beta (recombinant human FSH)

(3) **Menotropins** (purified combination of human FSH and LH)

d. ***Mechanism of action***

(1) Women: These agents replace deficient or abnormal FSH serum concentrations in patients experiencing ovulatory function impairment. They **mimic the actions of endogenous FSH** and directly stimulate **follicle recruitment, growth, and maturation.**

(2) Men: They **stimulate spermatogenesis** in men with hypogonadotropic hypogonadism.

e. ***Indications***

(1) Women: They are used in **controlled ovarian stimulation** in preparation for an assisted reproductive technology (in vitro fertilization).

(2) Men: They are used for **spermatogenesis** induction.

f. ***Adverse effects*** may include headache and abdominal cramps. Men may also experience breast pain and acne.

g. ***Precautions*** include an increased risk of **thromboembolic events.** Women are also at an increased risk for **OHSS** and **multiple births.**

(1) OHSS occurs about 10 days after using injectable medications to stimulate ovulation. Symptoms may include abdominal pain, bloating, weight gain, nausea, vomiting, and shortness of breath.

2. ***Human chorionic gonadotropin (hCG)***
   a. **hCG** is **produced by the placenta** and can be isolated and purified from the urine of pregnant women. It is nearly identical in activity to LH, but differs in sequence and carbohydrate content.
   b. ***Specific agents.*** Urine-derived or recombinant hCG.
   c. ***Mechanism of action***
      (1) Women: These agents **mimic the normal LH surge** and stimulate ovulation. They cause the **dominant follicle to release its egg.**
      (2) Men: They act like LH to **stimulate testosterone production** from Leydig cells. Stimulation of androgen production causes **development of secondary sex characteristics.**
   d. ***Indications***
      (1) Women: It is approved for **ovulation induction** with assisted reproductive technology. It is generally administered after FSH to stimulate the final maturation stages of the follicles. Ovulation will occur 36–72 hours after administration.
      (2) Men: It is used for the management of **hypogonadotropic hypogonadism** and **prepubertal cryptorchidism.**
   e. ***Adverse effects***
      (1) These agents may cause edema and headache. Men may also experience gynecomastia and precocious puberty.
   f. ***Precautions*** include an increased risk for **thromboembolism**. Women are also at an increased risk for **OHSS** and **multiple births.**

C. Thyroid-stimulating hormone

1. ***Structure and function***
   a. TSH is secreted from the anterior pituitary.
   b. It stimulates the **production** and release of **triiodothyronine (T_3)** and **thyroxine (T_4)** from the thyroid gland. The effect is mediated by stimulation of specific TSH receptors in the plasma membrane, thereby increasing intracellular cAMP.
2. ***Specific agent.*** **Thyrotropin α.**
3. ***Mechanism of action.*** Thyrotropin α binds to TSH receptors, which stimulates iodine uptake, organification, synthesis, and secretion of thyroglobulin (Tg), T_3, and T_4.
4. ***Indications***
   a. It is used for follow-up **diagnostic imaging** in patients with well-differentiated thyroid cancer who have previously undergone thyroidectomy.
      (1) When used as a diagnostic tool, the amount of Tg detected after administration can reveal whether a thyroidectomy or ablation was successful.
   b. It may also be used for thyroid tissue remnant ablation.
      (1) When used for cancer, it helps stimulate the uptake of radiolabeled iodine to destroy cancerous tissue.
5. ***Adverse effects*** may include nausea, headache, and paresthesias.

D. Adrenocorticotropic hormone (corticotropin) and cosyntropin

1. ***Actions and pharmacologic properties***
   a. ACTH is secreted from the anterior pituitary. It **stimulates the adrenocortical secretion of glucocorticoids** and, to a lesser extent, mineralocorticoids and androgens.
   b. Effects are mediated by specific membrane-bound ACTH receptors coupled to an increase in intracellular cAMP.
   c. The terminal sequence of ACTH is identical to α-melanocyte-stimulating hormone (α-MSH); excess ACTH levels may produce hyperpigmentation.
2. ***Specific agents*** include corticotropin injection and cosyntropin.
3. ***Indications***
   a. ACTH is used in the evaluation of primary or secondary hypoadrenalism. It is used to **screen for adrenocortical insufficiency.**
   b. ACTH may be used in special circumstances when an increase in glucocorticoids is desired. However, the direct administration of steroids is usually preferred.

4. ***Adverse effects and contraindications***
   a. The adverse effects associated with ACTH are similar to those of glucocorticoids.
   b. Allergic reactions, acne, hirsutism, and amenorrhea have been reported.

IV. THE POSTERIOR PITUITARY

A. Antidiuretic hormone (ADH; vasopressin)

1. ***ADH properties and actions***
   a. ADH is synthesized in the hypothalamus and stored in the posterior pituitary. It is released in response to increasing plasma osmolarity or a fall in blood pressure.
   b. Three types of receptors mediate the actions of ADH.
      (1) V_1 receptors are coupled to increased inositide turnover and increased intracellular calcium.
         (a) V_{1a} is located in the vascular smooth muscle, myometrium, and kidney.
         (b) V_{1b} is located in the CNS and adrenal medulla.
      (2) V_2 receptors are coupled to an increase in cAMP.
         (a) V_2 is located in renal tubules.
   c. Functions of ADH
      (1) In renal tubules, ADH increases the **permeability of water** through the insertion of **aquaporin-2** water channels into the apical and basolateral membranes.
      (2) It also increases the transport of urea in the inner medullary collecting duct, which increases the urine-concentrating ability of the kidney.
      (3) ADH causes **vasoconstriction** (via V_{1a} receptors) at higher doses.
      (4) It stimulates the hepatic synthesis of coagulation factor VIII and von Willebrand factor.
2. ADH analogues (see Chapter 3)
   a. ***Specific agents*** include vasopressin, desmopressin (DDAVP), lypressin, and terlipressin.
   b. ***Mechanism of action***
      (1) In vasodilatory shock, vasopressin stimulates the **V_1 receptor** (located on the vascular smooth muscles) **to increase systemic vascular resistance and mean arterial blood pressure**.
      (2) In central diabetes insipidus, stimulation of the **V_2 receptor** (located on the renal collecting ducts) increases cAMP, which **increases water permeability** at the renal tubule; this results in increased water reabsorption decreased **urine volume, and increased osmolality**.
      (3) In von Willebrand disease and hemophilia A, desmopressin increases plasma levels of von Willebrand factor, factor VIII, and tissue plasminogen activator (t-PA); this leads to a shortened activated partial thromboplastin time and bleeding time.
   c. ***Indications***
      (1) Synthetic vasopressin is approved for the treatment of **central diabetes insipidus** and to increase blood pressure in adults with **vasodilatory shock** (especially when standard treatments like epinephrine are ineffective). It has potential applications in the management of **esophageal variceal hemorrhage** and septic shock.
      (2) Desmopressin's V_2 activity is 3,000 times greater than its V_1 activity; it is effective for the treatment of central diabetes insipidus. It is also used for the treatment of nocturia, von Willebrand disease (type 1), and hemophilia A.
      (3) Terlipressin, a long-acting synthetic vasopressin analogue, is used in bleeding esophageal varices and hepatorenal syndrome in patients with cirrhosis (intravenous).
      (4) Lypressin is administered intranasally in patients with central diabetes insipidus but has been largely replaced by desmopressin due to latter's favorable safety profile.
   d. ***Adverse effects*** include **hyponatremia**.
3. **Selective vasopressin receptor antagonists** (aquaretics) (see Chapter 3)
   a. ***Specific agents*** include **tolvaptan** (oral) and **conivaptan** (intravenous).
   b. ***Mechanism of action***
      (1) These agents are **antagonists at the V_2 receptor**.

(2) They promote the **excretion of free water without loss of electrolytes**, which results in net fluid loss. The end effect is increased urine output, decreased urine osmolality, and **increased serum sodium** concentrations.

(3) Tolvaptan is selective for the V_2 receptor, whereas conivaptan blocks both V_{1a} and V_2 receptors.

c. ***Indications***. These agents are approved for the management of **euvolemic or hypervolemic hyponatremia** associated with conditions such as heart failure and cirrhosis including the syndrome of inappropriate secretion of antidiuretic hormone **(SIADH)**. It has been shown to increase serum sodium levels in such patients resulting in improved edema without affecting BP and heart rate.

d. ***Adverse effects and precautions***

(1) These agents can cause hypernatremia. Rapid correction of hyponatremia (>12 mEq/L/24 h) may cause **osmotic demyelination syndrome**. Symptoms of osmotic demyelination syndrome include paresis, behavioral disturbances, seizures, lethargy, confusion, and coma. In many cases, they are reversible or only partially reversible.

(2) Tolvaptan has been associated with idiosyncratic liver injury.

(3) Conivaptan may cause injection-related reactions, hypotension, and pyrexia.

4. Nonselective vasopressin receptor antagonist

a. ***Specific agent.*** **Demeclocycline**.

b. ***Mechanism of action***. This agent is a tetracycline antibiotic that also **inhibits the action of ADH**.

c. ***Indication***. It is used off-label for the management of SIADH.

d. ***Adverse effects*** may include photosensitivity and nephrogenic diabetes insipidus.

e. ***Precautions***. Use should be **avoided in young children** (younger than 8 years), since it can cause tissue hyperpigmentation and **tooth discoloration**.

B. Oxytocin

1. ***Actions and pharmacologic properties***

a. Oxytocin is synthesized in the hypothalamus and secreted by the posterior pituitary. It differs from ADH only by two amino acids.

b. **It elicits milk ejection from the breast and stimulates contraction of uterine smooth muscle.**

c. Oxytocin has been associated with parental, mating, and social behaviors.

2. ***Mechanism of action***. Oxytocin activates G protein–coupled receptors and triggers an **increase in intracellular calcium levels in uterine myofibrils**. It also increases local prostaglandin production, further stimulating uterine contraction.

3. ***Indications***. It can be used antepartum for **labor induction** and maintenance. It can be used to control **postpartum bleeding** or hemorrhage.

4. ***Adverse effects and precautions***

a. Oxytocin may produce **cardiovascular instability**, including hypotension and **tachycardia**.

b. Due to its structural similarity to ADH, high doses may have **antidiuretic effects**.

c. Oxytocin can cause uterine rupture and should not be used after uterine surgery or if signs of fetal distress are present.

V. DRUGS ACTING ON THE GONADAL AND REPRODUCTIVE SYSTEM

A. Estrogens

1. ***Structure and properties***

a. Natural estrogens

(1) Natural estrogens include 17β-estradiol (E2), estrone (E1), and estriol (E3).

(a) **Estradiol** is the major secretory product of the **ovary** and is the most potent natural estrogen.

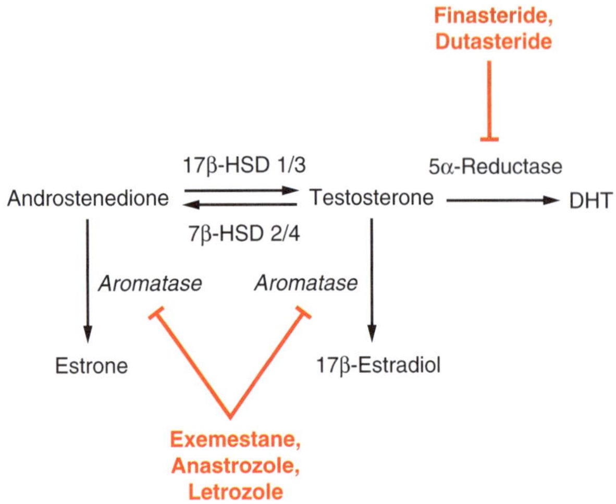

FIGURE 10.2. Enzymatic conversion of androgens to estrogens and dihydrotestosterone. 17β-HSD is hydroxysteroid dehydrogenase. There are multiple isoforms of this enzyme: types 1 and 3 catalyze reactions that make more active steroids; types 2 and 4 make less active metabolites. DHT, dihydrotestosterone.

(b) Estrone is the principal source of estrogen in postmenopausal women.
(c) Estriol is placental estrogen and is seen only during pregnancy.
(2) Natural estrogens are produced by the metabolism of cholesterol (Fig. 10.2).
(a) Testosterone is the immediate precursor of estradiol. **Conversion of testosterone to 17β-estradiol is catalyzed by the enzyme aromatase.**
(b) Estrone and estriol are produced in the liver and other peripheral tissues from 17β-estradiol.

b. Synthetic estrogens
(1) A variety of synthetic estrogens have been produced.
(2) Frequently used synthetic estrogens include **ethinylestradiol** and **mestranol**.
(3) They may be administered orally, topically, transdermally, or by injection.

2. *Metabolism*
a. 17β-Estradiol is extensively bound to sex steroid–binding globulin (SSBG) and serum albumin.
b. Natural estrogens are subject to a large first-pass effect.

3. *Mechanism of action* (see Fig. 10.1)
a. Estrogens bind to specific intracellular estrogen receptors (ER-α and ER-β).
(1) In general, ER-α has many growth-promoting properties, whereas ER-β has antigrowth effects.
b. The hormone–receptor complex interacts with specific DNA sequences and alters the transcription rates of target genes (see Fig. 1.1F) by recruiting coactivators and corepressors.
(1) This leads to a change in the synthesis of specific proteins within a target cell.

4. *Effects*
a. Growth and development
(1) Estrogens are required for the development and maturation of **female internal and external genitalia**, **growth of the breasts**, **linear bone growth** at puberty, and closure of the epiphyses.
(2) Estrogens also influence typical female distribution of subcutaneous fat and pubic and axillary hair.
(3) They are required in the uterus for growth of **myometrium** and for growth and development of the **endometrial lining**.
(a) Continuous exposure can lead to **endometrial hyperplasia** and bleeding.
b. Menstrual cycle
(1) Estrogens are required for ovarian **follicular development** and regulation of the **menstrual cycle**.
c. Systemic metabolism
(1) Estrogens **increase plasma triglycerides** and tend to **decrease serum cholesterol** by decreasing low-density lipoprotein (LDL) and increasing high-density lipoprotein (HDL) concentrations.

(2) They increase levels of transferrin, steroid- and thyroid-binding globulins (TBGs), plasminogen, fibrinogen, and coagulation factors II, VII, VIII, IX, and X. They decrease antithrombin III, protein C, and protein S.

(a) **Overall, estrogens increase the coagulability of blood.**

(3) Estrogens **decrease bone resorption**, with little effect on bone formation.

(4) They increase leptin release from adipose tissue.

d. Estrogens also influence libido and mood.

5. ***Indications***

a. Estrogens are used for **estrogen replacement** therapy in ovarian failure.

b. They are also used in **menopausal therapy.**

(1) Menopausal hormone therapy (MHT) can be achieved with oral, parenteral, topical (intravaginal), or transdermal estrogens, with or without progestins.

(a) Estrogens are usually administered in a **cyclical manner** to avoid long periods of continuous exposure.

(b) Concomitant use of **estrogen therapy with a progestin reduces the incidence of endometrial carcinoma.**

(2) Postmenopausal estrogen therapy **improves hot flashes, sweating, and atrophic vaginitis.** It also slows the rate of bone loss.

c. They are also used for menstrual abnormalities and oral contraception.

6. ***Adverse effects and contraindications***

a. Estrogens are associated with **nausea**, **headaches**, cholestasis, and hypertension.

b. They present an increased risk of **endometrial cancer** that is dose and duration dependent.

(1) Risk is **reduced by periodic withdrawal** of estrogen therapy and **replacement by progestin**, or concomitant treatment with both drugs.

c. Estrogen therapy is the major cause of **postmenopausal bleeding** and may mask bleeding due to endometrial cancer.

d. They are contraindicated in the presence of estrogen-dependent or estrogen-responsive carcinoma, liver disease, or thromboembolic disease.

B. Agents with antiestrogen activity

1. **Selective estrogen receptor modulator (SERM)**

a. SERMs are ligands for the estrogen receptor that have agonist activity in one tissue but may have antagonist activity or no activity in another tissue.

(1) **Agonist** activity is **preferred** in the **bone**, brain, and liver. It mimics the effects of estrogen providing beneficial effects, for example, maintaining bone density.

(2) **Antagonist** activity is **preferred** in the **breast** and **endometrium**, to prevent the development of cancer.

b. ***Specific agents.*** **Clomiphene, tamoxifen, raloxifene, bazedoxifene, ospemifene.**

2. **Clomiphene**

a. ***Mechanism of action*** (see Fig. 10.1)

(1) This agent is a SERM with **potent antiestrogen activity.**

(2) Clomiphene competes with estrogen for ER-binding sites and delays replenishment of ERs in cells. It inhibits the negative feedback effects of estrogen at hypothalamic and pituitary levels, leading to an **increase in gonadotropin release (FSH, LH).**

(3) This results in **enhanced follicular maturation and stimulation of ovulation.**

b. ***Indications.*** It is used for the treatment of **female infertility in women with ovulatory dysfunction.** It is not effective in women with ovarian or pituitary failure.

c. ***Adverse effects*** include **hot flashes** and **ovarian enlargement.**

d. ***Precautions*** include an increased risk for OHSS and ovarian cancer. It may also increase the risk for multiple births.

3. **Tamoxifen**

a. ***Mechanism of action***

(1) Tamoxifen exhibits antiestrogenic effects in breast tissue and estrogenic effects in the endometrium and bones.

b. ***Indications.*** **Estrogen receptor–positive breast cancer** in both premenopausal and postmenopausal women. It is also indicated for breast cancer risk reduction in high-risk women.

c. ***Adverse effects*** include **hot flashes**, weight gain, and gynecologic symptoms. Venous thromboembolic events and endometrial hyperplasia or cancer are also associated with tamoxifen.

4. **Raloxifene**
   a. ***Mechanism of action***
      (1) Acts as an estrogen agonist in the bone exerting an antiresorptive effect and exhibits antiestrogenic effects in breast and endometrial tissue exerting an antiproliferative effect on estrogen receptor–positive breast tumors
   b. ***Indications.*** Prevention and treatment of postmenopausal osteoporosis. It reduces risk of invasive breast cancer in postmenopausal women.
   c. ***Adverse effects*** include **hot flashes**, leg cramps, and increased risk of venous thromboembolism.
5. **Synthetic androgen**
   a. ***Specific agent.*** **Danazol.**
   b. ***Mechanism of action*** (see Fig. 10.1)
      (1) Danazol is a testosterone derivative with **antiandrogen, antiestrogenic, and antiprogestogenic properties.**
      (2) It inhibits several of the enzymes involved in steroidogenesis but does not inhibit aromatase.
      (3) It may also bind to estrogen and androgen receptors and inhibits gonadotropin release in both men and women.
      (4) Danazol **decreases pituitary output of FSH and LH**. It causes regression and atrophy of normal and ectopic endometrial tissue.
   c. ***Indications.*** It is used to treat **endometriosis** and **fibrocystic breast disease.**
   d. ***Adverse effects*** may include **weight gain**, **acne**, and **increased hair growth**.
   e. ***Precautions.*** It has the potential to cause several dangerous effects, including **hepatocellular disease**, intracranial hypertension, and thromboembolism.
   f. ***Contraindications.*** It should not be used in pregnant women and in patients with hepatic disease.
6. *Agents with antiestrogen activity that are used in the treatment of breast cancer are included in Chapter 12, which covers cancer chemotherapy. These include the following:*
   a. *Estrogen receptor antagonist (fulvestrant)*
   b. *SERMs (tamoxifen, raloxifene, toremifene)*
   c. *Aromatase inhibitors* (anastrozole, letrozole, exemestane)

C. Progestins

1. ***Structure and activity***
   a. The most important natural progestin is progesterone, which is synthesized by the ovaries, testes, and adrenals.
   b. Synthetic progestins include the 19-nor compounds, such as **norethindrone**, norgestrel, and **levonorgestrel**.
      (1) All of these agents are potent oral progestins derived from testosterone; some have androgenic activity.
   c. Several synthetic derivatives of progesterone have progestin activity, including **megestrol**, **medroxyprogesterone acetate**, and hydroxyprogesterone caproate.
   d. Gonanes include norgestimate and desogestrel; these agents have reduced androgenic activity.
   e. **Drospirenone is a spironolactone analogue** with antimineralocorticoid, antiandrogenic, and progestational activities.
2. ***Actions and pharmacologic properties*** (see Fig. 10.1)
   a. Progestins bind to intranuclear receptors (PR-A and PR-B) that alter the transcription of target genes.
   b. Progesterone is extensively bound to corticosteroid-binding globulin (CBG) in the plasma and is not administered orally because of rapid hepatic metabolism.
   c. Progestins are eliminated by hydroxylation to pregnanediol and conjugation with glucuronic acid and subsequent urinary excretion.

d. Progestins have multiple actions. They slow the mitotic activity of the estrogen-stimulated uterus, cause vascularization of the endometrium, and induce a more glandular appearance and function.
e. Progestins can decrease triglycerides and HDL, but may slightly increase LDL, depending on the preparation and dose. They also increase lipoprotein lipase.
f. Progestins increase basal and stimulated insulin secretion and stimulate appetite.

3. ***Indications***
a. Progestins are administered orally, by depot injection, as a vaginal gel, and as a slow-release intrauterine device.
b. **They are used for contraception, alone or in combination with estrogens.**
c. They can be used in the treatment of **endometrial cancer** and **endometrial hyperplasia**.
d. Progestins control **abnormal uterine bleeding** and can also be used to **delay menstruation** for surgical or postoperative reasons.
e. They may be used diagnostically to evaluate endometrial function in amenorrhea.

D. Agents with antiprogestin activity

1. ***Specific agent.*** **Mifepristone (RU-486)**.
2. ***Mechanism of action***
a. Mifepristone is a norethindrone derivative with potent antiprogestin and antiglucocorticoid activities.
b. It is a **competitive antagonist of progesterone** and glucocorticoid receptors (GR).
c. It blocks effects of progesterone and leads to **contraction-inducing activity** in the myometrium and sensitizes myometrium to prostaglandins eliciting cervical maturing.
3. ***Indications***
a. Mifepristone has been approved for use to induce **medical abortion** in the first trimester of pregnancy up to 9–10 weeks of gestation (in combination with misoprostol). It is administered as a single 200-mg oral dose followed by misoprostol 800 μg 24–48 hours later.
b. Mifepristone has emerged as one of the most effective hormonal methods for emergency contraception.
c. Antiglucocorticoid activity has potential therapeutic application in Cushing syndrome.
4. ***Adverse effects*** include nausea, diarrhea, **abdominal pain**, and **vaginal bleeding**.
5. ***Precautions.*** It has the potential to cause excessive bleeding and bacterial infections.

E. Hormonal contraceptives

1. **Combination oral contraceptives**
a. Specific agents include combinations of **estrogen and progestin**.
(1) The estrogen component is either **ethinylestradiol** or mestranol.
(2) The progestin component may include **norethindrone**, norgestrel, **levonorgestrel**, or drospirenone.
b. ***Mechanism of action*** (see Fig. 10.1)
(1) These **agents inhibit ovulation via negative feedback**. They **suppress the production of FSH to prevent follicle maturation** and **suppress the LH surge to prevent ovulation.**
(2) The **most important mechanism** for providing contraception is **inhibition of the midcycle LH surge**, so that **ovulation does not occur**.
(3) They also cause alterations in the genital tract, in which they induce endometrial decidualization and render the cervical mucosa thick and unfavorable for sperm penetration and produce an unfavorable environment for implantation of an embryo.
c. ***Indications.*** Other than their use in **contraception**, these agents are used for the management of **dysmenorrhea**, **polycystic ovary syndrome**, menorrhagia, **endometriosis**, acne, and hirsutism.
d. ***Administration***
(1) Most combination pills are taken continuously for 21 days, followed by a 7-day withdrawal (or placebo) period to induce withdrawal bleeding.
(2) Some oral contraceptives are given on an extended rather than monthly cycle.
(a) The number of episodes of withdrawal bleeding per year is reduced and can be completely eliminated.

(b) In addition, shortening the hormone-free interval may reduce symptoms associated with hormone withdrawal, such as headache or pelvic pain.

(3) Backup contraception is generally needed if two or more consecutive hormonal pills are missed.

e. ***Advantages*** of their use include a **decreased risk for endometrial, ovarian, and colon cancer**. They improve symptoms of premenstrual syndrome.

f. ***Adverse effects*** may include hypertension, increased triglycerides, and the potential for breakthrough bleeding.

g. ***Precautions***

(1) They increase the risk of **thromboembolism**.

(a) Estrogens increase levels of fibrinogen and coagulation factors II, VII, VIII, IX, and X, while decreasing concentrations of antithrombin III.

(2) They increase the risk of **breast cancer**.

(3) They are associated with an increase in morbidity and mortality due to **myocardial infarction** (may be age related).

(a) The risk of cardiovascular complications increases markedly in women **older than 35 years and in women who smoke**.

h. ***Contraindications***. These agents are contraindicated in cardiovascular disease, thromboembolic disease, estrogen-dependent cancer, impaired liver function, undiagnosed bleeding, and migraine.

i. ***Drug interactions***. Any drug that increases liver microsomal enzyme activity, such as rifampin and certain anticonvulsants, accelerates the metabolism of oral contraception and may decrease efficacy.

2. **Progestin-only preparations**

a. ***Specific agents***

(1) Norethindrone is available as an oral formulation ("minipill") and must be taken daily.

(2) Medroxyprogesterone acetate is available as a subcutaneous or intramuscular injection administered every 3 months.

(3) Etonogestrel is a subcutaneous implant that provides contraception for up to 3 years.

(4) Levonorgestrel is available as an intrauterine device that provides contraception for up to 5 years.

b. ***Mechanism of action***. The primary mechanism for progestin-only contraception is **thickening the mucus in the cervix, making it difficult for sperm to enter**. They also suppress ovulation, although they do not do this consistently; therefore, they may result in irregular fertile periods (see Fig. 10.1).

c. ***Indications***. These agents are ideal contraception for women in whom **estrogen is contraindicated** or causes additional health risks, including women who are **breastfeeding**, women with a **history of migraines** with aura, and women who **smoke**.

d. ***Administration***

(1) The oral formulation (minipill) must be taken at the **same time each day** to maximize contraceptive efficacy. Backup contraception should be used for at least 2 days if it is taken more than 3 hours late or missed.

e. ***Advantages***. It can **decrease the risk of endometrial cancer**.

f. ***Adverse effects*** may include irregular bleeding, **acne flairs**, and follicular cysts.

g. ***Precautions***. It can **increase the risk of breast cancer**.

h. ***Drug interactions***. Any drug that increases liver microsomal enzyme activity, such as rifampin and certain anticonvulsants, accelerates the metabolism of oral contraception, and may decrease efficacy.

3. **Postcoital (emergency) oral contraceptives**

a. ***Specific agent***. **Levonorgestrel**.

b. ***Mechanism of action***. The mechanism is not fully understood. It **alters sperm transport, inhibits ovulation, and prevents implantation**. It does not affect established pregnancies.

c. ***Indications***. It is used to **prevent unwanted pregnancy after unprotected intercourse or failure of a contraceptive method**. It is less effective than standard oral contraceptive regimens. It is most effective when taken within 72 hours after unprotected intercourse.

However, it can be taken up to 120 hours with decreased effectiveness. A single dose of 1.5 mg or two doses of 0.75 mg taken 12–24 hours apart is efficacious in preventing about 80% of pregnancies.

d. ***Administration.*** It can be offered **without regard to the day of the menstrual cycle** due to uncertainty in timing of ovulation. It must be taken within 72 hours of unprotected intercourse.

e. ***Adverse effects*** may include nausea, vomiting, and irregular bleeding.

f. Another available agent for emergency contraception is **ulipristal acetate.** It is more effective than levonorgestrel with sustained efficacy up to 120 hours after unprotected intercourse, but available only by prescription.

(1) This agent is a **progestin receptor modulator**. It prevents progestin from binding to the progesterone receptor and postpones follicular rupture when administered prior to ovulation; this can delay or inhibit ovulation.

F. Androgens and anabolic steroids

1. ***Testosterone***

a. Testosterone is synthesized primarily in the **Leydig cells** of the testes under the influence of LH.

b. It is **metabolized to the more potent 5α-dihydrotestosterone by 5α-reductase**.

c. Testosterone is extensively bound to SSBG and albumin.

d. Natural testosterone can be administered transdermally or intramuscularly.

2. ***Synthetic androgens***

a. The 17-substituted testosterone esters (testosterone propionate, testosterone enanthate, and testosterone cypionate) are administered by injection.

b. The 17-alkyl testosterone derivatives include methyltestosterone, fluoxymesterone, and oxymetholone.

c. Nandrolone and oxandrolone are testosterone derivatives with a higher anabolic-to-androgenic ratio than testosterone itself.

3. ***Actions*** (see Fig. 10.1)

a. Androgens form a complex with a specific intracellular receptor (a member of the nuclear-receptor family) and interact with specific genes to modulate differentiation, development, and growth (see Fig. 1.1F).

b. Androgenic actions

(1) Androgens stimulate the differentiation and development of Wolffian structures, including the **epididymis**, **seminal vesicles**, **prostate**, and **penis**.

(2) Androgens stimulate the development and maintenance of **male secondary sexual characteristics**.

c. Anabolic actions

(1) Anabolic steroids cause acceleration of **epiphyseal closure**, and they result in linear growth at puberty.

(2) Anabolic steroids cause an increase in muscle mass.

(3) Behavioral effects include **aggressiveness** and increased **libido**.

4. ***Indications***

a. Hypogonadism

(1) Androgens promote linear growth and sexual maturation and maintain male secondary sexual characteristics, libido, and potency.

b. Estrogen-dependent breast cancers

c. Wasting disorders in AIDS or after severe burns

5. ***Adverse effects and contraindications***

a. Androgens and anabolic steroids produce **decreased testicular function**, edema, and altered plasma lipids (increased LDL and decreased HDL levels).

b. These agents cause masculinization in women.

c. Androgens increase plasma fibrinolytic activity, causing severe bleeding with concomitant anticoagulant therapy.

d. **17-Alkyl substituted androgens** (but not testosterone ester preparations) are associated with **increases in hepatic enzymes**, hyperbilirubinemia, and cholestatic hepatitis, which may result in jaundice.

e. Androgens and anabolic steroids are contraindicated in pregnant women and in patients with carcinoma of the prostate or hepatic, renal, or cardiovascular disease.

6. ***Precautions.*** Athletes may use these agents inappropriately; large doses of androgens increase the extent and rate of muscle formation and may increase the intensity of training.

G. Agents with antiandrogen activity

1. **5α-Reductase inhibitors**
   a. ***Specific agents*** include **finasteride** and **dutasteride**.
   b. ***Mechanism of action.*** These agents **inhibit the conversion of testosterone to dihydrotestosterone**. They markedly suppress dihydrotestosterone levels and **decrease the size of the prostate gland** (see Fig. 10.1).
   c. ***Indications***
      (1) Both are approved for the treatment of **benign prostatic hyperplasia.**
         (a) They are more effective with larger prostates.
         (b) Treatment for 6–12 months may be needed to sufficiently reduce prostate size and improve symptoms.
         (c) Prostate-specific antigen (PSA) concentrations will decrease.
      (2) Finasteride is also approved for the treatment of **male pattern baldness**.
   d. ***Monitoring.*** After about 3–6 months of use, these agents reduce PSA concentrations. A new baseline PSA should be established; any patient with an increased PSA should be evaluated for prostate cancer.
   e. ***Adverse effects*** may include **sexual dysfunction**, including decreased libido and ejaculatory or erectile dysfunction.
   f. ***Precautions***
      (1) Although these agents reduce the overall incidence of prostate cancer, they may **increase the incidence of high-grade prostate cancers** in those that develop prostate cancer.
      (2) These agents **may affect the developing fetus**, including the potential for abnormalities of external male genitalia. Pregnant women should avoid contact with the medication, including exposure from the semen of a male partner who was exposed.
2. *Agents with antiandrogen activity that are used in the treatment of prostate cancer are included in Chapter 12, which covers cancer chemotherapy. This includes the following:*
   a. *Antiandrogen agents: Flutamide, bicalutamide, nilutamide*
   b. *Androgen synthesis inhibitors: Abiraterone and ketoconazole*

VI. ERECTILE DYSFUNCTION

Erectile dysfunction (ED) that affects men is characterized by the inability to achieve or maintain an erection sufficient and satisfactory for sexual intercourse.

A. Phosphodiesterase type 5 inhibitors (PDE-5i): Includes sildenafil, tadalafil, vardenafil, udenafil, and avanafil.

1. Act by blocking the degradation of cyclic guanosine monophosphate (cGMP), leading to increased cGMP levels and relaxation of penile smooth muscle cells.
2. Sildenafil needs to be taken one hour before sexual activity. Tadalafil can be taken 30 minutes to 12 hours before sexual activity.
3. **Common side effects** include headache, flushing, dyspepsia, and nasal congestion. Priapism may occur with improper dosage. Combination with nitrates and nitric oxide donors may be dangerous. **Topical application** is emerging as an alternative with fewer systemic side effects.
4. Patients with unstable angina, severe heart failure, or recent myocardial infarction should avoid these drugs. Dosage adjustments may be needed for men over 65 or those with hepatic or renal impairment.

B. Prostaglandins

1. Alprostadil is a prostaglandin analogue used to treat ED. It can be administered as an **intracavernosal injection** or a **urethral suppository**.
2. Alprostadil mimics the effects of prostaglandin E1, which induces **vasodilation** by increasing levels of cyclic adenosine monophosphate (**cAMP**) in smooth muscle cells, leading to relaxation of the smooth muscle in the corpus cavernosum and increased penile blood flow.
3. It is used when PDE-5 inhibitors fail.
4. Common adverse effects include pain at the injection site, penile fibrosis or curvature. Priapism and penile scarring are also observed.

C. Other Treatments

1. **Papaverine**, an opiate alkaloid and vasodilator may be useful in men who do not respond to oral medications like **PDE-5 inhibitors**. It is typically administered through **intracavernosal injection** into the penis, either alone or in combination with other drugs. Pain, scarring, and priapism are notable concerns. Topical formulations and combination therapies are promising alternatives to mitigate these risks.
2. **Yohimbine**, an α_2-adrenergic antagonist used less frequently due to variable efficacy and side effects.
3. **Apomorphine** acts as a dopamine receptor agonist, inducing and increasing penile erection responses via disinhibition following sexual stimulation.
4. Vacuum constriction devices
5. Penile prostheses

PDE5 inhibitors are recommended as first-line therapy for most men with ED who do not have specific contraindications to their use.

Intracavernosal injection therapy with alprostadil should be offered to patients as second-line therapy for ED. Intraurethral alprostadil is considered a less effective treatment than intracavernosal alprostadil for ED.

VII. THE ADRENAL CORTEX

A. Corticosteroids

1. ***Natural adrenocortical steroids***
   a. Glucocorticoids are synthesized under the control of ACTH.
   b. **Cortisol (hydrocortisone)** is the **predominant glucocorticoid** in humans (Fig. 10.3).
   c. The major **mineralocorticoid** of the adrenal cortex is **aldosterone** (Fig. 10.3).
   d. 11-Deoxycorticosterone, an aldosterone precursor, has both mineralocorticoid and glucocorticoid activities.
   e. The adrenals also synthesize various androgens, predominantly dehydroepiandrosterone and androstenedione.
2. ***Synthetic adrenocortical steroids***
   a. A wide array of steroid compounds with various ratios of mineralocorticoid to glucocorticoid properties has been synthesized (Table 10.1).
   b. A C_1–C_2 double bond, as in prednisolone and prednisone, increases glucocorticoid activity without increasing mineralocorticoid activity.
   c. The addition of a 9α-fluoro group increases activity (dexamethasone or fludrocortisone).
   d. Methylation or hydroxylation at the 16α position abolishes mineralocorticoid activity with little effect on glucocorticoid potency.
3. ***Mechanism of action.*** The effects of mineralocorticoids and glucocorticoids are mediated by two separate and specific intracellular receptors, the **mineralocorticoid receptor (MR)** and **GR**.
   a. Natural and synthetic steroids enter cells rapidly and interact with these intracellular receptors.
   b. The resulting complexes modulate the **transcription rate of specific genes** and lead to an increase or decrease in the levels of specific proteins.

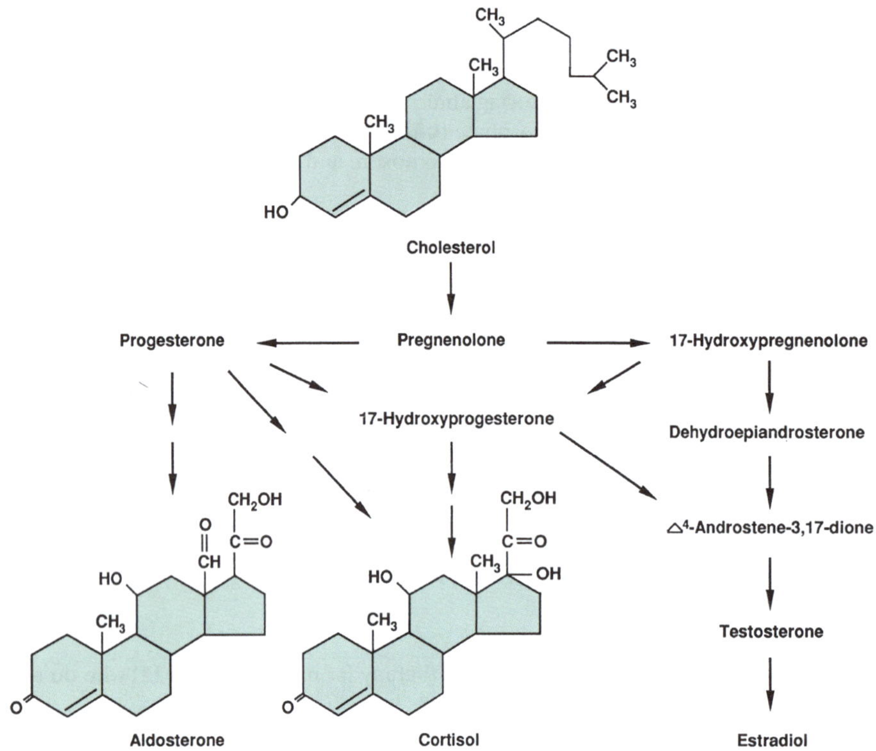

FIGURE 10.3. Biosynthesis of adrenal steroids.

TABLE 10.1 Properties of Adrenocortical Steroids

Agent	Equivalent Dose (mg)	Metabolic Potency	Anti-inflammatory Potency	Sodium-Retaining Potency
Oral glucocorticoids				
Cortisol	20	20	1	1
Cortisone	25	20	1	1
Prednisone	5	5	4	0.5
Prednisolone	5	5	4	0.5
Dexamethasone	0.75	1	30	0.05
Betamethasone	0.6	1.0–1.5	25–40	0.05
Triamcinolone	4	4	5	0.1
Aldosterone		0.3		3,000
Fludrocortisone	0.01	0.1		125–250
Topical glucocorticoids				
Betamethasone	Highest potency			
Clobetasol	Highest potency			
Halobetasol	Highest potency			
Amcinonide	High potency			
Fluocinonide	High potency			
Triamcinolone	High potency			
Beclomethasone	Medium potency			
Fluticasone	Medium potency			
Hydrocortisone	Medium potency			
Dexamethasone	Low potency			
Desonide	Low potency			

4. *Pharmacokinetic properties*

a. Most circulating cortisol is bound to CBG; some is also bound to plasma albumin.

(1) Some of the potent synthetic glucocorticoids, such as dexamethasone, do not bind to CBG, leaving all absorbed drug in a free state.

b. The kidney excretes both natural and synthetic steroids. Agents with the longest half-life tend to be the most potent.

(1) Short-acting agents such as cortisol are active for 8–12 hours.

(2) Intermediate-acting agents such as prednisolone are active for 12–36 hours.

(3) Long-acting agents such as dexamethasone are active for 39–54 hours.

c. There are a variety of different formulations, including oral, intravenous, intramuscular, subcutaneous, inhalation, otic, rectal, and topical.

5. *Administration*

a. In some cases, drug administration attempts to pattern the circadian rhythm: A double dose is given in the morning, and a single dose is given in the afternoon.

b. Alternate-day therapy may relieve clinical manifestations of the disease state while causing less severe suppression of the adrenal–hypothalamic–pituitary axis.

c. Patients removed from long-term glucocorticoid therapy **must be weaned off the drug over several days**, using progressively lower doses to allow recovery of adrenal responsiveness.

6. *Glucocorticoids*

a. Glucocorticoids affect virtually all tissues. Therapeutic actions and adverse effects are extensions of their physiologic effects.

(1) ***Physiologic effects***

(a) The physiologic effects of glucocorticoids are mediated by increased protein breakdown, leading to a **negative nitrogen balance**.

(b) They **increase blood glucose levels** by **stimulation of gluconeogenesis**.

(c) These agents increase the synthesis of several key enzymes involved in glucose and amino acid metabolism.

(d) Glucocorticoids **increase plasma fatty acids** and **ketone body formation** via increased lipolysis and decreased glucose uptake into fat cells and **redistribution of body fat**.

(e) These agents increase kaliuresis via increasing renal blood flow and glomerular filtration rate; increased protein metabolism results in release of intracellular potassium.

(f) Glucocorticoids decrease intestinal absorption of Ca^{2+} and inhibit osteoblasts.

(g) Glucocorticoids **promote Na^+ and water retention.**

(2) ***Anti-inflammatory effects.*** Glucocorticoids inhibit all of the classic signs of inflammation (erythema, swelling, soreness, and heat). Effects include the following:

(a) Inhibition of the antigenic response of macrophages and leukocytes

(b) Inhibition of vascular permeability by reduction of histamine release and the action of kinins

(c) **Inhibition of arachidonic acid and prostaglandin production** by inhibition of phospholipase A_2 (mediated by annexin 1) and the cyclooxygenase enzymes

(d) **Inhibition of cytokine production**, including IL-1, IL-2, IL-3, IL-6, tumor necrosis factor-α, and granulocyte-macrophage colony-stimulating factor

(3) ***Immunologic effects***

(a) Glucocorticoids **decrease circulating lymphocytes**, monocytes, eosinophils, and basophils.

(b) Glucocorticoids **increase circulating neutrophils.**

(c) Long-term therapy results in involution and **atrophy of all lymphoid tissues.**

(4) Other effects include the following:

(a) Inhibition of plasma ACTH and possible adrenal atrophy

(b) Inhibition of fibroblast growth and collagen synthesis

(c) Stimulation of acid and pepsin secretion in the stomach

(d) Altered CNS responses, influencing mood and sleep patterns

(e) Enhanced neuromuscular transmission

(f) Induction of surfactant production in the fetal lung at term

b. ***Indications***

(1) Glucocorticoids are used in **replacement therapy** for primary **(Addison disease)** or secondary (hypothalamic or pituitary disease) insufficiency; this therapy usually requires the use of both a mineralocorticoid and a glucocorticoid.

(2) **Inflammation and immunosuppression**

(a) Glucocorticoids are used to treat rheumatoid arthritis, gout, bursitis, lupus erythematosus, and other autoimmune diseases, asthma, nephrotic syndrome, inflammatory bowel disease, and ocular inflammation.

(b) These agents are also used in hypersensitivity and allergic reactions.

(c) Glucocorticoids can reduce organ or graft rejection.

(3) **Diagnosis of Cushing syndrome (dexamethasone suppression test)**

(a) This test measures the suppression of plasma cortisol following the administration of dexamethasone, which normally binds to GR in the pituitary and inhibits ACTH production. Failure to suppress cortisol may indicate primary Cushing syndrome or ectopic ACTH production.

(4) Other indications include sarcoidosis, dermatologic disorders, idiopathic nephrosis of children, neuromuscular disorders, such as Bell palsy, shock, adrenocortical hyperplasia, stimulation of surfactant production and acceleration of lung maturation in a preterm fetus, and neoplastic diseases including adult and childhood leukemia.

(5) Use of corticosteroids in infectious diseases has been a matter of debate, with evidence suggesting potential benefits in controlling excessive inflammatory response. Corticosteroids have shown efficacy in meningitis, septic shock, moderate to severe *Pneumocystis jirovecii* pneumonia and COVID-19. Use in miliary tuberculosis remains controversial. However, it is important to note that high doses of corticosteroids are associated with immunosuppression and enhanced risk of superinfections.

c. ***Adverse effects and contraindications***

(1) Adverse effects of glucocorticoids include the following:

(a) Suppression of the hypothalamo-pituitary–adrenal (HPA) axis

(b) Hyperglycemia and other metabolic disturbances, including steroid-induced diabetes mellitus and weight gain

(c) Osteoporosis and avascular necrosis

(d) Peptic ulcers

(e) Cataracts and increased intraocular pressure (leading to glaucoma)

(f) Edema

(g) Hypertension

(h) Increased susceptibility to infection

(i) Muscle weakness (steroid myopathy)

(j) Poor wound healing

(k) Thinning of skin

(2) Prolonged use may lead to iatrogenic Cushing disease characterized by moon face, buffalo hump, central obesity, and purple striae.

(3) Certain glucocorticoids have mineralocorticoid activity, potentially causing sodium retention, potassium loss, and eventual hypokalemic and hypochloremic alkalosis.

7. ***Mineralocorticoids***

a. ***Actions***. Mineralocorticoids primarily affect the kidney, regulating salt and water balance and increasing **sodium retention** and **potassium loss**.

b. ***Specific agent***. **Fludrocortisone** is the agent of choice for long-term mineralocorticoid replacement.

c. ***Indications***. Mineralocorticoids are used in **replacement therapy** to maintain electrolyte and fluid balance in **hypoadrenalism**.

d. ***Adverse effects*** include **sodium retention** and **hypokalemia**, edema, and **hypertension**.

B. Adrenocortical antagonists

1. **Mitotane**
   a. ***Mechanism of action.*** Mitotane is an adrenolytic agent. It suppresses the adrenal cortex and causes selective atrophy of the zona fasciculata and zona reticularis. It can reduce plasma cortisol levels in Cushing syndrome produced by adrenal carcinoma.
   b. ***Indication.*** It is used for **adrenocortical carcinoma.**
   c. ***Adverse effects*** may include GI distress, **confusion**, lethargy, and **rash**.
2. **Metyrapone** blocks the activity of 11-hydroxylase, thereby **reducing cortisol production**. It is used diagnostically to assess adrenal and pituitary function.
3. Ketoconazole is an antifungal agent that, at high doses, is a potent inhibitor of several of the P450 enzymes involved in steroidogenesis in the adrenals and gonads. It can be used for Cushing syndrome (see Fig. 10.1).

VIII. THE THYROID

A. Thyroid hormone receptor agonists

1. ***Synthesis of natural thyroid hormones***
   a. Natural **thyroid hormones are formed by the iodination of tyrosine residues** on the glycoprotein Tg.
   b. A tyrosine residue may be iodinated at one (monoiodotyrosine [MIT]) or two (diiodotyrosine [DIT]) positions.
   c. Two iodinated tyrosines are then coupled to synthesize **T_3 (formed from one molecule each of MIT and DIT) or T_4 (formed from two DIT molecules).**
   d. The thyroid hormones that are unbound in plasma are transported through the cell membrane into the cytoplasm.
   e. **T_4 has only minimal hormonal activity but is much longer lasting and can be converted to T_3, the more active form, by 5′ deiodinase.**
   f. TSH, which acts by a membrane-associated G protein-coupled receptor, increases follicular cell cAMP, and stimulates biosynthesis.
   g. I^- is a potent inhibitor of thyroid hormone release.
2. ***Thyroid hormone preparations***
   a. **Levothyroxine (synthetic T_4)**
      (1) This is the **preparation of choice**, although it takes 1–2 weeks before effects are seen.
   b. **Liothyronine (synthetic T_3)**
      (1) This agent is best for **short-term suppression of TSH.**
      (2) It is effective for the treatment of **myxedema coma.**
      (3) Since T_3 is the more potent form, it has an **increased risk for cardiotoxicity.**
   c. **Liotrix** is a 4:1 mixture of the above T_4 and T_3 preparations.
   d. **Desiccated thyroid (animal)** is prepared from animal thyroid glands and contains a mixture of T_4, T_3, MIT, and DIT.
      (1) The potency can vary. It also has the potential for protein antigenicity.
      (2) Given the availability of synthetics, it is not recommended for initial therapy.
3. ***Mechanism of action***
   a. Thyroid hormones interact with **specific nuclear receptor proteins** located in the nucleus of target cells. **T_3 is the most active form** in binding to the receptor.
   b. They alter the synthesis rate of specific mRNAs, leading to increased production of specific proteins.
   c. Thyroid hormones are **responsible for many life-sustaining actions**, including **optimal growth, development, function, and maintenance of body tissues.**
      (1) Increased ATP hydrolysis and oxygen consumption contribute to the effects of thyroid hormones on basal metabolic rate and thermogenesis.

4. ***Pharmacokinetic properties***
   a. More than 99% of circulating T_4 is bound to plasma proteins; only 5%–10% of T_3 is protein bound.
   b. Most T_3 and T_4 are bound to TBG.
5. ***Actions***
   a. Thyroid hormones are essential for **normal physical and mental development** of the fetus, including linear growth of the long bones, growth of the brain, and normal myelination.
      (1) **Hypothyroidism in infants leads to cretinism** (myxedema with physical and mental retardation).
   b. Thyroid hormones increase heart rate, peripheral resistance, basal metabolic rate, blood sugar levels, and synthesis of fatty acids.
   c. They **decrease plasma cholesterol** and triglyceride levels.
   d. They inhibit TRH and TSH release from the hypothalamus and pituitary, respectively.
   e. Thyroid hormones exert **maintenance effects** on the CNS, reproductive tract, GI tract, and musculature.
6. ***Indications***
   a. Primary, secondary, or tertiary hypothyroidism, including that caused by Hashimoto disease, myxedema coma, simple goiter, or following surgical ablation of the thyroid gland.
      (1) Hashimoto thyroiditis (chronic autoimmune thyroiditis): This is the most common cause of hypothyroidism in iodine-sufficient areas; it is characterized by gradual thyroid failure caused by autoimmune-mediated destruction of the thyroid gland.
      (2) Myxedema coma: This condition is a medical emergency; it is a life-threatening complication due to severe hypothyroidism. It can lead to hypothermia, slowing of organ function, and mental status changes.
   b. TSH-dependent carcinomas of the thyroid may be treated with thyroid hormones if other therapies are not feasible.
7. ***Adverse effects*** are directly related to hormone level.
   a. They may include **nervousness**, anxiety, and headache.
   b. High hormone levels may induce **arrhythmias,** angina, or **infarction.** Caution must be used in the elderly and in patients with underlying cardiovascular disease.
   c. Long-term therapy can **decrease bone mineral density** by causing an increase in bone turnover.
8. ***Drug interactions***. Medications such as sodium polystyrene, cholestyramine, calcium, multivitamins, and aluminum hydroxide may decrease absorption thyroid hormone.

B. Antithyroid drugs

1. Thioamides

a. ***Specific agents*** include the following:
   (1) **Propylthiouracil (PTU)**
      (a) Due to multiple daily dosing and the potential for causing severe hepatitis, its use is reserved for certain conditions, including:
         i. First trimester of **pregnancy** (it is more strongly protein bound than methimazole and less likely to cross the placenta)
         ii. **Thyroid storm** (since it is rapidly absorbed)
   (2) **Methimazole**
      (a) This agent is about 10 times more potent than PTU. **Carbimazole** is converted to methimazole in the body.
      (b) It is the **drug of choice** for hyperthyroidism since it can be administered once daily and has a **lower risk for liver injury**.

b. ***Mechanism of action*** (Fig. 10.4)
   (1) Thioamides interfere with the **organification and coupling of iodide by inhibiting the peroxidase** enzyme.
   (2) **PTU also inhibits the conversion of T_4 to T_3.**

c. ***Indications*** include the treatment of **hyperthyroidism** from a variety of causes, including **Graves disease** and **toxic goiter**. They are also used to control hyperthyroidism prior to thyroid surgery.

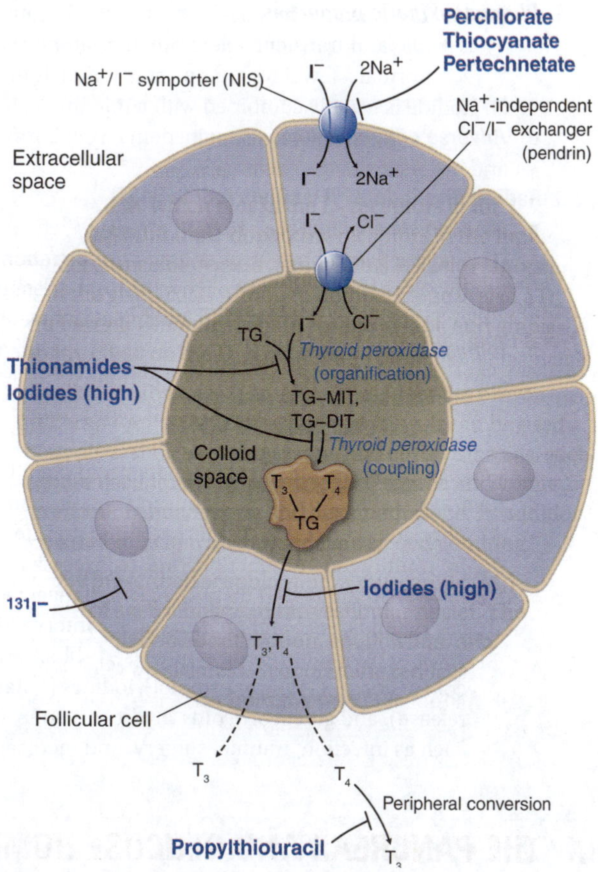

FIGURE 10.4. Medications affecting thyroid hormone synthesis. (Reprinted with permission from Golan D. Principles of Pharmacology. 4th ed. Philadelphia, PA: Wolters Kluwer Health, 2016, Fig. 28.5.)

(1) Graves disease is the leading cause of hyperthyroidism. It is an autoimmune disorder that results in overproduction of thyroid hormones.

(2) Toxic multinodular goiter is hyperthyroidism characterized by autonomously functioning thyroid nodules.

(3) Thyroid storm is a life-threatening condition associated with hyperthyroidism that is undertreated or untreated. Patients may experience increased body temperature, palpitations, chest pain, and anxiety.

d. ***Adverse effects*** may include **rashes**, headache, and nausea.

e. ***Precautions***. They have the potential to cause **agranulocytosis**.

2. Iodide

a. ***Specific agents*** include **potassium iodide** and iodine plus potassium iodide (**Lugol's iodine**—5% iodine in 10% potassium iodide).

b. ***Mechanism of action*** (Fig. 10.4)

(1) In high intracellular concentrations, iodide **inhibits several steps in thyroid hormone biosynthesis**, including iodide transport and organification (Wolff–Chaikoff effect).

(a) The **Wolff–Chaikoff effect** is a **protective downregulation** of **thyroid hormone** production in the presence of large amounts of iodine.

(2) Iodide inhibits the release of thyroid hormone.

(3) They **decrease the size and vascularity of the gland**.

c. ***Indications***

(1) **Lugol's iodine.** This agent is used **before thyroid surgery**, causing firming of thyroid tissues and decreased thyroid vascularity, thus decreasing intraoperative blood loss during thyroidectomy.

(2) It may also be used as an adjunct in thyroid storm.

(3) It is indicated only for **short-term use**.

(a) The negative feedback effect of the intrathyroidal iodide concentrations is reversible and transient; therefore, thyroid hormone synthesis and release will return to normal a few days after plasma iodide is increased.

(4) Iodide is usually combined with a thioamide; it is rarely used as sole therapy.

d. ***Adverse effects*** may cause angioedema, acneiform rash, a metallic taste on administration, and hypersensitivity reactions.

3. **Radioactive iodine ^{131}I (sodium iodide I-131)**

a. ***Mechanism of action*** (Fig. 10.4)

(1) Radioactive iodine ^{131}I, after **oral** administration, is transported and concentrated in the thyroid like the nonradioactive isotope. It **emits β particles** that are toxic to follicular cells, causing **selective and local destruction of the thyroid gland**.

b. ***Indications.*** It is used for the treatment of **hyperthyroidism** (toxic nodular goiter, Graves disease) and for some cases of **thyroid carcinoma**, via nonsurgical ablation of the thyroid gland or reduction of a hyperactive thyroid gland without damage to the surrounding tissue. This agent is also used to evaluate thyroid function.

c. ***Adverse effects*** include **hypothyroidism** and radiation thyroiditis.

d. ***Contraindicated*** in pregnancy and lactation. It should be used with caution in children.

(1) Thyroid storm is a life-threatening manifestation of thyrotoxicosis characterized by multiorgan dysfunction due to excessive thyroid hormone levels (hyperpyrexia, tachyarrhythmias, GI disturbances). Management includes supportive care (antipyretics, IV fluids, etc.) and pharmacologic interventions like thioamides (PTU and methimazole to inhibit hormone synthesis), β-blockers (propranolol which inhibits peripheral conversion of T_4 to T_3 or esmolol), iodides (potassium iodide to inhibit thyroid hormone release), and glucocorticoids (hydrocortisone or dexamethasone). Precipitating factors such as infection, trauma, surgery, and medications need to be identified and treated.

IX. THE PANCREAS AND GLUCOSE HOMEOSTASIS

A. Insulin

1. ***Structure and synthesis***

a. Insulin is a polypeptide hormone produced by the **pancreatic β cell**. It consists of two chains, A and B, linked by two disulfide bridges.

b. Insulin synthesis and release are modulated by the following:

(1) The most important stimulus is glucose. Amino acids, fatty acids, and ketone bodies also stimulate insulin release.

(2) The islets of Langerhans contain several cell types, other than β cells, which synthesize and release peptide humoral agents (including glucagon and SST) that help modulate insulin secretion.

(3) **α-Adrenergic pathways inhibit secretion of insulin**; this is the predominant inhibitory mechanism.

c. **β-Adrenergic stimulation increases insulin release.**

d. Elevated intracellular Ca^{2+} acts as an insulin secretagogue.

2. ***Mechanism of action*** (Fig. 10.5)

a. Insulin binds to the extracellular domain of specific high-affinity receptors (with tyrosine kinase activity) on the surface of liver, muscle, and fat cells.

(1) **When insulin binds, specific tyrosine residues of the insulin receptor become phosphorylated (autophosphorylation).** The phosphorylated receptor in turn phosphorylates other signaling proteins, which leads to a signal transduction cascade.

(2) Other substrates for phosphorylation include insulin receptor substrate-1 to -4.

(3) The increase in glucose transport in muscle and adipose tissue is mediated by the recruitment of **insulin-regulated glucose transporters** (GLUT-1 and GLUT-4) into the plasma membrane.

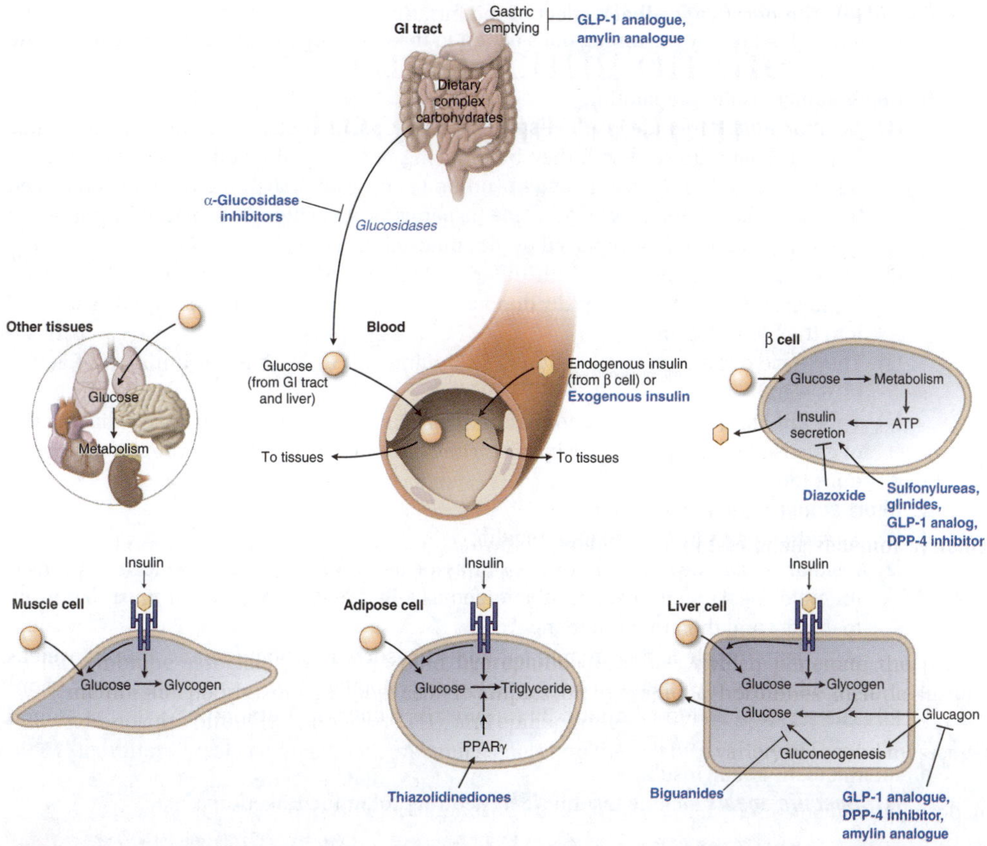

FIGURE 10.5. Physiologic and pharmacologic regulation of glucose homeostasis. DPP-4, dipeptidyl peptidase 4; GI, gastrointestinal; GLP-1, glucagon-like peptide-1. (Reprinted with permission from Golan D. Principles of Pharmacology. 4th ed. Philadelphia, PA: Wolters Kluwer Health, 2016, Fig. 31.1.)

(a) The effect of insulin on the glucose transporter distribution is reversible. Within an hour of insulin removal, GLUT-4 is removed from the membrane and restored in intracellular vesicles ready to be re-recruited to the surface by insulin.

b. Insulin alters the phosphorylation state of key metabolic enzymes, leading to enzymatic activation or inactivation.

c. **It induces the transcription of several genes involved in increasing glucose catabolism** and specifically inhibits transcription of other genes involved in gluconeogenesis.

3. *Physiologic actions of insulin*

a. Insulin promotes systemic **cellular K^+ uptake.**

b. Liver

(1) **Inhibits glucose production** and **increases glycolysis**

(2) **Inhibits glycogenolysis** and **stimulates glycogen synthesis**

(3) Increases the synthesis of triglycerides

(4) Increases protein synthesis

c. Muscle

(1) Increases glucose transport and glycolysis

(2) **Increases glycogen deposition**

(3) Increases protein synthesis

d. Adipose tissue

(1) Increases glucose transport

(2) Increases lipogenesis and lipoprotein lipase

(3) Decreases intracellular lipolysis

4. ***Insulin preparations*** (Table 10.2)
   a. Insulin is classified by the timing of its action in the body, including the onset of action and duration of action.
   b. **Rapid-acting** insulin preparations
      (1) ***Specific agents*** include insulin **lispro** (proline at position B28 and lysine at position B29 in the B-chain are reversed, thereby reducing tendency of insulin molecules to form dimers or hexamers), insulin **aspart** (proline at position B28 in the B-chain is replaced by aspartic acid), and insulin **glulisine** (asparagine at position B3 replaced by lysine and lysine at position B29 is replaced by glutamic acid).
      (2) These agents are modified with different amino acid residues to make them more soluble, allowing them to rapidly dissociate into monomers which are rapidly absorbed into the bloodstream.
      (3) They have a rapid onset of action (15–20 minutes), with a shorter duration of action (4–6 hours).
      (4) They are often injected minutes before a meal and provide better postprandial control of glucose levels than regular insulin. They have low incidence of hypoglycemic reactions too.
   c. **Short-acting** insulin preparations
      (1) ***Specific agents*** include **regular insulin.**
      (2) Regular crystalline insulin naturally self-associates into a hexameric molecule (six insulin molecules) when injected subcutaneously. Before it is absorbed, it must dissociate to dimers and then to monomers.
         (a) This principle is the premise for additives such as protamine and zinc, as well as modifications of amino acids for insulin analogues.
      (3) The onset of action is around 30 minutes to 1 hour; its duration of action is around 6–8 hours.
   d. **Intermediate-acting** insulin
      (1) ***Specific agents*** include insulin **NPH** (neutral protamine Hagedorn).

TABLE 10.2 Pharmacologic Properties of Insulin

	Onset	Peak	Duration	Directions
Rapid-acting insulin				
Insulin aspart Insulin glulisine Insulin lispro	10–30 minutes	30–90 minutes	3–5 hours	Usually taken immediately before a meal to cover the blood glucose elevation from eating Often used with longer-acting insulin
Short-acting insulin				
Regular insulin	30–60 minutes	2–4 hours	6–12 hours	Usually taken about 30 minutes before a meal to cover the blood glucose elevation from eating Often used with longer-acting insulin
Intermediate-acting insulin				
Insulin NPH	1–3 hours	4–8 hours	12–16 hours	Often combined with rapid- or short-acting insulin
Long-acting insulin				
Insulin detemir Insulin glargine	1–2 hours	Minimal	Up to 24 hours	Often combined with rapid- or short-acting insulin They lower blood glucose levels when rapid-acting insulin stops working
Ultra-long-acting insulin				
Insulin degludec	Not available	Minimal	Up to 42 hours	Often combined with rapid- or short-acting insulin They lower blood glucose levels when rapid-acting insulin stops working

(a) This insulin is modified with the addition of protamine, which prolongs the time required for absorption and increases the duration of action.

(2) The onset of action is typically within 1–2 hours, with a duration of action of more than 12 hours.

e. **Long-acting** insulin

(1) ***Specific agents*** include insulin **glargine**, insulin **detemir**, and insulin **degludec**.

(2) These agents were modified to **mimic basal insulin secretion** and have a **steady release with no peak effect**. The duration of action is up to 24 hours. They have more predictable effect and less or no weight gain. However, they cannot be mixed with any other insulins.

(a) Insulin degludec is considered an ultra-long-acting agent and has a longer duration of more than 40 hours. It can even be given three times a week with weekend-off dosing regimen. It offers improved glycemic control and reduced risk of hypoglycemia, especially nocturnal.

5. ***Indications***

a. Insulin is used to treat all manifestations of hyperglycemia, in **both type 1 (insulin-dependent)** and **type 2 (non-insulin-dependent) diabetes mellitus** administered subcutaneously.

(1) Most patients with type 2 diabetes are treated with dietary changes and oral hypoglycemic agents, although insulin can be used as first-line therapy in more severe cases.

6. ***Dosing considerations***

a. Patients with type 2 diabetes may require higher doses of insulin, due to insulin resistance.

b. ***Honeymoon phase*** (remission phase of diabetes)

(1) This may occur in patients recently diagnosed with type 1 diabetes.

(2) It occurs when β cells in the pancreas can still secrete enough endogenous insulin to aid in blood glucose control, resulting in a reduced exogenous insulin requirement.

c. ***Acute illness***

(1) Oftentimes with acute illness, there is an increase in cortisol, which causes an elevation in blood glucose.

(2) Patients with an acute illness may require higher insulin doses.

7. ***Adverse effects***

a. **Hypoglycemia** may occur. Symptoms include **tachycardia**, tremor, **sweating**, **confusion**, agitation, and, in more severe cases, loss of consciousness or coma.

b. Other adverse effects may include allergic reactions, **hypokalemia**, lipodystrophy, or hypertrophy of the subcutaneous fat at the injection site, and **weight gain**.

B. Sulfonylureas

1. ***Specific agents***

a. First-generation agents include tolbutamide, **chlorpropamide**, and tolazamide.

b. Second-generation agents include **glyburide (glibenclamide)**, **glipizide**, **gliclazide**, and **glimepiride**.

c. All are equally effective in lowering blood glucose.

d. Second-generation agents are prescribed more often; they are more potent and have fewer adverse effects and drug interactions.

2. ***Mechanism of action*** (Figs. 10.5 and 10.6)

a. These agents are oral **insulin secretagogues**; they cause insulin release from pancreatic β cells.

b. They bind to the sulfonylurea receptor (SUR_1) and **block ATP-sensitive potassium (K^+) channels**, resulting in depolarization. The voltage-gated calcium (Ca^{2+}) channels open, resulting in Ca^{2+} influx and triggering **insulin release**.

c. Long-term use also reduces serum glucagon, which may contribute to hypoglycemic effects.

3. ***Indications***. These agents are approved for the management of adults with **type 2 diabetes mellitus** (non-insulin-dependent diabetes mellitus).

a. Since they **require functional pancreatic β cells** to produce their effect on blood glucose, they cannot be used in patients with type 1 diabetes.

4. ***Adverse effects*** include **hypoglycemia** and **weight gain**. With some agents, such as chlorpropamide, alcohol consumption produces a disulfiram-like reaction.

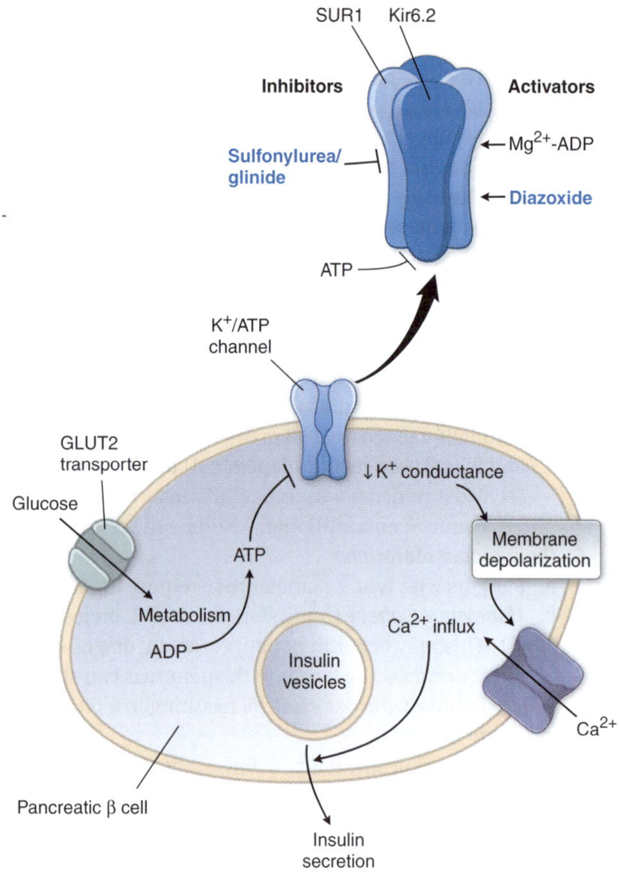

FIGURE 10.6. Physiologic and pharmacologic regulation of insulin release from pancreatic β cells. (Reprinted with permission from Golan D. Principles of Pharmacology. 4th ed. Philadelphia, PA: Wolters Kluwer Health, 2016, Fig. 31.3.)

5. ***Precautions***. Caution must be used in patients with hepatic or renal dysfunction. Caution must also be used in patients with a **sulfa allergy**.

C. Meglitinides

1. ***Specific agents*** include **repaglinide** and **nateglinide**.
2. ***Mechanism of action*** (see Fig. 10.5)
   a. These agents are oral **insulin secretagogues**.
   b. They have a similar mechanism to sulfonylureas, but they bind to distinct regions on the SUR_1 molecule.
   c. On binding, they **block ATP-sensitive potassium (K^+) channels**, resulting in depolarization. The voltage-gated calcium (Ca^{2+}) channels open, resulting in Ca^{2+} influx and triggering **insulin release**.
3. ***Indications***
   a. These agents are approved for the management of **type 2 diabetes mellitus**.
   b. Since they have a **fast onset** of action and **short duration** of action, they are recommended in patients with **irregular meal schedules**, and in patients who develop late postprandial hypoglycemia when taking a sulfonylurea.
   c. They are used instead of sulfonylureas in patients with a history of sulfa allergy.
4. ***Adverse effects*** include **hypoglycemia** (less risk compared with sulfonylureas). Repaglinide can cause weight gain.

D. Biguanides

1. ***Specific agent.*** **Metformin.**
2. ***Mechanism of action*** (see Fig. 10.5)
   a. Metformin **reduces hepatic glucose production and intestinal absorption of glucose**; it does not alter insulin secretion. These effects are believed to be due to an **increase in the activity**

of **AMP kinase**, a key intracellular regulator of energy homeostasis. Metformin also **increases peripheral insulin sensitivity**.

b. Its glucose-lowering action does not depend on functional pancreatic β cells.

3. ***Indications***. It is approved for the management of **type 2 diabetes mellitus**. It is used off-label to improve insulin resistance, reduce hyperinsulinemia, and reduce weight in women with polycystic ovary syndrome. It is used off-label in the management of obesity too.
4. ***Advantages***. It rarely causes hypoglycemia and weight gain.
5. ***Adverse effects*** include **GI distress**. It has the potential to cause **lactic acidosis**.
   a. Lactic acidosis is characterized by nonspecific symptoms, including GI distress (nausea, vomiting, abdominal pain), lethargy, hyperventilation, and hypotension.
6. ***Contraindications***
   a. Due to an increased risk of lactic acidosis, metformin should not be used in patients with congestive heart failure or renal impairment, or those who are seriously ill.
   b. In some cases, metformin should be temporarily discontinued before iodinated contrast, due to the potential for acute kidney injury and increased risk for lactic acidosis.

E. Thiazolidinediones

1. ***Specific agents*** include **pioglitazone** and **rosiglitazone**.
2. ***Mechanism of action*** (see Fig. 10.5)
   a. These agents are **insulin sensitizers**; they act to **decrease insulin resistance**.
   b. They bind to a specific intracellular receptor, **PPAR-γ** (peroxisome proliferator–activated receptor-gamma), a member of the nuclear-receptor family that regulates the transcription of various genes involved in lipid and glucose metabolism.
   c. They predominantly affect **liver, skeletal muscle**, and **adipose tissue**.
      (1) In the liver, thiazolidinediones **decrease glucose output** and insulin levels.
      (2) In muscle, thiazolidinediones **increase glucose uptake**.
      (3) In adipose tissue, these **drugs increase glucose uptake, decrease fatty acid release**, and may increase the release of hormones such as adiponectin and resistin.
   d. The actions of these drugs require the presence of insulin.
   e. Thiazolidinediones reduce plasma glucose and triglycerides.
3. ***Indications***. They are approved for the management of **type 2 diabetes mellitus**.
4. ***Adverse effects*** may include **edema** and **weight gain**.
5. ***Precautions***. They cause an increased risk for **fractures** and bladder cancer. They can cause or exacerbate **congestive heart failure**.
6. ***Contraindications*** include heart failure, liver disease, and bladder cancer.

F. α-Glucosidase inhibitors

1. ***Specific agents*** include **acarbose, voglibose**, and **miglitol**.
2. ***Mechanism of action*** (see Fig. 10.5)
   a. These agents act as competitive, **reversible inhibitors of pancreatic α-amylase and intestinal α-glucosidase enzymes**; they act in the lumen of the intestine.
   b. Inhibition of α-glucosidase **prolongs the digestion of carbohydrates** and reduces peak plasma glucose levels.
3. ***Indications***. They are approved for the management of **type 2 diabetes mellitus**. They are helpful in reducing postprandial glucose.
4. ***Adverse effects*** may include **GI distress** and flatulence.
5. ***Contraindications*** include intestinal diseases associated with disorders of digestion or absorption, such as intestinal obstruction and inflammatory bowel disease.

G. Glucagon-like peptide-1 (GLP-1) agonists

1. ***Specific agents*** include **exenatide, liraglutide**, lixisenatide, albiglutide, dulaglutide, and semaglutide.
2. ***Mechanism of action*** (see Fig. 10.5)
   a. These agents are **analogues of the hormone incretin (GLP-1)**.
   b. They **increase glucose-dependent insulin secretion**, **decrease inappropriate glucagon secretion**, **slow gastric emptying**, induce satiety through central actions, decrease food intake, and promote β-cell proliferation.

3. ***Indications***. They are approved for the management of **type 2 diabetes**. These agents also cause weight loss; therefore, liraglutide is also approved for weight management.
4. ***Adverse effects*** may include **GI distress**. Cholelithiasis has been reported.
5. ***Precautions***. They cause an increased risk for **acute pancreatitis** and **thyroid tumors**.

H. Dipeptidyl peptidase 4 (DPP-4) inhibitors

1. ***Specific agents*** include **sitagliptin, saxagliptin, alogliptin, linagliptin**, and **vildagliptin.**
2. ***Mechanism of action*** (see Fig. 10.5)
   a. **DPP-4 is responsible for the proteolysis of incretins, including GLP-1** and glucose-dependent insulinotropic peptide.
   b. These agents **inhibit DPP-4 to increase active incretins**. This leads to an increase in insulin synthesis and release and suppresses glucagon production in a glucose-dependent manner.
   c. They may also improve β-cell function.
3. ***Indication***. They are approved for the management of **type 2 diabetes.**
4. ***Adverse effects*** may include susceptibility to **nasopharyngitis** and upper respiratory infections. They may also cause **pancreatitis**.

I. Amylin analogues

1. ***Specific agent.*** **Pramlintide**.
2. ***Mechanism of action*** (see Fig. 10.5)
   a. Amylin is a polypeptide stored and secreted by β-cells of the pancreas; it is cosecreted with insulin to reduce blood sugar. Concentrations are abnormally low in patients with diabetes.
   b. Pramlintide can reduce postprandial glucose through prolongation of gastric emptying, reduction of postprandial glucagon secretion, and reduction of caloric intake through centrally mediated appetite suppression.
   c. It causes weight loss and reduces postprandial glucose levels.
3. ***Indications***. It is used in **combination with insulin** for **type 2 diabetes**. It is administered subcutaneously before meals.
   a. Long-acting newer amylin analogue cagrilintide has demonstrated potential as antiobesity medication.
4. ***Adverse effects*** may include nausea, hypoglycemia, injection site reactions, and gastroparesis.

J. Sodium–glucose cotransporter 2 (SGLT2) inhibitors

1. ***Specific agents*** include **canagliflozin**, **empagliflozin**, **dapagliflozin**, and **ertugliflozin**.
2. ***Mechanism of action***
   a. SGLT2 is the main site of filtered glucose reabsorption.
   b. These agents **inhibit SGLT2 in the proximal renal tubules**; this results in reduced reabsorption of filtered glucose from the tubular lumen and lowers the renal threshold for glucose (RTG).
   c. Reduction of filtered glucose reabsorption and lowering of RTG results in **increased urinary excretion of glucose**, thereby **reducing plasma glucose concentrations**.
3. ***Indications***. They are approved for the management of **type 2 diabetes** in patients with established cardiovascular disease.
   a. Dapagliflozin and canagliflozin have been approved for heart failure with reduced ejection fraction even in patients without type 2 diabetes. They have also demonstrated nephroprotective effects and used in patients with chronic kidney disease.
4. ***Advantages*** include **weight loss** and a **modest decrease in blood pressure**.
5. ***Adverse effects*** may include **genitourinary infections** and **increased serum potassium**.
6. ***Contraindications*** include severe renal impairment.

K. Agents that increase blood glucose (hyperglycemics)

1. **Glucagon**
   a. ***Structure and secretion***
      (1) Glucagon is **produced by the α cells of the pancreas.**
      (2) It is structurally similar to secretin, VIP, and gastric inhibitory peptide.

(3) Secretion is inhibited by elevated plasma glucose, insulin, and SST. It is stimulated by amino acids and sympathetic stimulation and secretion.

b. *Mechanism of action*

(1) Glucagon stimulates adenylate cyclase to produce increased cAMP.

(2) **It increases blood glucose by stimulating glycogenolysis and gluconeogenesis in the liver.** In general, its actions oppose the actions of insulin.

(3) Large doses produce marked relaxation of the smooth muscle in the stomach, intestines, and colon.

c. *Indications*

(1) Glucagon is used for the treatment of **severe hypoglycemia**. It rapidly increases blood glucose in insulin-induced hypoglycemia if hepatic glycogen stores are adequate.

(2) It can be used as a diagnostic aid, in which it provides intestinal relaxation prior to radiologic examination.

d. ***Adverse effects*** include a low incidence of nausea and vomiting.

2. Diazoxide

a. ***Mechanism of action.*** This agent **opens ATP-dependent potassium channels** on pancreatic β cells, resulting in **inhibition of insulin release.**

b. ***Indications*** include **hyperinsulinemic hypoglycemia.**

c. ***Adverse effects*** may include sodium retention, GI distress, and changes in circulating white blood cells.

X. THE CALCIUM HOMEOSTATIC SYSTEM

A. Drugs affecting calcium (Ca^{2+}) homeostasis

1. Parathyroid hormone (PTH)

a. *Secretion*

(1) PTH is secreted by the parathyroid glands in response to low serum Ca^{2+}.

(2) Agents such as β-adrenoceptor agonists, which increase cAMP in the parathyroid gland, cause an increase in PTH secretion.

b. *Physiologic effects of PTH*

(1) Bone

(a) PTH can increase the rate of both bone formation and bone resorption; this is mediated by cytokines produced by osteoblasts that regulate the number and activity of osteoclasts.

(b) Continuous exposure to PTH results in net bone resorption.

(c) Pulsatile exposure results in net bone formation.

(2) Kidney

(a) PTH increases the reabsorption of Ca^{2+} and magnesium (Mg^{2+}).

(b) It increases the production of 1,25-$(OH)_2D_3$ from 25-$(OH)D_3$ (1-hydroxylase step).

(c) It decreases reabsorption of phosphate, bicarbonate, amino acids, sulfate, sodium, and chloride.

(3) GI tract

(a) It increases intestinal absorption of Ca^{2+} indirectly by increasing 1,25-$(OH)_2D_3$.

c. ***Specific agent.*** **Teriparatide** (recombinant human PTH).

d. ***Mechanism of action.*** Similar to the physiologic effects of PTH, teriparatide stimulates osteoblast function, increases GI absorption of calcium, and increases renal tubular reabsorption of calcium. Intermittent exposure results in net bone formation.

e. ***Indications*** include the treatment of **osteoporosis.**

f. ***Adverse effects*** may include **hypercalcemia.**

g. ***Precautions.*** It is approved only for 2 years of use since it has been shown to increase the risk for osteosarcoma.

h. Abaloparatide is also a PTH analogue used for the treatment of osteoporosis.

2. Calcitonin

a. *Secretion*

(1) Calcitonin is secreted by perifollicular cells of the thyroid gland in response to elevated plasma Ca^{2+}.

(2) Gastrin, glucagon, cholecystokinin, and epinephrine can also increase calcitonin secretion.

b. *Physiologic actions*. Calcitonin **antagonizes the actions of PTH.**

(1) It interacts with specific receptors on osteoclasts to **decrease net reabsorption of Ca^{2+}**. Calcitonin may also stimulate bone formation.

(2) Calcitonin **increases renal excretion of Ca^{2+}**, Na^{+}, and phosphate.

c. *Specific agents* include synthetic calcitonin (salmon calcitonin).

d. *Indications*

(1) It can be used to reduce **hypercalcemia** due to **Paget disease**, hyperparathyroidism, idiopathic juvenile hypercalcemia, vitamin D intoxication, osteolytic bone disorders, and osteoporosis.

(a) Calcitonin can lower serum calcium by 1–2 mg/dL within 1–2 hours; therefore, it is a good choice for symptomatic hypercalcemia.

(b) **Tachyphylaxis**, a sudden decrease in the response to calcitonin after its administration, may develop within 48 hours; therefore, it is used for short-term therapy.

(2) It may also be used for **postmenopausal osteoporosis**.

e. *Administration*. It can be given via the intranasal route or by subcutaneous or intramuscular injection. Nasal application is not efficacious for the treatment of hypercalcemia.

f. *Adverse effects* may include flushing, rhinitis (with nasal application), hypocalcemia, and hypersensitivity reactions (due to salmon component).

3. Vitamin D and vitamin D metabolites (Table 10.3)

a. The calciferols include **vitamin D_3 (cholecalciferol)** and **vitamin D_2 (ergocalciferol)**.

(1) **Vitamin D_3 is produced in the skin** from cholesterol; this synthesis requires exposure to **ultraviolet light**.

(2) 25-(OH)D_3 (calcifediol)

(a) **Calcifediol is produced in the liver by hydroxylation of vitamin D_3.**

(b) It is the most abundant calciferol metabolite in the plasma.

(3) 1,25-$(OH)_2D_3$ (calcitriol)

(a) **Calcitriol is produced in the kidney by further hydroxylation of 25-(OH)D_3 by 1α-hydroxylase.** Regulation of 1α-hydroxylase activity determines the serum levels of **calcitriol.** Enzymatic activity is increased by PTH, estrogens, prolactin, and other agents, and it is decreased by 1,25-$(OH)_2D_3$, Fibroblast Growth Factor 23 (FGF23), and phosphate (direct effect).

(b) **Calcitriol is the most active metabolite of vitamin D.**

(4) Vitamin D_2 (ergocalciferol)

(a) Vitamin D_2 is derived from plant metabolism of ergosterol. It has a slightly different side chain, which does not alter its biologic effects in humans.

(b) In humans, vitamin D_2 is metabolized in the same manner as vitamin D_3 and appears to be bioequivalent.

TABLE 10.3 Pharmacologic Properties of Vitamin D Preparations

Agent	Metabolic Route	Onset of Action	Half-Life
Ergocalciferol (D_2)	Hepatic, renal	10–14 days	30 days
Cholecalciferol (D_3)	Hepatic, renal	10–14 days	30 days
Calcifediol	Renal	8–10 days	20 days
Calcitriol	None	10 hours	15 hours
Calcipotriene	Hepatic, renal	10 days	30 days
Doxercalciferol	Hepatic	5–8 hours	36 hours
Paricalcitol	None	Minutes (IV)	15 hours

(5) **Paricalcitol** (1,25-$(OH)_2$-19 norvitamin D_2) is a 1,25-hydroxylated vitamin D_2 derivative that reduces serum PTH levels without affecting serum Ca^{2+} or PO_4^{2-} levels. It is approved for the treatment of **hyperparathyroidism in patients with renal failure** who are on dialysis.

(6) Doxercalciferol (1α-(OH) vitamin D_2) is used for hyperparathyroidism secondary to renal failure. It does not increase intestinal Ca^{2+} absorption and does not cause hypercalcemia.

(7) Calcipotriene

(a) Calcipotriene is a 1,24-$(OH)_2D_3$ derivative for topical administration for the treatment of skin disorders such as psoriasis.

(b) It has reduced effects on calcium homeostasis.

b. ***Mechanism of action***

(1) Calcitriol **increases plasma levels of both Ca^{2+} and phosphate** by acting on several organ systems:

(a) **Intestine. Increases Ca^{2+} absorption** from the GI tract

(b) **Bone. Mobilizes Ca^{2+} and phosphate**, probably by stimulation of calcium flux out of osteoblasts

(c) **Kidney. Increases reabsorption of both Ca^{2+} and phosphate**

(2) All vitamin D metabolites bind to vitamin D–binding protein.

c. ***Indications***

(1) They are used to **elevate serum Ca^{2+}**.

(a) Vitamin D and vitamin D metabolites are used to treat hypocalcemia caused by a number of diseases, including vitamin D deficiency (nutritional rickets), hypoparathyroidism, renal disease, malabsorption, and osteoporosis.

(2) Reduce cellular proliferation.

(a) **Topical calcipotriene** has been approved for the treatment of **psoriasis**; it reduces fibroblast proliferation and induces differentiation of epidermal keratinocytes.

4. Bisphosphonates

a. ***Specific agents***

(1) Non-nitrogen-containing bisphosphonate: Etidronate.

(2) Nitrogen-containing bisphosphonates include **alendronate, ibandronate, risedronate, zoledronic acid**, and **pamidronate**.

b. ***Mechanism of action***

(1) Bisphosphonates are analogues of pyrophosphate that **bind directly to hydroxyapatite crystals in bone and impair reabsorption**.

(2) The non-nitrogenous bisphosphonates are internalized by osteoclasts and converted into an ATP analogue that cannot be hydrolyzed. This metabolite impairs various functions and induces apoptosis in osteoclasts.

(3) The nitrogen-containing bisphosphonates have a different mechanism. They work through the **inhibition of farnesyl diphosphate synthase**, part of the cholesterol biosynthetic pathway. This **impairs post-translational modification of a number of regulator proteins critical for osteoclast function**, including Ras, Rho, and Rac. They may also induce a unique ATP analogue that causes osteoclast apoptosis.

c. ***Indications*** include **osteoporosis**, Paget disease, and hypercalcemia.

d. ***Administration***

(1) After oral administration, all bisphosphonates have **very poor (<10%) oral absorption** that is decreased by food.

(a) They should be taken on an empty stomach with a full glass of water.

(b) Patients must also sit upright for 30 minutes after oral administration, to prevent esophageal and gastric irritation.

(2) Intravenous administration allows for a larger amount of drug to enter the body and markedly reduces the frequency of administration.

e. ***Adverse effects*** may include **esophageal or gastric irritation**.

f. ***Precautions***. They can cause **osteonecrosis of the jaw** and atypical femur fractures.

5. **Denosumab**
   a. ***Mechanism of action***
      (1) Osteoblasts secrete receptor activator of nuclear factor kappa-B ligand (RANKL), which activates osteoclast precursors and subsequent osteolysis.
      (2) Denosumab is a **monoclonal antibody** that binds to RANKL and **blocks the interaction between RANKL and RANK** (a receptor located on osteoclast surfaces); this **prevents osteoclast formation**.
      (3) The end effect is **decreased bone resorption** and **increased bone mass**.
   b. ***Indications***
      (1) It is approved for the treatment of **osteoporosis** and for **reducing the risk of bone loss** and bone metastasis in patients with **cancer**.
   c. ***Adverse effects*** may include hypocalcemia.
   d. ***Precautions:*** Similar to bisphosphonates, denosumab may cause osteonecrosis of the jaw.
6. **Calcimimetic**
   a. ***Specific agent.*** **Cinacalcet.**
   b. ***Mechanism of action***
      (1) The parathyroid gland senses Ca^{2+} via the action of the calcium-sensing receptor (**CaSR**); activation of CaSR **reduces the amount of PTH synthesized and released by the gland**.
      (2) Cinacalcet increases the sensitivity of the CaSR and lowers PTH and serum calcium and phosphorus levels.
   c. ***Indications*** include **hyperparathyroidism** and parathyroid carcinoma.
   d. ***Adverse effects*** may include GI distress, paresthesias, and arthralgias.
   e. ***Contraindications*** include hypocalcemia.
7. **Calcium supplements**
   a. Calcium supplements are available in a variety of Ca^{2+} concentrations and in parenteral and oral formulations.
   b. ***Indications***. They are useful as dietary supplements for the treatment or prevention of osteoporosis and for the immediate treatment of acute hypocalcemia and hypocalcemic tetany.
   c. ***Adverse effects***. Long-term use may cause hypercalcemia.

XI. RETINOIC ACID AND DERIVATIVES

A. Topical tretinoin (all-*trans* retinoic acid)

1. Tretinoin is a naturally occurring metabolite of **vitamin A**.
2. ***Mechanism of action***
   a. It may modify epithelial growth and differentiation.
   b. It can decrease the cohesiveness of follicular epithelial cells.
   c. It may stimulate mitotic activity and increase turnover of follicular epithelial cells.
3. ***Indications***. As a topical preparation, it is used for the treatment of **acne** and **photoaged skin** including palliation of fine wrinkles, spotty hyperpigmentation, and facial skin roughness.
4. ***Adverse effects*** of tretinoin include tenderness, erythema, and burning. It can cause an increased risk of **sunburn**.
5. ***Precautions***. It should not be used in pregnant women or those attempting to conceive, due to the risk for birth defects.
6. *More information about its use in acute promyelocytic leukemia can be seen in Chapter 12 on Cancer Chemotherapy.*

B. Isotretinoin

1. ***Mechanism of action***. Isotretinoin reversibly reduces the size of sebaceous glands and hence the production of sebum.
2. ***Indications***. It is an oral agent used for the treatment of **severe cystic acne** and the symptomatic management of keratinization disorders.

3. ***Adverse effects*** of isotretinoin include inflammation of mucous membranes (most often the lips), rash, and alopecia. Less common adverse effects include arthralgia and myalgia. Retinoids tend to inhibit lipoprotein lipase, which leads to an increase in serum triglycerides.
4. ***Precautions***. Isotretinoin is **teratogenic** and should not be used in women who are pregnant or trying to conceive.

C. Acitretin

1. ***Mechanism of action***. This agent binds to and activates retinoid X receptors and retinoic acid receptors to inhibit the expression of the proinflammatory cytokines, including interleukin-6 and interferon-gamma. This leads to anti-inflammatory and antiproliferative activity (keratinocyte differentiation is normalized).
2. ***Indications*** include the treatment of severe **psoriasis**.
3. ***Adverse effects*** include **skin and nail abnormalities**.
4. ***Precautions***. It is **teratogenic** and cannot be used in women who are pregnant or trying to conceive.

D. Other retinoic acid derivatives. Other retinoic acid derivatives include alitretinoin (used in skin disorders associated with Kaposi syndrome), tazarotene (used for psoriasis, photoaging, and acne), and adapalene (used for acne).

DRUG SUMMARY TABLE

Hypothalamic/Pituitary Agents
Bromocriptine
Cabergoline
Cetrorelix
Conivaptan
Corticorelin
Corticotrophin injection gel
Cosyntropin
Desmopressin acetate
Ganirelix
Goserelin
Histrelin
Leuprolide
Nafarelin
Octreotide
Oxytocin
Pegvisomant
Thyrotropin α
Tolvaptan
Triptorelin
Vasopressin

Gonadotropins
Follitropin alfa
Follitropin β
Human chorionic gonadotropin (recombinant hCG)
Menotropins
Urofollitropin

Estrogens and Progestins
Equine estrogens (conjugated)
Estradiol
Ethinylestradiol
Ethinylestradiol and desogestrel
Ethinylestradiol and drospirenone
Ethinylestradiol and levonorgestrel
Ethinylestradiol and norelgestromin
Ethinylestradiol and norethindrone
Ethinylestradiol and norgestimate
Hydroxyprogesterone caproate
Levonorgestrel
Medroxyprogesterone acetate
Megestrol
Mestranol and norethindrone
Norethindrone

Progestin Receptor Modulator
Ulipristal acetate

Antiestrogens
Clomiphene
Fulvestrant
Danazol

SERMs
Raloxifene
Tamoxifen
Toremifene

Aromatase Inhibitors
Anastrozole
Exemestane
Letrozole

Antiprogestin
Mifepristone

Androgens
Fluoxymesterone
Methyltestosterone
Oxandrolone
Oxymetholone
Testosterone
Testosterone cypionate
Testosterone enanthate
Testosterone propionate

Antiandrogens
Bicalutamide
Dutasteride
Finasteride
Flutamide
Ketoconazole
Nilutamide
Spironolactone

Corticosteroids
Amcinonide
Beclomethasone
Betamethasone
Clobetasol
Cortisone acetate
Desonide
Dexamethasone
Fludrocortisone
Fluocinonide
Fluticasone
Halobetasol
Hydrocortisone
Prednisolone
Prednisone
Triamcinolone

Ultra-Short-Acting Insulin
Insulin aspart
Insulin glulisine
Insulin lispro

Short-Acting Insulin
Insulin regular

Intermediate-Acting Insulin
Insulin NPH

(Continued)

Long-Acting Insulin
Insulin detemir
Insulin glargine

Ultra-Long-Acting Insulin
Insulin degludec

Sulfonylureas
Chlorpropamide
Glimepiride
Glipizide
Glyburide
Tolazamide
Tolbutamide

Meglitinides
Nateglinide
Repaglinide

Biguanide
Metformin

α-Glucosidase Inhibitors
Acarbose
Miglitol

Thiazolidinediones
Pioglitazone
Rosiglitazone

Glucagon and Glucagon-Like Peptide-1 (GLP-1) Receptor Agonists
Albiglutide
Dulaglutide
Exenatide
Liraglutide
Lixisenatide
Glucagon

DPP-IV Inhibitors
Linagliptin
Saxagliptin
Sitagliptin

Sodium–Glucose Cotransporter 2 (SGLT2) Inhibitors
Canagliflozin
Dapagliflozin
Empagliflozin

Agents that Increase Blood Glucose
Diazoxide
Glucagon

Agents Affecting Ca^{2+} Homeostasis
Abaloparatide
Calcifediol
Calcitonin
Calcitriol
Calcipotriene
Denosumab
Doxercalciferol
Ergocalciferol (vitamin D_2)
Paricalcitol
Teriparatide

Bisphosphonates
Alendronate
Etidronate
Ibandronate
Pamidronate
Risedronate
Zoledronic acid

Calcimimetic
Cinacalcet

Retinoic Acid Derivatives
Acitretin
Adapalene
Alitretinoin
Bexarotene
Isotretinoin
Tazarotene
Tretinoin

Review Test

Directions: Select the best answer for each question.

1. A 49-year-old woman presents to her primary care physician with complaints of sweating profusely nearly every night. She has a history of a transvaginal hysterectomy 5 years ago but has intact ovaries. She has a BMI of 22. On physical examination, all her vital signs are within normal limits. Which of the following would best manage her symptoms?

(A) Calcitriol
(B) Conjugated estrogens
(C) Levonorgestrel
(D) Raloxifene

2. A 42-year-old woman is admitted to the intensive care unit with symptoms of mental status changes and hypothermia. On physical examination, her blood pressure is 80/55 mm Hg and her heart rate is 50 beats/min. She is diagnosed with myxedema coma and started on intravenous fluids. Which of the following medications would also be appropriate to start at this time?

(A) Liothyronine
(B) Methimazole
(C) Radioactive iodine
(D) Teriparatide

3. A 71-year-old man presents to his doctor with complaints of back pain, difficulty urinating, and blood in his urine. After further testing, he is diagnosed with prostate cancer and started on leuprolide therapy. Three days later, the man returns to the office with complaints of increased difficulty with urination and increased pain. Why are his symptoms worse?

(A) Direct effect of leuprolide on the prostate
(B) Reduced conversion of testosterone to dihydrotachysterol
(C) Prostatic resistance to leuprolide
(D) Transient agonist action of leuprolide

4. A 62-year-old woman presents to her physician for the treatment of osteoporosis. She is started on a new medication that is an estrogen receptor agonist in the bone and an antagonist in the breast. What are the potential adverse effects of this medication?

(A) Acneiform rash
(B) Arrhythmias
(C) Hot flashes
(D) Rhinitis

5. A 36-year-old woman complains of hot flashes, feelings of weakness, and increased appetite. Physical examination reveals that the patient is tachycardic and has a prominent pulse pressure. Laboratory tests are positive for anti-TSH antibodies. Which of the following would be the most appropriate treatment for this patient?

(A) Ketoconazole
(B) Liotrix
(C) Methimazole
(D) Thyrotropin α

6. A 45-year-old woman is diagnosed with type 2 diabetes by her endocrinologist. She is started on a new medication, in which the side effects may include hypoglycemia and weight gain. What medication was most likely prescribed?

(A) Canagliflozin
(B) Exenatide
(C) Glyburide
(D) Pramlintide

7. A 55-year-old woman complains to her dentist about swelling, pain, and redness in her gums and two loose teeth. She has a recent history of a tooth extraction. Her past medical history is positive for osteoporosis and hypertension. Which of the following medications may have caused this patient's symptoms?

(A) Cinacalcet
(B) Ibandronate
(C) Raloxifene
(D) Propylthiouracil

8. A 55-year-old man with a 10-year history of alcoholism presents to his family physician for his annual history and physical examination. On physical examination, his doctor notes icterus and yellow sclerae. The patient's serum bilirubin levels are elevated, and liver function tests are abnormal. In addition, his serum calcium is abnormally low. The doctor prescribes a vitamin D derivative to correct his calcium level. Which of the following would be most appropriate for this patient?

(A) Calcitriol
(B) Cholecalciferol
(C) Dihydrotachysterol
(D) Ergosterol

9. A 59-year-old woman presents to the emergency department with symptoms of confusion and difficulty breathing. On physical examination, the doctor notes that she is tachycardic, is tachypneic, and appears very disoriented. She does not remember the day of the week. The patient has a history of type 2 diabetes and vaguely remembers taking her "sugar medicine" earlier in the day. Which of the following drugs is most likely responsible for her condition?

(A) Acarbose
(B) Glipizide
(C) Glucagon
(D) Metformin

10. A 60-year-old man with a history of type 2 diabetes presents to his endocrinologist for a follow-up appointment 3 months after starting glipizide and metformin for the management of type 2 diabetes. Laboratory tests reveal a fasting blood glucose of 182 mg/dL and a HbA1c level of 7.9%. Since his A1c target was not achieved after several months of dual therapy, the doctor prescribes a medication that increases insulin sensitivity in adipose tissue and muscle. Which of the following medications was prescribed?

(A) Dapagliflozin
(B) Miglitol
(C) Nateglinide
(D) Rosiglitazone

11. A 50-year-old woman underwent thyroidectomy for papillary thyroid carcinoma. The tumor was confined to the thyroid gland with no evidence of any metastasis. The treating oncologist considers treatment with radioactive iodine after 6 weeks of surgery. Which of the following statement about radioactive iodine is false?

(A) It is taken up by thyroid and thyroid cancer cells.
(B) It is given to ablate any remaining thyroid tissue and potential microscopic disease.
(C) It has to be given by intravenous infusion with proper monitoring.
(D) It can cause dry mouth and altered taste as side effects.

12. A 35-year-old male who is a known case of type 1 diabetes mellitus presents to the emergency department with nausea, vomiting, and altered mental status. He is dehydrated too. His random blood sugar is 750 mg/dL. Urine examination confirms the presence of ketone bodies. The most appropriate initial treatment in this patient would be:

(A) Oral glibenclamide
(B) Subcutaneous regular insulin
(C) Intravenous insulin lispro
(D) Intravenous insulin glargine

13. A 55-yrear-old man who is a known case of type 2 diabetes mellitus was prescribed metformin. Despite lifestyle modifications and adequate dose of metformin, his HbA1C remained elevated at 8.5% after 2 years. The diabetologist decided to start him on glibenclamide. After two weeks, he presented to the emergency department with sweating, tachycardia, and confusion. The most likely cause of his symptoms would be:

(A) Hyperosmolar hyperglycemic state
(B) Diabetic ketoacidosis
(C) Lactic acidosis
(D) Hypoglycemia

14. A 28-year-old lady with uncreative colitis requires a high-dose, long-term corticosteroid for the remission of an acute exacerbation of the disease. To minimize the HPA axis suppression, all of the following measures are useful in this patient EXCEPT:

(A) Prescribing a long-acting corticosteroid like dexamethasone
(B) Administration of two-thirds of the dose in the morning and one-third in the evening
(C) Administration of the corticosteroid on alternate days
(D) Prescribing the lowest dose for the least duration as possible

15. A 70-year-old woman with a history of osteoporosis presents with recent vertebral compression fracture despite being on a bisphosphonate for the past three years. Her physician considers to put her on teriparatide. The following statement regarding teriparatide is incorrect:

(A) It is administered as a daily subcutaneous injection.
(B) It may be used to treat hypoparathyroidism.
(C) It is contraindicated in patients with Paget's disease.
(D) It primarily stimulates osteoclastic activity and inhibits osteoblastic activity.

Answers and Explanations

1. **The answer is B.** Vasomotor symptoms are the most common complaint of perimenopausal women. Estrogen is the only effective treatment for these symptoms. Since there is no concern of endometrial cancer, a progestin is not indicated. Raloxifene makes hot flashes worse; and while a vitamin D analogue might help maintain Ca^{2+}, it would not have any effect on the vasomotor symptoms.

2. **The answer is A.** Myxedema coma is a severe form of hypothyroidism that can occur due to long-standing decrease in thyroid hormone levels. Liothyronine (synthetic T_3) is effective for short-term suppression of TSH and is useful in the treatment of myxedema coma. Methimazole and radioactive iodine are used for the management of hyperthyroidism. Teriparatide is a parathyroid hormone analogue used for severe osteoporosis.

3. **The answer is D.** Leuprolide and the other GnRH agonists may cause "tumor flare," due to a transient increase in gonadal steroid production before downregulation of receptors occurs. During the first 2 weeks of therapy, an initial increase in serum testosterone may cause worsening of symptoms, such as bone pain, hematuria, or bladder outlet obstruction.

4. **The answer is C.** The patient was started on raloxifene, which is an estrogen receptor agonist in the bone and an antagonist in the breast. Adverse effects of raloxifene include hot flashes, peripheral edema, and an increased risk of thrombosis. The other adverse effects listed are not common with this medication.

5. **The answer is C.** The patient's symptoms and anti-TSH antibodies indicate that she most likely has hyperthyroidism. Methimazole blocks the initial oxidation of iodine as well as the coupling of monoiodotyrosine and diiodotyrosine into T_4. Liotrix is a thyroid hormone preparation and would be contraindicated. Ketoconazole inhibits a number of P450-catalyzed reactions, but not the production of thyroid hormone.

6. **The answer is C.** Sulfonylureas such as glyburide increase the release of insulin from the pancreas. They have the potential to cause hypoglycemia and weight gain. Exenatide (GLP-1 agonist), pramlintide (amylin analogue), and canagliflozin (SLG2 inhibitor) can cause weight loss.

7. **The answer is B.** The patient most likely has osteonecrosis of the jaw, a rare but serious adverse effect of bisphosphonate therapy, such as ibandronate. The risk is higher after dental procedures, such as implants or extractions. The other medications do not cause osteonecrosis of the jaw.

8. **The answer is A.** Calcitriol would be the most effective agent for hypocalcemia in a patient with impaired liver function. The liver provides the required 25-hydroxylation of dihydrotachysterol, cholecalciferol, and ergosterol.

9. **The answer is B.** Sulfonylureas, such as glipizide, can cause hypoglycemia. Symptoms of hypoglycemia may include confusion, dizziness, sweating, increased heart rate, and weakness. Metformin and α-glycosidase inhibitors, such as acarbose, rarely cause hypoglycemia. Glucagon would raise plasma glucose.

10. **The answer is D.** Rosiglitazone is a thiazolidinedione, which works by increasing sensitivity to insulin in adipose, skeletal muscle, and liver. The α-glucosidase inhibitors, such as miglitol, inhibit intestinal hydrolysis of complex saccharides and thereby reduce glucose absorption. SLG2 inhibitors, such as dapagliflozin, decrease reabsorption of filtered glucose from the tubular lumen in the kidney, allowing for increased urinary excretion of glucose and reducing plasma glucose concentrations. Nateglinide, a meglitinide, stimulates insulin release by closing the potassium channels in pancreatic β cells.

11. **The answer is C.** Radioactive iodine is taken up primarily by thyroid and thyroid cancer cells, sparing other tissues. Common side effects include dry mouth, eye inflammation, altered taste and smell, especially with higher doses. The key difference is that radioactive iodine is admin-

istered orally as a capsule or liquid, not by injection. It is given to ablate any remaining thyroid tissue and potential microscopic disease.

12. **The answer is C.** The patient has diabetic ketoacidosis (DKA), a known life-threatening complication of type 1 diabetes mellitus. Intravenous rapid-acting insulins like insulin lispro, insulin aspart, or regular insulin are the most appropriate in the management of this condition. Oral medications like sulfonylureas and metformin are not effective in DKA. Subcutaneous insulins do not reduce the blood glucose fast enough. Insulin glargine cannot be given intravenously.
13. **The answer is D.** Glibenclamide is a sulfonylurea which is an insulin secretagogue. It is known to cause hypoglycemia. Sweating, tachycardia, and confusion are the symptoms of hypoglycemia. Hyperosmolar hyperglycemic state and diabetic ketoacidosis are both conditions caused by hyperglycemia. Lactic acidosis is caused by metformin and not sulfonylureas.
14. **The answer is A.** To minimize the HPA axis suppression, a short-acting corticosteroid like hydrocortisone or an intermediate-acting agent like prednisolone has to be prescribed. Long-acting agents like betamethasone and dexamethasone cause more suppression of HPA axis. Other measures to prevent HPA axis suppression are administration of two-thirds of the dose in the morning and one-third in the evening and administration of the corticosteroid on alternate days (giving drug holidays) and prescribing the lowest dose for the least duration as possible.
15. **The answer is D.** Teriparatide is administered as a subcutaneous injection into the thigh or abdomen, typically at a dosage of 20 μg once daily. Despite its lack of approval, teriparatide has been explored as a treatment option for patients with chronic hypoparathyroidism, especially in those who do not respond adequately to conventional therapies such as calcium and vitamin D supplementation. It is contraindicated in patients with Paget's disease. Paget's disease is characterized by abnormal bone remodeling, leading to enlarged and weakened bones. The use of teriparatide, which stimulates bone formation, could exacerbate these abnormalities and potentially lead to further complications, including the risk of osteosarcoma in already affected bone tissue. It primarily stimulates osteoblastic activity and stimulates bone formation.

Chapter 11

Drugs Used in Treatment of Infectious Diseases

Competencies Addressed: PH1.42–PH1.48

I. INFECTIOUS DISEASE THERAPY

Infectious disease therapy is based on the principle of selective toxicity, in which the intent is to destroy the infecting organism without damage to the host. This can be accomplished by exploiting basic biochemical and physical differences between the two organisms.

A. Choice of appropriate antibacterial agent

1. The preferred drug is usually the most active drug against the pathogen and/or the least toxic of several alternative drugs.
2. Antimicrobials are often used prophylactically to prevent infections; for example, antimicrobials are given prior to surgery to prevent surgical-site infections.
3. The mechanism of action may play an important role in choosing the most appropriate drug, in which antibiotics can (Fig. 11.1):
   a. Inhibit bacterial cell wall biosynthesis
   b. Inhibit DNA synthesis and integrity
   c. Inhibit protein synthesis (transcription and translation)

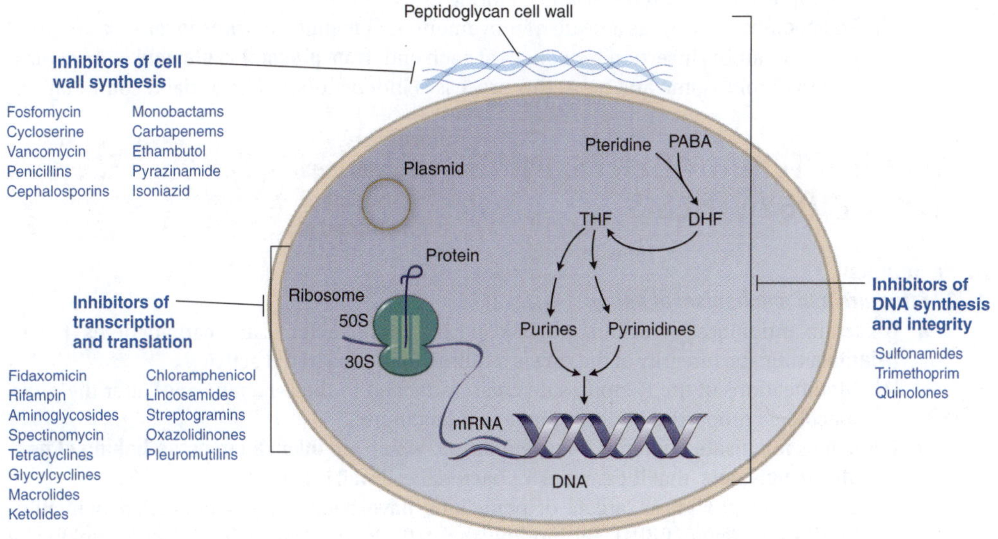

FIGURE 11.1. Antibacterial drug classes. (Reprinted with permission from Golan D. Principles of Pharmacology, 4th edition. Philadelphia, PA: Wolters Kluwer Health, 2016, Fig. 33.1.)

B. Bactericidal and bacteriostatic agents

1. **Bactericidal** agents cause the **death of the microorganism**. They eradicate the infection in the absence of host defense mechanisms. These agents include the following:
   a. Inhibitors of cell wall synthesis
      (1) Penicillins, cephalosporins, carbapenems, aztreonam, vancomycin
   b. Inhibitors of DNA synthesis and integrity
      (1) Fluoroquinolones, antifolate drugs, such as cotrimoxazole
   c. Aminoglycosides (lead to misreading of the genetic code)
2. **Bacteriostatic** agents **temporarily inhibit the growth** of the microorganism. They do not kill the organism; therefore, they require the host defense mechanisms to eradicate the infection. These agents include the following:
   a. Inhibitors of protein synthesis
      (1) Macrolides, tetracyclines, clindamycin, and linezolid
3. This distinction between bacteriostatic and bactericidal antimicrobials is restricted to the in vitro setting, with less relevance to a clinical setting, especially in immunocompetent patients with uncomplicated infections.

C. Antibiotic resistance

1. **Resistance** is the lack of sensitivity of pathogenic bacteria to antimicrobials. The minimum inhibitory concentration is greater than the plasma concentration of the drug.
2. **Intrinsic resistance (insensitivity)** is the **natural ability** of bacteria **to resist activity** from certain antibacterial drugs; this may occur due to different functional or structural features, such as the production of enzymes that metabolize the drug or inability of the drug to enter the bacteria.
3. **Acquired resistance** occurs when the bacteria **develop the ability to resist** activity from certain antimicrobial agents.
   a. **Spontaneous, random chromosomal mutations** in the bacteria may result in change in a protein receptor for an antibiotic or a protein involved in drug transport. Mutation in bacterial targets ensures that the antimicrobial no longer effectively binds to the target or the drug is inactivated or is expelled from the bacteria.
   b. Acquired resistance may be **propagated** by extrachromosomal transfer of drug-resistant genes:
      (1) **Transformation.** Transfer of naked DNA between cells of the same species.
      (2) **Transduction via R plasmids**. Asexual transfer of plasmid DNA in a bacterial virus between bacteria of the same species.
      (3) **Conjugation** is the **passage of genes from bacteria to bacteria** via direct contact through a sex pilus or bridge. It occurs primarily in gram-negative bacilli and is the principal mechanism of acquired resistance among Enterobacteriaceae.
      (4) **Transpositions** occur as a result of movement or **"jumping" of transposons** (stretches of DNA containing insertion sequences at each end) **from plasmid to plasmid** or from plasmid to chromosome and back; this process is independent of bacterial recombination.

II. ANTIBACTERIAL AGENTS: INHIBITORS OF BACTERIAL CELL WALL BIOSYNTHESIS

A. Penicillins

1. ***Structure and mechanism of action*** (Fig. 11.2)
   a. β-Lactam antibiotics (penicillins, cephalosporins, monobactams, and carbapenems) have a **β-lactam ring**; the integrity of the ring is required for antibacterial activity.
      (1) Modifications of the R-group side chain (attached to the β-lactam ring) alter the pharmacologic properties and resistance to β-lactamase.
   b. Penicillins **inactivate bacterial transpeptidases**, which are **involved in cross-linking of peptidoglycan polymers**, that is essential for bacterial cell wall integrity.
      (1) These transpeptidase targets of penicillins have been collectively called penicillin-binding proteins (PBPs). By binding these PBPs, penicillins inhibit cross-linking of peptidoglycans thus inhibiting cell wall synthesis
      (2) This results in loss of rigidity of the cell wall and a susceptibility to rupture.

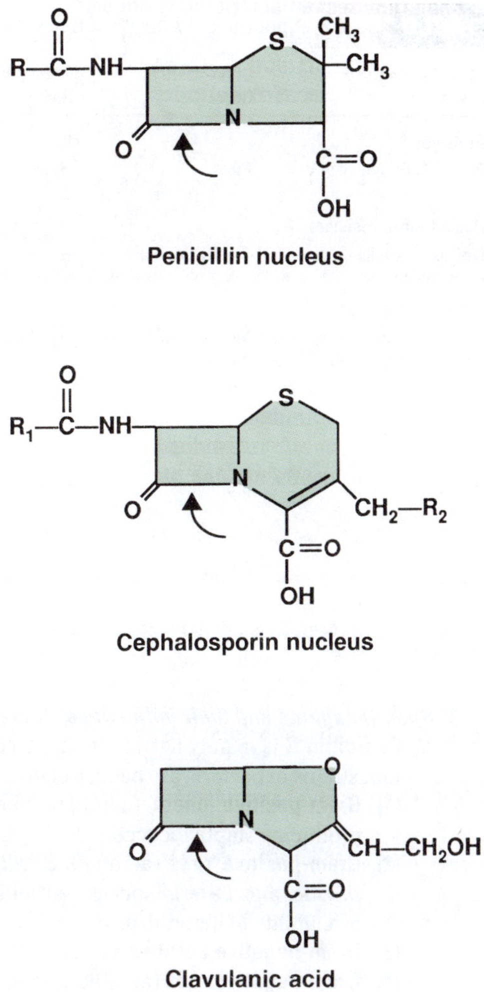

FIGURE 11.2. Structures of penicillin, cephalosporin, and clavulanic acid nuclei. *Arrows* indicate bond attacked by β-lactamases.

c. Penicillins are **bactericidal** for growing cells. **Gram-positive bacteria** with thick external cell walls are particularly susceptible.

d. There are three causes for development of **resistance**.

(1) The production of **β-lactamases (penicillinases)**: The genes for β-lactamases can be transmitted during conjugation or as small plasmids (minus conjugation genes) via transduction. Common organisms capable of producing penicillinase include *Staphylococcus aureus, Escherichia coli, Pseudomonas aeruginosa, Neisseria gonorrhoeae,* and *Bacillus, Proteus,* and *Bacteroides* species.

(2) Resistance may also occur because bacteria develop modified PBPs. A sensitive strain may acquire resistance via mutations that decrease the affinity of PBPs for the antibiotic or by acquiring the ability to express new, low-affinity PBPs.

(3) Some bacteria are impermeable to penicillins, have active efflux pumps, lack cell walls, or are metabolically inactive.

2. *Pharmacologic properties*

a. Penicillins are absorbed rapidly after oral administration (although erratically) and parenteral administration. Gastrointestinal (GI) absorption may be decreased in the presence of food.

b. They are distributed throughout body fluids. They penetrate the cerebrospinal fluid (CSF) and ocular fluid to a significant extent only during inflammation.

c. Probenecid slows the renal tubular secretion of penicillins.

TABLE 11.1 Spectrum of Activity of Penicillins

Classification and Drugs	Gram-positive Cocci	Gram-positive Rods	Gram-negative Cocci	Gram-negative Rods	Anaerobes
Prototype					
Penicillin G, penicillin V	**Most**	*Bacillus*	Gonococci and meningococci[a]	None	Most (except *B. fragilis*)
Penicillinase resistant					
Nafcillin, oxacillin, dicloxacillin	**Staphylococci[b]**	—	—	—	—
Extended spectrum					
Ampicillin, amoxicillin, ampicillin/sulbactam, amoxicillin/clavulanic acid	Most penicillinase-producing staphylococci[b]	*Bacillus*	Gonococci and meningococci[c]	*Salmonella, H. influenzae, Protons,* and *enterococci*	—
Antipseudomonal					
Ticarcillin/clavulanic acid, piperacillin	Less potent than prototypes	Less potent than prototypes	Less potent than prototypes	*Proteus, E. coli, Salmonella, Pseudomonas, Enterobacter,* and *Klebsiella*	—

[a]Nonpenicillinase producing.
[b]Not effective against methicillin-resistant staphylococcal infections.
[c]Penicillinase producing.

3. ***Specific agents and their indications*** (Table 11.1)
   a. **Penicillin G** is mainly used to treat infections with the following organisms (although resistant strains of bacteria are being isolated more frequently):
      (1) **Gram-positive cocci** (aerobic). Pneumococci, streptococci, and non-penicillinase-producing staphylococci.
      (2) **Gram-positive rods** (aerobic). *Bacillus* species, also *Clostridium perfringens, C. diphtheriae,* and *Listeria* species, although the use of these agents is declining due to the availability of better drugs.
      (3) **Gram-negative aerobes**. Gonococci (nonpenicillinase producing) and meningococci.
      (4) **Gram-negative rods** (aerobic). None.
      (5) **Anaerobes**. Most, except *Bacteroides fragilis*; it is used for oral anaerobes.
      (6) **Other**. *Treponema pallidum* (syphilis) and *Leptospira* species. These are common pathogens for which first-generation penicillins are used.
   b. **Penicillin V** is an oral form of penicillin G with poor bioavailability. It has a narrower spectrum of activity.
   c. **Penicillin G benzathine and penicillin G procaine** are suspensions of penicillin G that prolong its half-life allowing a reduced frequency of injections.
   d. **Penicillinase-resistant penicillins** (**oxacillin, dicloxacillin, methicillin**, and **nafcillin**) are used predominantly for penicillinase-producing **staphylococcal infections**.
      (1) Their use is declining due to the increased incidence of **methicillin-resistant *S. aureus* (MRSA)** that also confers resistance to cephalosporins.
   e. **Extended-spectrum penicillins**
      (1) These agents have more **gram-negative** coverage than penicillin G. Like many other penicillin agents, resistance has become a more common problem as they are inactivated by β-lactamases.
         (a) **Ampicillin** is useful for infections caused by *Haemophilus influenzae, Streptococcus pneumoniae, Streptococcus pyogenes, Neisseria meningitidis, Proteus mirabilis,* and *Enterococcus faecalis.*
         (b) **Amoxicillin** is similar to ampicillin but has **better oral absorption**, consequently necessitating a **thrice-daily administration and lower rate of diarrhea**. It is commonly used for endocarditis prophylaxis before major procedures.
         (c) **Piperacillin** has good activity against *Pseudomonas* and *Enterobacter.*

f. **β-Lactamase inhibitors** irreversibly **inhibit β-lactamase** and **increase stability of penicillin** agents, resulting in an extended spectrum of activity.
   (1) They are structurally related to penicillin but have **no antimicrobial properties on their own** (Fig. 11.2).
   (2) ***Specific agents*** include **clavulanic acid**, **sulbactam**, and **tazobactam**.
      (a) Clavulanic acid is used in combination with amoxicillin.
      (b) Sulbactam is used in combination with ampicillin; it is most commonly used for gram-negative bacteria as well as most anaerobes.
      (c) Tazobactam is used in combination with piperacillin and is effective against most gram-negative organisms, including ***Pseudomonas*** species.

4. ***Adverse effects***
   a. Penicillin agents may cause **hypersensitivity** reactions (type 1—IgE mediated); symptoms may include urticaria, severe pruritus, fever, or anaphylaxis.
      (1) Cross-sensitivity with cephalosporins and other β-lactam agents must be considered.
   b. **GI disturbances**, such as nausea and diarrhea, may occur.

B. Cephalosporins (Table 11.2)

1. ***Structure and mechanism of action***
   a. Cephalosporins also have a β-lactam ring (Fig. 11.2).
      (1) Substitutions at R_1 determine antibacterial activity.
      (2) Substitutions at R_2 determine pharmacokinetics.
   b. Cephalosporins have the same mechanisms of action as penicillins. They also bind to, and inactivate, **PBPs** involved in cell wall synthesis. They inactivate bacterial transpeptidases and **prevent the cross-linking of peptidoglycan polymers** that is essential for bacterial cell wall integrity.
      (1) This results in loss of rigidity and a **susceptibility to rupture**.
2. ***Pharmacologic properties***
   a. Cephalosporins are widely distributed in body fluids; selected agents (**cefuroxime**, **cefotaxime**, and **ceftizoxime**) penetrate CSF.
   b. Probenecid slows the renal tubular secretion of cephalosporins.
   c. Each newer generation of cephalosporins is increasingly **resistant to penicillinases.**

TABLE 11.2 Properties of Cephalosporins

Drugs and Route of Administration	Spectrum of Activity	Enters CNS	Resistance to β-Lactamase: *Plasmid*	Resistance to β-Lactamase: *Chromosomal*
First generation				
Cephalexin (O) Cefadroxil (O) Cefazolin (P)	Gram-positive and some gram-negative organisms Use: *Escherichia coli, Klebsiella, Proteus mirabilis,* penicillin- and sulfonamide-resistant **UTI, surgical prophylaxis**	No	Yes	No
Second generation				
Cefaclor (O) Cefotetan (P) Cefoxitin (P) Cefuroxime (P, O)	Spectrum extends to indole-positive ***Proteus***, and **anaerobes** Use: **UTI, respiratory tract infections, surgical prophylaxis**	No	Yes	Relatively
Third and fourth generations				
Ceftizoxime (P) Cefotaxime (P) Ceftriaxone (P) Cefdinir (P) Ceftazidime (P) Cefixime (O) Cefepime (P)	Reduced gram-positive activity; ***Pseudomonas*** (cefoperazone and ceftazidime only), *N. gonorrhoeae, N. meningitidis, H. influenzae, Enterobacter, Salmonella,* indole-positive *Proteus, Serratia, E. coli*; moderate **anaerobe** activity Use: Serious **nosocomial infections, gonorrhea, meningitis**	Yes, especially ceftriaxone (but not cefoperazone)	Yes	Relatively (most)

CNS, central nervous system; O, oral administration; P, parenteral administration; UTI, urinary tract infection.

d. Third-generation cephalosporins are sensitive to the **cephalosporinases** (genes are generally located on chromosomes as opposed to plasmids).

3. ***Specific agents and their indications***. Cephalosporins are categorized by their antibacterial spectrum. All are inactive against enterococci and methicillin-resistant staphylococci.
   a. **First-generation cephalosporins**
      (1) First-generation cephalosporins include **cephalexin, cefazolin**, and cefadroxil.
      (2) These agents have good activity against some gram-positive organisms (streptococci) and some gram-negative organisms.
      (3) They are used mainly for **skin and soft-tissue infections** and mild **upper respiratory tract infections**. They may also be used in ***E. coil*** and ***Klebsiella*** infections and penicillin- and sulfonamide-resistant **urinary tract infections.**
      (4) They are also used prophylactically in various surgical procedures.
      (5) These agents **do not penetrate CSF**.
   b. **Second-generation cephalosporins**
      (1) Second-generation cephalosporins include **cefoxitin**, cefaclor, **cefuroxime**, **cefotetan**, and cefprozil.
      (2) These agents have a somewhat wider spectrum of activity than first-generation drugs.
      (3) They are used in the treatment of **streptococcal** infections. Most **anaerobes** (with exception of *Clostridium difficile*) are covered as well. Third-generation cephalosporins have mostly replaced them in the treatment of gram-negative infections.
      (4) Second-generation cephalosporins are used primarily in the management of **respiratory tract, bone, and soft-tissue infections** and prophylactically in various surgical procedures.
      (5) With the **exception of cefuroxime**, these agents **do not penetrate the CSF**.
   c. **Third-generation cephalosporins**
      (1) Third-generation cephalosporins include **cefdinir**, cefixime, **cefotaxime**, ceftazidime, and **ceftriaxone**.
      (2) These agents have **enhanced activity against gram-negative** organisms. They demonstrate high potency against ***H. influenzae, N. gonorrhoeae, N. meningitides, Enterobacter, Salmonella,*** **indole-positive** *Proteus* and ***Serratia*** species, and ***E. coli***; and **moderate activity against anaerobes.**
         (a) **Cefoperazone** and **ceftazidime** have excellent activity against ***P. aeruginosa***.
         (b) **Ceftriaxone** is used for sexually transmitted infections caused by **gonorrhea**, as well as in enteric fever and empiric therapy for community-acquired **meningitis**.
      (3) These agents **penetrate the CSF** (except cefoperazone).
      (4) Most are excreted by the kidney, except **cefoperazone** and **ceftriaxone**, which are excreted through the biliary tract.
   d. **Fourth-generation cephalosporin**
      (1) **Cefepime** has powerful coverage against ***Pseudomonas*** species, as well as **other gram-negative bacteria**.
   e. **Fifth-generation cephalosporin**
      (1) **Ceftaroline** is active against **methicillin-resistant staphylococci** and is used to treat skin infections and community-acquired pneumonia.
         (a) It has limited activity against β-lactamase-producing bacteria.

4. ***Adverse effects and drug interactions***
   a. Cephalosporins may cause **hypersensitivity** reactions (type 1—IgE mediated); symptoms may include urticaria, severe pruritus, fever, or anaphylaxis.
      (1) Cross-sensitivity with penicillins and other β-lactam agents must be considered.
   b. **GI disturbances**, such as nausea and diarrhea, may occur, especially with cefoperazone.
   c. Alcohol intolerance (**disulfiram-like**) is seen with **cefotetan, cefoperazone**, and **ceftriaxone.**
   d. Some agents can cause vitamin K deficiency.

C. Carbapenems

1. ***Specific agents*** include **imipenem–cilastatin, ertapenem, meropenem**, and **doripenem**.
2. ***Mechanism of action***
   a. Similar to other β-lactam agents, carbapenems inhibit bacterial cell wall synthesis by binding to one or more of the **PBP**.

   b. They inhibit the final transpeptidation step of peptidoglycan synthesis in bacterial cell walls.
   c. **Cilastatin is an inhibitor of renal dehydropeptidase** I (which inactivates imipenem).
   d. Carbapenems are relatively **resistant to β-lactamases.** In general, they do not demonstrate cross-resistance with other antibiotics.
3. ***Pharmacologic properties and indications***
   a. They are useful for infections caused by **penicillinase-producing *S. aureus*,** *E. coli*, *Klebsiella* species, ***Enterobacter*** species, and ***H. influenzae***, among others.
   b. They are also used for ***Pseudomonas*** infections (except ertapenem).
4. ***Adverse effects***
   a. GI distress such as nausea and vomiting may occur.
   b. They have the potential to cause central nervous system (CNS) effects, including **seizures**. Imipenem has the highest risk for seizures.
   c. They may cause **hypersensitivity** reactions (type 1—IgE mediated); symptoms may include urticaria, severe pruritus, fever, or anaphylaxis.
      (1) Cross-sensitivity with other β-lactam agents must be considered.

D. Monobactam

1. ***Specific agent.*** **Aztreonam**
2. ***Mechanism of action***
   a. Although aztreonam has a **monobactam ring**, the mechanism of action is similar to β-lactam agents, in which it **inhibits bacterial cell wall synthesis** by binding to one or more of the **PBP**.
   b. It inhibits the final transpeptidation step of peptidoglycan synthesis in bacterial cell walls.
3. ***Pharmacologic properties and indications***
   a. Aztreonam lacks the thiazolidine ring that is **highly resistant to β-lactamases.**
   b. It has **good activity against gram-negative organisms**, including *P. aeruginosa*, but it **lacks activity against anaerobes and gram-positive organisms**.
   c. Aztreonam is useful for various types of infections caused by ***E. coli, Klebsiella pneumoniae, H. influenzae, P. aeruginosa, Enterobacter*** species, ***Citrobacter*** species, and ***P. mirabilis.***
4. ***Adverse effects*** may include skin rash and increased serum liver transaminases.
   a. It **does not have cross-sensitivity** to other β-lactam agents. Hence, it may be used to treat gram-negative infections in patients hypersensitive to β-lactams.

E. Glycopeptides

1. ***Specific agents*** include **vancomycin**, **telavancin**, dalbavancin, and oritavancin.
2. ***Mechanism of action***
   a. These agents **bind to the terminal end (D-alanyl-D-alanine)** of the growing peptidoglycan; they prevent further elongation and cross-linking due to **inhibition of transglycosylase.**
   b. This results in decreased cell membrane activity and increased cell lysis.
   c. Telavancin, dalbavancin, and oritavancin have a lipophilic side chain giving them additional mechanisms; they can cause disruption of membrane potential and changes in cell permeability.
3. ***Pharmacologic properties and indications***
   a. Vancomycin only penetrates CSF during inflammation.
   b. Vancomycin is only active against **gram-positive organisms**, including **MRSA** infections.
   c. Oral vancomycin is used for the treatment *C. difficile* colitis.
   d. Telavancin, dalbavancin, and oritavancin are used to treat skin and skin-structure infections.
4. ***Adverse effects***
   a. Rapid infusion of vancomycin may cause **red man syndrome**, which is an infusion-related reaction caused by the release of histamine. It is not considered a drug allergy.
      (1) Prolonging the infusion to 1–2 hours will prevent this reaction.
   b. High levels of vancomycin may cause **nephrotoxicity**.
   c. Telavancin and dalbavancin are potentially teratogenic.

F. Lipopeptide

1. ***Specific agent.*** **Daptomycin**
2. ***Mechanism of action***

a. Daptomycin binds to the cell membrane via calcium-dependent insertion of its lipid tail; this results in depolarization of the cell membrane with potassium efflux and rapid cell death.

3. ***Pharmacologic properties and indications***

a. Daptomycin has antibacterial actions similar to those of vancomycin.

b. It **covers only gram-positive bacteria** and may be **active against MRSA** and vancomycin-resistant strains.

c. It **cannot be used for the treatment of pneumonia**; it is inactivated by pulmonary surfactant and does not achieve sufficient concentrations in the respiratory tract.

4. ***Adverse effects and drug interactions***

a. Daptomycin may cause **myopathy (rhabdomyolysis)**; for this reason, caution must be used with HMG-CoA reductase inhibitors (statins).

b. Its use may result in eosinophilic pneumonia.

G. Miscellaneous cell wall inhibitors

1. **Bacitracin**

a. ***Mechanism of action***

(1) Bacitracin prevents the transfer of mucopeptides into the growing cell wall.

(2) It inhibits dephosphorylation and reuse of the phospholipid required for acceptance of *N*-acetylmuramic acid pentapeptide, the building block of the peptidoglycan complex.

b. ***Pharmacologic properties and indications***

(1) Bacitracin is most active against **gram-positive** bacteria.

(2) It can be **used topically** in combination with **neomycin** or **polymyxin** for minor infections.

c. ***Adverse effects*** may include allergic reactions.

2. **Fosfomycin**

a. ***Mechanism of action***

(1) Fosfomycin inactivates pyruvyl transferase, an enzyme that is critical in the synthesis of bacterial cell walls.

b. ***Pharmacologic properties and indications***

(1) This agent is active against both gram-positive and gram-negative organisms.

(2) It is used to treat simple lower **urinary tract infections.**

c. ***Adverse effects*** may include headache and GI distress.

III. ANTIBACTERIAL AGENTS: INHIBITORS OF BACTERIAL PROTEIN SYNTHESIS

A. Aminoglycosides

1. ***Structure and mechanism of action***

a. Aminoglycosides passively diffuse via porin channels through the outer membrane of gram-negative aerobic bacteria.

(1) Transport across the inner membrane requires active uptake that is dependent on electron transport (**gram-negative aerobes only**).

b. They interact with receptor proteins on the **30S ribosomal subunit** (Fig. 11.3).

(1) They interfere with the initiation complex of peptide formation.

(2) They cause misreading of mRNA, causing incorporation of incorrect amino acids into the peptide and resulting in nonfunctional proteins.

(3) They lead to a buildup of nonfunctional monosomes.

c. Aminoglycosides lead to misreading of the genetic code, which is why they are bactericidal (other drugs that inhibit protein synthesis are bacteriostatic).

d. Resistance generally results from bacterial enzymes that inactivate the drugs, or due to failure to penetrate the bacterial cell. The resistance contained on plasmids is transmitted by conjugation.

2. ***Pharmacologic properties***

a. These agents do not penetrate the CSF.

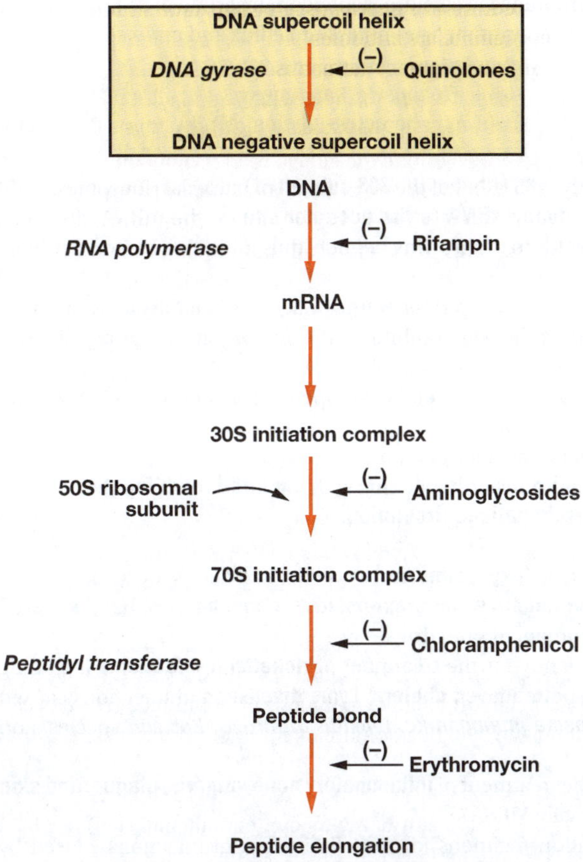

FIGURE 11.3. Antimicrobial action on bacterial nucleic acid and protein synthesis.

b. Aminoglycosides have a **narrow therapeutic range**; it is necessary to monitor serum concentrations and individualize the dose.

3. ***Specific agents and their indications***

a. Streptomycin can be used for the **plague** (*Yersinia pestis*), **severe cases of brucellosis**, and as an adjunct to the treatment of **mycobacterial infections.**

b. Gentamicin and **tobramycin**

(1) Gentamicin and tobramycin are active against ***Enterobacter,*** **indole-positive *Proteus, Pseudomonas, Klebsiella***, and ***Serratia*** species, among other gram-negative organisms.

(2) These agents are often used **synergistically** in combination with β-lactam antibiotics or vancomycin for serious infections that require broad coverage.

c. Amikacin is used in the treatment of **severe gram-negative infections**, especially those resistant to gentamicin or tobramycin.

d. Neomycin is administered topically for **minor soft-tissue infections** (often in combination with **bacitracin** and **polymyxin**).

e. Oral neomycin is used for hepatic encephalopathy.

(1) GI bacteria by-products result in large amounts of ammonia, which is normally cleared by the liver; use of neomycin temporarily inactivates the intestinal flora.

f. The role for aminoglycosides has decreased substantially due to their narrow spectrum of activity, potential for toxicity, and the availability of other agents.

4. ***Adverse effects***

a. Aminoglycosides are **ototoxic,** affecting either vestibular (streptomycin, gentamicin, and tobramycin) or cochlear auditory function (neomycin, amikacin, gentamicin, and tobramycin).

b. They are **nephrotoxic** and may cause **acute tubular necrosis;** this can lead to a reduction in the glomerular filtration rate and a rise in serum creatinine and blood urea nitrogen. Damage is usually reversible.

c. At high doses, these agents produce a curare-like **neuromuscular blockade** with respiratory paralysis. Calcium gluconate and neostigmine are antidotes.
d. When applied topically, neomycin can cause contact dermatitis.

B. Tetracyclines

1. ***Structure and mechanism of action***
   a. Tetracyclines bind reversibly to the 16S rRNA of the **30S subunit** of bacterial ribosomes.
   b. They **prevent the binding of aminoacyl tRNA to the acceptor site** on the mRNA–ribosome complex and **addition of amino acids** to the growing peptide, thus inhibiting bacterial protein synthesis.
   c. Resistance is plasmid mediated and results primarily from a decreased ability to accumulate in the bacteria and from the production of an inhibitor of the binding site for tetracyclines.
2. ***Pharmacologic properties***
   a. Tetracyclines are distributed throughout body fluids; therapeutic concentrations in the brain and CSF can be achieved with minocycline.
   b. The primary route of elimination for most tetracyclines is the kidney.
      (1) **Doxycycline** is the **safest** to administer in patients with **impaired renal function**.
   c. Many tetracyclines undergo **enterohepatic recirculation**.
3. ***Specific agents and indications***
   a. Specific agents include **tetracycline, doxycycline**, minocycline, and demeclocycline.
   b. They are active against both **gram-negative** and **gram-positive organisms**; use has decreased due to resistance and the development of safer drugs.
   c. Tetracyclines are used predominantly for the treatment of **rickettsial infections**, including scrub typhus, Rocky Mountain spotted fever, **cholera, Lyme disease**, and infections caused by ***Chlamydia*** **species**, ***Mycoplasma pneumoniae***, *Bacillus anthracis, Borrelia* species, and ***Plasmodium*** species.
   d. These agents may be useful for the treatment of **inflammatory acne vulgaris, plague, and skin and soft-tissue infections** (especially MRSA).
   e. They are also used in combination regimens for the elimination of infections caused by ***Helicobacter pylori***.
   f. **Demeclocycline** interferes with the action of ADH at the renal collecting duct and can be used in refractory cases of **syndrome of inappropriate secretion of antidiuretic hormone (SIADH)**.
4. ***Adverse effects***
   a. Tetracyclines cause GI distress, including nausea, vomiting, and diarrhea.
   b. They have the potential to cause **photosensitivity** reactions.
   c. Tetracyclines can **complex with calcium in teeth and bones**. They are contraindicated in young children and in pregnancy.
      (1) Children can develop **tooth discoloration**.
      (2) They can reduce bone growth in neonates.
   d. **Nephrotoxicity** may be precipitated in patients with preexisting renal impairment. Fanconi syndrome with damage to proximal tubules has been associated with consumption of outdated tetracyclines.
   e. At high doses, they can cause hepatic damage, particularly in pregnant women and renal failure.
5. ***Food and drug interactions***
   a. Dairy products, antacids, and multivitamins that contain **calcium** may impair oral absorption. Diuretics may augment renal damage.

C. Glycylcycline

1. ***Specific agent.*** Tigecycline.
2. ***Mechanism of action.*** The mechanism is similar to that of tetracyclines, in which it binds to the **30S ribosomal subunit** of bacteria and inhibits protein synthesis.
3. ***Pharmacologic properties and indications***
   a. Tigecycline is a derivative of minocycline.
   b. It has activity against a variety of gram-positive and gram-negative bacteria, including **MRSA**.

c. Indications include community-acquired pneumonia, complicated intra-abdominal infections, and complicated skin infections.

4. ***Adverse effects*** are similar to those of the tetracyclines and include GI distress and photosensitivity.

D. Macrolides

1. ***Structure and mechanism of action*** (Fig. 11.3)
   a. These agents bind reversibly to the 23S rRNA of the **50S subunit**.
   b. They **inhibit aminoacyl translocation** and the **formation of initiation complexes** by blocking the exit tunnel from which the growing peptide emerges.
   c. Resistance is plasmid encoded and is prevalent in most strains of staphylococci and, to some extent, in streptococci. It is due primarily to increased **active efflux** or **ribosomal protection** by increased methylase production.
2. ***Pharmacologic properties***
   a. Erythromycin distributes into all body fluids, except the brain and CSF.
3. ***Specific agents and their indications***
   a. Specific agents include **erythromycin**, clarithromycin, **azithromycin**, and telithromycin.
   b. Erythromycin is active against gram-positive organisms. It is useful in patients with an allergy to β-lactam antibiotics. It is the most effective drug for **Legionnaires disease** (*Legionella pneumophila*); it is also useful for the treatment ***M. pneumoniae***, corynebacterial infections (e.g., **diphtheria**), and ***Bordetella pertussis*** **disease (whooping cough)**.
   c. Azithromycin with a once-daily dosing is commonly used for **community-acquired pneumonia, chlamydial infections**, and **sinusitis**. A single dose of 1 g is combined with ceftriaxone to treat **chancroid and gonorrhea**.
   d. Clarithromycin or azithromycin is effective in the multidrug-regimen treatment of disseminated ***Mycobacterium avium–intracellulare*** **complex (MAC) infections**.
4. ***Adverse effects*** include GI distress. They may also cause **QT prolongation**.
5. ***Drug interactions***
   a. Erythromycin and clarithromycin inhibit the metabolism of hepatic **cytochrome P450 3A4 substrates.**
6. Fidaxomicin is a macrolide antibiotic used for the treatment of *C. difficile* infection. It has less adverse effects and drug interactions.

E. Lincosamide

1. ***Specific agent.*** Clindamycin.
2. ***Mechanism of action.*** It has a mechanism similar to that of the macrolides. It binds reversibly to the 23S rRNA of the **50S subunit** and **inhibits peptide bond formation.**
3. ***Pharmacologic properties and indications***
   a. Clindamycin is well distributed throughout body fluids, except for the CNS.
   b. It has **good anaerobic coverage** and can be used for the treatment of gynecologic infections, intra-abdominal infections, and skin and bone infections.
   c. Topical preparations of the drug are used for the treatment of **acne**.
4. ***Adverse effects***
   a. **Diarrhea** is common with clindamycin. It has a high risk for causing ***C. difficile*** **infections (pseudomembranous colitis)**.

F. Oxazolidinones

1. ***Specific agent.*** **Linezolid.**
2. ***Mechanism of action.*** Linezolid inhibits bacterial protein synthesis by binding to the 23S rRNA of the **50S subunit**; this **prevents the formation of a functional 70S initiation complex**, which is essential for bacterial translation.
3. ***Indications***
   a. Linezolid can only be used for **gram-positive infections.**
   b. It is commonly used for the treatment of **vancomycin-resistant enterococci** (VRE) infections, hospital-acquired pneumonia, and skin and soft-tissue infections.
   c. It is a reserve drug for **drug-resistant tuberculosis (TB)**.

4. ***Adverse effects***
   a. Linezolid may cause **thrombocytopenia**, headache, and GI distress.
   b. It is not preferred for prolonged therapy due to the potential for serious hematologic and neurologic toxicity (optic and peripheral neuritis).
5. ***Drug interactions*** include serotonergic agents, in which it may increase the risk for **serotonin syndrome**.

G. Miscellaneous inhibitors of bacterial protein synthesis

1. **Chloramphenicol**
   a. ***Structure and mechanism of action*** (Fig. 11.3)
      (1) Chloramphenicol inhibits bacterial protein synthesis by binding to the bacterial **50S ribosomal subunit** to **block the action of peptidyl transferase** and thus prevents amino acid incorporation into newly formed peptides.
      (2) High concentrations inhibit eukaryote mitochondrial protein synthesis.
      (3) Resistance results from the production of a plasmid-encoded acetyltransferase capable of inactivating the drug.
   b. ***Pharmacologic properties***
      (1) Chloramphenicol is absorbed rapidly and distributed throughout body fluids.
         (a) Therapeutic levels can be obtained in the CSF.
   c. ***Indications***
      (1) Chloramphenicol is a broad-spectrum, bacteriostatic antibiotic that is active against most **gram-negative organisms**, many **anaerobes**, **clostridia**, ***Chlamydia***, *Mycoplasma*, and *Rickettsia*.
      (2) Due to the potential for **severe and potentially fatal adverse effects, use is limited** to the treatment of infections that cannot be treated with other drugs, such as **anaerobic infections** due to *B. fragilis*, **meningitis** due to *H. influenzae*, not responding to first-line drugs, and topically for conjunctivitis.
   d. ***Adverse effects and drug interactions***
      (1) Chloramphenicol causes dose-related **bone marrow suppression**, resulting in pancytopenia that may lead to **irreversible aplastic anemia**.
         (a) It may also cause **hemolytic anemia** in patients with low levels of **glucose 6-phosphate dehydrogenase**.
      (2) Use in neonates may lead to **gray baby syndrome**, which results from the inadequacy of both cytochrome P450 and glucuronic acid conjugation systems to detoxify the drug.
         (a) Symptoms include cyanosis, abdominal distention, and vasomotor collapse.
      (3) Chloramphenicol inhibition of cytochrome P450 isozymes can result in elevated and toxic levels of other drugs.
2. **Quinupristin plus dalfopristin**
   a. ***Mechanism of action.*** Similar to clindamycin and erythromycin, this combination binds the **50S ribosomal subunit** and is bactericidal against most organisms.
   b. ***Indications.*** It is used to treat severe infections caused by **VRE, MRSA**, and **multidrug-resistant streptococci**.
   c. ***Adverse effects*** include a complex arthralgia–myalgia.

IV. ANTIBACTERIAL AGENTS: INHIBITORS OF DNA SYNTHESIS AND INTEGRITY

A. Antifolate agents

1. ***Specific agents.*** Trimethoprim plus sulfamethoxazole (**cotrimoxazole**).
2. ***Structure and mechanism of action*** (Fig. 11.4)
   a. **Sulfamethoxazole** is a sulfonamide; it is a structural analogue of *para*-aminobenzoic acid (PABA).
      (1) It is a bacteriostatic agent that competes with endogenous bacterial PABA to **inhibit the activity of dihydropteroate synthase**.

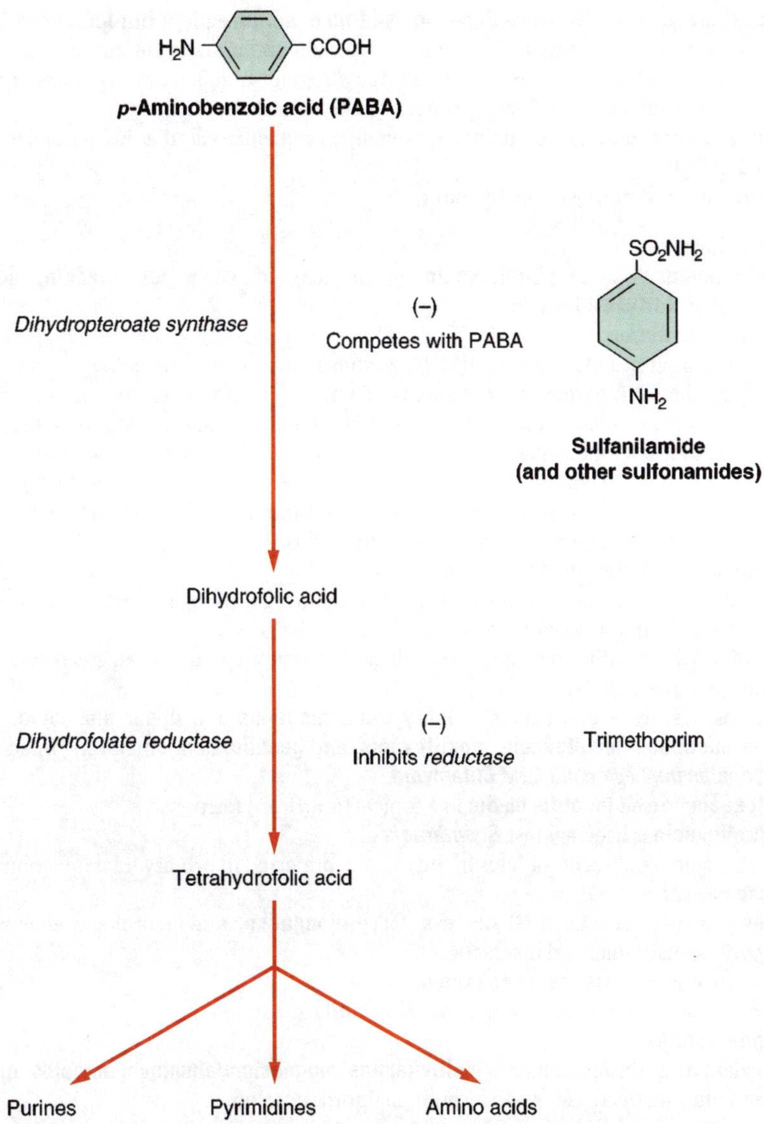

FIGURE 11.4. Sulfonamides and trimethoprim inhibition of tetrahydrofolic acid synthesis.

(2) It prevents the synthesis of dihydrofolic acid.

b. **Trimethoprim inhibits dihydrofolate reductase**, which prevents the synthesis of tetrahydrofolic acid.

c. The combination provides **synergistic activity** due to sequential inhibition of folate synthesis. They inhibit the production of nucleic acid (purines and pyrimidines) and amino acids and thus inhibit bacterial growth. Bacteria that synthesize folic acid de novo are susceptible.

3. *Indications*

a. Trimethoprim–sulfamethoxazole has many indications, including **urinary tract infections** due to *E. coli*, *Klebsiella*, *Enterobacter*, and *Proteus* species, acute otitis media, shigellosis, traveler diarrhea, and the prophylaxis and treatment of ***Pneumocystis* pneumonia** (PCP).

b. Topical sulfonamides, such as silver sulfadiazine, are used for burn treatment.

4. *Adverse effects*

a. Sulfamethoxazole

(1) This agent may cause **hypersensitivity** reactions, including rash.

(2) It rarely causes **Stevens–Johnson syndrome**, an infrequent but fatal form of erythema multiforme associated with lesions of the skin and mucous membranes.
(3) Patients with glucose-6-phosphate dehydrogenase deficiency are more susceptible to adverse effects, manifested primarily as **hemolytic reactions**.

b. Trimethoprim may cause anemia, especially in the elderly and at higher doses as the ones used in PCP.
c. GI distress and photosensitivity may occur.

B. Fluoroquinolones

1. ***Specific agents*** include **ciprofloxacin**, norfloxacin, ofloxacin, **levofloxacin**, **moxifloxacin**, gemifloxacin, and prulifloxacin.
2. ***Mechanism of action***
   a. Fluoroquinolones block bacterial DNA synthesis and are bactericidal.
   b. They **inhibit DNA gyrase** (topoisomerase II) mainly in gram-negative bacteria and prevent relaxation of positively supercoiled DNA required for normal transcription and replication.
   c. They also **inhibit topoisomerase IV** mainly in gram-positive bacteria and interfere with separation of replicated chromosomal DNA into the respective daughter cells during cell division.
   d. Resistance and cross-resistance are due to point mutations in the target enzyme or due to changes in the organism's permeability to the drugs.
3. ***Pharmacologic properties and indications***
   a. Ciprofloxacin and ofloxacin are highly active against gram-negative bacteria and moderately active against gram-positive bacteria.
   b. Levofloxacin, moxifloxacin, gemifloxacin, and prulifloxacin have even greater activity against gram-positive organisms.
   c. Quinolones are useful against **urinary tract infections** and **upper and lower respiratory tract infections** (**levofloxacin, moxifloxacin**, and **gemifloxacin**), including infections due to ***Mycoplasma***, *Legionella*, and ***Chlamydia***.
   d. **Ofloxacin** is used for **otitis media** in a topical (otic drop) form.
   e. **Ciprofloxacin** is used against ***B. anthracis***.
   f. Norfloxacin which accumulates in the urine is preferred in urinary tract infections.
4. ***Adverse effects***
   a. These agents can cause GI distress, **QT prolongation**, and neurologic effects, including dizziness, insomnia, and headache.
   b. They increase the **risk of tendon rupture**.
   c. Use has been strongly associated with ***C. difficile*** infections.
5. ***Drug interactions***
   a. Divalent and trivalent cations (**multivitamins, magnesium/aluminum antacids**, mineral supplements) can decrease the absorption of fluoroquinolones.

V. ANTIBACTERIAL AGENTS: MISCELLANEOUS DRUGS

A. Miscellaneous inhibitors of bacterial nucleic acid synthesis

1. ***Specific agent.*** **Nitrofurantoin**.
   a. ***Mechanism of action.*** Bacterial flavoproteins reduce nitrofurantoin to reactive metabolites; these metabolites inhibit the action of bacterial ribosomal proteins, as well as protein and cell wall synthesis.
   b. ***Pharmacologic properties and indications***
      (1) Nitrofurantoin is concentrated in urine and is used solely for the treatment of **urinary tract infections**.
   c. ***Adverse effects*** include nausea and vomiting, headache, and **hemolytic anemia** in glucose-6-phosphatase-deficient patients. It can turn **urine brown**.
2. ***Specific agent.*** **Metronidazole**.
   a. ***Mechanism of action***
      (1) Metronidazole, a prodrug, is **bactericidal** against most **anaerobic bacteria**, as well as other organisms, including **anaerobic protozoal parasites**.

(2) Transport proteins (such as ferredoxin) transfer electrons to the nitro group of metronidazole forming a nitroso **free radical**, which interacts with intracellular DNA resulting in the **inhibition of DNA synthesis and degradation** and ultimately bacterial death.

b. ***Indications***

(1) It is used for many anaerobic infections, including ***Trichomonas vaginalis*** and ***C. difficile*** **colitis**.

(2) It is also used in protozoal infections like **amoebiasis** and **giardiasis**.

c. ***Adverse effects***

(1) Metronidazole may cause GI distress, headache, and **peripheral neuropathy**.

(2) It can cause a **disulfiram-like reaction**; therefore, alcohol should be avoided.

B. Miscellaneous antibiotics

1. Polymyxins

a. Polymyxin is a polypeptide that acts as a deterrent to **disrupt the cell membrane** functions of **gram-negative** bacteria (bactericidal).

b. It has substantial **nephrotoxicity** and **neurotoxicity** and is therefore indicated only for ophthalmic, otic, or topical use.

c. Polymyxin B is often applied as a topical ointment in combination with bacitracin or neomycin.

2. **Mupirocin** is used topically for ***S. aureus*** infections such as **impetigo** and **furunculosis**.

VI. ANTIMYCOBACTERIAL AGENTS

A. First-line drugs used in the treatment of tuberculosis

1. Isoniazid (INH)

a. ***Structure and mechanism of action***

(1) INH is an analogue of pyridoxine (vitamin B_6).

(2) Its active metabolite inhibits synthesis of the **mycobacterial cell wall**, by inhibiting the enzyme enoyl-ACP reductase required for the synthesis of **mycolic acid** (which is unique to mycobacteria).

b. ***Pharmacologic properties***

(1) INH **penetrates most body fluids and accumulates in caseated lesions.** It enters host cells and has access to intracellular forms of mycobacteria.

(2) It is active against ***Mycobacterium tuberculosis*** but is not active against most atypical mycobacteria.

(3) It does not demonstrate cross-resistance with other first-line drugs.

(4) INH is acetylated in the liver.

c. ***Indications***

(1) INH is administered in combination with three other first-line drugs to counter the development of resistance, which occurs due to mutations that result in decreased conversion of INH to its active metabolite.

(2) For **prophylaxis**, INH is used alone.

d. ***Adverse effects***

(1) INH may produce allergic reactions, including rash or fever.

(2) The metabolites of INH may be **hepatotoxic**; fast acetylators are more susceptible. Jaundice may be observed.

(3) High serum concentrations of this agent may result in **peripheral neuropathy**; slow acetylators are more susceptible. This effect is minimized by the coadministration of **pyridoxine**.

2. **Rifampin** (and its analogues: rifapentine and rifabutin)

a. ***Mechanism of action***

(1) Rifampin **inhibits RNA synthesis** by binding selectively to the β-subunit of bacterial DNA-dependent RNA polymerase (Fig. 11.3).

(a) Most **atypical mycobacteria** are sensitive.

(2) Rifapentine and rifabutin are analogues of rifampin. Their pharmacologic properties are similar to those of rifampin.

(3) Resistance, a change in affinity of the polymerase, develops rapidly when the drug is used alone.

b. ***Pharmacologic properties***

(1) It is widely distributed, including the CSF.

c. ***Indications***

(1) Rifampin is active against **most gram-positive organisms, *Neisseria* species**, and **mycobacteria**, including *M. tuberculosis* (in combination with other drugs such as **INH, pyrazinamide, and ethambutol**).

(2) It is also used in combination with other drugs for the treatment of most **atypical mycobacteria**, including *Mycobacterium leprae.*

(3) Rifampin is also **used prophylactically for meningitis** from meningococci or *H. influenzae*, among contacts.

d. ***Adverse effects***

(1) Rifampin may cause nausea and vomiting, fever, and jaundice. Excretions, including urine, sweat, and tears, may become an orange-red color.

(2) **Hepatotoxicity** is dose-related and is reversible on discontinuation.

e. ***Drug interactions***

(1) Rifampin enters enterohepatic circulation and may induce the metabolism of several drugs, including anticonvulsants and contraceptives.

3. **Ethambutol**

a. ***Mechanism of action***

(1) It inhibits **arabinosyl transferases** involved in cell wall biosynthesis.

b. ***Indications***

(1) It is active against ***M. tuberculosis*** and *M. kansasii.*

(2) Ethambutol is administered orally in **combination with INH, rifampin, and pyrazinamide** to limit the development of resistance.

c. ***Adverse effects***

(1) It produces **visual disturbances**, resulting from reversible retrobulbar neuritis. It should be discontinued immediately in any patient with changes in vision, including color blindness.

(2) It may also cause GI distress.

4. **Pyrazinamide**

a. ***Mechanism of action***

(1) Pyrazinamide is a prodrug that is converted to pyrazinoic acid, which inhibits mycobacterial cell function.

(2) It is inactive at a neutral pH but **inhibits tubercle bacilli in the acidic (pH 5)** phagosomes of macrophages.

(3) Pyrazinamide primarily acts on **extracellular tubercle bacilli**.

b. ***Indications*** include TB.

c. ***Adverse effects***

(1) It may cause GI distress.

(2) **Hepatotoxicity**, including jaundice or liver atrophy, may occur.

(3) It decreases urate secretion and may precipitate gout.

5. **Streptomycin** may be administered in combination with other antimycobacterial agents, including resistant strains of TB.

a. It is not preferred as a first-line drug because it must be administered intramuscularly and has adverse effects like ototoxicity and nephrotoxicity.

b. It may be administered in TB meningitis or when any of the first-line drugs need to be replaced due to adverse effects.

B. Second-line drugs used in the treatment of tuberculosis

1. **Group A**

a. **Levofloxacin**.

b. **Moxifloxacin**.

c. **Bedaquiline** is a diarylquinoline that targets mycobacterial ATP synthase.

(1) It is used only in adult, nonpregnant patients with pulmonary multidrug resistant TB (MDR-TB).

(2) Adverse effects include QTc prolongation and hepatotoxicity.

d. **Linezolid**

2. **Group B**

a. **Clofazimine**, generally used in leprosy. It is also one of the components of combination regimen for drug-resistant TB.

b. **Cycloserine** is an analogue of D-alanine that **inhibits cell wall biosynthesis.**

(1) ***Adverse effects*** include **CNS toxicity**, including seizures and peripheral neuropathy; alcohol increases the possibility of seizures. Pyridoxine administered with cycloserine reduces the incidence of neuropathies.

c. **Terizidone.**

3. **Group C**

a. **Delamanid** is a nitro-dihydro-imidazo-oxazole for the treatment of MDR-TB.

(1) It is bactericidal drug with two different mechanisms of action. It blocks the synthesis of mycolic acids as well as releases nitric oxide which is toxic to the bacilli.

b. **Imipenem–cilastatin.**

c. **Meropenem.**

d. **Amikacin.**

e. **Ethionamide**

(1) Similar to INH, this agent blocks the **synthesis of mycolic acid.**

(2) Resistance develops rapidly, but there is no cross-resistance to INH.

(3) ***Adverse effects*** include severe GI disturbances, peripheral neuropathy (when not given with pyridoxine), and hepatotoxicity.

f. ***para*-Aminosalicylic acid (aminosalicylate)**

(1) This agent is an analogue of PABA; it works similar to sulfonamides but **penetrates** only **mycobacteria.**

(2) It may produce GI disturbances.

C. Commonly used drug regimen for TB

1. In general, **6-month regimens** are used for patients with drug-sensitive TB.

a. The regimen consists of **INH, rifampin, pyrazinamide, and ethambutol.**

b. All **four agents** are used daily for the initial **2 months.**

c. The **continuation phase is 4 months and consists of INH, rifampin, and ethambutol.**

(1) This phase is extended for an additional 3–6 months in patients who at presentation had cavitary lesions, CNS TB, skeletal TB, disseminated TB, or cavitary lesions on a follow-up chest X-ray or are culture positive at the 2-month point.

2. Second-line agents can be used when there is resistance to first-line agents.

D. Drugs used in the treatment of *M. leprae* (leprosy)

1. **Dapsone**

a. ***Mechanism of action.*** Dapsone is structurally related to sulfonamides; it competitively **inhibits dihydropteroate synthase to prevent folic acid biosynthesis.**

b. ***Indications***

(1) It is more effective against ***M. leprae*** than against *M. tuberculosis*; it is also used as a **second-line** agent to treat **PCP.**

(2) It is used in combination with rifampin and clofazimine to delay the development of resistance and shorten the course of therapy.

(3) A daily dose of 100 mg is given for **6 months for paucibacillary leprosy** and **12 months for multibacillary leprosy.**

c. ***Adverse effects*** include **hemolysis, methemoglobinemia,** nausea, rash, and headache.

2. **Clofazimine** is leprostatic. It is used as a component of the multidrug regimen for multibacillary leprosy for 12 months.

a. It is also used in **lepra reaction,** owing to its anti-inflammatory property.

b. **Adverse effects** include dark pigmentation of the skin and conjunctiva, as well as abdominal distress.

E. Management of Lepra reactions

1. Lepra reactions are immunological reactions that usually occur on initiation of leprosy therapy. The clinical presentation of these reactions may range from mild to severe.

2. Mild reactions are treated with Clofazimine 200 mg, daily till symptoms subside.
3. Severe reactions are treated by administering prednisolone 1 mg/kg/day. Prednisolone treatment may be tapered over 2-3 months. Thalidomide may also be added at a dose of 100–400 mg/day.

F. Drugs used against atypical mycobacteria

1. Atypical, noncommunicable mycobacteria include *M. kansasii, M. marinum,* MAC, *M. scrofulaceum,* and others.
2. A combination of rifampin, ethambutol, and INH is used to treat *M. kansasii.*
3. MAC is treated by a combination of agents, such as clarithromycin, ethambutol, and ciprofloxacin, to prevent the emergence of resistance. The treatment for this infection may be lifelong.

VII. ANTIFUNGAL AGENTS

A. Drugs that affect fungal membranes

1. Amphotericin B

a. *Structure and mechanism of action*

(1) Amphotericin B **binds to ergosterol**, a major component of fungal cell membranes. Bacteria are not susceptible because they lack ergosterol.

(2) It forms "amphotericin pores" that alter membrane stability and allow **leakage of cellular contents.**

(3) Amphotericin B binds to mammalian cholesterol with much lower affinity, but this action may explain some adverse effects.

b. *Pharmacologic properties*

(1) It has poor penetration into the CNS but can be administered intrathecally for CNS infections that do not respond to other agents.

c. *Indications*

(1) Amphotericin B has a **broad spectrum of activity**.

(2) It can be used for the treatment of severe systemic fungal infections, including those caused by ***Candida albicans, Histoplasma capsulatum, Cryptococcus neoformans, Coccidioides immitis, Blastomyces dermatitidis, Aspergillus* species, and *Sporothrix schenckii.***

(3) In some cases, combination therapy with **flucytosine** is advantageous for the treatment of cryptococcal meningitis.

(4) It is also used in resistant cases of leishmaniasis.

d. *Adverse effects*

(1) Conventional amphotericin B can cause **infusion-related reactions** that may include nausea, vomiting, chills, and rigors. Premedications, such as diphenhydramine, acetaminophen, and/or hydrocortisone are administered to minimize these effects.

(2) It can also cause **nephrotoxicity, anemia due to bone marrow suppression**, and **electrolyte abnormalities**.

(3) **Lipid formulations** have been developed to reduce the toxicities associated with conventional amphotericin B, including nephrotoxicity, thus enabling administration of higher doses. They also achieve targeted delivery ensuring better efficacy.

2. Azole antifungal agents

a. *Specific agents* include **itraconazole**, ketoconazole, miconazole, **fluconazole**, clotrimazole, **voriconazole**, and posaconazole.

b. *Mechanism of action*

(1) These agents selectively **inhibit** the **cytochrome P450**-mediated sterol **demethylation of lanosterol to ergosterol** in fungal membranes by **inhibiting the activity of lanosterol 14-α-demethylase**.

(2) The affinity for the mammalian P450-dependent enzyme is significantly lower.

c. ***Indications***

(1) These agents are **broad-spectrum** antifungals; they also inhibit some protozoa.

(2) Indications for **itraconazole** include **aspergillosis**, **blastomycosis**, candidiasis, histoplasmosis, and onychomycosis.

(3) Voriconazole is used for the treatment of **invasive aspergillosis, *Candida* infections**, and infections due to *Scedosporium apiospermum* and *Fusarium* species (including *Fusarium solani*).

(4) **Fluconazole** is used for ***Candida* infections**, **cryptococcal meningitis**, and antifungal prophylaxis in patients with allogeneic bone marrow transplant.

(5) **Posaconazole** is indicated for prophylaxis of *Aspergillus* and *Candida* infections as well as for the treatment of oropharyngeal candidiasis. It is also used to treat **mucormycosis**.

(6) Miconazole, clotrimazole, and ketoconazole are available for topical application. They are useful for many dermatophyte infections, including tinea pedis, ringworm, and cutaneous and vulvovaginal candidiasis.

d. ***Adverse effects***

(1) They may cause GI distress and have the potential to cause **hepatotoxicity**.

e. ***Drug interactions***

(1) Itraconazole, voriconazole, and posaconazole cause inhibition of CYP3A4 enzyme and may decrease metabolism of certain drugs.

B. Echinocandins

1. ***Specific agents*** include **caspofungin**, **micafungin**, and anidulafungin.
2. ***Mechanism of action.*** These agents are noncompetitive **inhibitors of β-D-glucan synthesis**. They disrupt the fungal cell wall by depleting cell wall glucan cross-linking, resulting in cell death.
3. ***Indications.*** Due to a better safety profile, these agents are preferred in invasive **candidiasis** and **aspergillosis**.
4. ***Adverse effects.*** Overall, they are well tolerated. Adverse effects may include elevations in liver enzymes and occasional GI distress.

C. Other antifungal agents

1. **Griseofulvin**

a. ***Mechanism of action.*** This agent inhibits fungal cell mitosis during metaphase. It binds to microtubules and **prevents spindle formation and mitosis in fungi**. It also binds filament proteins such as keratin.

b. ***Pharmacologic properties.*** It accumulates in the skin, hair, and nails.

c. ***Indications*** include **hair, nail**, and **dermatophyte infections**.

d. ***Adverse effects.*** Griseofulvin is generally well tolerated but may cause GI distress and rash. Rarely, CNS effects and hepatotoxicity occur.

2. **Flucytosine**

a. ***Mechanism of action.*** Flucytosine is actively transported into fungal cells and is converted to **5-fluorouracil** and subsequently to **5-fluorodeoxyuridylic acid**, which inhibits thymidylate synthetase and pyrimidine and **nucleic acid synthesis**.

(1) Human cells lack the ability to convert large amounts of flucytosine to the uracil form.

b. ***Indications***

(1) It is often used in combination with other agents in the treatment of **cryptococcal meningitis** and candidiasis.

(2) **Resistance develops rapidly** and limits its use.

c. ***Adverse effects*** include **bone marrow depression** and hair loss.

3. Nystatin can be used locally for cutaneous and mucocutaneous fungal infections, including oral candidiasis. It works by binding to sterols in fungal cell membrane, which causes changes in the permeability of the cell wall and cell contents to leak.

4. Topical agents used for the treatment of dermatophyte infections of the skin, hair, and nails include tolnaftate, naftifine, terbinafine, and butenafine.

VIII. ANTIPARASITIC DRUGS

A. Agents active against protozoal infections

1. *Agents active against malaria*

a. Malaria parasite life cycle

(1) In the primary state of infection, sporozoites are injected into the host by the female *Anopheles* mosquito. In this pre-erythrocytic stage, the sporozoites are resistant to drug therapy.

(2) The sporozoites migrate to the liver (primary exoerythrocytic stage) and then sporulate.

- **(a)** *Plasmodium vivax* and *P. ovale* may not develop to mature liver stages for up to 2 years (hypnozoites).

(3) The merozoites that emerge infect erythrocytes (erythrocytic stage), where asexual division leads to cell lysis and causes clinical symptoms.

(4) In *P. vivax* and *P. ovale*, the merozoites released can reinfect other red blood cells (secondary erythrocytic stage) or reinfect the liver.

- **(a)** Elimination of parasites from erythrocytes and the liver requires multidrug therapy effect as cure.
- **(b)** *P. malariae* and *P. falciparum* differ from the other plasmodia in that the merozoites cannot reinfect the liver to produce a secondary exoerythrocytic stage. The lack of a tissue reservoir makes therapy somewhat easier.

(5) The merozoites differentiate into sexual forms (gametocytes) that can reproduce in the gut of another female mosquito.

- **(a)** Gametocidal drugs help reduce such transmission.

b. Treatment of malaria

(1) Chloroquine is used for the control of acute, recurrent attacks, but it is not radically curative.

- **(a)** For chloroquine-resistant plasmodia, artemisinin combination therapy (ACT) is used.
- **(b)** ACTs include **artesunate–sulfadoxine + pyrimethamine, artemether–lumefantrine,** and **artesunate–mefloquine**, among others.
- **(c)** Quinine may be used as an alternative to ACT.

(2) In prophylaxis, chloroquine/mefloquine is used in a weekly dose to suppress erythrocytic forms either before or during exposure.

- **(a)** Primaquine is added after exposure to treat exoerythrocytic forms.
- **(b)** In regions with chloroquine-resistant strains, mefloquine or atovaquone/proguanil is used for prophylaxis.
- **(c)** Tetracyclines and doxycycline are used daily for short-term prophylaxis in areas with multiresistant strains of plasmodia.

c. Chloroquine

(1) ***Mechanism of action.*** Chloroquine concentrates in acidic parasite vacuoles, raising their pH, and **inhibits the activity of heme polymerase**, which converts host hemoglobin toxic by-products to nontoxic polymerized material.

(2) ***Indications***

- **(a)** Chloroquine is used for malaria treatment and prophylaxis.
- **(b)** It is used in the control of **acute, recurrent attacks**, but it is not radically curative.
- **(c)** It is effective against all plasmodia (*P. falciparum, P. vivax, P. malariae,* and *P. ovale*).
- **(d)** Many species of *P. falciparum* are resistant to chloroquine.
- **(e)** Other indications include extraintestinal amebiasis and lupus erythematosus.

(3) ***Adverse effects.*** Nausea, vomiting, and pruritis are common. Rarely, **hemolysis** can develop in patients with glucose-6-phosphate dehydrogenase deficiency.

- **(a)** Rapid parenteral administration of a single high dose may be fatal.

d. Primaquine (8-aminoquinoline)

(1) ***Mechanism of action.*** This agent disrupts mitochondria and binds to DNA.

(2) ***Indications***

(a) Primaquine is used in the treatment of malaria. In combination with chloroquine, it is used specifically to eliminate liver hypnozoites after exposure to *P. vivax* or *P. ovale* for terminal prophylaxis and (radical) cure from malaria.

(b) It is **gametocidal**, and helps prevent onward transmission into mosquitoes.

(c) It can be also be used for prophylaxis before exposure (casual prophylaxis) when other drugs are ineffective or unavailable.

(3) ***Adverse effects***

(a) **Blood dyscrasias** or **arrhythmias** may rarely occur.

(b) Primaquine may result in **intravascular hemolysis or methemoglobinemia** in African Americans and dark-skinned Caucasians with glucose-6-phosphate dehydrogenase deficiency.

(c) Due to the relative deficiency of glucose-6-phosphate dehydrogenase, use of this agent is not advised during the first trimester of **pregnancy**.

e. **Artemether**

(1) ***Mechanism of action***

(a) Artemisinin and its derivatives **interact with heme** in plasmodia, leading to the release of free radicals that cause protein damage.

(2) ***Indications***

(a) They are highly efficacious and rapidly acting, used against both **complicated and uncomplicated *falciparum* malaria**.

(b) Due to their short duration of action, they are always combined with long-acting antimalarials and are not used in prophylaxis.

f. **Quinine**

(1) ***Mechanism of action***

(a) Quinine **inhibits nucleic acid synthesis and protein synthesis** and decreases carbohydrate metabolism in *P. falciparum*. In addition, it binds to hemozoin in parasitized erythrocytes.

(2) ***Indications***

(a) It is used in the treatment of malaria and is active against the **erythrocytic stage**. It is used to treat chloroquine-resistant *P. falciparum,* often in combination with doxycycline, as an alternative to ACT.

(3) ***Adverse effects***

(a) Quinine has a **low therapeutic index**.

(b) It produces **curare-like effects** on the skeletal muscle and may cause headache, nausea, visual disturbances, dizziness, and tinnitus **(cinchonism)**.

(c) **Hypoglycemia**, which can be fatal, and (rarely) hypotension may occur.

(d) Quinine is associated with **"blackwater fever"** in previously sensitized patients; although rare, it has a fatality rate of 25% due to intravascular coagulation and renal failure.

(4) Quinidine is an agent with similar properties and is active against *P. vivax* and *P. malaria.*

g. **Mefloquine**

(1) ***Mechanism of action.*** This agent causes destruction of the asexual blood forms of malarial pathogens.

(2) ***Indications***

(a) It is useful for prophylaxis and treatment of chloroquine-resistant *P. falciparum* and for prophylaxis against *P. vivax* and *P. ovale.*

(b) It acts specifically on the **erythrocytic stage** of infection. For eradication of *P. falciparum,* it is used with artesunate.

(c) For eradication of *P. ovale* and *P. vivax,* it is used with primaquine.

(3) ***Adverse effects.*** Mefloquine causes GI disturbances at therapeutic doses. Seizures and other CNS manifestations are also seen.

(4) ***Contraindications.*** Use is contraindicated in patients with **epilepsy** and **psychiatric disorders**, and in patients using drugs that alter cardiac conduction.

h. **Atovaquone** and **atovaquone/proguanil**
   (1) ***Mechanism of action***
      (a) Atovaquone inhibits electron transport to reduce the membrane potential of mitochondria. Resistance develops rapidly.
      (b) The mechanism of antimalarial action of proguanil is uncertain. Its metabolite, cycloguanil, selectively inhibits plasmodia **dihydrofolate reductase/thymidylate synthetase** to inhibit DNA synthesis.
   (2) ***Indications***
      (a) Coadministration of atovaquone with proguanil is effective for the treatment and prophylaxis of *P. falciparum.*
      (b) Atovaquone is used as an alternative treatment for *P. jirovecii* pneumonia.
   (3) ***Adverse effects*** include GI dysfunction, headache, and rash.

i. **Pyrimethamine**
   (1) ***Mechanism of action.*** Pyrimethamine and its prodrug analogue, **proguanil**, **inhibit dihydrofolate reductase** of plasmodia at concentration less than that needed to inhibit the host enzyme.
   (2) ***Indications.*** Pyrimethamine is used in combination with sulfadoxine, a sulfonamide with similar pharmacologic properties. The pyrimethamine–sulfadoxine combination is used along with artesunate.
   (3) ***Adverse effects.*** It is associated with **megaloblastic anemia** and **folate deficiency** (at high doses).

j. **Lumefantrine** is formulated with artemether.
   (1) ***Mechanism of action.*** These agents inhibit nucleic acid and protein synthesis to reduce and eliminate parasites.
   (2) ***Indications.*** Lumefantrine–artemether combination is used for the treatment of uncomplicated malaria. It is used as first-line therapy to treat the erythrocytic stage of *P. falciparum,* in the northeastern parts of India, where strains resistant to artesunate-SP have been detected.
   (3) ***Adverse effects*** may include GI distress, weakness, and dizziness.

2. ***Agents active against amebiasis***

a. The major infecting organism in amebiasis is *Entamoeba histolytica,* which is ingested in cyst form, divides in the colon, and can invade the intestinal wall to cause severe dysentery.

b. **General drug characteristics**
   (1) The **tissue amebicides (metronidazole** and **tinidazole)** are active against organisms in the intestinal wall, **liver**, and other **extraintestinal tissues**.
   (2) The **luminal amebicides (iodoquinol, paromomycin**, and **nitazoxanide)** act effectively in the **intestinal lumen**.

c. **Metronidazole and tinidazole**
   (1) ***Mechanism of action.*** These agents form free radicals that damage DNA and prevent further DNA synthesis.
   (2) ***Indications***
      (a) Metronidazole and tinidazole are used for **intestinal amebiasis** as well as for **amebic liver abscesses**, generally in combination with a luminal amebicide **iodoquinol** or **paromomycin** to eradicate luminal disease.
      (b) These agents are also active against ***Giardia intestinalis*** (formerly *G. lamblia*) and ***T. vaginalis***.
      (c) Metronidazole shows activity against many **anaerobic bacteria**.
   (3) ***Adverse effects***
      (a) **Metronidazole** has a **disulfiram-like action**; therefore, alcohol should be avoided. Tinidazole appears to be better tolerated.
      (b) **Metronidazole** should be avoided in the **first trimester of pregnancy** due to possible teratogenic effects.

d. **Paromomycin** is a broad-spectrum antibiotic, related to neomycin and streptomycin, which is useful as an alternative treatment for **mild-to-moderate luminal infections** or in **asymptomatic carriers**. It may cause GI distress.

3. ***Agents active against leishmaniasis***
   a. **Stibogluconate sodium**
      (1) ***Mechanism of action.*** It is an antimonial agent; the mechanism is unknown.
      (2) ***Indications.*** It is effective against all ***Leishmania*** (cutaneous, visceral).
      (3) ***Adverse effects.*** GI disturbances are common, and electrocardiogram changes may occur with continued therapy.
   b. **Pentamidine**
      (1) ***Mechanism of action.*** It interferes with microbial nuclear metabolism through inhibition of DNA, RNA, phospholipid, and protein synthesis.
      (2) ***Indications.*** It can be used to treat ***L. donovani*** infections when antimonials have failed or are contraindicated. It is also indicated for the treatment of **PCP**.
      (3) ***Adverse effects*** may include **nephrotoxicity** and **hypoglycemia**.
   c. **Nitazoxanide** is used to treat *G. lamblia and C. parvum.* It inhibits the pyruvate-ferredoxin metabolic pathway. Overall, it is well tolerated.
4. ***Agents used in the treatment of trypanosomiasis***
   a. **Nifurtimox** is used to treat South American trypanosomiasis caused by *Trypanosoma cruzi* **(Chagas disease)**.
   b. **Suramin**, the mechanism of which is unknown, is useful for the treatment of early stage **African trypanosomiasis**, or **sleeping sickness**, caused by *T. brucei rhodesiense.* Adverse effects include GI disturbances and rarely rash, among others.
   c. **Eflornithine**, an alternative for late-stage West African trypanosomiasis, is an ornithine decarboxylase inhibitor.
   d. **Pentamidine** is standard therapy for the disease caused by *T. rhodesiense;* it can be used as an alternative to **suramin** in the early stage of the disease.
5. ***Drug therapy for other protozoal infections***
   a. **Giardiasis. Metronidazole** and **tinidazole** are the drugs of choice. **Nitazoxanide** is also used.
   b. **Toxoplasmosis** is treated with a combination of **pyrimethamine** and **sulfadiazine** (or clindamycin). This is a common opportunistic infection in immune-compromised patients.

B. Agents active against metazoan infections (anthelmintics)

1. ***Agents effective against nematode (roundworm) infections***
   a. **Albendazole** and **mebendazole**
      (1) ***Mechanism of action***
         (a) These agents **bind with high affinity to parasite-free β-tubulin** to inhibit its polymerization and microtubule assembly.
         (b) They also irreversibly **inhibit glucose uptake by nematodes**; the resulting glycogen depletion and decreased ATP production **immobilize the intestinal parasite**, which is then cleared from the GI tract.
      (2) ***Indications***
         (a) Albendazole is the drug of choice for **cysticercosis** and **cystic hydatid disease**.
         (b) Mebendazole and albendazole are used to treat **roundworm infections** caused by *Ascaris lumbricoides, Capillaria philippinensis, Enterobius vermicularis* (pinworm), *Necator americanus* (hookworm), and *Trichuris trichiura* (whipworm).
         (c) They are also recommended for infections caused by the cestodes, *E. granulosus* and *E. multilocularis.*
      (3) ***Adverse effects*** may include GI distress during short-term therapy. They are potentially **teratogenic**.
   b. **Pyrantel pamoate**
      (1) ***Mechanism of action.*** It selectively produces **depolarizing neuromuscular blockade** and **inhibition of acetylcholinesterase (AChE)** of the worm, resulting in **paralysis**; intestinal nematodes are flushed from the system.
      (2) ***Indications*** include the treatment of infections caused by **roundworm**, **hookworm**, and **pinworm**.
      (3) ***Adverse effects*** may include dizziness, headache, and GI distress.

c. **Diethylcarbamazine**

(1) ***Mechanism of action.*** This agent **decreases microfilariae muscular activity**, causing their dislocation. It also disrupts their membranes, making them susceptible to host defense mechanisms.

(2) ***Indications.*** It is the drug of choice to treat **loiasis**, despite host response-induced toxicity, and it is a first-line agent for the treatment of **lymphatic filariasis** and **tropical pulmonary eosinophilia** caused by *Wuchereria bancrofti* and *Brugia malayi*.

(3) ***Adverse effects.*** Host destruction of parasites may result in **severe but reversible reactions**, including leukocytosis, retinal hemorrhages, and ocular complications. Tachycardia, rash, fever, encephalitis, and lymph node enlargement may also occur.

d. **Ivermectin**

(1) ***Mechanism of action.*** It causes **paralysis** of the organism's **musculature** by activation of **invertebrate-specific glutamate-gated Cl^- channels.**

(2) ***Indications.*** It is the drug of choice for the oral treatment of **onchocerciasis**, and it is also used for the oral treatment of **scabies**.

(3) ***Adverse effects.*** In onchocerciasis, the destruction of the microfilariae can cause bronchospasm, hypotension, and high fever.

2. ***Agents effective against cestode (tapeworm) and trematode (fluke) infections***

a. **Praziquantel**

(1) ***Mechanism of action.*** Praziquantel causes **paralysis** of the worm due to increased cell membrane permeability of calcium.

(2) ***Indications.*** It is the most effective drug against all types of **fluke infections**, including blood fluke infections **(schistosomiasis)**, intestinal and liver fluke infections, and lung fluke infections **(paragonimiasis)**. It is also useful in the treatment of **tapeworm infections**.

(3) ***Adverse effects*** include fever and rashes. Use is contraindicated in ocular cysticercosis because of host-defense-induced **irreversible eye damage**.

b. **Bithionol** inhibits parasite respiration. It is an alternative for *Fasciola hepatica* (sheep liver fluke infection) and is also used as an alternative to praziquantel for acute pulmonary paragonimiasis.

IX. ANTIVIRAL DRUGS

A. Antiherpetic drugs

1. **Acyclovir** and **valacyclovir**

a. ***Mechanism of action***

(1) **Acyclovir** is a **purine analogue** that needs to be converted to nucleoside triphosphate for activity.

(2) It **requires viral thymidine kinase** to be selectively converted to monophosphate; it then uses cellular enzymes to be **converted to a triphosphate form** that competitively **inhibits the activity of viral DNA polymerase.**

(3) Acyclovir triphosphate is also incorporated into viral DNA, where it acts to compete with deoxy-GTP for viral DNA polymerase and as a chain terminator.

(4) It **does not eradicate latent virus.**

(5) **Valacyclovir** is a **prodrug** that is converted rapidly and completely in the intestine and liver to acyclovir.

(6) Resistance generally develops due to decreased viral thymidine kinase activity or an alteration in DNA polymerase.

b. ***Indications***

(1) These agents are active against **herpes simplex virus (HSV)** types I and II and to a lesser extent against **Epstein–Barr virus (EBV), varicella-zoster virus (VZV),** and **cytomegalovirus (CMV).**

(2) Chronic oral administration provides suppression and **shortening of duration of symptoms** in recurrent genital herpes.

(3) Ophthalmic application is used to treat **herpes simplex dendritic keratitis** and topical application is used for **mucocutaneous herpetic infections** in immunosuppressed patients.
(4) They may be used to **prevent reactivation of HSV** infections.

c. ***Adverse effects***
(1) Reversible **renal insufficiency** (crystalline nephropathy) or **neurotoxicity**, including tremor, delirium, and seizures, may develop without adequate patient hydration.

d. **Famciclovir** is a prodrug that is well absorbed and then converted by deacetylation to **penciclovir**, which has activity similar to that of acyclovir except that it does not cause chain termination.

2. **Penciclovir**, **docosanol**, and **trifluridine** are used as topical creams to treat herpes infections.
a. **Docosanol prevents fusion of the HSV envelope with cell plasma membranes**, thereby inhibiting viral penetration.
b. Host cell phosphorylated **trifluridine inhibits viral DNA polymerase** with inhibition of DNA synthesis.

3. **Ganciclovir** and **valganciclovir**
a. ***Mechanism of action***
(1) Ganciclovir is a deoxyguanosine analogue that, as the **triphosphate** (like acyclovir), **inhibits replication of CMV** (also HSV, but not as well); monophosphorylation in CMV is catalyzed by a viral phosphotransferase (in HSV by a viral thymidine kinase).
(2) Resistance is primarily the result of impaired phosphorylation due to a point mutation or a deletion in the viral phosphotransferase.

b. ***Indications***
(1) Ganciclovir is used to treat **CMV retinitis, colitis, esophagitis**, and **pneumonitis** in immunocompromised patients.

c. ***Adverse effects*** include **reversible neutropenia** and **thrombocytopenia**.
d. **Valganciclovir** is an ester prodrug that is converted to ganciclovir by intestinal and liver enzymes. Its uses are similar to those of ganciclovir.

4. **Foscarnet**
a. ***Mechanism of action***
(1) Foscarnet inhibits **viral DNA and RNA polymerase and human immunodeficiency virus (HIV) reverse transcriptase** directly by binding to the pyrophosphate-binding site.
(2) Resistance is due to point mutations in viral DNA polymerase and HIV reverse transcriptase.
(a) Foscarnet is **not cross-resistant** with most other antivirals.

b. ***Indications.*** Foscarnet is approved for use in the treatment of **CMV infections** and **acyclovir-resistant HSV infections.**
c. ***Adverse effects.*** Use is limited by **nephrotoxicity** and **electrolyte wasting**, which may lead to paresthesias, arrhythmias, and seizures.

5. **Cidofovir**
a. ***Mechanism of action.*** This agent is a **cytosine analogue active against CMV**. It does not require viral enzymes for phosphorylation and subsequent **inhibition of DNA polymerase** and DNA synthesis.
b. ***Indications*** include **CMV** infections, including CMV **retinitis**.
c. ***Adverse effects*** include **nephrotoxicity** and **neutropenia**.

B. Agents used for influenza

1. **Amantadine** and **rimantadine**
a. ***Mechanism of action.*** Amantadine and rimantadine interact with the M2 protein of the proton channel of the virus to **inhibit the uncoating and replication of the viral RNA in infected cells.** The point mutation development of resistance is common (Fig. 11.5).
b. ***Indications.*** Amantadine and rimantadine are used to treat **influenza A** infections (when **administered within the first 48 hours of symptoms**) and as **prophylaxis during flu season**. These agents do not suppress the immune response to the influenza A vaccine.
c. ***Adverse effects.*** They cause mild **CNS effects (insomnia, nervousness)** and some GI dysfunction. Patients with a history of seizures require close monitoring. **Teratogenic** effects have been noted.

2. **Zanamivir** and **oseltamivir**
   a. ***Mechanism of action.*** These agents are **neuraminidase inhibitors**; they potentially alter particle aggregation and release (Fig. 11.5).
   b. ***Indications.*** They are used for the treatment and prophylaxis of **acute uncomplicated influenza infection**. The agents are effective against both **influenza A and B**.
   c. ***Adverse effects.*** **Abdominal pain** and **GI dysfunction** are common with **oseltamivir** (an oral agent). **Zanamivir** (an intravenous agent) may cause **bronchospasm**.

X. ANTIRETROVIRAL DRUGS

A. Nucleoside reverse transcriptase inhibitors

1. ***Specific agents*** include **tenofovir**, abacavir, **zidovudine**, **emtricitabine**, **lamivudine**, didanosine, and stavudine.
2. ***Mechanism of action*** (Fig. 11.5)
   a. Nucleoside reverse transcriptase inhibitors (NRTIs) act by **competitively inhibiting HIV-encoded RNA-dependent DNA polymerase (reverse transcriptase)** to cause chain termination that decreases viral DNA synthesis and virus replication. They prevent infection, but do not clear cells already infected.
   b. NRTIs must first **undergo intracellular phosphorylation** to be active.
3. ***Indications***
   a. These agents are used for the treatment of HIV-1 and -2 in combination with other antiretroviral agents; they are referred to as the backbone of antiretroviral therapy.
      (1) They are often administered in pairs; **combination therapy** is used for treatment and to **reduce the likelihood of the development of resistance**.
      (2) Some agents, like **lamivudine**, are used as part of the combination regimen for **postexposure prophylaxis** and for the **prevention of perinatal HIV** transmission.
4. ***Adverse effects.*** NRTIs may cause **leukopenia**, **neuropathies**, **pancreatitis**, and hepatic steatosis. They also have the potential to cause lactic acidosis.

B. Non-nucleoside reverse transcriptase inhibitors (NNRTIs)

1. ***Specific agents*** include **efavirenz**, nevirapine, rilpivirine, etravirine, and delavirdine.
2. ***Mechanism of action*** (Fig. 11.5)
   a. These agents are **noncompetitive inhibitors** of **HIV-encoded RNA-dependent DNA polymerase (reverse transcriptase)**. Similar to NRTIs, they cause chain termination that decreases viral DNA synthesis and virus replication. They prevent infection, but do not clear cells already infected.
   b. They **do not require phosphorylation** for their activity but rather act directly.
3. ***Indications.*** **Efavirenz** combined with NRTI backbone is an alternative regimen used for the treatment of HIV-1.
4. ***Adverse effects*** may include **GI dysfunction**, hepatitis, and **skin reactions**, including Stevens–Johnson syndrome.
   a. Efavirenz and rilpivirine may cause neurologic and psychiatric side effects.

C. HIV-1 protease inhibitors

1. ***Specific agents*** include **ritonavir**, **darunavir**, **atazanavir**, and **lopinavir**. Rarely used agents include indinavir, nelfinavir, saquinavir, fosamprenavir, and tipranavir.
2. ***Mechanism of action*** (Fig. 11.5)
   a. These agents are **HIV-1 protease inhibitors** (PIs) that competitively **inhibit viral-induced Gag-Pol polyprotein cleavage by HIV-1 protease**, a step necessary for virion maturation; this leads to clearance of the immature virion.
3. ***Indications***
   a. These agents are used for the treatment of HIV-1 and -2. They are used in **combination with nucleoside analogues**.

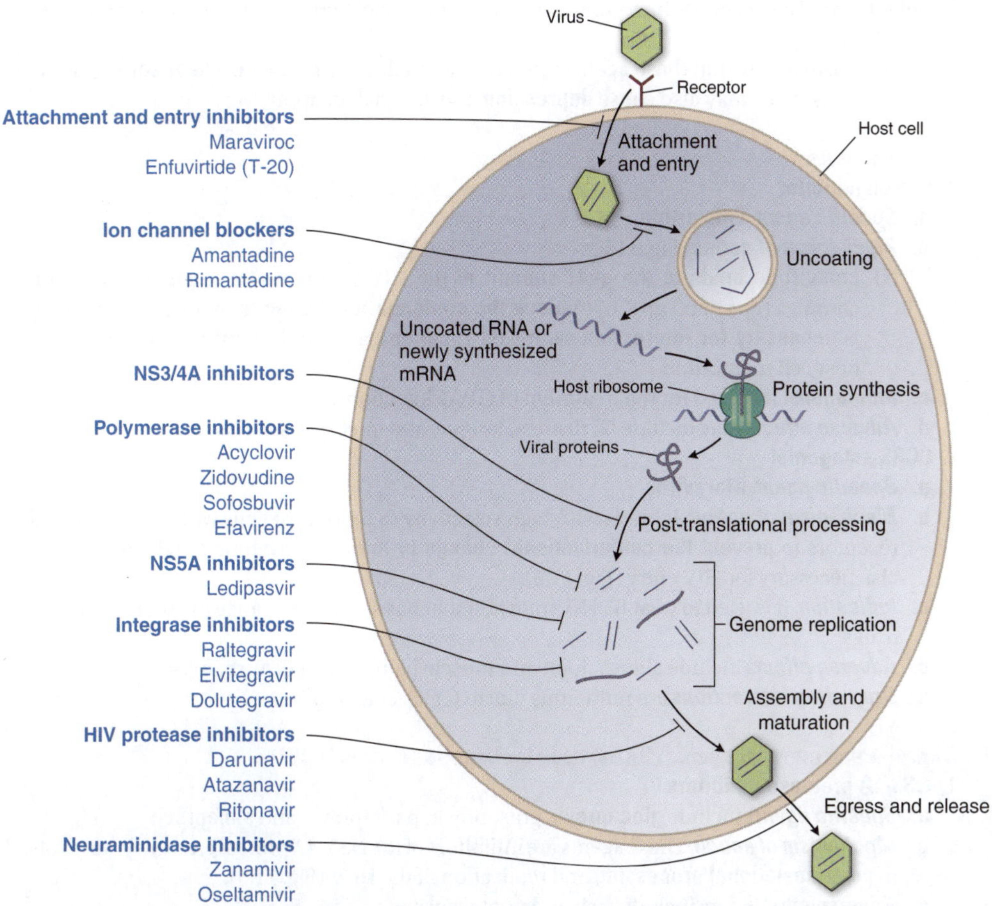

FIGURE 11.5. Sites of action of antiviral drugs. (Reprinted with permission from Golan D. Principles of Pharmacology. 4th ed. Philadelphia, PA: Wolters Kluwer Health, 2016, Fig. 33.2.)

4. ***Pharmacologic properties***
   a. Bioavailability of most PIs is increased with a **high-fat meal**.
   b. Resistance due to changes in the protease gene may occur.
5. ***Adverse effects***
   a. These agents may cause many **metabolic effects**, including **hyperglycemia**, **hyperlipidemia**, **lipodystrophy**, and hepatotoxicity. Some agents also have the potential to cause cardiac arrhythmias.
6. Significant **drug–drug interactions** have been noted that are due to inhibition or induction of CYP isoforms.
   a. Ritonavir extensively **inhibits many liver CYP enzymes**; it may be used as a pharmacokinetic "booster" in combination with other PI.

D. Integrase strand transfer inhibitors (INSTIs)

1. ***Specific agents*** include **raltegravir**, elvitegravir, **dolutegravir**, and bictegravir.
2. ***Mechanism of action*** (Fig. 11.5)
   a. HIV integrase is essential for HIV replication; it is an enzyme that catalyzes the process in which viral DNA is integrated into the genome of the host cell.
   b. These agents **bind to the viral enzyme integrase to prevent HIV replication and viral integration into the host cell.**
   c. They target the strand transfer step of viral DNA integration and prevent the binding of the preintegration complex to the host cell DNA.

3. ***Indications.*** These agents in combination with NRTI backbone are the first-line treatment of HIV-1 and -2.
4. ***Adverse effects.*** Overall these agents are well tolerated. They may cause **headache**, insomnia, or dizziness. They may also cause **depression** and suicidal ideation.

E. Entry inhibitors

1. **Fusion inhibitor**
   a. ***Specific agent.*** **Enfuvirtide.**
   b. ***Mechanism of action*** (Fig. 11.5)
      (1) **Enfuvirtide binds to the gp41 subunit of** the HIV-1 viral envelope gp160 glycoprotein complex (gp41 and gp120) to **block the conformational change** in the glycoprotein that is **necessary for interaction with CD4 receptors** and viral membrane fusion with the host cell membrane.
   c. ***Indications.*** It is used for the treatment of HIV-1 infections.
   d. ***Adverse effects*** may include GI distress, fatigue, and infection-site reactions.
2. **CCR5 antagonist**
   a. ***Specific agent.*** **Maraviroc.**
   b. ***Mechanism of action.*** It binds with high selectivity to those host cells with **CCR5 chemokine** receptors to **prevent the conformational change** in the viral envelope **gp120 subunit** that is also necessary for HIV entry (Fig. 11.5).
   c. ***Indication.*** It is used to treat R5 HIV infection that has shown resistance to other antiretroviral drugs.
   d. ***Adverse effects*** include allergy, joint and muscle pain, and GI disturbances.
   e. ***Drug–drug interactions*** are numerous due to CYP3A metabolism.

F. Direct-acting antiviral agents (DAAs) used for hepatitis C virus (HCV)

1. **NS3/4A protease inhibitors**
   a. ***Specific agents*** include **glecaprevir,** grazoprevir, paritaprevir, and **simeprevir**.
   b. ***Mechanism of action.*** These agents are inhibitors of the NS3/4A protease, an enzyme involved in **posttranslational processing** and replication of the HCV (Fig. 11.5).
   c. ***Adverse effects*** may include rash and photosensitivity.
   d. ***Drug interactions***. CYP inducers and inhibitors may affect drug levels.
2. **NS5A protein inhibitors**
   a. ***Specific agents*** include **daclatasvir**, elbasvir, **ledipasvir**, ombitasvir, pibrentasvir, and velpatasvir.
   b. ***Mechanism of action.*** They interfere with viral replication and assembly of the HCV virus by binding to the N-terminus of HCV nonstructural protein 5A (NS5A) (Fig. 11.5).
   c. ***Adverse effects*** may include GI distress, headache, and fatigue.
   d. ***Drug interactions*** vary by agent; P-glycoprotein and CYP inducers and inhibitors may affect drug levels.
3. **NS5B polymerase inhibitors**
   a. ***Specific agents***
      (1) Nucleoside/nucleotide polymerase inhibitor (NPI): **Sofosbuvir**.
      (2) Non-nucleoside polymerase inhibitor (NNPIs): **Dasabuvir**.
   b. ***Mechanism of action***
      (1) NS5B is a RNA-dependent RNA polymerase; it is active in **post-translational processing**, which is needed for HCV replication.
         (a) Sofosbuvir (NPI) binds to the catalytic site of NS5B, leading to chain termination.
         (b) Dasabuvir (NNPI) is an allosteric inhibitor of NS5B.
   c. ***Adverse effects*** may include headache, fatigue, and GI distress.

G. Agents used for hepatitis B

1. **Lamivudine** is an NRTI (see above) used for hepatitis B virus (**HBV**) infections, providing effective and rapid response in most patients. It is a cytosine analogue that competes with deoxycytidine triphosphate to subsequently **inhibit HBV DNA polymerase**. This agent **slows progression to liver fibrosis**. It has only minor adverse effects at doses used for HBV infections.

2. **Adefovir**
   a. ***Mechanism of action.*** It is a nucleotide analogue that is phosphorylated to its active metabolite. It interferes with HBV viral RNA-dependent DNA polymerase to inhibit viral replication.
   b. ***Indication.*** It is used for the treatment of **HBV**.
   c. ***Adverse effect.*** Dose-related **nephrotoxicity** may occur.
3. **Interferon alpha**
   a. ***Mechanism of action.*** This agent binds to cell membrane receptors to initiate a series of reactions that lead to inhibition of viral activity, including replication.
   b. ***Indications.*** It may be used for both **HBV** and **HCV**.
      (1) Combination with **ribavirin** leads to synergistic effects.
   c. ***Adverse effects*** include an **influenza-like syndrome** after injection, **thrombocytopenia** and **granulocytopenia**, as well as **neuropsychiatric effects.**
4. **Entecavir**
   a. ***Mechanism of action.*** This agent **inhibits HBV DNA polymerase**. It is a nucleoside analogue that is phosphorylated to its active metabolite.
   b. ***Indications.*** It is used for the treatment of HBV infections.
   c. ***Adverse effects.*** It is generally well tolerated with headache and fatigue being the most common effects.
5. **Tenofovir** is also used to treat HBV infections.

H. Other antivirals

1. **Ribavirin**
   a. ***Mechanism of action.*** The mechanism is not clear. It is a guanosine analogue that alters the synthesis of guanosine triphosphate and appears to inhibit capping of the viral messenger RNA and inhibit viral RNA polymerases.
   b. ***Indications.*** Ribavirin is administered as an aerosol to treat respiratory syncytial virus (RSV).
   c. ***Adverse effects.*** It may cause **hemolytic anemia** and is potentially teratogenic.
2. **Palivizumab** is a humanized **monoclonal antibody** directed against the F glycoprotein on the surface of RSV. It is used for the prevention of **RSV** in children and premature infants and children. Adverse effects include respiratory infection, rash, and GI dysfunction.
3. **Imiquimod** is a topical cream used for **anal and genital warts** caused by human papillomavirus. The exact mechanism of action is not well elucidated. Skin reactions are a common effect.

DRUG SUMMARY TABLE

Penicillins
Amoxicillin
Amoxicillin/clavulanate
Ampicillin
Ampicillin/sulbactam
Dicloxacillin
Nafcillin
Oxacillin
Penicillin G
Penicillin G benzathine
Penicillin G procaine
Penicillin V
Piperacillin/tazobactam

Cephalosporins
First generation
Cefadroxil
Cefazolin
Cephalexin
Second generation
Cefaclor
Cefotetan
Cefoxitin
Cefprozil
Cefuroxime
Third generation
Cefdinir
Cefditoren
Cefixime
Cefotaxime
Cefpodoxime
Ceftazidime
Ceftibuten
Ceftriaxone
Fourth generation
Cefepime
Fifth generation
Ceftaroline
Cephalosporin combinations
Ceftazidime/avibactam
Ceftolozane/tazobactam

Carbapenems
Doripenem
Ertapenem
Imipenem–cilastatin
Meropenem
Meropenem and vaborbactam

Monobactam
Aztreonam

Glycopeptides
Dalbavancin
Oritavancin
Telavancin
Vancomycin

Lipopeptide
Daptomycin

Other Cell Wall Inhibitors
Bacitracin
Fosfomycin

Aminoglycosides
Amikacin
Gentamicin
Neomycin
Streptomycin
Tobramycin

(Continued)

Tetracyclines
Demeclocycline
Doxycycline
Minocycline
Tetracycline

Glycylcycline
Tigecycline

Macrolides
Azithromycin
Clarithromycin
Erythromycin
Fidaxomicin
Telithromycin

Oxazolidinones
Linezolid
Tedizolid

Streptogramin
Quinupristin/dalfopristin

Lincosamide
Clindamycin

Miscellaneous Antimicrobials
Chloramphenicol
Metronidazole
Mupirocin
Nitrofurantoin
Polymyxin B

Antifolate Agents
Mafenide
Silver sulfadiazine
Sulfacetamide
Sulfasalazine
Trimethoprim
Trimethoprim/sulfamethoxazole

Pyrimethamine

Fluoroquinolones
Ciprofloxacin
Delafloxacin
Gemifloxacin
Levofloxacin
Moxifloxacin
Norfloxacin
Ofloxacin

Antivirals
Antiherpetic agents
Acyclovir
Cidofovir
Docosanol
Famciclovir
Foscarnet
Ganciclovir
Penciclovir
Trifluridine
Valacyclovir
Valganciclovir
Anti-influenza agents
Amantadine
Oseltamivir
Peramivir
Rimantadine
Zanamivir
Antiretroviral agents
Abacavir
Atazanavir
Darunavir
Delavirdine
Didanosine
Efavirenz
Emtricitabine
Enfuvirtide
Etravirine
Fosamprenavir
Indinavir
Lamivudine
Lopinavir/ritonavir
Maraviroc
Nelfinavir
Nevirapine
Raltegravir
Rilpivirine
Ritonavir
Saquinavir
Stavudine
Tenofovir
Tipranavir
Zidovudine
Combination antiretroviral agents
Abacavir and lamivudine
Abacavir, lamivudine, and zidovudine
Atazanavir and cobicistat
Bictegravir, emtricitabine, and tenofovir alafenamide
Darunavir and cobicistat
Darunavir, cobicistat, emtricitabine, and tenofovir alafenamide
Dolutegravir, abacavir, and lamivudine
Dolutegravir and rilpivirine
Efavirenz, emtricitabine, and tenofovir disoproxil fumarate
Efavirenz, lamivudine, and tenofovir disoproxil fumarate
Elvitegravir, cobicistat, emtricitabine, and tenofovir alafenamide
Elvitegravir, cobicistat, emtricitabine, and tenofovir disoproxil fumarate
Lamivudine and tenofovir disoproxil fumarate
Lopinavir and ritonavir
Rilpivirine, emtricitabine, and tenofovir alafenamide
Rilpivirine, emtricitabine, and tenofovir disoproxil fumarate
Tenofovir alafenamide and emtricitabine
Tenofovir disoproxil fumarate and emtricitabine
Zidovudine and lamivudine
Antihepatitis agents
Adefovir
Daclatasvir
Elbasvir and grazoprevir
Entecavir
Glecaprevir and pibrentasvir
Interferon alpha-2b
Lamivudine
Ledipasvir and sofosbuvir
Ombitasvir, paritaprevir, ritonavir, plus dasabuvir
Pegylated interferon alfa-2b
Simeprevir
Sofosbuvir
Sofosbuvir and velpatasvir
Tenofovir disoproxil fumarate
Velpatasvir
Miscellaneous antiviral agents
Imiquimod
Palivizumab
Ribavirin

Antifungal Agents
Amphotericin B—conventional
Amphotericin B—lipid complex
Amphotericin B—liposomal
Butenafine
Butoconazole
Caspofungin
Clotrimazole
Econazole
Fluconazole
Flucytosine
Griseofulvin
Isavuconazole
Itraconazole
Ketoconazole
Miconazole
Micafungin
Naftifine
Nystatin
Oxiconazole
Posaconazole
Sertaconazole
Sulconazole
Terbinafine
Terconazole
Tioconazole
Tolnaftate
Voriconazole

Antimycobacterial Agents
Capreomycin
Cycloserine
Ethambutol
Ethionamide
Isoniazid
Pyrazinamide
Rifabutin
Rifampin
Rifapentine
Rifaximin

Drugs for *Mycobacterium leprae*
Clofazimine
Dapsone

Antiparasitic Agents
Albendazole
Artemether/lumefantrine
Artesunate[a]
Atovaquone
Atovaquone/proguanil
Chloroquine
Diethylcarbamazine[a]
Eflornithine[a]
Ivermectin
Mebendazole
Mefloquine
Nitazoxanide
Paromomycin
Pentamidine
Praziquantel
Primaquine
Pyrantel pamoate
Quinine
Sodium stibogluconate[a]
Tinidazole

[a]Available from the CDC, WHO, or other distribution programs.

Review Test

Directions: Select the best answer for each question.

1. A 27-year-old man presents to his primary care physician with complaints of a painless ulcer on his penis. The patient admits to having unprotected intercourse 2 weeks prior. Visualization of the lesion by dark-field microscopy demonstrates spirochetes, and he is diagnosed with syphilis. The patient has no known drug allergies. Which of the following medications would be most appropriate for the treatment of this patient?

(A) Bacitracin
(B) Doxycycline
(C) Erythromycin
(D) Penicillin G

2. A 19-year-old man presents to the emergency room with a severe headache, photophobia, and a stiff neck. After a lumbar puncture, the patient is diagnosed with bacterial meningitis. Which of the following cephalosporins is most appropriate for empiric treatment?

(A) Cefazolin
(B) Cefepime
(C) Ceftriaxone
(D) Cefuroxime

3. A 27-year-old woman with a history of intravenous drug abuse is admitted to the hospital for fever and shortness of breath. Multiple blood cultures are positive for *S. aureus* with resistance to methicillin. A transesophageal echocardiogram is positive for tricuspid vegetations consistent with endocarditis. Which of the following is an appropriate antibiotic to treat this condition?

(A) Aztreonam
(B) Ceftriaxone
(C) Gentamicin
(D) Imipenem
(E) Vancomycin

4. A 16-year-old boy presents to his pediatrician with a rash on the palms and soles of his feet as well as fever and headache. His mother reports that a tick bit him while camping the week prior. His Weil–Felix test result is positive, suggesting Rocky Mountain spotted fever. What agent should be given to treat this condition?

(A) Bacitracin
(B) Ciprofloxacin
(C) Doxycycline
(D) Erythromycin
(E) Streptomycin

5. A 27-year-old woman presents to the emergency room with complaints of urinary frequency, urgency, and dysuria. A urinalysis demonstrates bacteria and white blood cells; therefore, she is started on trimethoprim/sulfamethoxazole for empiric treatment. Three days later, she returns with a fever and blisters around, and inside, her mouth and nose. What should be included in the differential diagnosis?

(A) Aplastic anemia
(B) Glucose-6-phosphate dehydrogenase deficiency
(C) Red man syndrome
(D) Stevens–Johnson syndrome

6. A 43-year-old woman with a history of HIV presents to the emergency room with shortness of breath. Laboratory results reveal a $CD4^+$ count of 150, and an arterial blood gas indicates hypoxia. A chest X-ray shows bilateral interstitial infiltrates. The emergency room physician suspects *Pneumocystis jirovecii* pneumonia, which is confirmed with bronchoscopy and silver staining of bronchial washings. Which of the following medications should be started?

(A) Azithromycin
(B) Clindamycin
(C) Isoniazid
(D) Miconazole
(E) Trimethoprim/sulfamethoxazole

7. A 35-year-old woman with a history of type 2 diabetes presents to her primary care physician with fever and dysuria. She is started on a medication that has the potential to cause tendon rupture. What is the mechanism of action for the drug that was started?

(A) Inhibition of bacterial cell wall synthesis
(B) Inhibition of DNA gyrase
(C) Inhibition of RNA synthesis
(D) Inhibition of the 30S ribosome
(E) Inhibition of the 50S ribosome

8. A 35-year-old man presents to his family physician for a physical examination after his mother is diagnosed with tuberculosis (TB). Although a purified protein derivative (PPD) is negative, the physician recommends prophylaxis against TB. Which of the following medications is most appropriate for TB prophylaxis in this patient?

(A) Ethambutol
(B) Isoniazid
(C) Pyrazinamide
(D) Rifampin
(E) Streptomycin

9. A 12-year-old girl with a history of acute lymphoblastic leukemia is admitted to the hospital for a bone marrow transplant. Seven days after her transplant, she develops a fever. Blood cultures reveal a resistant strand of *Candida albicans*, and she is started on appropriate treatment. After her first infusion, the patient develops hypotension, fever, and rigors. The next day, labs reveal that her serum creatinine is increased. Which medication was most likely administered?

(A) Amphotericin B
(B) Fluconazole
(C) Griseofulvin
(D) Micafungin
(E) Nystatin

10. A 23-year-old man with a history of AIDS presents to the emergency room with fever, neck pain, and photophobia. A lumbar puncture is performed and the cerebrospinal fluid is positive for *Cryptococcus neoformans* on India ink stain. Which of the following agents is preferred for the treatment of this condition?

(A) Cycloserine
(B) Flucytosine
(C) Fluconazole
(D) Griseofulvin
(E) Tolnaftate

11. A 23-year-old man is planning to spend a year in Africa to work in the Peace Corps. He is counseled about malaria prevention and is prescribed a medication for chemoprophylaxis, which concentrates in acidic parasite vacuoles and inhibits the activity of heme polymerase. What medication is prescribed for chemoprophylaxis?

(A) Atovaquone
(B) Chloroquine
(C) Doxycycline
(D) Pyrimethamine
(E) Quinine

12. A 14-year-old boy returns from a Boy Scout backpack trip with foul-smelling watery diarrhea. On further questioning, he admits to drinking water from a mountain brook without boiling it first. Stool is sent for ova and parasites. He is eventually diagnosed with a *Giardia lamblia* infection. Which of the following drugs is the most appropriate treatment?

(A) Mebendazole
(B) Metronidazole
(C) Nifurtimox
(D) Suramin
(E) Thiabendazole

13. A 42-year-old man, with a history of myelodysplastic syndrome, presents to the emergency room with mental status changes and a headache. A computed tomography scan is ordered and demonstrates a ring-enhancing lesion. He is started on empiric treatment for a *Toxoplasmosis gondii* abscess. Which agent should be included in his treatment?

(A) Ivermectin
(B) Niclosamide
(C) Praziquantel
(D) Pyrimethamine
(E) Pyrantel pamoate

14. A 23-year-old woman with a history of non-Hodgkin lymphoma presents to the hospital for her next cycle of chemotherapy. A week after treatment, she complains of abdominal pain, bloody diarrhea, and low-grade fevers. Cultures are positive for CMV, and the infectious disease team starts treatment with empiric therapy for CMV colitis. Two days later, the patient requires supplementation with most electrolytes, including potassium. Which medication was most likely started for the treatment of CMV colitis?

(A) Amantadine
(B) Docosanol
(C) Foscarnet
(D) Ganciclovir
(E) Trifluridine

15. A 23-year-old woman presents to an appointment with her obstetrician after she discovers that she is 6 weeks pregnant. The patient has a history of HIV and is concerned about the potential consequences. The doctor counsels her about a medication that may be used to decrease the risk of transmission to the unborn child. What is the mechanism of action for this medication?

(A) CCR5 antagonist
(B) Fusion inhibitor
(C) Integrase strand transfer inhibitor
(D) Nucleoside reverse transcriptase inhibitor
(E) Protease inhibitor

Answers and Explanations

1. **The answer is D.** Patients with primary syphilis require a single intramuscular dose of benzathine penicillin G. Oral preparations of penicillin G or penicillin V are insufficient. Doxycycline for 14 days is an alternative treatment in penicillin-allergic patients. Bacitracin is indicated only for topical use and insufficient for syphilis. Erythromycin is not indicated for syphilis.
2. **The answer is C.** Ceftriaxone is a third-generation cephalosporin that has excellent CNS penetration. Most third-generation cephalosporins enter the CNS. The first- and second-generation agents, cefazolin and cefuroxime, respectively, do not enter the CNS. There are limited data on the effectiveness of cefepime in meningitis.
3. **The answer is E.** Vancomycin is the drug of choice for serious infections due to methicillin-resistant *S. aureus* (MRSA). In the case of endocarditis, the treatment is usually 6 weeks. The resistance of MRSA is often due to altered penicillin-binding proteins, not β-lactamases. Aztreonam, imipenem, and ceftriaxone do not treat MRSA. Gentamicin is often used in conjunction with penicillins in a non-MRSA setting.
4. **The answer is C.** Doxycycline, a tetracycline (30S ribosome inhibitor), is the antibiotic of choice to treat Rocky Mountain spotted fever, a rickettsial disease. Streptomycin can be used to treat plague and brucellosis. Bacitracin is used only topically. Ciprofloxacin can be used to treat anthrax, and erythromycin is the most effective drug for the treatment of Legionnaires disease.
5. **The answer is D.** Stevens–Johnson syndrome is a form of erythema multiforme, rarely associated with sulfonamide use. Signs and symptoms may include fever and a red or purple rash that spreads. The rash is often painful and may cause blisters on mucous membranes, such as the mouth, nose, and genital areas. Patients with glucose-6-phosphate dehydrogenase deficiency are at risk of developing hemolytic anemia. Red man syndrome is associated with vancomycin.
6. **The answer is E.** Trimethoprim/sulfamethoxazole not only is the treatment for *Pneumocystis jirovecii* pneumonia but should also be considered for prophylaxis in patients undergoing immunosuppressive therapy or with HIV. Azithromycin can be of use in *Mycobacterium avium-intracellulare* (MAC complex). Isoniazid is used for tuberculosis (TB). Miconazole is an antifungal used for vulvovaginal candidiasis.
7. **The answer is B.** The patient was most likely started on a fluoroquinolone, such as ciprofloxacin, a group of antibiotics that inhibit bacterial topoisomerase II (DNA gyrase). Fluoroquinolones cause an increased risk of tendon rupture. The antibiotic classes that inhibit the 30S ribosome include aminoglycosides and tetracycline. Inhibitors of the 50S ribosome include chloramphenicol, erythromycin, and clindamycin. Bacterial cell wall inhibitors include penicillins, cephalosporins, and vancomycin. Rifampin inhibits DNA-dependent RNA polymerase (RNA synthesis).
8. **The answer is B.** Isoniazid can be used alone for the prophylaxis of tuberculosis (TB) in the case of such exposure. All the other agents are important in the treatment of a known TB infection and are often used in combination with isoniazid. Often rifampin, ethambutol, streptomycin, isoniazid, and pyrazinamide are used for months together, as many strains are multidrug resistant.
9. **The answer is A.** Amphotericin B is used in the treatment of severe disseminated candidiasis. It often causes severe adverse effects, which is why its use is reserved for more resistant infections. Adverse effects may include fevers and chills on infusion and nephrotoxicity. Toxicity has been decreased with liposomal preparations. Nystatin is used as a "swish and swallow" treatment for oral candidiasis. Micafungin and fluconazole are used for the treatment of candidiasis but do not cause nephrotoxicity and infusion-related reactions. Griseofulvin is a topical agent used in dermatophyte infections.

10. **The answer is C.** Fluconazole is the best agent to treat cryptococcal meningitis and has good central nervous system (CNS) penetration. Flucytosine penetrates the CNS and is often used with other antifungals, as resistance to flucytosine commonly develops. Tolnaftate and griseofulvin are topical agents used in dermatophyte infections. Cycloserine is an alternative drug used for mycobacterial infections, is nephrotoxic, and causes seizures.

11. **The answer is B.** The patient was most likely prescribed chloroquine, which concentrates in acidic parasite vacuoles, raising their pH. It also inhibits the activity of heme polymerase, which converts host hemoglobin toxic by-products to nontoxic polymerized material. For malaria prophylaxis, it is used weekly.

12. **The answer is B.** Metronidazole is used to treat protozoal infections due to *Giardia*, *Entamoeba*, and *Trichomonas* species. Nifurtimox is used to treat Chagas disease (due to *Trypanosoma cruzi*). Suramin is used to treat African trypanosomiasis. Mebendazole is used to treat roundworm infections, and thiabendazole is used to treat *Strongyloides* infection.

13. **The answer is D.** Toxoplasmosis is treated with a combination of pyrimethamine and sulfadiazine. Ivermectin is used to treat filariasis, whereas praziquantel is used to treat schistosomiasis. Niclosamide can be used to treat tapeworm infections, and pyrantel pamoate is used to treat many helminth infections.

14. **The answer is C.** Foscarnet is indicated for the treatment of CMV infections. Adverse effects include electrolyte wasting and nephrotoxicity. In most cases, electrolytes need to be supplemented during foscarnet therapy. Ganciclovir is used for the treatment of CMV but does not have the same adverse effect profile; it causes neutropenia. The other agents are not used for the management of CMV.

15. **The answer is D.** Zidovudine is the only agent approved to prevent fetal transmission of HIV as it crosses the placenta. It is a non-nucleoside reverse transcriptase inhibitor that causes chain termination, which decreases viral DNA synthesis and virus replication.

Chapter 12

Cancer Chemotherapy

Competency Addressed: PH1.49

I. PRINCIPLES OF CANCER CHEMOTHERAPY

A. General principles for cancer and antineoplastic therapy

1. Cancers **arise from a single mutated cell**. As the tumor grows, it develops more mutations, where it becomes more **heterogeneous** and more difficult to treat.
   a. The greater the tumor burden, the more difficult it is to treat; therefore, early treatment is critical.
2. **Metastasis** occurs when cancer cells **break away from the location of the primary cancer** and travel through the blood or lymphatic system to form new tumors in other parts of the body.
   a. Metastatic cancer has the same name and the same type of cancer cells as the original, or primary, cancer. For example, breast cancer that spreads to the lung is not considered lung cancer (it is considered breast cancer).
3. The **growth fraction** is the **proportion** of cells in a tumor population that are **actively dividing**.
   a. Most cancers have a **high growth fraction**.
   b. Slow-growing tumors with a small growth fraction are less responsive to cell cycle–specific (CCS) drugs.
4. The **log-cell kill model** states that cell destruction caused by chemotherapy is a **first-order process**, in which each dose of chemotherapy **kills a constant fraction of malignant cells** rather than a constant number.
5. There are many different sites of action for cancer chemotherapeutic drugs (Fig. 12.1).
6. Cancer treatment now engages many **modalities**, which may be used either used alone or in combination:
   a. Cytotoxic chemotherapy
   b. Hormonal therapy
   c. Immunotherapy
   d. Targeted therapy
   e. Surgery
   f. Radiotherapy
7. Multimodality approach to cancer treatment
   a. **Adjuvant chemotherapy:** Cytotoxic chemotherapy follows surgery and/or radiotherapy to eliminate the remaining cancer cells.
   b. **Neoadjuvant chemotherapy:** Cytotoxic chemotherapy is administered prior to surgery, to reduce the size of a large tumor for ease of surgical resection.
8. Many malignancies cannot be cured; however, with the recent use of a multimodality approach, survival has been prolonged. Hence, palliative treatment of pain/symptom control and treatment of adverse effects like vomiting and myelosuppression are equally important.

B. The cell cycle (Fig. 12.2)

1. Many chemotherapy drugs act only on cells that are actively reproducing; they do not kill cells that are in the resting phase (G_0).

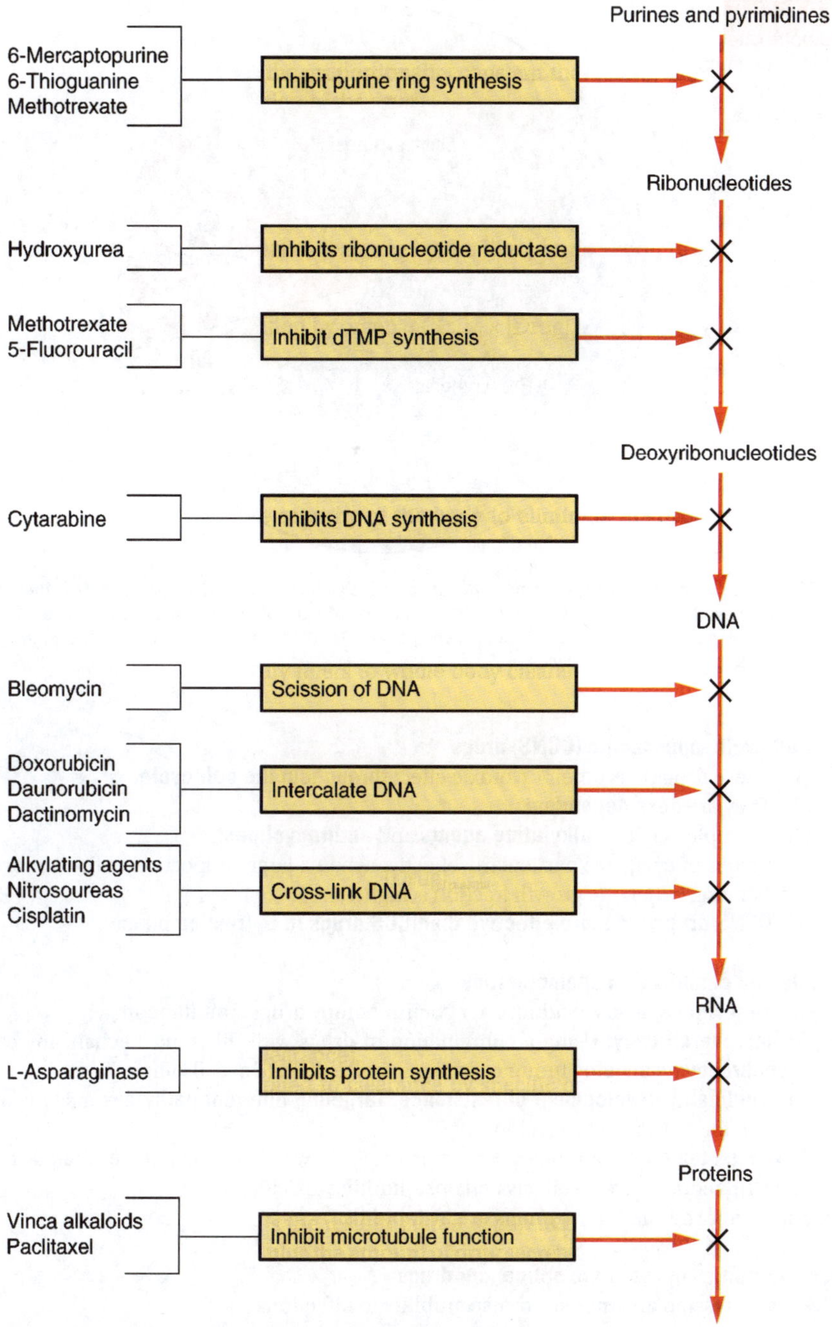

FIGURE 12.1. Sites of action for cancer chemotherapeutic drugs.

2. Cancer drugs can be divided into two general classes:

a. CCS drugs

(1) These drugs are toxic to the proportion of cells in the part of the cell cycle in which the agent is active.

(2) Examples include **antimetabolites (S phase), taxanes (M phase),** and **vinca alkaloids (M phase)**. (Fig. 12.2).

(3) They are **schedule dependent** and are generally more effective when given as a longer, or continuous, infusion.

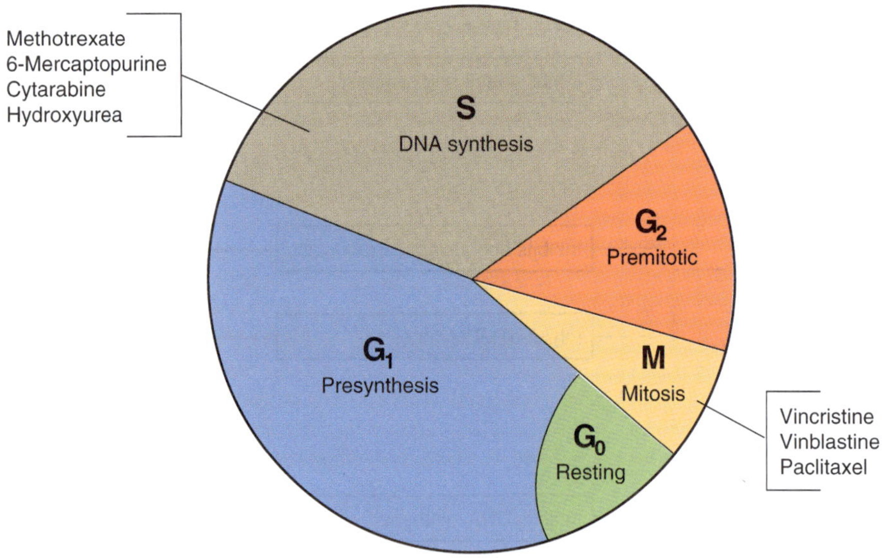

FIGURE 12.2. Cell cycle specificity of some antitumor drugs. *S* is the phase of DNA synthesis; G_2 is the premitotic phase for synthesis of essential components for mitosis; *M* is the phase of mitosis in which cell division occurs; G_1 is the phase for synthesis of essential components for DNA synthesis; G_0 is a "resting" phase that cells may enter when they do not divide.

- **b. Cell cycle–nonspecific (CCNS) drugs**
  - **(1)** These drugs exert their cytotoxic effect **throughout the cell cycle**.
  - **(2)** They are **dose dependent**.
  - **(3)** Examples include **alkylating agents** and **anthracyclines**.
- **c.** Both types of drugs are particularly effective when a large proportion of the tumor cells are proliferating (when the growth fraction is high).
  - **(1) CCNS drugs are more effective than CCS drugs in G_0 (resting phase).**

C. Principles for combination chemotherapy

1. There are several reasons to administer chemotherapy drugs simultaneously.
   - **a. To improve efficacy:** Using a combination of drugs with different mechanisms can **target asynchronously dividing** tumor cells to maximize the rate of cell killing.
   - **b. To avoid/delay development of resistance: Targeting different pathways** may make it more difficult for resistance to develop.
   - **c. To reduce toxicity:** Combination regimens may allow for the use of **lower drug doses**, which can help reduce adverse effects and dose-limiting toxicities.
2. Examples of combination regimens are in Table 12.1.

D. General toxicities of cytotoxic anticancer drugs

1. Myelosuppression and increased susceptibility to infections
2. Damage to gastrointestinal (GI) mucosa
3. Nausea and vomiting
4. Alopecia
5. Impaired wound healing
6. Carcinogenicity
7. Sterility
8. Teratogenicity

E. Resistance

1. Resistance may occur due to the inability of chemotherapeutic agents to reach sufficient "kill" levels in certain tissues (e.g., brain, ovaries, testes).

TABLE 12.1 Examples of Common Combination Regimens

Acronym	Drugs Combined	Indication
ABVD	Adriamycin (doxorubicin), bleomycin, vinblastine, dacarbazine	Hodgkin lymphoma
BEP	Bleomycin, etoposide, platinum (cisplatin)	Testicular
CHOP	Cyclophosphamide, hydroxydaunorubicin (doxorubicin), vincristine, prednisone	Non-Hodgkin lymphoma
CAF	Cyclophosphamide, Adriamycin (doxorubicin), 5-FU	Breast
CMF	Cyclophosphamide, methotrexate, 5-FU	Breast
FOLFOX	5-FU, oxaliplatin, leucovorin	Colorectal
MOPP	Mechlorethamine, vincristine, prednisone, procarbazine	Hodgkin lymphoma
MVAC	Methotrexate, vinblastine, Adriamycin, cisplatin	Bladder
R-CHOP	Rituximab, cyclophosphamide, hydroxydaunorubicin (doxorubicin), vincristine, prednisone	Non-Hodgkin lymphoma
PVB	Platinum (cisplatin), vinblastine, bleomycin	Testicular
VAD	Vincristine, Adriamycin (doxorubicin), dexamethasone	Multiple myeloma

5-FU, 5-fluorouracil.

2. ***Primary resistance***
   a. Primary resistance is seen in tumor cells that **do not respond to initial therapy**.
   b. It is related to the **frequency of spontaneous mutation**.
   c. There is less likelihood that a small tumor burden has resistant cells.
3. ***Acquired resistance***
   a. Acquired resistance **develops or appears during therapy.**
   b. Acquired resistance can result from the **amplification of target genes.**
   c. Gene amplification also occurs in the **multidrug resistance phenotype** (*MDR1*).
4. ***Mechanisms for drug resistance***
   a. **Reduced intracellular concentration** of a drug can occur through several methods; this results in an insufficient amount of drug to reach the target. It can occur by the following:
      (1) **Preventing uptake of a drug**; for example, decreased methotrexate (MTX) entry may occur due to decreased expression of the reduced folate carrier.
      (2) **Promoting efflux of a drug**; for example, classical **multidrug resistance (MDR)** occurs as a consequence of increased expression of drug efflux pumps such as P-glycoprotein or MDR-associated proteins. This causes resistance to many drug classes including **taxanes**, **anthracyclines**, and **vinca alkaloids** (Table 12.2).
      (3) Drugs may also be inactivated (or prodrugs may not be activated).

TABLE 12.2 The Multidrug Resistance (*MDR*) Gene: Drug Specificity and Tissue Distribution

Drugs Affected by *MDR*	Drugs Not Affected by *MDR*
Adriamycin	Methotrexate
Daunomycin	6-Thioguanine
Dactinomycin	Cytarabine
Plicamycin	Cyclophosphamide
Etoposide	BCNU
Vinblastine	Bleomycin
Vincristine	Cisplatin
VP-16	
Tissues with High *MDR* Expression	**Tissues with Low *MDR* Expression**
Colon	Bone marrow
Liver	Breast
Pancreas	Ovary
Kidney	Skin
Adrenal	Central nervous system

b. **Target-based mechanisms** can cause drug resistance through **altered drug transport** or **bypassing metabolic requirements** for the drug target.
   (1) An example is the expression of a mutant dihydrofolate reductase (DHFR), which alters the drug target for MTX, preventing it from binding.
c. Some mutations in proteins cause **insensitivity to apoptosis**.
   (1) For example, mutations in key proteins associated with control of apoptosis, such as **p53** and **Bcl-2**, can result in failure to induce the apoptotic response to DNA damage and can thereby reduce the sensitivity of tumor cells to anticancer drugs.
   (2) The p53 protein is crucial in multicellular organisms, where it regulates the cell cycle and functions as a tumor suppressor. Loss of activity of p53 commonly occurs in pancreatic, lung, and colon cancers.
d. **Cellular repair of drug effect** is another mechanism for drug resistance.

II. ALKYLATING AGENTS

A. General characteristics of alkylating agents

1. ***Mechanism of action***
   a. Cytotoxicity from alkylating agents results from directly damaging DNA, including inhibition of DNA replication and transcription, mispairing of DNA, and strand breakage.
      (1) They have an **electrophilic center** that becomes covalently linked to the nucleophilic centers of target molecules.
      (2) Most agents target the **nitrogens** and **oxygens of purines and pyrimidines** in DNA. This may lead to abnormal DNA strand cross-links.
      (3) They **directly damage DNA** to prevent cancer cells from reproducing.
   b. They are CCNS agents and **work in all phases** of the cell cycle.
2. ***Adverse effects***
   a. The dose-limiting adverse effect is **myelosuppression**.
   b. **Carcinogenesis:** Since they damage DNA, they may cause long-term damage to the bone marrow and can lead to **secondary leukemia**.
   c. **Nausea and vomiting** are common adverse effects of alkylating agents.
   d. They are also highly toxic to dividing mucosal cells, causing oral and **GI ulcers**.
   e. They may cause **infertility** and **alopecia**.

B. Nitrogen mustards

1. ***Specific agents*** include **cyclophosphamide** and **ifosfamide**.
2. ***Mechanism of action.*** These agents are **prodrugs** and require activation by hepatic cytochrome **P450 enzymes** before being metabolized to their respective cytotoxic species, phosphoramide mustard and ifosfamide mustard. They cause cross-linking within DNA strands, thus preventing replication.
3. ***Indications***
   a. Cyclophosphamide is a component of many combination treatments for a variety of cancers, such as non-Hodgkin lymphoma, breast carcinoma, and ovarian carcinoma. It is also used in certain autoimmune conditions, such as lupus nephritis.
   b. Ifosfamide is used for the treatment of various cancers as well, including non-Hodgkin lymphoma, testicular cancer, and sarcoma.
4. ***Adverse effects***
   a. Myelosuppression is common.
   b. **Hemorrhagic cystitis** may occur due to **acrolein**, a by-product of the activation of cyclophosphamide or ifosfamide.
      (1) This is characterized by **diffuse bladder mucosal inflammation with hemorrhage** involving the entire bladder. Symptoms may occur such as bladder pain, irritative bladder symptoms, and blood in urine.
      (2) It can be **prevented** by coadministration of the sulfhydryl compound 2-mercaptoethanesulfonate **(mesna)**, which complexes with acrolein to form a nontoxic product eliminated in urine. Ample hydration is also important.

c. Ifosfamide can cause encephalopathy, which may include symptoms of confusion, hallucinations, or blurred vision.

C. Alkyl sulfonate

1. ***Specific agent.*** **Busulfan.**
2. ***Indications.*** It is used in the conditioning regimen (in combination with cyclophosphamide) prior to allogeneic hematopoietic progenitor cell transplantation for chronic myeloid leukemia (CML).
3. ***Adverse effects***
   a. Busulfan causes severe myelosuppression.
   b. In high doses, it produces a rare but sometimes fatal **pulmonary fibrosis.**
   c. It has been associated with skin **hyperpigmentation**.

D. Nitrosoureas

1. ***Specific agents*** include **carmustine** and **lomustine**.
2. ***Mechanism of action.*** These agents are highly lipophilic and **cross the blood–brain barrier**. They require biotransformation, which occurs by **nonenzymatic decomposition**, to metabolites with both alkylating and carbamoylating activities.
3. ***Indications.*** Since they **cross the blood–brain barrier**, they are useful for the treatment of brain tumors.
4. ***Adverse effects***
   a. These agents are markedly **myelosuppressive** but with **delayed effect**, possibly up to 6 weeks.
   b. They can also cause **pulmonary toxicity** and central nervous system (CNS) toxicity, including ataxia and dizziness.

E. Platinum analogues

1. ***Specific agents*** include **cisplatin**, **carboplatin**, and **oxaliplatin**.
2. ***Indications***
   a. Cisplatin and carboplatin are used to treat various types of cancer, including lung, ovarian, bladder, and testicular cancer.
   b. Oxaliplatin is used to treat colorectal cancer.
3. ***Adverse effects***
   a. **Cisplatin** can cause dose-limiting **nephrotoxicity** and **peripheral neuropathy**.
      (1) **Amifostine** can help reduce the cumulative renal toxicity associated with repeated administration of cisplatin in patients with advanced ovarian cancer.
         (a) Its active metabolite detoxifies reactive metabolites of cisplatin.
         (b) It can also act as a scavenger of free radicals that may be generated (by cisplatin or radiation therapy) in tissues; therefore, it is also indicated to reduce xerostomia in patients with head and neck cancer.
   b. **Cisplatin is known to cause severe nausea and vomiting.**
   c. **Carboplatin** causes dose-limiting **myelosuppression**.
   d. Both **cisplatin** and **carboplatin** can cause **ototoxicity**, which may manifest as tinnitus or hearing loss in high-frequency range.
   e. **Oxaliplatin** may cause two types of dose-limiting **peripheral sensory neuropathy**.
      (1) The first type is an acute presentation, which is reversible. Peripheral symptoms are often exacerbated by cold; therefore, exposure to cold temperatures or cold food and beverages should be avoided.
      (2) The second type is dose dependent and often interferes with activities of daily living, such as buttoning a shirt, writing, or even swallowing.

III. ANTIMETABOLITES

A. General characteristics of antimetabolites

1. Antimetabolites are often **structurally related to naturally occurring compounds** found in the body (amino acids, DNA, RNA).

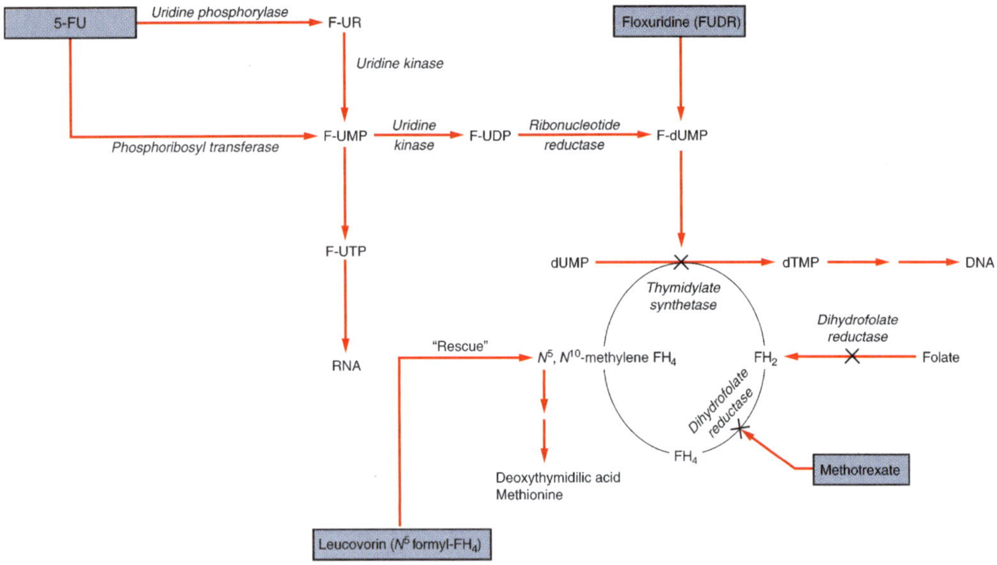

FIGURE 12.3. Mechanism of action of fluorouracil, floxuridine, methotrexate, and leucovorin. 5-FU, 5-fluorouracil; dUMP, deoxyuridine monophosphate; FH_2, dihydrofolate; FH_4, tetrahydrofolate.

2. They usually exert damage to DNA by competing for binding sites on enzymes or incorporating directly into DNA or RNA. The net effect is inhibition of cell growth and proliferation.
3. Generally, these agents induce cell death in the **S phase** of the cell cycle.
4. **Myelosuppression** is the dose-limiting toxicity for most drugs in this class.

B. Methotrexate

1. ***Mechanism of action.*** MTX is a **folic acid analogue** that irreversibly binds to and **inhibits DHFR**, thereby inhibiting the formation of reduced folates and thymidylate synthetase (Fig. 12.3).
   a. It reduces the pool of tetrahydrofolate required for the conversion of deoxyuridine monophosphate (dUMP) to deoxythymidylic acid (dTMP), and consequently, N^5,N^{10}-methylenetetrahydrofolate is not formed.
   b. The net result is **indirect inhibition of DNA synthesis**.
2. ***Indications.*** MTX has many different indications. It is used for the treatment of **acute lymphoblastic leukemia (ALL)** in children. It is also useful for the treatment of different types of leukemia and lymphoma in adults, as well as for the management of a variety of **immune disorders**, including **refractory rheumatoid arthritis** and Crohn disease.
3. ***Adverse effects***
   a. Common adverse effects of MTX include **myelosuppression** and GI toxicity, including **mucositis**.
   b. **Nephrotoxicity** may occur at high doses because of precipitation (crystalluria) of the 7-OH metabolite of MTX.
   c. Long-term use may lead to hepatotoxicity and pulmonary toxicity.
4. ***Leucovorin rescue*** with high-dose MTX (Fig. 12.3)
   a. Leucovorin (folinic acid) is a reduced form of folic acid. It **supplies the necessary cofactor blocked by MTX** and **restores active folate stores** required for DNA/RNA synthesis.
   b. It is used to reduce the toxic effects of high-dose MTX.
5. ***Precautions***
   a. Clearance of MTX is delayed in the presence of **third-space fluids**, such as **pleural effusions or ascites**.
6. ***Drug interactions***
   a. Some Non-steroidal anti-inflammatory drugs (NSAIDs) like aspirin may decrease renal excretion of MTX.

C. Pemetrexed

1. ***Mechanism of action.*** The primary action of pemetrexed is **inhibition of thymidylate synthetase**, although it also inhibits other enzymes involved in folate metabolism and DNA synthesis. These actions result in inhibition of purine and thymidine nucleotide and protein synthesis.
2. ***Indications.*** It is approved for the treatment of **mesothelioma** and **non–small cell lung cancer (NSCLC)**.
3. ***Adverse effects***
   - **a.** The dose-limiting side effect is **myelosuppression.**
   - **b.** It has the potential to cause mucositis and **severe cutaneous reactions.** Pretreatment with dexamethasone is necessary to prevent dermatologic toxicity.
   - **c.** Supplementation with folic acid and vitamin B_{12} may reduce the severity of toxicities.

D. 5-Fluorouracil (5-FU) and capecitabine

1. ***Mechanism of action.*** 5-FU is a **pyrimidine antagonist** that must be converted to an active metabolite. 5-Fluoro-2′-deoxyuridine-5′-monophosphate (F-dUMP) inhibits **thymidylate synthetase** and thus the production of dTMP and DNA. Fluorouridine monophosphate (F-UMP) is incorporated into RNA to replace uracil and inhibit cell growth. Capecitabine is the oral prodrug of fluorouracil that undergoes hydrolysis in the liver and tissues to form fluorouracil (Fig. 12.3).
2. ***Indications***
   - **a.** These agents are used in the treatment of colorectal cancer and breast cancer.
   - **b.** 5-FU is also used in pancreatic and gastric cancer.
   - **c.** Topical 5-FU is used to treat premalignant keratosis and superficial basal cell carcinomas.
3. ***Adverse effects***
   - **a.** Both agents cause **myelosuppression** and GI toxicity.
   - **b.** They have the potential to cause **hand-and-foot syndrome**, which is characterized by **numbness**, **paresthesias**, tingling, swelling, and **erythema.** They may also lead to blistering and severe pain.
   - **c.** 5-FU may cause neurotoxicity.
   - **d.** Capecitabine may cause hyperbilirubinemia.

E. Cytarabine

1. ***Mechanism of action.*** Cytarabine is a structural analogue of the pyrimidine nucleoside, cytidine. It must undergo conversion to the triphosphate nucleotide (Ara-CTP), which then acts as competitive inhibitor of DNA polymerase, resulting in decreased DNA synthesis and repair.
2. ***Indications.*** It is used for the management of various types of leukemia, including **acute myelogenous leukemia** (AML).
3. ***Adverse effects***
   - **a.** It is highly **myelosuppressive** and can produce severe leukopenia, thrombocytopenia, and anemia.
   - **b.** It can also produce severe GI disturbances.
   - **c.** At high doses, cytarabine can cause **cerebellar toxicity**.

F. Gemcitabine

1. ***Mechanism of action.*** Gemcitabine is a **pyrimidine antagonist** that inhibits DNA synthesis via chain termination and other mechanisms.
2. ***Indications.*** It is used for the treatment of pancreatic cancer, NSCLC, breast cancer, and ovarian cancer.
3. ***Adverse effects.*** **Myelosuppression** is the main dose-limiting effect.

G. 6-Mercaptopurine (6-MP) and 6-thioguanine

1. ***Mechanism of action***
   - **a.** 6-MP and 6-thioguanine are **purine antagonists** (analogues of hypoxanthine and guanine, respectively). They act as false metabolites and are incorporated into DNA and RNA to eventually inhibit synthesis.

2. ***Pharmacologic properties***
   a. ***6-MP*** is metabolized to an **inactive metabolite** by **xanthine oxidase.**
      (1) In the presence of a xanthine oxidase inhibitor, such as allopurinol, the dose must be decreased significantly to avoid drug toxicity.
3. ***Indications***
   a. 6-MP is useful in the treatment of ALL.
   b. 6-Thioguanine is used to treat ALL and AML.
4. ***Adverse effects***
   a. **Myelosuppression** is the dose-limiting toxicity.
   b. Hepatotoxicity and GI distress may also occur.

H. Cladribine

1. ***Mechanism of action.*** Cladribine is a **purine antagonist**. The active form, 5'-triphosphate derivative (2-CaAMP), incorporates into DNA to result in the breakage of DNA strand and prevent DNA synthesis and repair. It also results in the depletion of nicotinamide adenine dinucleotide and adenosine triphosphate (ATP). It is CCNS.
2. ***Indications.*** This agent is used for **hairy cell leukemia**.
3. ***Adverse effects.*** Cladribine is transiently myelosuppressive. It may also cause neurotoxicity and nephrotoxicity.

IV. MICROTUBULE DAMAGING AGENTS

A. Vinca alkaloids

1. ***Specific agents*** include **vinblastine**, **vincristine**, and vinorelbine.
2. ***Mechanism of action***
   a. Vinca alkaloids interfere with microtubule assembly and block cells in mitosis by **inhibiting microtubule polymerization**.
   b. They bind to tubulin and inhibit microtubule formation and disrupt formation of the mitotic spindle.
   c. These agents are most active during mitosis at **metaphase (M phase)**, blocking chromosomal migration and cell division.
3. ***Indications***
   a. Vincristine and vinblastine are used for various types of cancer, including lymphoma.
   b. Vinorelbine is used for NSCLC.
4. ***Adverse effects***
   a. **Vinblastine** and **vinorelbine** cause dose-limiting **myelosuppression**.
   b. **Vincristine** can cause dose-limiting **peripheral neuropathy**, which may manifest as paresthesias, or even lead to bilateral foot drop. It can also cause **constipation** or paralytic ileus.
   c. They are potent **vesicants**, in which leakage of these drugs out of a vein into the tissue may cause blistering or lead to tissue necrosis.

B. Taxanes

1. ***Specific agents*** include **paclitaxel**, **docetaxel**, and cabazitaxel.
2. ***Mechanism of action.*** These agents bind to and **stabilize microtubules** by **enhancing tubulin polymerization** (inhibit microtubule depolymerization); this arrests cells in mitosis and eventually leads to apoptosis. They interfere with the late G_2 and mitotic phases of the cell cycle.
3. ***Indications***
   a. Paclitaxel is used in breast cancer, ovarian cancer, and NSCLC.
   b. Docetaxel is used in breast cancer, prostate cancer, and NSCLC.
   c. Cabazitaxel is used for prostate cancer.
4. ***Adverse effects***
   a. **Myelosuppression** is the dose-limiting toxicity. They also cause **peripheral neuropathy**.
   b. **Paclitaxel** causes **hypersensitivity** reactions due to the vehicle in which it is solubilized; premedications are required.
   c. **Docetaxel** causes **fluid retention** and peripheral edema; premedications are required.

V. TOPOISOMERASE INHIBITORS

A. General characteristics of topoisomerase inhibitors

1. ***Actions of topoisomerase***
   a. Regulation of DNA supercoiling is essential to transcription and replication.
   b. Topoisomerase is an enzyme that alters the supercoiling of double-stranded DNA. It cuts one or both strands of the DNA to relax the coil and extend the DNA molecule.
2. ***Mechanism of action***
   a. Topoisomerase inhibitors **bind to topoisomerase I or topoisomerase II.**
   b. They stabilize the cleavable complex so that religation of the cleaved DNA strand cannot occur, which results in the accumulation of cleavable complexes and **single- or double-strand DNA breaks that are never repaired.** This leads to cell death.
      (1) Topoisomerase I inhibitors cause single-strand DNA breaks.
      (2) Topoisomerase II inhibitors cause double-strand DNA breaks.

B. Camptothecins: Topoisomerase I inhibitors

1. ***Specific agents*** include **topotecan** and **irinotecan.**
2. ***Indications.*** Topotecan is used for ovarian cancer. Irinotecan is used for colorectal cancer.
3. ***Adverse effects***
   a. Both agents can cause **secondary leukemia.**
   b. **Topotecan** can cause dose-limiting **myelosuppression.**
   c. **Irinotecan** can cause **early and late forms of diarrhea.**
      (1) The **early form** occurs within the **first 24 hours** of treatment. It is thought to be a **cholinergic effect** and can be treated with **atropine.**
      (2) The **delayed form** is due to the release of an active metabolite, SN-38, which induces direct mucosal damage with water and electrolyte malabsorption and mucus hypersecretion. It can be life threatening and should be treated with **loperamide.**
4. ***Precautions***
   a. SN-38 is metabolized by UDP-glucuronosyltransferase 1A1 (UGT1A1) to form an inactive metabolite. Patients with abnormalities in this enzyme (Gilbert syndrome) are highly susceptible to irinotecan toxicity.

C. Epipodophyllotoxins: Topoisomerase II inhibitors

1. ***Specific agent.*** **Etoposide (VP-16).**
2. ***Indications*** include small cell lung cancer, testicular cancer, and lymphoma.
3. ***Adverse effects*** include dose-limiting **myelosuppression** (primarily leukopenia). It can also cause hypotension with rapid administration and must be infused slowly.

VI. ANTITUMOR ANTIBIOTICS

A. General characteristics of antitumor antibiotics

1. These drugs are isolated from various strains of the soil microbe *Streptomyces.*

B. Anthracyclines

1. ***Specific agents*** include **doxorubicin, daunorubicin,** idarubicin, and epirubicin.
2. ***Mechanism of action***
   a. These agents **inhibit topoisomerase II** and prevent religation of DNA during replication, causing DNA strand breaks.
   b. They also form **intercalations between DNA base pairs,** causing additional DNA breaks.
   c. They are metabolized in the liver to form **oxygen free radicals,** which adds to the cytotoxicity (and adverse effects).
3. ***Indications.*** These agents are used for various types of cancer, including leukemia, lymphoma, breast cancer, and ovarian cancer.

4. ***Adverse effects***
   a. Anthracyclines can cause dose-limiting **myelosuppression** (primarily leukopenia).
   b. They can also cause dose-limiting **cardiotoxicity.**
      (1) The acute form may occur immediately after a single dose. It is uncommon and transient. It may lead to arrhythmias or, more rarely, pericarditis.
      (2) The **chronic form** is **dose dependent** and is more common.
         (a) Its onset is usually within a year of receiving anthracycline therapy, although it can occur several years after therapy.
         (b) It may be life threatening and can lead to **dilated cardiomyopathy associated with heart failure.**
         (c) The exact mechanism is unknown, but it may be the result of increased production of free radicals within the myocardium.
      (3) **Dexrazoxane** is a cardioprotectant that is a potent intracellular chelating agent. It interferes with iron-mediated oxygen free radical generation.
5. ***Precaution***
   a. These agents may cause red or orange discoloration of the urine.

C. Dactinomycin

1. ***Mechanism of action.*** Dactinomycin binds to the guanine portion of DNA intercalating between base pairs. It inhibits DNA and RNA synthesis.
2. ***Indications.*** It is often used in **pediatric cancers**, such as Wilms tumor, Ewing sarcoma, or rhabdomyosarcoma.
3. ***Adverse effects*** may include nausea and vomiting, myelosuppression, and hepatotoxicity.
4. ***Precautions.*** It is a potent **vesicant** and may lead to extravasation without correct catheter placement.

D. Bleomycin

1. ***Mechanism of action.*** Bleomycin binds to DNA producing single- and double-strand DNA breaks through the generation of **oxygen free radicals.**
2. ***Indications*** include **testicular cancer** and Hodgkin lymphoma.
3. ***Adverse effects.*** **Pulmonary toxicity**, such as pulmonary fibrosis, is the dose-limiting toxicity. It can also cause **hyperpigmentation** of the skin.
4. ***Precautions.*** Although rare, it may cause severe idiosyncratic reaction, which may lead to hypotension, fever, chills, wheezing, and confusion.

VII. MISCELLANEOUS ANTINEOPLASTIC AGENTS

A. Hydroxyurea

1. ***Mechanism of action.*** Hydroxyurea inhibits **ribonucleoside diphosphate reductase** (during the S phase of the cell cycle), which catalyzes the conversion of ribonucleotides to deoxyribonucleotides and is crucial for the **synthesis of DNA.**
2. ***Indications.*** It is primarily used in the management of **chronic granulocytic leukemia** and other myeloproliferative disorders. It is also used for the management of **sickle cell anemia**.
3. ***Adverse effects*** include **myelosuppression** and **GI distress.**

B. L-Asparaginase

1. ***Mechanism of action.*** L-Asparaginase is an enzyme that catalyzes the deamidation of asparagine to aspartic acid and ammonia. It helps decrease circulating levels of asparagine. Leukemia cells are unable to synthesize asparagine; this agent results in cytotoxicity by **reducing the exogenous asparagine source** for those cells.
2. ***Indication.*** This agent is used for the treatment of **ALL**.
3. ***Adverse effects***
   a. This agent may be toxic to the liver and pancreas.
   b. **Hypersensitivity** and anaphylactic shock to the protein may develop.
   c. Hemorrhaging may occur due to the inhibition of clotting factor synthesis.

C. Bortezomib

1. ***Mechanism of action.*** Bortezomib **inhibits the 26S proteasome and downregulates the nuclear factor kappa B (NF-κB) signaling pathway**; this leads to cell cycle arrest and apoptosis.
2. ***Indication.*** It is approved for the treatment of **multiple myeloma.**
3. ***Adverse effects*** include GI distress and **peripheral neuropathy.**

D. Tretinoin (all-*trans* retinoic acid [ATRA])

1. ***Mechanism of action.*** Tretinoin binds to one or more nuclear receptors. It decreases proliferation and **induces differentiation of acute promyelocytic leukemia** (APL) cells. It initially produces maturation of primitive promyelocytes and repopulates the marrow and peripheral blood with normal hematopoietic cells to achieve complete remission.
2. ***Indication.*** It is used to treat APL.
3. ***Adverse effects*** include **differentiation syndrome** (formerly called retinoic acid–APL syndrome), signs and symptoms of which may include fever, dyspnea, edema, and the potential for multiorgan failure. Treatment includes administration of glucocorticoids (dexamethasone). It can also cause **leukocytosis** due to a rapid maturation of a large mass of leukemic cells. It may result in **leukostasis.**

VIII. TARGETED THERAPY

A. Sites of action for targeted agents

1. Targets for small molecule compounds, such as tyrosine kinase inhibitors, are typically located inside the cell. These agents enter cells relatively easily.
2. Since monoclonal antibodies are relatively large and cannot enter cells, their targets are outside cells or on the cell surface.

B. Monoclonal antibodies

1. **Rituximab**
   a. ***Mechanism of action.*** Rituximab is a chimeric (human/mouse) **antibody to IgG** directed against the **CD20 antigen on B lymphocytes.** This leads to cell lysis, possibly secondary to antibody-dependent cytotoxicity or complement-dependent cytotoxicity.
   b. ***Indications.*** This agent is used for the treatment of **CD20-positive non-Hodgkin lymphoma** and **CD20-positive chronic lymphocytic leukemia.** It is also indicated for the management of rheumatoid arthritis.
   c. ***Adverse effects***
      (1) Rituximab may cause GI distress and neutropenia.
      (2) It can cause **infusion-related reactions** that may include fever, chills, and hypotension. Premedications are required.
   d. ***Precautions***
      (1) It can cause **mucocutaneous reactions**, such as Stevens–Johnson syndrome or toxic epidermal necrolysis.
      (2) **Hepatitis B reactivation** may occur.
      (3) Progressive multifocal leukoencephalopathy (PML) due to an infection from the John Cunningham (JC) virus has been reported.
2. **Brentuximab vedotin**
   a. ***Mechanism of action.*** Brentuximab vedotin is an antibody drug conjugate **directed at CD30** that contains a **microtubule-disrupting agent** (MMAE). It binds to cells that express CD30 and forms a complex, which is internalized. MMAE is released and binds to the tubules to induce cell cycle arrest and apoptosis.
   b. ***Indications*** include **Hodgkin lymphoma** and anaplastic large cell lymphoma.
   c. ***Adverse effects*** include **peripheral neuropathy**, neutropenia, and infusion-related reactions.
   d. ***Precautions.*** PML and Stevens–Johnson syndrome have been reported.

3. **Trastuzumab**
   a. ***Mechanism of action.*** Trastuzumab is a humanized IgG antibody against the **human epidermal growth factor receptor 2 (HER2) protein**. It mediates antibody-dependent cellular cytotoxicity by inhibiting proliferation of cells that overexpress the HER2 protein.
   b. ***Indications.*** This agent is used in treating **HER2-positive breast cancer** and **HER2-positive gastric cancer.**
   c. ***Adverse effects***
      (1) Diarrhea, rash, myelosuppression, and infusion reactions may occur.
      (2) **Cardiomyopathy** is a dose-limiting toxicity, in which trastuzumab may be associated with reductions in left ventricular ejection fraction and heart failure.
4. **Cetuximab**
   a. ***Mechanism of action.*** Cetuximab is a chimeric human–mouse IgG antibody that binds to the **epidermal growth factor receptor (EGFR)**. It competitively inhibits the binding of epidermal growth factor and other ligands, blocking activation. This results in inhibition of cancer cell growth and induction of apoptosis.
   b. ***Indications.*** Cetuximab is used in the management of **KRAS wild-type, EGFR-expressing metastatic colorectal cancer** (as determined by approved tests). It is also used in treatment of squamous cell cancer of the head and neck.
   c. ***Adverse effects.*** It can cause GI distress and a **rash** that may be severe.
5. **Bevacizumab**
   a. ***Mechanism of action.*** Vascular endothelial growth factor (VEGF) normally initiates angiogenesis. Bevacizumab is a recombinant humanized monoclonal antibody that **prevents VEGF-A from binding** to target VEGF receptors. This causes **inhibition of microvascular growth**, which is believed to retard the growth of all tissues, including metastatic tissue.
   b. ***Indications.*** This agent is used in the management of colorectal cancer, NSCLC, and renal cell cancer.
   c. ***Adverse effects***
      (1) **Hypertension** is a dose-limiting toxicity.
      (2) Its use has been associated with **thrombotic events**, including myocardial infarction (MI), pulmonary embolism (PE), and deep vein thrombosis (DVT).
   d. ***Precautions***
      (1) Bevacizumab has been associated with **GI perforation, wound healing complications,** and **hemorrhage**.
6. **Ipilimumab**
   a. ***Mechanism of action.*** Cytotoxic T-lymphocyte–associated antigen 4 (CTLA-4) is a downregulator of T-cell activation pathways. Ipilimumab is a recombinant human IgG1 monoclonal antibody that **binds to CTLA-4**, which allows for enhanced **T-cell activation and proliferation**. It may indirectly enhance and mediate T-cell immune responses against tumors.
   b. ***Indications.*** It is used for the treatment of **melanoma** and renal cell carcinoma.
   c. ***Adverse effects*** include GI distress and rash.
   d. ***Precautions.*** This agent may cause severe and **fatal immune-mediated reactions**, including enterocolitis, hepatitis, dermatitis (including toxic epidermal necrolysis), neuropathy, and endocrinopathy. Any organ system may be involved. Close monitoring is essential.

C. Tyrosine kinase inhibitors

1. **Imatinib**, dasatinib, nilotinib, and ponatinib
   a. ***Mechanism of action.*** These agents **inhibit the BCR–ABL tyrosine kinase**. Inhibition blocks proliferation and promotes apoptosis in BCR–ABL-positive cell lines. They also inhibit platelet-derived growth factor (PDGF) and c-Kit.
   b. ***Indications.*** They are used for the treatment of **Philadelphia chromosome-positive (Ph+)** CML and ALL and c-Kit-positive GI stromal tumors.
      (1) The Ph+ chromosome **[t(9;22)(q34;q11)]** results in the formation of a unique gene product (BCR–ABL), which is a constitutively active tyrosine kinase.

c. ***Adverse effects*** may include **peripheral edema**, nausea and vomiting, and **elevated transaminases.** They may also cause dose-limiting myelosuppression.

d. ***Drug interactions.*** Imatinib, dasatinib, and nilotinib are major substrates of CYP3A4; therefore, inhibitors or inducers of CYP3A4 should be used with caution.

2. **Gefitinib** and **erlotinib**

a. ***Mechanism of action.*** These agents are inhibitors of **EGFR tyrosine kinase** that is overexpressed in many types of cancer.

b. ***Indications.*** They are approved for use in EGFR-positive metastatic NSCLC. Erlotinib is also used in pancreatic cancer.

c. ***Adverse effects*** include GI distress, **acne**, and rash.

d. ***Drug interactions.*** These agents are major substrates of CYP3A4; therefore, inhibitors or inducers of CYP3A4 should be used with caution.

3. **Vemurafenib**

a. ***Mechanism of action.*** Vemurafenib is a **BRAF kinase inhibitor**. It inhibits tumor growth in melanomas by inhibiting kinase activity of certain mutated forms of BRAF (V600E mutation).

b. ***Indication.*** It is used for the treatment of unresectable or metastatic **melanoma** in patients with a **BRAFV600E mutation**.

c. ***Adverse effects*** may include rash, arthralgia, and QT prolongation.

d. ***Precautions.*** It may cause **photosensitivity** and **squamous cell carcinoma**.

D. Immunomodulators

1. **Thalidomide** and **lenalidomide**

a. ***Mechanism of action.*** These agents have immunomodulatory, antiangiogenic, and antineoplastic effects through various mechanisms.

(1) Both agents **inhibit secretion of proinflammatory cytokines**, such as tumor necrosis factor-alpha.

(2) They **enhance cell-mediated immunity** by increasing interleukin-2 and interferon-gamma secretion.

(3) They cause immune modulation (increase T-helper cells).

b. ***Indications.*** Both agents can be used for the treatment of **multiple myeloma**. Lenalidomide is also used in the treatment of mantle cell lymphoma and myelodysplastic syndrome.

c. ***Adverse effects*** include **hematologic toxicity** (neutropenia and thrombocytopenia). Thalidomide can cause constipation and **peripheral neuropathy**.

d. ***Precautions***

(1) Both agents are associated with an increased risk of arterial and venous **thromboembolic events**, including MI, DVT, and PE.

(2) These agents should **not be taken during pregnancy**; they may cause severe **birth defects** or **embryo–fetal death**.

IX. CORTICOSTEROIDS

Mechanism, adverse effects, and other properties of corticosteroids are covered in Chapter 10. Their use in malignancy is considered here.

1. ***Specific agents*** include **prednisone** and **dexamethasone.**
2. They are **lymphocytic** and **antimitotic** agents.
3. These agents are useful in treating acute leukemia in children, malignant lymphoma, and both Hodgkin and non-Hodgkin lymphoma.
4. They also alleviate some adverse effects of anticancer drugs and are used as adjuvants in treating chemotherapy-induced vomiting.
5. Corticosteroids have significant systemic effects, and their long-term use is not recommended.

X. HORMONE THERAPY

A. Selective estrogen receptor modulators

1. ***Specific agents*** include **tamoxifen**, toremifene, and **raloxifene**.
2. ***Mechanism of action***
   a. Selective estrogen receptor modulators (SERMs) are drugs that have estrogen receptor (ER) agonist or antagonist properties depending on the target tissue.
   b. In the **breast**, all three agents have **antiestrogenic activity**.
      (1) They inhibit estrogen-dependent cellular proliferation and may increase the production of the growth inhibitor, transforming growth factor-beta (TGF-β).
3. ***Indications***
   a. Tamoxifen and toremifene are used in **hormone receptor–positive breast cancer treatment**.
   b. Tamoxifen and raloxifene are used for **risk reduction** for women at a high risk of breast cancer.
   c. **Raloxifene** can also be used for **osteoporosis** due to its estrogenic activity in bone.
4. ***Adverse effects*** may include **hot flashes**. Toremifene can cause QT prolongation.
5. ***Precautions***
   a. **Tamoxifen** has estrogenic activity in the endometrium and can increase the risk for **endometrial cancer**.
   b. These agents also carry the risk for **thromboembolic events**.

B. Estrogen receptor antagonist

1. ***Specific agent.*** **Fulvestrant**.
2. ***Mechanism of action.*** Fulvestrant **competitively binds to the ER** on tumors. The nuclear complex causes a dose-related downregulation of ERs and **blocks the action of estrogen** to inhibit tumor growth.
3. ***Indication.*** It is approved for **hormone-positive breast cancer** in postmenopausal females who have progressed on tamoxifen.
4. ***Adverse effects*** may include **hot flashes** and increased liver enzymes.

C. Aromatase inhibitors

1. ***Specific agents***
   a. Competitive inhibitors: **Anastrozole**, letrozole
   Noncompetitive inhibitor: Exemestane
2. ***Mechanism of action***
   a. Aromatase is the enzyme that catalyzes the final step in the production of estrogens from androgenic precursors within the ovary or in peripheral tissues.
   b. It is responsible for the conversion of adrenal androgens and gonadal androstenedione and testosterone to the estrogens, estrone, and estradiol, respectively.
   c. These agents **inhibit the aromatase enzyme** and **prevent the conversion of androstenedione to estrone and testosterone to estradiol**.
   d. They decrease tumor mass and delay tumor progression.
3. ***Indications.*** These agents are used for the treatment of **breast cancer** in postmenopausal females.
4. ***Adverse effects*** may include **decreased bone mineral density**, hot flashes, and nausea. Anastrozole and letrozole may cause **hypercholesterolemia**.
5. ***Precautions***
   a. Anastrozole may increase the risk for ischemic cardiovascular events in patients with preexisting ischemic cardiac disease.
   b. These agents **do not benefit premenopausal women**.

D. Gonadotropin-releasing hormone (GnRH) agonists

1. ***Specific agents*** include **leuprolide**, triptorelin, **goserelin**, and histrelin.
2. ***Mechanism of action***
   a. These agents are potent inhibitors of gonadotropin secretion.
   b. Long-term administration results in the **suppression of luteinizing hormone (LH)** and **follicle-stimulating hormone (FSH)** secretion from the pituitary.
   c. This leads to a **subsequent decrease in levels of testosterone, dihydrotestosterone**, and **estrogen**.

- **d.** The use of these agents results in **castration levels of testosterone** in men and **postmenopausal levels of estrogen** in women.

3. ***Indications***
   - **a.** All agents are used in the management of **advanced prostate cancer.**
   - **b.** Goserelin can be used for the management of advanced breast cancer.
   - **c.** Leuprolide, triptorelin, and histrelin can be used for central precocious puberty.
   - **d.** Leuprolide and goserelin are indicated for endometriosis; leuprolide is also approved for the treatment of uterine fibroids.
4. ***Adverse effects*** may include **hot flashes**, **gynecomastia**, **sexual dysfunction**, and decreased bone mineral density.
5. ***Precautions***
   - **a. Tumor flare. Initial administration** of these agents, before pituitary receptor desensitization occurs, may result in **increased LH and FSH release,** with a **transitory increase in testosterone** and an **exacerbation of disease.**
     - **(1)** They are often administered with the antiandrogens (**flutamide, bicalutamide**, or **nilutamide**), which **block the translocation of androgen receptors to the nucleus** and thereby prevent testosterone action.
     - **(2)** Tumor flare can also occur in patients with breast cancer, due to an increase in estrogen.
   - **b.** Androgen-deprivation therapy (ADT) may increase the risk for cardiovascular disease, including MI, sudden cardiac death, and stroke.

E. Gonadotropin-releasing hormone antagonist

1. ***Specific agent.*** **Degarelix.**
2. ***Mechanism of action.*** It **blocks GnRH receptors** to **decrease secretion** of **LH** and **FSH**. This results in **rapid androgen deprivation** by decreasing testosterone production. It acts more quickly than GnRH agonists.
3. ***Indication.*** It is used for the treatment of **advanced prostate cancer.**
4. ***Adverse effects*** may include **hot flashes**, weight gain, increased liver enzymes, and decreased bone mineral density.
5. ***Precautions.*** ADT may increase the risk for cardiovascular disease, including MI, sudden cardiac death, and stroke. It does not cause tumor flare.

F. Androgen synthesis inhibitors

1. ***Specific agents*** include **abiraterone** and ketoconazole.
2. ***Mechanism of action***
   - **a.** CYP17 (17α-hydroxylase and 17,20-lyase) is required for androgen biosynthesis. **Inhibiting CYP17 will inhibit the formation of the testosterone precursors.**
   - **b.** Abiraterone selectively and irreversibly inhibits CYP17.
   - **c.** Ketoconazole also inhibits CYP17 but is less specific.
3. ***Indications.*** These agents can be used for **metastatic castration-resistant prostate cancer.** Ketoconazole is an antifungal agent that is used off-label for this indication.
4. ***Adverse effects***
   - **a.** Abiraterone may cause edema and fatigue.
   - **b.** Ketoconazole may cause nausea and vomiting and skin rash.
5. ***Precautions***
   - **a.** Both agents carry the risk of **hepatotoxicity** and adrenocortical insufficiency.

G. First-generation antiandrogens

1. ***Specific agents*** include **flutamide**, bicalutamide, and nilutamide.
2. ***Mechanism of action.*** These agents **inhibit the binding of androgens to the androgen receptor.** They **block testosterone effects** at the androgen receptor and prevent testosterone stimulation of cell growth in prostate cancer.
3. ***Indications.*** They are used for the treatment of **advanced prostate cancer** in combination with GnRH agonist or surgical castration.
4. ***Adverse effects*** are due to decreased androgen activity and include fatigue, gynecomastia, **loss of libido**, and **impotence**.

5. ***Precautions***
   a. Flutamide may cause hepatic failure.
   b. Nilutamide may cause interstitial pneumonitis.
   c. ADT may increase the risk for cardiovascular disease, including MI, sudden cardiac death, and stroke.

H. Second-generation antiandrogen

1. ***Specific agent.*** **Enzalutamide**.
2. ***Mechanism of action.*** This agent is a **pure androgen receptor signaling inhibitor**. It inhibits androgen receptor nuclear translocation, DNA binding, and coactivator mobilization, which leads to cellular apoptosis and decreased prostate tumor volume.
3. ***Indication.*** It is used in **metastatic castration-resistant prostate cancer**.
4. ***Adverse effects*** may include fatigue, hot flashes, back pain, and **seizures**.
5. ***Precautions***
   a. Enzalutamide may cause **impaired male fertility**.
   b. ADT may increase the risk for cardiovascular disease, including MI, sudden cardiac death, and stroke.

DRUG SUMMARY TABLE

Alkylating Agents
Busulfan
Carboplatin
Carmustine
Chlorambucil
Cisplatin
Cyclophosphamide
Dacarbazine
Ifosfamide
Lomustine
Mechlorethamine
Melphalan
Oxaliplatin
Procarbazine
Streptozocin
Temozolomide
Thiotepa

Antimetabolites
5-Fluorouracil
6-Mercaptopurine
6-Thioguanine
Capecitabine
Cladribine
Cytarabine
Floxuridine
Fludarabine
Gemcitabine
Methotrexate
Pemetrexed

Microtubule Damaging Agents
Vinca alkaloids
Vinblastine
Vincristine
Vinorelbine
Taxanes
Cabazitaxel
Docetaxel
Nab-paclitaxel
Paclitaxel

Topoisomerase Inhibitors
Etoposide
Irinotecan
Topotecan

Antitumor Antibiotics
Bleomycin
Dactinomycin
Daunorubicin
Doxorubicin
Epirubicin
Idarubicin
Mitomycin
Mitoxantrone
Valrubicin

Monoclonal Antibodies
Bevacizumab
Brentuximab vedotin
Cetuximab
Ipilimumab
Panitumumab
Rituximab
Trastuzumab

Tyrosine Kinase Inhibitors
Dasatinib
Erlotinib
Gefitinib
Imatinib
Nilotinib
Pazopanib
Sorafenib
Vemurafenib

Immunomodulators
Interferon alfa-2b
Lenalidomide
Thalidomide

Miscellaneous Antineoplastic Agents
Aldesleukin
Asparaginase
Bortezomib
Hydroxyurea
Megestrol
Mitotane
Tretinoin (all-*trans* retinoic acid [ATRA])

Selective Estrogen Receptor Modulators
Raloxifene
Tamoxifen
Toremifene

Estrogen Receptor Antagonist
Fulvestrant

Aromatase Inhibitors
Anastrozole
Letrozole
Exemestane

Gonadotropin-Releasing Hormone Antagonist
Degarelix

Gonadotropin-Releasing Hormone Agonist
Leuprolide
Goserelin
Histrelin
Triptorelin

Antiandrogens
Bicalutamide
Enzalutamide
Flutamide
Nilutamide

Adjunct Agents
Allopurinol
Amifostine
Darbepoetin alfa
Dexrazoxane
Epoetin alfa
Filgrastim
Mesna
Leucovorin
Pegfilgrastim
Sargramostim

Review Test

Directions: Select the best answer for each question.

1. A 64-year-old man is admitted to the hospital for the management of non-Hodgkin lymphoma. He did not respond to his first round of treatment and is now started on the RICE chemotherapy regimen, which includes rituximab, ifosfamide, carboplatin, and etoposide. The next day, the patient complains of a sudden onset of hematuria and bladder pain. Which of the following medications may have prevented this patient presentation?

(A) Amifostine
(B) Dexrazoxane
(C) Filgrastim
(D) Leucovorin
(E) Mesna

2. A 21-year-old man starts the VIP regimen (etoposide, ifosfamide, cisplatin, mesna) for the treatment of metastatic testicular cancer. The regimen also includes ondansetron for the prevention of nausea and vomiting. Three days into the first cycle, the patient complains of ringing in his ears and difficulty hearing. The oncologist is concerned that the patient may be experiencing an adverse effect due to one of the medications. Which of the following medications caused this patient's symptoms?

(A) Cisplatin
(B) Etoposide
(C) Ifosfamide
(D) Mesna
(E) Ondansetron

3. A 53-year-old woman is started on the hyper-CVAD regimen (cyclophosphamide, vincristine, doxorubicin, dexamethasone, methotrexate, cytarabine) for the treatment of acute lymphoblastic leukemia. The nurse is required to administer leucovorin to reduce the potential for dangerous adverse effects from one of the chemotherapy agents. What is the mechanism of action for the medication that requires leucovorin administration?

(A) Blocks chromosomal migration and cell differentiation
(B) Carbamylate intracellular macromolecules
(C) Complexes with DNA to form cross-links
(D) Indirectly inhibits DNA synthesis
(E) Inhibits topoisomerase

4. A 53-year-old man presents with changes in bowel frequency and pencil-thin stools with occasional bright red blood in his stool. Further evaluation leads to a diagnosis of colon cancer with metastasis in the liver. His oncologist starts him on a topoisomerase I inhibitor that has the potential to cause severe diarrhea. Which of the following agents was prescribed?

(A) 5-Fluorouracil
(B) Carmustine
(C) Epirubicin
(D) Irinotecan
(E) Vincristine

5. A 53-year-old woman with breast cancer undergoes a breast-conserving lumpectomy and lymph node biopsy. Following radiation therapy, a chemotherapy regimen is started that includes paclitaxel. Which adverse effect may the patient experience due to this drug?

(A) Arrhythmias
(B) Hematuria
(C) Hot flashes
(D) Peripheral neuropathy
(E) Shortness of breath

6. A 74-year-old man with a 100-pack/year history of smoking is evaluated for hemoptysis. A computed tomography (CT) scan of the chest shows numerous pulmonary nodules. The patient undergoes a CT-guided biopsy, which is positive for small cell carcinoma of the lung. He is started on a chemotherapy regimen that includes a topoisomerase II inhibitor. Which of the following medications has this mechanism of action?

(A) Busulfan
(B) Capecitabine
(C) Etoposide
(D) Topotecan
(E) Vinorelbine

7. A 56-year-old woman is diagnosed with stage IV metastatic breast cancer. Her oncologist starts her on a chemotherapy regimen that includes a drug that may cause dose-dependent cardiomyopathy associated with heart failure. What is the mechanism of action for this particular agent?

(A) Activates complement-dependent cytotoxicity
(B) Inhibits dihydrofolate reductase
(C) Inhibits thymidylate synthetase
(D) Inhibits topoisomerase II
(E) Promotes microtubule assembly

8. A 32-year-old man is diagnosed with metastatic testicular cancer with lesions in both his lung and brain. He is a professional cyclist and refuses the standard treatment after he learns that it may compromise his pulmonary function. Which of the following drugs may cause this complication?

(A) Bleomycin
(B) Cisplatin
(C) Cyclophosphamide
(D) Topotecan
(E) Vinorelbine

9. A 35-year-old man presents to his physician with complaints of fullness in the inguinal region. A computed tomography (CT) scan demonstrates several confluent enlarged lymph nodes. Biopsy specimens demonstrate malignant CD20-positive B cells. He is diagnosed with diffuse large B-cell lymphoma. Which of the following agents will likely be effective for the treatment of his cancer?

(A) Bevacizumab
(B) Brentuximab
(C) Ipilimumab
(D) Rituximab
(E) Trastuzumab

10. A 17-year-old girl sees her physician for swollen lymph nodes in the supraclavicular region. A core biopsy demonstrates Reed–Sternberg cells and fibrotic bands, a finding characteristic of nodular sclerosis Hodgkin disease. She is started on a medication that targets CD30-positive cancer cells and inhibits microtubule polymerization. What is a potential adverse effect of this medication?

(A) Arrhythmias
(B) Gastrointestinal perforation
(C) Peripheral neuropathy
(D) Photosensitivity
(E) Thrombotic event

11. A 63-year-old postmenopausal woman is diagnosed with early stage estrogen receptor–positive breast cancer, which is initially managed by partial mastectomy and radiation therapy. Her oncologist also prescribes a medication to prevent relapse. Which of the following medications was prescribed?

(A) Anastrozole
(B) Carboplatin
(C) Goserelin
(D) Hydroxyurea
(E) Leuprolide

12. A 56-year-old man complains of fatigue and malaise. On physical examination, he has significant splenomegaly. His white blood cell count is dramatically elevated, and the physician suspects leukemia. Chromosomal studies indicate a (9:22) translocation, the Philadelphia chromosome, confirming the diagnosis of chronic myelocytic leukemia (CML). Which of the following might be used in his treatment?

(A) Amifostine
(B) Anastrozole
(C) Gefitinib
(D) Imatinib
(E) Rituximab

13. A 37-year-old man presents with changes in bowel habits for the last several months. He complains of narrow stools along with occasional blood in his stool. After further evaluation, including a colonoscopy, he is diagnosed with stage IV colon cancer with metastatic lesions in his liver. The oncologist recommends the use of a medication that blocks signaling by vascular endothelial growth factor. What is a common side effect of this medication?

(A) Cardiomyopathy
(B) Hypertension
(C) Hepatitis
(D) Neuropathy
(E) Photosensitivity

14. A 54-year-old woman is diagnosed with chronic myeloid leukemia. She also has a history of gout, for which she takes allopurinol. Her hematologist would like to start chemotherapy within the next couple of days. A significant dose reduction is required for one of the chemotherapy agents due to a drug interaction that prevents its metabolism. Which of the following drugs will require a large dose reduction?

(A) Capecitabine
(B) Cisplatin
(C) Fluorouracil
(D) Mercaptopurine
(E) Thalidomide

15. A 63-year-old man with a history of prostate cancer presents to his oncologist with complaints of back pain. Laboratory tests reveal that his prostate-specific antigen levels are increased, and a computed tomography scan reveals enlarged para-aortic lymph nodes and osteoblastic lesions of his lumbar spine. Therapy with which agent should be started?

(A) Anastrozole
(B) Leuprolide
(C) Mitotane
(D) Prednisone
(E) Tamoxifen

16. A 56-year-old woman with a history of pancreatic cancer presents to her oncologist with complaints of pain, swelling, and tingling in her feet. She told her doctor that it began shortly after she went for a long walk. Her physical examination is positive for plantar erythema that looks like a sunburn. What chemotherapy agent most likely caused this patient presentation?

(A) 5-Fluorouracil
(B) Etoposide
(C) Irinotecan
(D) Thalidomide
(E) Vinorelbine

17. A 42-year-old premenopausal woman undergoes a partial mastectomy and radiation therapy for stage II estrogen receptor–positive breast cancer. After completing the treatment, her oncologist explains that there is little advantage to adding systemic chemotherapy in such an early stage cancer and recommends treatment with tamoxifen. Which of the following is a concerning side effect of this medication?

(A) Aplastic anemia
(B) Bowel perforation
(C) Hypotension
(D) Myelosuppression
(E) Thromboembolism

18. A 73-year-old woman with an advanced, incurable cancer requests therapy to improve quality of life by symptom control. Which of the following modalities would be most suitable for her?

(A) Adjuvant therapy
(B) Neoadjuvant therapy
(C) Cytotoxic chemotherapy
(D) Palliative therapy
(E) Targeted therapy

Answers and Explanations

1. **The answer is E.** The patient may be experiencing hemorrhagic cystitis due to ifosfamide therapy. Symptoms of hemorrhagic cystitis usually occur within 48 hours of treatment and may include hematuria (blood in the urine), pain, and trouble voiding. It occurs due to acrolein, a by-product of the activation of ifosfamide. The drug sodium 2-mercaptoethanesulfonate (mesna) has been used to prevent hemorrhagic cystitis. Mesna forms a complex with the terminal methyl group of acrolein; it forms a nontoxic thioether that is rapidly removed from the urinary tract. The other medications do not prevent the incidence of hemorrhagic cystitis.
2. **The answer is A.** The patient is most likely experiencing ototoxicity due to cisplatin therapy. Symptoms of ototoxicity may include tinnitus or loss of high-frequency hearing and, occasionally, deafness. The other medications do not cause ototoxicity.
3. **The answer is D.** Methotrexate requires leucovorin administration when it is given at high doses. It inhibits the enzyme dihydrofolate reductase, which ultimately decreases the availability of thymidylate to produce DNA. Nitrosoureas can carbamylate intracellular molecules. Vinca alkaloids, such as vinblastine, block chromosomal migration and cellular differentiation. Cisplatin works primarily by complexing with DNA to form cross-links. Agents like etoposide can inhibit topoisomerase.
4. **The answer is D.** Irinotecan is a topoisomerase I inhibitor indicated for the management of colorectal cancer. It has the potential to cause life-threatening diarrhea. The diarrhea can occur in an early phase (within the first 24 hours of chemotherapy), which can be treated with atropine, or in a late phase (more than 24 hours after chemotherapy), which can be treated with loperamide. The other agents are not topoisomerase inhibitors. While diarrhea is a common side effect of many chemotherapy agents, it can be much more severe with irinotecan.
5. **The answer is D.** Common adverse effects of paclitaxel include myelosuppression and peripheral neuropathy. The neuropathy usually manifests as numbness and tingling in the distal extremities. Hematuria, or blood in the urine, can indicate hemorrhagic cystitis, a complication of cyclophosphamide use. Arrhythmias may occur with acute cardiac toxicity due to anthracycline therapy. Hot flashes are a common complaint in patients using tamoxifen. Shortness of breath can result from pulmonary fibrosis secondary to busulfan or bleomycin use.
6. **The answer is C.** Etoposide is used in the treatment of small cell lung carcinomas as well as testicular tumors. Its mechanism of action is related to its ability to inhibit topoisomerase II. Busulfan is an alkylating agent. Capecitabine is an antimetabolite. Topotecan is a topoisomerase I inhibitor. Vinorelbine is a vinca alkaloid that inhibits microtubule polymerization.
7. **The answer is D.** Anthracyclines, such as doxorubicin, are associated with dose-limiting cardiomyopathy. Before using this agent, a thorough cardiac evaluation is required, including an echocardiogram or nuclear medicine scan of the heart. Anthracyclines have several different mechanisms. They inhibit topoisomerase II and prevent religation of DNA during replication. In addition, they also form intercalations between base pairs and cause cytotoxicity through the formation of oxygen free radicals.
8. **The answer is A.** Bleomycin is included in the treatment of metastatic testicular neoplasms and can cause pulmonary fibrosis. The other agents do not cause pulmonary dysfunction.
9. **The answer is D.** Rituximab is a monoclonal antibody directed against the CD20 antigen on B lymphocytes. It can be used for the management of CD20-positive non-Hodgkin lymphoma or CD20-positive chronic lymphocytic leukemia. Bevacizumab is a monoclonal antibody that prevents vascular endothelial growth factor (VEGF-A) from interacting with the target receptors. Brentuximab vedotin is a monoclonal antibody directed at CD30. Ipilimumab is a monoclonal antibody that causes CTLA-4 inhibition, allowing T-cell proliferation. Trastuzumab is a monoclonal antibody that binds to the human epidermal growth factor receptor 2 (HER2) protein.

10. **The answer is C.** Brentuximab vedotin is a monoclonal antibody directed at CD30. It is used in the treatment of Hodgkin lymphoma and anaplastic large cell lymphoma. Common adverse effects may include peripheral neuropathy, neutropenia, and infusion-related reactions. It does not normally cause the other adverse effects listed.

11. **The answer is A.** Anastrozole is an aromatase inhibitor used to inhibit estrogen synthesis in the adrenal gland, a principal source in postmenopausal women. It is used for the treatment of breast cancer. Hydroxyurea is used in the treatment of some leukemias as well as myeloproliferative disorders. Leuprolide and goserelin are GnRH antagonists used to treat prostate cancer. Carboplatin is used in the treatment of ovarian cancer.

12. **The answer is D.** Imatinib is an orally active small molecule inhibitor of the oncogenic BCR–ABL kinase produced as a result of the Philadelphia chromosome. It is used to treat CML. Anastrozole is used in the management of breast cancer. Rituximab is an antibody used in the treatment of non-Hodgkin lymphoma. Gefitinib is an orally active small molecule inhibitor of the EGF receptor used in the treatment of some lung cancers. Amifostine is used as a radioprotectant with or without cisplatin.

13. **The answer is B.** Bevacizumab is a monoclonal antibody against vascular endothelial growth factor (VEGF) interaction with its receptor. Adverse effects may include hypertension, thrombotic events, decreased wound healing, and gastrointestinal perforation. The other adverse effects listed are not commonly caused by bevacizumab.

14. **The answer is D.** 6-Mercaptopurine (6-MP) is a structural analogue of guanine that is incorporated into DNA to prevent purine synthesis. It is metabolized to an inactive metabolite by xanthine oxidase. Allopurinol is a xanthine oxidase inhibitor and prevents the metabolism of 6-MP to its active metabolite. Significant dose reductions (up to 75%) are required for 6-MP when it is given in combination with xanthine oxidase inhibitors like allopurinol.

15. **The answer is B.** Leuprolide is used to treat metastatic prostate cancer by decreasing the secretion of luteinizing hormone (LH) and follicle-stimulating hormone (FSH) from the pituitary, leading to decreased testosterone (which is used by the tumor cells to grow). Anastrozole is used in breast cancer in postmenopausal women to decrease estrogen levels. Tamoxifen is also used in the treatment of breast cancer to inhibit estrogen-mediated gene transcription. Mitotane is used in the treatment of inoperable adrenocortical carcinomas. Prednisone is used in the treatment of leukemias and lymphomas.

16. **The answer is A.** The patient most likely has hand–foot syndrome, a dose-limiting toxicity of 5-fluorouracil (5-FU). This syndrome is characterized by paresthesias in a sock-and-glove distribution. It occurs when small amounts of drug leak out of capillaries in the palms of the hands and soles of the feet. Exposure to heat and friction increases the amount of drug in the capillaries and increases the amount of drug leakage. Signs and symptoms may include redness, numbness, tenderness, and possibly peeling of the palms and soles. The other agents listed do not cause hand–foot syndrome.

17. **The answer is E.** Patients with estrogen receptor–positive tumors benefit from tamoxifen adjunct treatment. It carries a risk of thromboembolism, as well as the potential to develop endometrial cancer. Bevacizumab has been associated with the risk of bowel perforation. Alkylating agents and topoisomerase I inhibitors may cause secondary leukemia and myelosuppression. Many of the therapeutic monoclonal antibodies can cause hypotension due to infusion-related reactions.

18. **The answer is D.** Patients with incurable cancer are best treated with palliative care, to reduce pain and for symptom control. A clear risk–benefit assessment is needed and the risk of drug toxicity is justified only if there is a realistic expectation of cure or substantial prolongation of life.

Chapter 13

Miscellaneous

Competencies Addressed: PH1.51–PH1.53, PH1.58

I. PRINCIPLES AND TERMINOLOGY

A. Toxicology

Toxicology is concerned with the deleterious effects of physical and chemical agents (including drugs) in humans (Table 13.1).

1. ***Occupational toxicology*** is concerned with chemicals encountered in the workplace.
2. ***Environmental toxicology*** is concerned with substances encountered in food, air, water, and soil.
3. ***Ecotoxicology*** is concerned with the toxic effects of physical and chemical agents on populations and organisms in a defined ecosystem.
   a. For many of these agents (air pollutants and solvents), the **threshold limit values** (TLVs) are defined in either parts per million (ppm) or milligrams per cubic meter (mg/m^3) (Table 13.2). These limits are described as follows:
      (1) **Time-weighted averages (TLV-TWA)** reflect concentrations for a workday or workweek.
      (2) **Short-term exposure limits (TLV-STEL)** reflect the maximum concentration that should not be exceeded in a 15-minute interval.
      (3) **Ceilings (TLV-C)** are the concentrations to which a worker should never be exposed.
      (4) Some chemicals that enter the food chain are defined in terms of their **acceptable daily intake (ADI)**, the level at which they are considered safe, even if taken daily.

B. The dose–response relationship

1. The dose–response relationship implies that higher doses of a drug or toxicant in an *individual* can result in a **graded response**.
   a. Higher doses in a *population* result in a larger percentage of individuals responding to the agent (**quantal dose–response**).
2. The most commonly used index of toxicity for drugs used therapeutically is the **therapeutic index** (TI). This is defined as the ratio of the dose of drug that produces a toxic effect (TD_{50}) or a lethal effect (LD_{50}) to the dose that produces a therapeutic effect (ED_{50}) in 50% of the population.

C. Risk and hazard

1. **Risk** is defined as the **expected frequency of occurrence of unwanted effects** of a physical or chemical agent. The benefit-to-risk ratios influence the acceptability of compounds.
2. **Hazard** is defined as the **ability of a toxicant to cause harm in a specific setting**. It relates to the amount of a physical or chemical agent to which an individual will be exposed.
3. **No-observable-effect level** (NOEL) is defined as the **highest dose of a chemical that does not produce an observable effect in humans**. This value, based on animal studies, is used for chemicals for which a full dose-response curve for toxicity in humans is unknown or unattainable.

TABLE 13.1 Acute and Evident Changes in the Poisoned Patient and Possible Causes

Changes	Causes
Cardiorespiratory Abnormalities	
Hypertension, tachycardia	Amphetamines, cocaine, phencyclidine (PCP), nicotine, antimuscarinic drugs
Hypotension, bradycardia	Opioids, clonidine, β-blockers, sedative–hypnotics
Hypotension, tachycardia	Tricyclic antidepressants, phenothiazines, theophylline
Rapid respiration	Sympathomimetics (including amphetamines), salicylates, carbon monoxide, any toxin that produces metabolic acidosis (including alcohol)
Hyperthermia	Sympathomimetics, salicylates, antimuscarinic agents, most drugs that induce seizures or rigidity
Hypothermia	Alcohol, phenothiazines, sedatives
Central Nervous System Effects	
Nystagmus, dysarthria, ataxia	Phenytoin, alcohol, sedatives
Rigidity, muscular hypertension	Phencyclidine, haloperidol, sympathomimetics
Seizures	Tricyclic antidepressants, theophylline, isoniazid, phenothiazines
Flaccid coma	Opioids and sedative hypnotics
Hallucinations	Lysergic acid diethylamide, poisonous plants (nightshade, jimsonweed)
Gastrointestinal Changes	
Ileus	Antimuscarinics, opioids, sedatives
Cramping, diarrhea, increased bowel sounds	Organophosphates, arsenic, iron, theophylline, *Amanita phalloides*
Nausea, vomiting	*A. phalloides*
Visual Disturbances	
Miosis (pupil constriction)	Clonidine, opioids, phenothiazines, cholinesterase inhibitors (including organophosphate insecticides)
Mydriasis (pupil dilation)	Amphetamines, cocaine, LSD, antimuscarinic agents
Nystagmus	Phenytoin, alcohol, sedatives (including barbiturates), phencyclidine
Ptosis, ophthalmoplegia	Botulism
Skin Changes	
Flushed, hot, dry skin	Antimuscarinics (including atropine)
Excessive sweating	Nicotine, sympathomimetics, organophosphates
Cyanosis	Drugs that induce hypoxemia or methemoglobinemia
Icterus	Hepatic damage from paracetamol or *A. phalloides*
Mouth and Taste Alterations	Caustic substances
Burns	Arsenic, organophosphates
Odors	Garlicky breath: Arsenic, organophosphates
	Bitter almond breath: Cyanide
	Rotten egg odor: Hydrogen sulfide
	Pear-like odor: Chloral hydrate
	Chemical smell: Alcohol, hydrocarbon solvents, paraldehyde, gasoline, ammonia
Green tongue	Vanadium
Metallic taste	Lead, cadmium

4. According to the World Health Organization, the ADI of a chemical is the "daily intake of a chemical, which during the entire lifetime appears to be without appreciable risk on the basis of all known facts at that time."

a. ADI values are calculated from NOELs and other "uncertainty" factors, including estimated differences in human and animal sensitivity to the toxic agent.

TABLE 13.2 Threshold Limit Values for Selected Air Pollutants and Solvents

	Threshold Limit Values	
	TWA	STEL
Air Pollutant		
Carbon monoxide	25	—
Nitrogen dioxide	3	5
Ozone	0.05	—
Sulfur dioxide	2	5
Solvent		
Benzene	0.5	2.5
Carbon tetrachloride	5	10
Chloroform	10	—
Toluene	50	—

STEL, short-term exposure limit; TWA, time-weighted average.

D. Classification of toxic response

1. The **duration of exposure** is used to **classify toxic response.**
   a. **Acute exposure** resulting in a toxic reaction represents a single exposure or multiple exposures over 1–2 days.
   b. **Chronic exposure** resulting in a toxic reaction represents multiple exposures over longer periods of time.
   c. **Delayed toxicity** represents the appearance of a toxic effect after a delayed interval following exposure.

E. Route of exposure

1. The rate of exposure can determine the extent of toxicity and outcomes.
2. Most toxicants (e.g., **heavy metals**) cause toxic effects directly, including binding to functional groups on proteins containing oxygen (O), sulfur (S), and nitrogen (N) atoms.
3. In other instances, in a process referred to as **toxication** (or bioactivation), a substance may be converted in the body to a chemical form that is directly toxic or participates in reactions that generate other highly reactive toxic species.
   a. Examples include **superoxide anion (O_2^-)**, **hydroxyl (OH) free radicals**, and **hydrogen peroxide (H_2O_2)**, which can cause DNA, protein, and cell membrane damage and loss of function.
   b. Endogenous **glutathione** plays a central role in detoxication of these reactive species either directly or coupled to **superoxide dismutase** and **glutathione peroxidase**.
   c. Superoxide dismutase coupled to **catalase** is also involved in detoxication pathways.
   d. Endogenous metallothionein offers some limited protection from metal toxicity.

II. AIR POLLUTANTS

A. General characteristics

1. Air pollutants enter the body primarily through **inhalation** and are either absorbed into the blood (e.g., gases) or eliminated by the lungs (e.g., particulates).
   a. Ozone is also of special concern in certain geographic locations.
2. Air pollutants are characterized as either **reducing types** (sulfur oxides) or **oxidizing types** (nitrogen oxides, hydrocarbons, and photochemical oxidants).

B. Carbon monoxide

1. ***Properties and mechanism of action***
   a. Carbon monoxide (CO) is a colorless, odorless, nonirritating gas produced from the incomplete combustion of organic matter. It is a neutral oxide.

b. It competes for and **combines with the oxygen-binding site of hemoglobin to form carboxyhemoglobin**, resulting in a **functional anemia**.
   (1) The binding affinity of CO for hemoglobin is 220 times higher than that of oxygen itself.
   (2) Carboxyhemoglobin also interferes with the dissociation in tissues of the remaining oxyhemoglobin.
c. CO also binds to cellular respiratory cytochromes.
d. CO concentrations of 0.1% (1,000 ppm) in air will result in 50% carboxyhemoglobinemia.
   (1) Smokers may routinely exceed normal carboxyhemoglobin levels of 1% by up to 10 times.

2. ***Poisoning and treatment***
   a. It is the **most frequent cause of death from poisoning** (see Table 13.2 for TLVs).
   b. CO intoxication (>15% carboxyhemoglobin) results in **progressive hypoxia**.
      (1) Symptoms include **headache**, **dizziness**, nausea, **vomiting**, syncope, and seizures.
      (2) A cherry-red appearance and coma may occur with carboxyhemoglobin concentrations greater than 40%.
   c. Chronic low-level exposure may be harmful to the cardiovascular system.
      (1) Populations at special risk include smokers with ischemic heart disease or anemia, the elderly, and the developing fetus.
   d. Treatment includes removal from the source of CO, maintenance of respiration, and administration of oxygen. Hyperbaric oxygen may be required in severe poisoning.

C. Sulfur dioxide

1. ***Properties and mechanism of action***
   a. Sulfur dioxide (SO_2) is a colorless, irritant gas produced by the combustion of sulfur-containing fuels (see Table 13.2 for TLVs).
   b. It can be converted in the atmosphere to **sulfuric acid** (H_2SO_4), which has irritant effects similar to those of SO_2.
2. ***Poisoning and treatment***
   a. At low levels (5 ppm), SO_2 has **irritant effects on exposed membranes** (eyes, mucous membranes, skin, and upper respiratory tract with bronchoconstriction).
      (1) Patients with asthma are more susceptible; **delayed pulmonary edema** may be observed after severe exposure.
   b. SO_2 poisoning is treated by therapeutic interventions that reduce irritation in the respiratory tract.

D. Nitrogen dioxide

1. ***Properties and mechanism of action***
   a. Nitrogen dioxide (NO_2) is an irritant brown gas produced in **fires** and from **decaying silage**. It is also produced from a reaction of nitrogen oxide (from **auto exhaust**) with oxygen (O_2) (see Table 13.2 for TLVs).
   b. It causes the degeneration of alveolar type I cells, with **rupture of alveolar capillary endothelium**.
2. ***Poisoning and treatment***
   a. Acute symptoms include **irritation of eyes and nose**, coughing, dyspnea, and chest pain.
   b. Severe exposure for 1–2 hours may result in **pulmonary edema** that may subside and then recur more than 2 weeks later.
   c. Chronic low-level exposure may also result in pulmonary edema.
   d. NO_2 poisoning is treated with therapeutic interventions that reduce pulmonary irritation and edema.

E. Ozone

1. ***Properties and mechanism of action***
   a. Ozone (O_3) is an irritating, naturally occurring bluish gas found in high levels in **polluted air** and around high-voltage equipment (see Table 13.2 for TLVs).
   b. It is formed by a complex series of reactions involving NO_2 absorption of ultraviolet light with the generation of free oxygen.
   c. O_3 causes **functional pulmonary changes** similar to those with NO_2.
   d. Toxicity may result from **free radical formation**.

2. ***Poisoning and treatment***
   a. O_3 **irritates mucous membranes** and can cause **decreased pulmonary compliance**, pulmonary edema, and increased sensitivity to bronchoconstrictors.
   b. Chronic exposure may cause decreased respiratory reserve, bronchitis, and pulmonary fibrosis.
   c. Treatment is similar to that used in NO_2 poisoning.

F. Hydrocarbons

1. Hydrocarbons are oxidized by sunlight and by incomplete combustion to short-lived aldehydes such as **formaldehyde** and **acrolein**; aldehydes are also found in, and can be released from, certain construction materials.
2. Hydrocarbons **irritate the mucous membranes of the respiratory tract and eyes**, producing a response similar to that seen with SO_2 exposure.

G. Particulates

1. Inhalation of particulates can lead to **pneumoconiosis**, most commonly caused by **silicates (silicosis)** or **asbestos (asbestosis).**
   a. **Bronchial cancer** and **mesothelioma** are associated with asbestos exposure, particularly in conjunction with cigarette smoking.
2. Particulates **adsorb other toxins**, such as polycyclic aromatic hydrocarbons, and **deliver them to the respiratory tract.**
3. They also increase susceptibility to pulmonary dysfunction and disease and may yield **fibrotic masses in the lungs** that develop over years of exposure.

H. Particulate matter (PM) consists of solid and liquid particles that remain suspended in air.

1. These can enter the respiratory system and can cause respiratory diseases as well as premature death.
2. Dust from road and construction site contains coarse PM. Vehicular smoke contains fine PM.
3. **$PM_{2.5}$** are solid particles or droplets in the air with a width ≤ 2.5 μm. PM ≤ 10 μm in width is **PM_{10}**.

III. SOLVENTS

A. Aliphatic and halogenated aliphatic hydrocarbons

1. Aliphatic and halogenated aliphatic hydrocarbons include fuels and industrial solvents such as ***n*-hexane, gasoline, kerosene, carbon tetrachloride, chloroform**, and **tetrachloroethylene** (see Table 13.2 for TLVs).
2. These agents are **central nervous system (CNS) depressants** and cause neurologic, liver, and kidney damage. Cardiotoxicity is also possible. All of these effects may be mediated by **free radical interaction** with cellular lipids and proteins.
   a. **Polyneuropathy** from cytoskeletal disruption predominates with ***n*-hexane** poisoning.
   b. **Neural effects**, such as memory loss and peripheral neuropathy, predominate with **chloroform** and **tetrachloroethylene** exposure.
   c. **Chloroform** also causes **nephrotoxicity** and can sensitize the heart to **arrhythmias**.
   d. **Hepatotoxicity** (delayed) and **renal toxicity** are common with **carbon tetrachloride** poisoning.
   e. **Carcinogenicity** has been associated with **chloroform, carbon tetrachloride**, and **tetrachloroethylene**.
3. Aspiration with **chemical pneumonitis** and **pulmonary edema** is common.
4. ***Treatment*** is primarily supportive and is oriented to the organ systems involved.

B. Aromatic hydrocarbons

1. **Benzene** poisoning is the **most common**.
   a. **CNS depression** is the major acute effect.
   b. Chronic exposure can result in severe **bone marrow depression**, resulting in aplastic anemia and other blood dyscrasias.
   c. Low-level benzene exposure has been linked to leukemia.
   d. No specific treatment is available for benzene poisoning.

2. **Toluene** and **xylene** can depress the CNS.
   a. They can cause **fatigue** and **ataxia** at relatively low levels and loss of consciousness at high levels (10,000 ppm).

C. Polychlorinated biphenyls

1. Polychlorinated biphenyls (PCBs) are stable, highly lipophilic agents that, although not used since 1977, still persist in the environment.
2. **Dermatologic disorders** are the most common adverse effect.
3. Possible reproductive dysfunction and carcinogenic effects linked to PCBs may be largely due to other contaminating polychlorinated agents such as the dioxin, 2,3,7,8-tetrachlorodibenzo-*p*-dioxin (TCDD).

IV. INSECTICIDES AND HERBICIDES

A. Organophosphorus insecticides (see Chapter 2)

1. ***Properties and mechanism of action***
   a. Organophosphorus insecticides include **parathion, malathion**, and **diazinon.**
      (1) They have replaced **organochlorine pesticides** (except for a very restricted use in the United States of dichlorodiphenyltrichloroethane, i.e., **DDT**), which persist in the environment and have been associated with an increased risk of cancer.
      (2) Organophosphorus insecticides do not persist in the environment; however, their potential for acute toxicity is higher.
   b. Organophosphorus insecticides are characterized by their ability to **phosphorylate the active esteratic site of acetylcholinesterase (AChE).**
      (1) Toxic effects result from **acetylcholine (ACh) accumulation.**
   c. These agents are well absorbed through the skin and via the respiratory and gastrointestinal (GI) tracts.
   d. Some other organophosphate insecticide compounds (e.g., **triorthocresyl phosphate**) also phosphorylate a "neuropathy target esterase," which results in **delayed neurotoxicity** with sensory and motor disturbances of the limbs.
2. ***Treatment of poisoning***
   a. Assisted respiration and decontamination are needed as soon as possible to **prevent the irreversible inhibition ("aging") of AChE,** which involves strengthening of the phosphorus-enzyme bond.
   b. **Atropine** reverses all muscarinic effects but does not reverse neuromuscular activation or paralysis.
   c. **Pralidoxime** (2-PAM) **reactivates AChE,** particularly at the neuromuscular junction. It is often used as an **adjunct to atropine** (may reverse some toxic effects). It is very effective in parathion poisoning.

B. Carbamate insecticides (see Chapter 2)

1. Carbamate insecticides include **carbaryl, carbofuran, isolan,** and **pyramat.**
2. These agents are characterized by their ability to **inhibit AChE by carbamoylation.**
3. Carbamate insecticides produce toxic effects similar to those of the phosphorus-containing insecticides.
   a. Generally, the toxic effects of carbamate compounds are **less severe** than those of the organophosphorus agents because carbamoylation is **rapidly reversible.**
4. Treatment for carbamate poisoning is similar to that used for organophosphate poisoning except that pralidoxime therapy is not an effective antidote because it does not interact with carbamoylated AChE.

C. Botanical insecticides

1. **Nicotine** stimulates nicotinic receptors and results in membrane depolarization.
   a. Symptoms of poisoning may include **salivation, vomiting,** muscle weakness, **seizures,** and respiratory arrest. Treatment includes anticonvulsants and symptomatic relief.

2. **Pyrethrum**, a common household insecticide, is toxic only at high levels.
   a. Allergic manifestations and **irritation of the skin and respiratory tract** are the most common adverse effects; treatment includes symptomatic relief.
3. **Rotenone** poisoning is rare in humans and generally results in **GI disturbances** that are treated symptomatically.

D. Herbicides

1. **Glyphosate** is widely used worldwide; it is a relatively safe herbicide that does not persist in the environment. Adverse effects are **irritation of the skin and eyes**.
2. **Paraquat** causes acute GI irritation with bloody stools, followed by delayed respiratory distress and the development of **congestive hemorrhagic pulmonary edema**, which is thought to be caused by superoxide radical formation and subsequent cell membrane disruption.
   a. Death may ensue several weeks after ingestion.
   b. Treatment consists of prompt gastric lavage; administration of cathartics and adsorbents benefits some victims.
3. **2,4-Dichlorophenoxyacetic acid** (2,4-D) causes **neuromuscular paralysis** and coma. Long-term toxic effects are rare.

E. Fumigants and rodenticide: cyanide

1. **Cyanide** possesses a high affinity for ferric iron; it **reacts with iron and cytochrome oxidase** in mitochondria to **inhibit cellular respiration**, thereby blocking oxygen use.
2. It is absorbed from all routes (except alkali salts, which are toxic only when ingested).
3. Poisoning is signaled by **bright red venous blood** and a characteristic **odor of bitter almonds**.
4. Cyanide causes transient CNS stimulation followed by **hypoxic seizures** and death.
5. Treatment must be immediate with administration of 100% oxygen.
   a. **Amyl or sodium nitrite**, which oxidizes hemoglobin and produces methemoglobin (compete for cyanide ion), can also be administered.
   b. **Sodium thiosulfate** can be administered to accelerate the conversion of cyanide to nontoxic thiocyanate by mitochondrial rhodanese (sulfurtransferase).
   c. Activated charcoal may also be used.
   d. Hydroxocobalamin, which binds with cyanide, is also available as an antidote.

V. HEAVY METAL POISONING AND MANAGEMENT

A. Inorganic lead poisoning

1. Organic lead poisoning is increasingly rare due to phased elimination of tetraethyl and tetramethyl lead (antiknock components in gasoline).
   a. Historically, paint and gasoline were major sources of lead exposure and still can be found in the environment.
   b. Other sources include home crafts, such as pottery and jewelry making.
2. Inorganic metallic lead oxides and salts are slowly absorbed through all routes except the skin. Organic lead compounds are well absorbed across the skin.
   a. The **GI route** is the **most common** route of exposure in **nonindustrial** settings (children absorb a higher fraction than do adults).
   b. The **respiratory route** is more common for **industrial** exposure.
3. Inorganic lead **binds to hemoglobin in erythrocytes**, with the remainder distributing to soft tissues such as the brain and kidney. Through redistribution, it later accumulates in bone, where its elimination half-life is 20–30 years.
4. **CNS effects** (**lead encephalopathy**) are common after chronic exposure to lead, particularly in children, for whom no threshold level has been established.
   a. Early signs of poisoning include vertigo, ataxia, headache, restlessness, and irritability; **wrist drop** is a common sign of **peripheral neuropathy**.
   b. Projectile vomiting, delirium, and seizures may occur with the progression of encephalopathy with lead concentrations of 100 μg/dL.

c. **Mental deterioration with lowered intelligence quotient (IQ) and behavioral abnormalities** may be a consequence of **childhood exposure**.

5. GI upset, including epigastric distress, is also seen, particularly in adults.
6. Constipation and a metallic taste are early signs of exposure to lead. Intestinal spasm with severe pain (lead colic) may become evident in advanced stages of poisoning.
7. Renal fibrosis may occur with chronic exposure.
8. Lead may increase spontaneous abortion and is associated with altered production of sperm.
9. Treatment includes the use of parenteral sodium calcium edetate (calcium disodium ethylenediaminetetraacetic acid [EDTA]) or, in less severe cases, oral succimer. Dimercaprol and penicillamine can be used as adjuvants to calcium disodium EDTA.

B. Inorganic arsenic

1. ***Properties and mechanism of action***
   a. Inorganic arsenic can be found in coal and metal ores, herbicides, seafood, and drinking water. It is absorbed through the GI tract and lungs.
   b. Trivalent forms (arsenites) are generally more toxic than the pentavalent forms (arsenates). Methylated metabolites may account for their adverse effects.
      (1) **Arsenites inhibit sulfhydryl enzymes** (pyruvate dehydrogenase/glycolysis is especially sensitive), resulting in damage to the epithelial lining of the GI and respiratory tracts and damage to tissues of the nervous system, liver, bone marrow, and skin.
      (2) **Arsenates uncouple mitochondrial oxidative phosphorylation** by "substituting" for inorganic phosphate.
2. Symptoms of **acute poisoning** include the following:
   a. **Severe nausea**, vomiting, abdominal pain, laryngitis, and bronchitis may occur.
   b. Capillary damage with dehydration and shock may occur.
   c. **Diarrhea** is characterized as **"rice-water stools."**
   d. There is often a **garlicky breath** odor.
   e. Initial episodes of arsenic poisoning may be fatal; if the individual survives, bone marrow depression, severe neuropathy, and encephalopathy may occur.
3. Symptoms of **chronic poisoning** include the following:
   a. **Weight loss** due to GI irritation, perforation of the nasal septum, **hair loss**, sensory neuropathy, **depression of bone marrow function**, and kidney and liver damage may occur.
   b. The **skin often appears pale and milky ("milk and roses" complexion)** because of anemia and vasodilation.
      (1) Skin pigmentation, hyperkeratosis of the palms and soles, and white lines over the nails may be observed after prolonged exposure.
   c. Inorganic arsenicals have been implicated in cancers of the respiratory system.
4. Treatment is primarily supportive after acute poisoning and involves termination of exposure, emesis, gastric lavage, rehydration, and restoration of electrolyte imbalance.
   a. Chelation therapy with **dimercaprol** or its analogue, unithiol, is indicated in severe cases.
   b. **Succimer**, another derivative of dimercaprol, may also be used.
5. Treatment of chronic poisoning is supportive, including termination of exposure.
6. Organic arsenicals are excreted more readily and are less toxic than inorganic forms; poisoning is rare.
7. **Arsine gas** (AsH_3) poisoning may occur in industrial settings.
   a. The effects are **severe hemolysis** and subsequent renal failure; symptoms include jaundice, dark urine, and severe abdominal pain.
   b. Treatment includes **transfusion** and **hemodialysis** for renal failure. Chelation therapy is ineffective.

C. Mercury

1. ***Inorganic mercury***
   a. ***Properties and mechanism of action***
      (1) **Inorganic mercury** occurs as a potential hazard primarily because of occupational or industrial exposure. The major source of poisoning is by **consumption of contaminated food**.

(2) Elemental mercury (Hg) is poorly absorbed by the GI tract but is volatile and can be absorbed by the lungs.
   (a) Hg itself causes CNS effects; the ionized form, **Hg^{2+}**, accumulates in the kidneys and causes **damage in the proximal tubules** by combining with sulfhydryl enzymes.
(3) Mercuric chloride ($HgCl_2$) is well absorbed by the GI tract and is toxic.
(4) Mercurous chloride (HgCl) is also absorbed by the GI tract but is less toxic than $HgCl_2$.

b. ***Acute poisoning and treatment***

(1) **Mercury vapor** poisoning produces chest pain, shortness of breath, nausea, vomiting, and a metallic taste. Chemical pneumonitis and gingivostomatitis may also occur. Muscle tremor and psychopathology can develop.
(2) **Inorganic mercury salts**
   (a) Inorganic mercury salts cause hemorrhagic gastroenteritis producing intense pain and vomiting. Hypovolemic shock may also occur.
   (b) **Renal tubular necrosis** is the most prevalent and serious systemic toxicity.
(3) Treatment involves removal from exposure, supportive care, and chelation therapy with **dimercaprol,** unithiol, or **succimer**. Hemodialysis may be necessary.

c. ***Chronic poisoning***

(1) **Mercury vapor** poisoning may lead to a **fine tremor** of the limbs that may progress to choreiform movements, and **neuropsychiatric symptoms** that may include insomnia, fatigue, anorexia, and memory loss, as well as changes in mood and affect. **Gingivostomatitis** is also common. Erethism (a combination of excessive perspiration and blushing) may also occur.
(2) **Inorganic mercury salts. Renal injury** predominates. Erythema of extremities **(acrodynia)** is often coupled with anorexia, tachycardia, and GI disturbances.
(3) For the treatment, unithiol or succimer may be helpful. Dimercaprol should be avoided as it will redistribute mercury to the CNS.

2. ***Organic mercurials (methylmercury)***

a. Organic mercurials are found in seed dressings and fungicides.
b. They can be absorbed from the GI tract and often distribute to the CNS, where they exert their toxic effects, including paresthesias, ataxia, and hearing impairment. **Visual disturbances** often predominate.
c. Exposure of the fetus to methylmercury in utero may result in mental retardation and a syndrome resembling cerebral palsy.
d. Treatment is primarily supportive. Unithiol or succimer may be helpful.

D. Iron (see Chapter 7)

E. Metal-chelating agents

1. ***General properties***

a. Metal-chelating agents usually contain two or more electronegative groups that **form stable coordinate–covalent complexes with cationic metals,** which can then be excreted from the body.
   (1) The greater the number of metal–ligand bonds, the more stable is the complex and the greater is the efficiency of the chelator.
b. These agents contain functional groups such as –OH, –SH, and –NH, which compete for metal binding with similar groups on cell proteins.
c. Their effects are generally greater when administered soon after exposure.

2. ***Edetate calcium disodium (sodium calcium edetate) and EDTA***

a. EDTA is an efficient chelator of many transition metals. Since it can also chelate body calcium, EDTA is administered intramuscularly or by intravenous (IV) infusion as the disodium salt of calcium.
b. It is used primarily in the treatment of **lead poisoning**.
c. EDTA is rapidly excreted by glomerular filtration.
d. It is nephrotoxic, particularly at renal tubules, at high doses. Maintenance of urine flow and short-term treatment can minimize this effect.

3. ***Dimercaprol***

a. Dimercaprol is an oily, foul-smelling liquid administered intramuscularly as a 10% solution in peanut oil.

b. Dimercaprol interacts with metals, reactivating or **preventing the inactivation of cellular sulfhydryl-containing enzymes**. It is most effective if administered immediately following exposure.
c. This agent is useful in **arsenic, inorganic mercury, and lead poisoning** (with EDTA).
d. Adverse effects include tachycardia, hypertension, gastric irritation, and pain at the injection site.
e. **It should not be used in cadmium, iron, or selenium poisoning**. The resulting chelate metal complex is more toxic, particularly to the kidneys, than the metal alone.
f. **Succimer** is a derivative of dimercaprol that can be taken orally and is approved for use in children to treat **lead poisoning**. It is also used to treat **arsenic** and **mercury** poisoning. Adverse effects are generally minor and include nausea, vomiting, and anorexia. A rash indicating hypersensitivity may require the termination of therapy.
g. **Unithiol** is another analogue of dimercaprol used to treat acute **arsenic** and **inorganic mercury** poisoning. Skin reactions are its most common adverse effect.

4. ***Penicillamine***
a. Penicillamine, a derivative of penicillin, is used primarily to chelate excess copper in individuals with **Wilson disease**.
b. It is also useful in mercury and chronic lead poisoning.
c. Apart from metal toxicity, it has been used to treat cystinuria (to prevent cystine stone formation) and scleroderma.
d. Allergic reactions, **bone marrow toxicity** and **renal toxicity,** are the major adverse effects.

5. ***Deferoxamine (desferrioxamine), deferasirox,* and deferiprone**
a. Deferoxamine is a specific **iron-chelating agent** that **binds with ferric ions to form ferrioxamine**; it **also binds to ferrous ions.**
(1) It can also remove iron from ferritin and hemosiderin outside the bone marrow, but it does not capture iron from hemoglobin, cytochromes, or myoglobin.
b. It is metabolized by plasma enzymes and excreted by the kidney, turning the urine red.
c. Rapid IV infusion of deferoxamine may result in hypotensive shock due to the release of histamine.
d. Deferoxamine may cause allergic reactions and, rarely, **neurotoxicity** or **renal toxicity**. It is contraindicated in patients with renal disease or renal failure.
e. Deferasirox and deferiprone are oral iron chelators approved for the treatment of iron overload.

VI. DRUG POISONING

A. General management of the poisoned patient
1. Observe vital signs.
2. Obtain history.
3. Perform a toxicologically oriented physical examination.

B. Symptoms
1. The symptoms of most drug and chemical poisonings are extensions of their pharmacologic properties.
2. The common causes of death include CNS depression with respiratory arrest, seizures, cardiovascular abnormalities with severe hypotension and arrhythmias, cellular hypoxia, and hypothermia.

C. Treatment
1. Measures to support vital functions, slow drug absorption, and promote excretion are generally sufficient treatment. If available, specific antidotes can also be used.
2. **Vital function support**
a. In the presence of severe CNS depression, it is important to clear the **airway** and maintain adequate **breathing** and **circulation (ABC)**. Comatose patients may die as a result of airway obstruction, respiratory arrest, or aspiration of gastric contents into the tracheobronchial tube.
b. Other important supportive measures include **maintaining electrolyte balance** and **maintaining vascular fluid volume** with IV crystalloid infusion.

3. **Drug absorption**
   a. Drug absorption may be slowed or prevented by decontamination of the skin.
   b. **Emesis is contraindicated if corrosives have been ingested** (reflux may perforate the stomach or esophagus), petroleum distillates have been ingested (may induce chemical pneumonia if aspirated), the patient is comatose or delirious and may aspirate gastric contents, or CNS stimulants have been ingested (may induce seizure activity with stimulation of emesis).
   c. **Gastric lavage** is performed only when the airway is protected by an endotracheal tube.
   d. **Chemical adsorption with activated charcoal**
      (1) Activated charcoal will bind many toxins and drugs, including **salicylates, acetaminophen**, and **antidepressants**.
      (2) This procedure can be used in combination with gastric lavage.
   e. **Laxatives**, such as a **polyethylene glycol electrolyte solution**, are used occasionally to speed up the removal of toxins from the GI tract.
4. **Promotion of elimination** may be achieved by the following:
   a. **Enhancing urinary excretion.** Administration of agents such as **sodium bicarbonate** raises the urinary pH and decreases the renal reabsorption of certain organic acids, such as aspirin and phenobarbital.
   b. **Hemodialysis** is an efficient way to remove certain low-molecular-weight, water-soluble toxins and restore electrolyte balance.
      (1) Salicylates, methanol, ethanol, ethylene glycol, paraquat, and lithium poisonings are effectively treated with hemodialysis.
      (2) Hemoperfusion may enhance the whole-body clearance of some agents, including carbamazepine, phenobarbital, and phenytoin.
      (3) Drugs and poisons with large volumes of distribution are not effectively removed by dialysis.
5. **Antidotes** are available for some poisons and should be used when a specific toxin is identified.
   a. Some examples include the following:
      (1) Acetylcysteine (for paracetamol poisoning)
      (2) Atropine (to reverse cholinergic effects; for organophosphate or carbamate insecticide or nerve agent poisoning)
      (3) Digoxin immune Fab (for digoxin toxicity)
      (4) Ethanol (for methanol or ethylene glycol overdose)
      (5) Flumazenil (for benzodiazepine overdose)
      (6) Fomepizole (for methanol or ethylene glycol overdose)
      (7) Metal chelators
      (8) Naloxone (for opioid overdose)
      (9) Pralidoxime (for anticholinesterase overdose; for organophosphate poisoning)
      (10) Physostigmine (to reverse anticholinergic effects)
      (11) Phytonadione (vitamin K_1) (for warfarin overdose)

VII. COMMON STINGS AND BITES

A. **Insect/scorpion sting:** Insect stings are common and can cause severe local reactions. However, these do not require any specific treatment unless there are systemic symptoms which are uncommon.
   1. Multiple stings can result in systemic symptoms. Treatment generally involves local wound care, antihistamines, analgesics, and, in case of severe allergic reactions, (anaphylaxis) adrenaline.
   2. Scorpion sting (Indian red scorpion [*Mesobuthus tamulus*]) can produce systemic effects, particularly cardiovascular, besides the severe local pain at the stung site.
      a. It can produce autonomic storm: initial cholinergic stimulation followed by adrenergic stimulation.
   3. Treatment:
      a. General measures include washing the site of sting with soap and water, cold compress, and analgesic.

b. Prazosin (α1-adrenergic antagonist) to reverse the venom-induced cardiovascular changes.
c. Scorpion antivenom administered intravenously neutralizes circulating scorpion toxin. Hypersensitivity reactions can occur.

B. Snake bite: The clinical presentation of snake bite envenomation depends on the species of snake. Cobra (*Naja Naja*) and krait (*Bungarus caeruleus*) venom are primarily neurotoxic whereas viper (Russells' Viper [*Daboia russalie*] and Saw scaled viper [*Echis carinatus*]) venom is hematotoxic.

Treatment

1. General measures involve immobilization of the affected limb and maintaining airway, breathing, and circulation.
2. Antisnake venom
   a. Polyvalent equine antisnake venom is infused intravenously until signs of envenomation subside. Hypersensitivity reactions can occur.
3. Depending on the type of snake bite, specific treatment may be required.
   a. Fresh frozen plasma to counteract coagulopathy due to viper bite.
   b. Neostigmine (with atropine to counteract the muscarinic adverse effects) for cobra bite induced muscle paralysis.
   c. Calcium gluconate in case of krait bite.
4. Due to absence of antibodies, antisnake venom is not indicated in sea snake and pit viper bite.

C. Dog bite: Depending on the type of exposure (extent of damage to the skin), the bites are categorized into I (no exposure), II (minimal exposure), and III (severe exposure).

Treatment

1. General measures including local wound care, antimicrobials, administration of tetanus toxoid (If not received in the past 5 years).
2. Post-exposure prophylaxis with rabies vaccine
   a. Indicated in category II and III exposures.
   b. Administered intradermally (8 doses, injected at 2 sites on day 0, 3, 7, and 28) or intramuscularly (5 doses, injected on day 0, 3, 7, 14, and 28).
   c. Intradermal route should not be used in those on chloroquine, hydroxychloroquine, or immunosuppressants due to possibility of reduced response.
3. Since antibody production following the anti-rabies vaccination takes a few days, in category III exposures, human or equine rabies immunoglobulin is infiltrated into or close to the wound to provide passive immunity.

VIII. ANTIGLAUCOMA DRUGS

1. **Glaucoma** is an ocular disorder characterized by progressive damage of the optic nerve due to raised IOP (Table 13.3).
   a. It is a leading cause of permanent blindness.
   b. Pharmacotherapy aims at lowering the raised IOP by decreasing the synthesis of aqueous humor or increasing its drainage (via trabecular meshwork or uveoscleral outflow).
   c. **Open-angle glaucoma** is an insidious, chronic disease.
   d. **Narrow-angle glaucoma** (angle-closure glaucoma) is an ophthalmologic emergency.
2. **Indications**
   a. Open-angle glaucoma: Topical prostaglandin analogues or β-blockers are the first-line drugs. Other topical drugs are used if there is inadequate response with the combination of these or discontinuation due to adverse effects.
   b. Narrow-angle glaucoma: IOP is reduced using a systemic drug (mannitol and acetazolamide). This is accompanied with topical agents which are continued after the fall in IOP until a definitive measure is instituted (surgical or laser iridotomy).

TABLE 13.3 Mechanism of Action of Antiglaucoma Drugs

Target	Action	Effect	Drugs
α_1-Receptor agonist	Vasoconstriction of ciliary blood vessels	↓ aqueous humor formation	Dipivefrine (prodrug of adrenaline)
α_2-Receptor agonist	Ciliary epithelium	↓ aqueous humor formation	Dipivefrine, apraclonidine, brimonidine
β_2-Receptor antagonist	Ciliary epithelium	↓ aqueous humor formation	Timolol, betaxolol, levobunolol
M_3 agonist	Constriction of sphincter pupillae	↑ trabecular outflow	Pilocarpine; physostigmine and echothiophate (act indirectly by anticholinesterase action)
FP receptor agonist	Increased permeability of ciliary muscle tissue	↑ uveoscleral outflow	Latanoprost, bimatoprost, travoprost
Carbonic anhydrase enzyme inhibitor	Reduces bicarbonate secretion from ciliary epithelium	↓ aqueous humor formation	Acetazolamide[a], dorzolamide, brinzolamide
–	Osmotic action—extracts water	↓ volume of aqueous humor	Mannitol[a], glycerin[a]

[a]Administered systemically; used only in acute angle-closure glaucoma to immediately reduce intraocular pressure (IOP).

3. **Adverse effects**
   a. Most of the topical agents cause burning and stinging sensation in the eye.
   b. Prostaglandin analogues can cause increased pigmentation of the iris and periorbital tissue, thickening and darkening of the eyelashes, and macular edema.
   c. α-Receptor agonists can cause lid edema, conjunctivitis, foreign body sensation, and dry mouth.
   d. Carbonic anhydrase inhibitors can cause corneal edema and bitter taste.
   e. Cholinergic agonists can decrease visual acuity and cause headache.
   f. Topical ocular drugs can sometimes get absorbed systemically and cause adverse effects.

DRUG SUMMARY TABLE

Amyl nitrite	Dimercaptosuccinic acid	Unithiol
Atropine	Edetate calcium disodium	Sodium nitrite
Deferasirox	Ethylenediaminetetraacetic acid (EDTA)	Sodium thiosulfate
Deferoxamine	Penicillamine	
Dimercaprol	Pralidoxime	

Review Test

Directions: Select the best answer for each question.

1. What treatment would be appropriate in a 3-year-old boy with a dramatically elevated blood level of lead?

(A) Deferoxamine
(B) Digoxin immune Fab
(C) Sodium calcium edetate
(D) Glucagon
(E) Pyridoxine

2. A 56-year-old man with a history of chronic alcohol abuse is brought to the emergency room with an altered mental status and vision changes. During the history and physical examination, the patient complains of vision loss. He also reveals that he ran out of whiskey and ingested locally produced alcohol instead. His laboratory test results demonstrate a severe anion gap and acute renal failure. Which of the following would be an appropriate therapy?

(A) Ethylene glycol
(B) Fomepizole
(C) Hyperbaric oxygen
(D) Lidocaine
(E) Methylene blue

3. An 18-year-old man is brought to the emergency room by ambulance. His friends called the emergency telephone number after he passed out at a party and was unresponsive. They tell the physician that the patient consumed two or three beers and took several diazepam tablets. On examination, the patient is unresponsive, with decreased respirations (8 per minute). What is an appropriate treatment?

(A) Carbon tetrachloride
(B) Dextrose
(C) Ethyl alcohol
(D) Flumazenil
(E) Strychnine

4. A 23-year-old woman is brought to the emergency room unresponsive. According to her boyfriend, she became unresponsive shortly after taking multiple pills to help her back pain. On physical examination, she is found to have pinpoint pupils and respiratory depression. What is the most appropriate agent to administer at this point?

(A) Atropine
(B) Dimercaprol
(C) Insulin
(D) Naloxone
(E) Penicillamine

5. A 2-year-old girl is brought to the emergency room after ingesting numerous ferrous sulfate tablets that her mother was taking for anemia. The child complains of severe abdominal pain. She has bloody diarrhea, nausea, and vomiting. Her serum iron is dramatically elevated. What should be given to treat this toxicity?

(A) Activated charcoal
(B) Deferoxamine
(C) Mercury vapor
(D) Penicillamine
(E) Succimer

6. The chelating agent that would be suitable to treat iron overload in a child undergoing repeated blood transfusions for a blood disorder is:

(A) Calcium disodium edetate
(B) Deferasirox
(C) Dimercaprol
(D) Succimer
(E) Penicillamine

7. Mesothelioma is associated with exposure to:

(A) Asbestos
(B) Benzene
(C) Formaldehyde
(D) Paraquat
(E) Sulfur dioxide

8. Which of the following toxic agents would pose a systemic problem with dermal exposure?

(A) Cadmium
(B) Inorganic arsenic
(C) Inorganic lead
(D) Organophosphate insecticide
(E) Silicates

9. Dimercaprol is contraindicated in which of the following metal poisoning?

(A) Antimony
(B) Arsenic
(C) Bismuth
(D) Iron
(E) Mercury

10. Atropine can be used as an antidote for the treatment of poisoning by which toxic agent?

(A) Carbaryl
(B) Chlorophenothane
(C) Methanol
(D) Parathion
(E) Rotenone

11. A 68-year-old woman is prescribed ophthalmic timolol for the treatment of elevated intraocular pressure due to open-angle glaucoma. Topical application of this medication to the eye would be expected to induce which of the following effects?

(A) Decreased formation of aqueous humor
(B) Miosis
(C) Mydriasis
(D) Increased outflow of aqueous humor
(E) Increased ciliary blood flow

12. A 26-year-old female presents to the emergency with severe pain in the right eye and blurring of vision. The intraocular pressure is elevated. The drug that would be most useful in decreasing the intraocular pressure in this patient is:

(A) Betaxolol
(B) Dorzolamide
(C) Homatropine
(D) Latanoprost
(E) Mannitol

Answers and Explanations

1. **The answer is C.** Sodium calcium edetate is a chelator used in the treatment of inorganic lead poisoning. The drug is given intravenously for several days along with dimercaprol. Deferoxamine is used in cases of iron toxicity. Pyridoxine is used in a toxicology setting to reverse seizures due to isoniazid overdose. Digoxin immune Fab is a Fab fragment antibody used in cases of digoxin toxicity. Glucagon has been used to treat beta-blocker toxicity.
2. **The answer is B.** Fomepizole is an inhibitor of alcohol dehydrogenase, the enzyme that converts methanol (present in adulterated alcohol) to formic acid. Formic acid causes severe adverse effects, such as blindness and high anion gap acidosis. Ethylene glycol (antifreeze) toxicity is also treated with fomepizole. Hyperbaric oxygen is used in the treatment of carbon monoxide poisoning. Lidocaine can be used to help manage arrhythmias in the case of digoxin toxicity. Methylene blue is used in the treatment of methemoglobinemia.
3. **The answer is D.** Flumazenil is a benzodiazepine antagonist used in the management of benzodiazepine overdose. Ethyl alcohol can be used to treat ingestion of both methanol and ethylene glycol; however, such use often results in ethanol intoxication; therefore, fomepizole is preferred as it does not cause the same effects. Dextrose is an effective treatment for altered mental status due to hypoglycemia in a diabetic patient. Strychnine is a rat poison that can cause seizures when ingested, which are managed by giving diazepam. Carbon tetrachloride is an industrial solvent that can cause fatty liver and kidney damage.
4. **The answer is D.** The patient is most likely experiencing an opioid overdose. The drug of choice for treatment is naloxone, an opioid-receptor antagonist. Insulin is used to treat hyperglycemia, which is less likely to cause altered mental status than is hypoglycemia. Dimercaprol is a chelator used in many cases of heavy metal toxicity (i.e., lead). Penicillamine is used in the treatment of copper toxicity, as in Wilson disease. Atropine is used to treat cholinergic toxicity, which can cause miosis, although it is an unlikely cause in this clinical presentation.
5. **The answer is B.** Deferoxamine is an iron chelator that is given systemically to bind iron and promote its excretion. Although activated charcoal is useful in reducing the absorption of numerous toxic ingestions, it does not bind iron. Succimer is an orally available substance related to dimercaprol and is used for treating lead toxicity. Mercury vapor is toxic, and its ingestion is treated with dimercaprol or penicillamine. The latter is also the drug of choice for treating copper toxicity.
6. **The answer is B.** Deferasirox is an oral iron chelator useful to tackle iron overload in patients undergoing repeated blood transfusions, as in case of thalassemia. Calcium disodium edetate is not the suitable drug in this case. Similarly, penicillamine is not useful to treat iron overload. Dimercaprol and succimer are also not useful; in fact, the dimercaprol–iron complex is itself toxic.
7. **The answer is A.** Mesothelioma and bronchial malignancies are associated with exposure to asbestos. Exposure to formaldehyde and sulfur dioxide causes respiratory symptoms due to their irritant effects. Benzene is a solvent which has been linked to the development of leukemia. Paraquat is an herbicide, poisoning due to which can result in congestive hemorrhagic pulmonary edema.
8. **The answer is D.** In contrast to the organophosphate insecticides, inorganic forms of arsenic and lead are poorly absorbed through the skin. Dermal exposure is not significant for cadmium and silicates.
9. **The answer is D.** Dimercaprol is contraindicated in iron poisoning because the complex it forms with iron is toxic. It is useful in the treatment of arsenic, bismuth, antimony, and mercury poisoning.
10. **The answer is D.** If administered early in poisoning, atropine reverses the muscarinic cholinoceptor effects of organophosphate insecticides such as parathion, which inhibit acetylcholinesterase (AChE). Pralidoxime (2-PAM) is often used as an adjunct to atropine. Inhibition of AChE by carbamate insecticides such as carbaryl is reversed spontaneously. The toxicity of methanol, chlorophenothane (DDT), and rotenone is unrelated to acetylcholine action.

11. **The answer is A.** β-Adrenoceptor blocking agents, such as timolol, reduce aqueous humor formation.

12. **The answer is E.** Timolol is a nonselective β-adrenergic receptor blocker. It is used topically in the treatment of glaucoma. However, some amount of the drug can enter the systemic circulation via the nasolacrimal duct and block the β_2-receptors which mediate bronchodilation. In a patient with asthma, the drug can precipitate an attack of bronchospasm.

Index

Note: Page numbers followed by *t* and *f*, indicate table and figure respectively.

A

B

C

D

E

F

G

H

I

K

L

M

N

O

P

Q

R

U

V

W

Y

Z